Realities in Childbearing

MARY LOU MOORE, R.N., M.A.

Instructor, Neonatal Intensive Care Nursing Program,
Bowman Gray School of Medicine
Winston-Salem, North Carolina

With a contribution by
ORA STRICKLAND DAVIS, R.N., Ph.D.

Assistant Professor of Maternal-Infant Nursing and
Research and Evaluation; School of Nursing,
University of North Carolina at Greensboro

1978

W. B. SAUNDERS COMPANY   Philadelphia · London · Toronto

W. B. Saunders Company: West Washington Square
Philadelphia, Pa. 19105

1 St. Anne's Road
Eastbourne, East Sussex BN21 3UN, England

1 Goldthorne Avenue
Toronto, Ontario M8Z 5T9, Canada

Realities in Childbearing   ISBN 0-7216-6497-0

Last digit is the print number: 9   8   7   6   5   4   3   2   1

To My Parents

MARY BLACKWELL HANSON
and
HAROLD EPHRAIM HANSON

PREFACE

The bearing of children is of major importance to every society, for therein lies the survival of that society. Thus the nursing care of childbearing families is also highly significant.

In caring for families during that time of life in which children are born, nurses must constantly be aware not only of physiologic realities but also of the cultural, emotional, developmental, and environmental context of childbearing.

Our knowledge is constantly expanding. Much that we write here today may be revised by what we learn tomorrow. We hope that the students and professional nurses who read this book will challenge the ideas found here when they discover still better ways of caring for families, and then share their ideas with all of us.

We are aware that many student nurses who study the nursing care of childbearing families in the undergraduate curriculum will never practice in this area. Yet we believe that the understanding they gain from such a course and from this book will enhance their care of families, whatever their nursing specialty.

And so this book is written for all nurses, student and professional, in order that we may all, each in our own way, contribute to the quality of care, and of life, in our society.

MARY LOU MOORE

ACKNOWLEDGMENTS

It is impossible to acknowledge all of the individuals who are a part of a book such as this one. The families for whom we have cared, the students we have taught, professional colleagues in nursing, medicine, nutrition and the social sciences—each has contributed and continues to contribute to the knowledge we share with you here.

We would be remiss, however, if we did not give special recognition to those who have made particular contributions to this volume: Brenda McBride, R.N., who both shared ideas and read portions of the manuscript; Charlene Miller, R.N. and Susan Stevens, M.S.W., who shared their knowledge of adolescents who are pregnant; Diane Kerwin, R.D., M.P.H., who so carefully evaluated the nutrition information and made many helpful suggestions; Kathy Auerbach, Ph.D., who read and commented upon several chapters; Robert Dillard, M.D., and Richard Weaver, M.D., who have shared so many ideas with us; George Lynch and Joe Roselli, who prepared the original illustrations; Sandy Harmon, Barbara Laughinghouse, and Jan Phipps, who not only typed the manuscript but offered advice and counsel. To Ora Strickland Davis, R.N., Ph.D., our special thanks for the chapters she wrote. To Susan and Bob Stevens and Alice, Carolyn and John Ashburn and Sharon, Lynne and Neil Carter and Todd, and Sharon Howell and Brooklyn, and Brenda McBride, R.N., and Dr. Robert Dillard, our thanks for allowing us to photograph them. We appreciate the response of the American Nurses' Association, the Nurses Association of the American College of Obstetricians and Gynecologists, the Arizona Nurses' Association, and all of those companies and agencies that allowed us to reproduce material. Our deepest gratitude to Helen Dietz, Senior Nursing Editor at W. B. Saunders, and Robert E. Wright, former Nursing Editor, whose guidance and faith made this book possible.

CONTENTS

QUESTIONNAIRE

We are very interested in your comments concerning *Realities in Childbearing* and your suggestions for its next edition. Your answers to any or all of the following questions and your comments will aid our evaluation and in this way, we believe, contribute to continually improving the ways in which nurses assist and care for families during childbearing.

1. What are the strongest features in *Realities in Childbearing?*

2. What parts of the book should be revised, expanded, shortened, etc. to make it more helpful to you?

3. What topics should be added?

4. What topics should be deleted?

Additional comments:

Please return to Mary Lou Moore, 701 Austin Lane, Winston-Salem, North Carolina, 27106.

Chapter 1

CHILDBEARING IN TODAY'S WORLD

Student nurses, like all of us, have accumulated many attitudes and feelings about childbearing long before they take a course or meet their first patient. These feelings and attitudes do make a difference in the meaning that a course in "maternity nursing" will have for them. This is the first reality each of us must consider.

Think back to the first time you were aware of pregnancy or of birth. What were the circumstances? How did you feel? Did you discuss your feelings with your family or your friends? Think about women you have known who were pregnant—their feelings and your reactions. Have you ever seen an infant during the process of birth or a film of the birth process? Have you ever seen a baby who was nursing at his mother's breast? What did you think? What did you feel?

REALITY VERSUS "THE MYTH"

There is a popular myth in the United States, and probably in the rest of the world to a certain extent, that babies are born to couples who are married, who want them, and who are able to care for them, perhaps with a little help from us. For some of the families we meet as we participate in maternity care, the myth appears to be close to the truth, although as we come to know these families more intimately, we find that even for them there are adjustments to be made and stresses that they may not have anticipated, which are not always readily apparent at first glance.

For many others, the myth bears little resemblance to the reality of their experience. There may be no husband or mate, only a mother alone. This does not mean that the baby is necessarily unwanted (just as marriage by no means guarantees a wanted baby), nor does it mean that there is not support from others (such as a grandmother), but this may be true. Poverty, poor health, inadequate nutrition, and family disorganization often coexist with pregnancy and birth. The disappointment of infertility or of the birth of a child who is less than normal may happen in any family.

THE PREGNANT WOMAN AND HER FAMILY

Throughout this text we will talk about the pregnant woman and her family. Who is her family? For some women,

1

family means a husband and perhaps other children. But for many pregnant women—more than half the women met in some agencies—there is no husband. The father may have a close, ongoing relationship with the mother, or he may have a very tentative relationship with her. The mother, or mother-to-be, may be living with her own mother and may have a close relationship with her, or she may be totally alienated from that family. The term *significant other(s)* is used by behavioral scientists to refer to the individual(s) who have a close, meaningful relationship with a particular person. Because significant other is a somewhat unwieldy term to use over and over throughout a text, we have used the words "father" or "family" frequently, while recognizing that for some women the significant person in her life may be neither of these.

The needs of each woman and the significant people in her life must be assessed and met on an individual basis. Families don't fit into neat boxes—husbands and wives in this one, unmarried mothers in a second, and the like—a theme that will be repeated throughout this text.

CARE AND CONFLICT IN CONTEMPORARY CHILDBEARING

Caring for childbearing families often places nurses in situations of conflict. This is one of the realities we must face each day. Three major areas of conflict, breifly discussed here, are recurrent themes, occurring in actual practice and referred to throughout this volume:

1. The conflict that may result between nurses and physicians because of their differing perspectives about care

2. The conflict in values that may occur both among professionals and between professionals and patients over issues such as out-of-wedlock pregnancy and abortion

3. The conflict between consumer desire and traditional practice.

Conflict: Nursing Support Versus Obstetric Care

Does obstetric care, which we will define as the *medical* care of the obstetric patient, differ from the nursing care of the childbearing family? Although there are obvious variations in individual practice settings, some specific, very important differences do exist.

Certain aspects of care, namely medical care *per se* with its primarily physiologic orientation, are physician-directed. The care itself is often delegated to a nurse-midwife or to another designated nurse, but physician consultation is available and physician back-up is usually decreed by the nurse-practice acts and by standards of care (see, for example, the discussion of the nurse-midwife in Chapter 23).

Nursing care is concerned with much more than the physiologic process of pregnancy. Recognition of the changes in both the mother and father as individuals and in the dynamics of family interaction at each stage of pregnancy is significant for nurses.

Closely related are those skills that offer support to the family in coping with these changes. The importance of understanding the physiologic aspects of the maternity cycle is not ignored; such understanding is, however, considered insufficient in itself.

In these areas, nurses frequently function in an independent role. For example, nurses may teach classes in preparation for childbirth or postpartal classes on a fee-for-service basis quite independently of any medical practice. Even within institutions (clinics or hospitals, for example) this component of care is planned and organized by nurses. Supporting the family during labor, teaching the mother and father to care for their new baby, assessing the need for help from other professionals (a nutritionist or a social worker, for example), and referring the family to a professional are but a few examples of ways in which *nurses* care for childbearing families.

The difference in emphasis may lead to conflict between professionals (particularly between nurses and physicians) or may result in combining the strengths of both professions to offer the best talents of both for the care of patients. The physician who sees the nurse's role as one of a "handmaiden" who is available to prepare supplies for him, but never to counsel *his* patient, does not understand the role of nursing. The nurse who practices to meet this kind of expectation deprives her patient of comprehensive care.

Nurses who are knowledgeable about the total process of childbearing—its physiologic, emotional, and social components—have much to offer families that is unique and essential. It is toward this concept of care that this book is directed.

Conflicts in Values

Childbearing is important to every society; it is the means by which the society is perpetuated. So it should not be surprising that in every society there are strongly held values and beliefs about activities related to childbearing—sexual intercourse, abortion, and infanticide, for example.

Because we live in a society that is (1) pluralistic, i.e., with many cultural traditions, and (2) undergoing rapid social change, there are many conflicts about cultural beliefs.

Nurses who care for childbearing families are often caught in the conflict between their own values (marriage should occur before pregnancy; abortion is "murder"; or abortion is a woman's right, for example) and the values or beliefs of their patients or coworkers.

Conflict: Traditional Practice Versus Consumer Desire

In few areas of nursing practice is there as much conflict about the way in which patient and family needs should be met as there is in maternity nursing. A growing number of families are searching for new and more meaningful experiences surrounding pregnancy and birth—experiences that do not separate families at one of the significant times of their lives and experiences that they feel are oriented in favor of human dignity. Research data support many of their contentions.

Meanwhile, in many hospitals, in an attempt to meet the needs of those mothers who are at high risk of complication, an increasing level of technology surrounds birth. Examples of this technology are the use of fetal monitors, amniocentesis, fetal scalp sampling, and the like. Such technology is not bad in itself; under certain circumstances it contributes significantly to the care of certain mothers. There is, however, a concern about the extension of such technology to all mothers as a safety precaution. For example, some workers now suggest that soon fetal monitors will, and should, be a part of every labor. If this should occur, will it be counterproductive in that it will drive some couples from hospitals to delivery under circumstances that are perhaps less than ideal?

The 1970's have seen a rise in consumer activism in all areas of life, including the way in which maternity care is provided. Among the lay and lay-professional organizations that have been active (through conferences, publications, and the efforts of individuals) in bringing about changes in the care of childbearing families are the International Childbirth Education Association (ICEA), the American Society for Psychoprophylaxis in Obstetrics (ASPO), the American Academy of Husband Coached Childbirth, and the La Leche League. (The addresses of these and similar organizations are found in Appendix J.) These organizations, which we will term advocacy groups, have played a part in bringing about changes toward a more family-oriented system of maternity care in some areas of the United States.

Nurses may feel "caught" between two adversaries when advocacy groups and institutional policies conflict. On the one side are families who view nurses as implementers of institutional policy. On the other are administrators and physicians who are resistant to change and against whom nurses may feel quite powerless in effecting the changes that families desire. Student nurses at times feel very antagonistic toward staff nurses who fulfill traditional roles and who are not able to bring about changes.

Why should there be such conflict? Unlike most areas of practice, both outpatient and hospital, maternity nursing largely involves "patients" who are well, rather than ill. The healthy mother, with no complications, does not really fit into a "medical model" designed primarily for individuals who are sick. Yet often she is treated within the framework of illness.

A major function of nurses who care for childbearing families is the exami-

nation of both traditional practices and the desires of families in relation to knowledge currently available to us—knowledge of both the biologic and the psychosocial needs of parents and infants—in order to chart the most appropriate course for contemporary maternity nursing.

Not every encounter between nurses and advocacy groups is helpful to either, especially in the beginning. Sometimes the clash is a matter of individual personalities. Often nurses feel that their professional competency is being attacked. If members of advocacy groups are demanding change, then they are obviously dissatisfied with current care.

Many nurses, of course, are a part of advocacy groups or maintain close associations with members of these groups. They have discovered that their nursing role as an advocate for families can often best be served by working along with families to bring about changes that both feel are desirable.

For example, in one community there was a strong desire on the part of a group of mothers, many of whom were members of the La Leche League, for "rooming-in" (i.e., allowing the baby to spend most of his day in his mother's room rather than in a central nursery). Over the period of a year, conversations between individual mothers and nurses resulted in a shared enthusiasm for a change in policy within the hospital. Nurses began to look at the practical aspects of the changes within the framework of safe and acceptable maternal and newborn care. Their professional expertise was essential before the desires of the families could become reality. Mothers and fathers were encouraged to communicate their feelings to the hospital administration, a factor also seen as significant to success. This feedback was continued after a trial period of rooming-in was established.

During the trial, data were collected from both mothers and staff to assess both good and bad aspects of the change. By the conclusion of a 3 month trial period, the change was firmly established, and within the year a similar change occurred in the community's other hospital.

Moreover, the bridges built between the La Leche group and the staff nurses have resulted in cooperation in other aspects of care. Money was raised by the group to purchase a breast pump for the hospital. There has been cooperation in the teaching of prenatal classes in the community. Hospital nurses more frequently refer mothers to La Leche leaders for help after they return home from the hospital. Undoubtedly, further enhancement of care will occur as a result of future cooperation.

Nurses can also become effective advocates of other aspects of care at local, state, and federal levels.

PROBLEM: FRAGMENTATION OF CARE

Who cares for, nurtures, and supports the family during pregnancy? At least part, and often a major part, of that support comes from people other than nurses, physicians, or other professionals. It is well that it does, for professional care is frequently fragmented, divided among many professional people.

Consider just the number of nurses the woman (and her family) meets. One or more are in the antepartal clinic or the physician's office. If the woman attends prenatal classes, she meets another. Still another nurse may teach a specific class in preparation for labor. Within the hospital there are often a variety of nurses in the labor room and

nursery and on the postpartal unit. Upon discharge, the mother may be referred to a public health nurse and/or a family planning nurse and/or a follow-up clinic.

In addition, she must cope with a variety of physicians, nutritionists, social workers, and others. Even if she is the patient of a physician in private practice, the physician is probably in a group practice, and she may see a different member of the group at each visit.

If childbearing were a purely biologic occurrence, if all that were required were checks of hemoglobin and blood pressure and urine, such a fragmented approach to care might possibly suffice. But childbearing is a complex biologic psychosocial process that is best served by a continuous relationship between the patient, the family, and the provider of care. Nurses, of all the potential providers, are in the best position to supply that care.

In order to provide this kind of comprehensive care, nurses are developing new roles and expanding established ones (Chapter 23).

PROBLEM: PERINATAL MORTALITY

Perinatal mortality is the term used to describe the death of a fetus or infant between 20 weeks of gestational age (i.e., age since the mother's last menstrual period) and 28 days after birth (Chapter 10).

In the United States perinatal mortality is higher than it is in much of the rest of the industrialized world. This difference appears to be not merely a matter of the way in which statistics are kept, but an actual difference in the number of deaths.

Much of the technological development described above has been in an effort to reduce this mortality. The problem is complex and is discussed more fully in the chapters on the high risk infant.

NURSING ROLES IN TRANSITION

The problems described above— the desires and needs of families for meaningful, humanistic, family-centered childbearing; the proliferation of technology at least in part to deal with the very real issue of high perinatal mortality with its own special demands, and fragmentation of care— have put diverse pressures on nurses.

Nurses have found the need to increase their skills in assessment, in communication, and in support of families, for example, and also to increase their skills in technical areas, such as the vaginal examination of the woman in labor and the administration of intravenous fluids to preterm infants weighing 2 pounds.

What is the role of nurses who care for childbearing families? Some nurses suggest that the supportive, teaching roles are paramount for the professional nurse and that the purely technical tasks may best be performed by someone else. To us this seems a further fragmentation of care, and so we emphasize, both in our practice and in this text, a nursing role that to us combines the best of both worlds. For example, the nurse most intimately concerned with the minute-by-minute care of a sick newborn infant, care that is in some aspects highly technical, has the best opportunity, we believe, to foster attachment of parents and baby, to help parents grieve (Chapter 22), and, in short, to give the comprehensive care that the family needs. Other professionals and paraprofessionals, such as physicians,

social workers, nutritionists, and respiratory therapists, play a part in that care, but the nurse devises and implements the comprehensive nursing plan.

How Do Nurses Improve Care by Developing New or Expanded Roles?

If fragmentation of care and the desire of families for a human experience are major issues, what answers can nurses offer?

Many nurses are now practicing in settings that enable them to care for families throughout a childbearing cycle. They see women and families in the antenatal period, both individually and in classes that prepare them for childbearing. They may coach the mother or couple during labor, counsel both parents following delivery about self-care and care of their baby and family, and make one or more home visits. If the nurse is a certified nurse-midwife, she may also deliver the baby if the delivery is expected to be uncomplicated.

While there are barriers to this kind of care, it is a possibility in every community if nurses make a real commitment to achieving it.

What Must Nurses Know to Care for Childbearing Families?

How much and what must a nurse know to adequately care for childbearing families? Until fairly recently, much nursing knowledge was set in a medical model. The body of knowledge that might be described as pertaining purely to nursing was relatively small.

We view the knowledge needed for the nursing care of families as:

1. A body of basic knowledge derived from the physical and psychosocial sciences, important to all who care for parents and their babies.

2. A body of knowledge specifically related to reproduction, important to all who care for parents and infants.

3. A body of concepts derived from the humanities, to assist in developing a philosophy that helps one cope with the value issues of childbearing, issues such as abortion and the care of a dying, malformed newborn.

4. Specific knowledge that is chiefly or entirely a part of nursing practice.

From the biologic sciences we gain an understanding of the anatomy and physiology of the male and female reproductive tracts, of genetics, and of embryology, for example. From social science we must understand concepts such as individual and family developmental tasks, the dynamics of changing roles, and the way in which culture influences our lives.

Examples of knowledge of reproduction include the circumstances of conception; the body's reaction to pregnancy, labor, birth, and recovery; the meaning of pregnancy for men and women; and their reaction to it.

All of these types of knowledge serve as the basis from which nursing knowledge has developed—the specific ways in which we, as nurses, care for families and enable familes to care for themselves and to cope physically, emotionally, and socially with childbearing.

Nurses who specialize in the care of childbearing families frequently seek additional educational preparation. Some are nurse-midwives; others are obstetric, neonatal, family planning, or family nurse practitioners. Some participate in continuing education programs to enhance their knowledge. Some earn advanced degrees in maternal-child health care (Chapter 23).

For all nurses a basic course in the care of childbearing families is a foun-

dation, a beginning, not the sum total of knowledge.

NURSING RESEARCH AND CHILDBEARING

In *The Logic of Scientific Discovery,* Karl Popper states:

... it is not in the *possession* of knowledge, of irrefutable truth, that makes the man of science, but his persistent and recklessly critical *quest* for truth. . . Science never pursues the illusory aim of making its answers final, or even probable. Its advance is, rather, towards the infinite yet attainable aim of ever discovering new, deeper and more general problems, and of subjecting its very tentative answers to ever renewed and ever more rigorous tests.[1]

Nursing is barely a generation away from rigid proscriptions about how care should be given. Many nurses practicing today were educated by rigid models. In our student years, mothers who had delivered not only were confined to bed for several days but were given bedpans only at specific intervals, the rationale being that this would help them to void regularly! (To our credit we, as students, provided bedpans on request, an activity that required considerable stealth lest our unlawful activities be discovered.)

We know that there are always, as Popper suggests, better ways of doing what we do—better ways of helping families cope, better ways of facilitating care. Many of the suggestions in this book will be improved upon, through nursing research, by those of you now reading it as undergraduate students or as practicing nurses. Some of this research will be formal, supported perhaps by grants; other projects will be on a smaller scale but nevertheless valuable. Several nursing research projects that we feel have made significant contributions to care have been described in some detail in this volume (for example, study of the newborn's temperature under the warmer and on his mother's abdomen, in Chapter 15).

We hope that readers—both nursing students and professional nurses—will consider the ideas in this volume, use them as a springboard to develop new concepts and ideas, and share their new ideas with us and with nurses everywhere. In this way our nursing care of childbearing families will continue to grow and improve, to their benefit and to our own satisfaction in a nursing job well done.

REFERENCE

1. Popper, K.: *The Logic of Scientific Discovery.* New York, Basic Books, Inc., 1959.

Chapter 2

BIOLOGIC POTENTIAL:
The Genetic Basis of Reproduction

The links between parents (represented biologically by a single egg and a single sperm) and their child are hundreds of thousands of genes. Located on the chromosomes, genes are the blueprint for the developing human being.

An understanding of the basic principles of genetics is essential for any nurse who cares for persons during their childbearing years. Some of these men and women will be met in obstetric practice—as visitors to family planning clinics, as expectant mothers and fathers, or as parents following the birth of a child with an anomaly. Others may be parents of a child with a genetic disorder, such as cystic fibrosis; a teenager with hemophilia; or a young wife who has been found to have sickle cell trait following a visit to a screening clinic.

Some nurses are part of genetic counseling teams, while others recognize the need for counseling in their practice and know how to make appropriate referrals. Because genetic problems are so far reaching, all of us, at one time or another, are likely to be involved with people whose lives are affected by such problems. Genetic counseling is discussed as one aspect of family planning in Chapter 5. The support of a family who give birth to an infant with a genetic disorder is discussed in Chapter 22.

THE GENETIC BASIS OF DEVELOPMENT

The genetic potential of all organisms is encoded in genes. Genes are made up of nucleoproteins that are, in turn, composed of nucleic acid and protein. The principal substance in nucleic acid is deoxyribonucleic acid (DNA), with the exception of some of the simplest viruses in which DNA is replaced by ribonucleic acid (RNA).

Molecules of DNA are double helices of polynucleotide chains (Fig. 2-1). Each single segment of the helical strand, called a *nucleotide,* consists of a phosphate, deoxyribose (a special kind of sugar), one of two purines (adenine or guanine), and one of two pyrimidines

Figure 2–1   Replication of DNA. Note that the original molecule (top) unwinds, and the halves separate. The new half molecules of DNA are formed on the old halves by adenine *(A)* pairing with thymine *(T)* and by guanine *(G)* pairing with cytosine *(C)*.

(thymine or cytosine). The purines and the pyrimidines serve as bases.

The chains of the helix are held together by hydrogen bonds between the bases. Each chain is the exact complement of the other. An adenine base in one chain is always linked to a thymine base in the other; guanine is always bonded to cytosine. Thus, when the double helix separates into two single threads, each is able to re-form an exact copy of the original by coupling the proper bases. *It is this ability to re-form exact copies that makes replication (self-reproduction) possible.*

Since from 200 to 2000 nucleotides make up a single gene and as many as 3000 genes make up a single chromosome, in man each cell division involves more than 27 million nucleotide repli-

cations, an estimate that is probably conservative. When one considers the number of cell divisions that takes place each day from conception to death, the intricacies of our biologic heritage are truly overwhelming.

It is in the arrangement of the bases (adenine, guanine, cytosine, and thymine) that genes differ from one another. The DNA molecule is the "blueprint" that directs all of development. If the DNA arrangement in a part of a particular gene varies, the wrong message may be delivered to the developing cell and a variation in development may occur. For example, sickle cell anemia is produced by a single gene, one that is probably different in one or a few nucleotides. This variation in the gene molecule causes a different message to be sent to the developing hemoglobin molecule. The red blood cell develops differently than it normally would, and the cell then behaves abnormally.

OVUM AND SPERM

The genetic potential of an individual is present in every cell of his body, but it is transferred from generation to generation through specialized cells, the female ovum (egg) and the male sperm. Understanding the development of these cells and their division is essential background for understanding the action of genes and chromosomes.

Oogonia and *spermatogonia*, the forerunners of mature ova and sperm, originate as large, spherical *primordial germ cells* during the fourth week of intrauterine life. The processes by which they develop into mature ova and sperm *(oogenesis* and *spermatogenesis)* are described below and are summarized in Table 2–1.

Table 2–1 PROCESS OF OOGENESIS AND SPERMATOGENESIS

Oogenesis			Spermatogenesis			
Germ Cell			Germ Cell			
(Mitosis)			(Mitosis)			
Oogonium			Spermatogonium			
(Develops)			(Develops)			
Primary Oocyte			Primary Spermatocyte)			
(First Meiotic Division)			(First Meiotic Division)			
Secondary Oocyte	First Polar Body		Secondary Spermatocyte		Secondary Spermatocyte	
(Second Meiotic Division)			(Second Meiotic Division)			
Ovum	Second Polar Body	Polar Bodies	Spermatid	Spermatid	Spermatid	Spermatid

Oogenesis

Ova develop from oogonia located in the cortical tissue of the ovary. During early fetal development, oogonia divide by *mitosis* (see below) to form additional oogonia. By the fifth to sixth month of fetal life, all of the oogonia for a woman's lifetime have been produced; many will degenerate before sexual maturity is reached.

The differentiation of the oogonium into a *primary oocyte* also occurs during fetal life, as does the first *meiotic division* (see below) of the primary oocyte. Then development ceases until after puberty, when a second meiotic division occurs for certain ova at some time in the years that follow. It will be 40 years or more before some of the primary oocytes resume meiotic division; many never will. The completion of the development of a mature ovum is described below in the discussion of meiosis.

Spermatogenesis

In contrast to the oogonia, in which the process of development of the mature ova begins during fetal life, the spermatogonia present in the newborn's testes at birth disappear until puberty. From that time, spermatogenesis continues throughout life.

Spermatogenesis begins as the germ cells lining the seminiferous tubules of the testes (Chapter 3) divide by mitosis to form spermatogonia, which in turn grow into primary spermatocytes. Two meiotic divisions result first in two secondary spermatocytes and, shortly afterward, in four spermatids (Fig. 2–2). Spermatogenesis occurs simultaneously in hundreds of thousands of spermatogonia in order to produce the millions of sperm that are constantly present in the adult male reproductive tract. Before the spermatid can become a functioning sperm, still other changes, described in Chapter 3, must occur.

CELL DIVISION: MITOSIS AND MEIOSIS

In order to understand the way in which chromosomes affect inheritance, it is necessary to review the two proc-

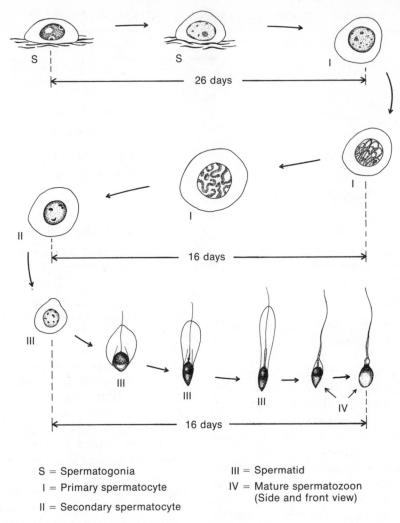

S = Spermatogonia   III = Spermatid

I = Primary spermatocyte   IV = Mature spermatozoon
                                          (Side and front view)
II = Secondary spermatocyte

Figure 2–2   Spermatogenesis.

esses of cell division: *mitosis* and *meiosis.*

Mitosis is the process by which all cells divide, except those that produce the ovum and sperm after the stage of the primary oocyte and primary spermatocyte. The stages of mitosis are diagrammed in Figure 2–3. Observe that when all the chromosomes are aligned in the equatorial plane of the cell (Fig. 2–3C), the nuclear membrane is no longer present. It is at this point that the *centromere* of the chromosome (i. e., the point at which the strands, called *chromatids,* are joined) splits to complete the chromosome separation. The chromosomes are pulled to the opposite ends (poles) of the cell with the centromeres leading (Fig. 2–3D). This gives each chromosome a special shape during anaphase that aids in the recognition of the different types of chromosomes. After the chromosomes arrive at the poles, they fade from sight, nuclear

Figure 2–3   The stages of mitosis. Only two of the 23 chromosome pairs are shown. Chromosomes from one parent are shown in outline; chromosomes from the other parent are in black. *A*, Interphase; *B*, prophase; *C*, metaphase; *D*, anaphase; *E*, telophase; and *F*, interphase. (From Thompson and Thompson: *Genetics in Medicine.* 2nd Edition. Philadelphia, W. B. Saunders Co., 1973.)

membranes form, and cell division is completed. *Two* cells now exist in place of one.

A second process of cell division, meiosis, is reserved for the *gametes* (i.e., sex cells). In meiosis the chromosomes split once, as in mitosis, but the cell divides *two times,* so that *four* cells result, each with one-half the number of chromosomes of the parent cell.

Consider what would happen if this did not occur. At the end of mitosis, each cell in humans has 46 chromosomes, as did the original cell. (See section on Chromosomes, below.) If the ovum and sperm were each to have 46 chromosomes, the resulting zygote would have

92 chromosomes. Meiosis gives the ovum and sperm 23 chromosomes each, so the the resulting zygote has 46 chromosomes, the correct number for humans.

Figures 2–4 and 2–5 diagram meiotic division; compare them with Figure 2–3. Note first that the pairs of homologous chromosomes come together in the first phase (prophase). This process is called *synapse* (which means "coming together"). The chromosomes of each pair are aligned so that the loci for specific genes are next to each other and often touch. As in mitosis, the chromosomes are split, so that each of the 23 pairs consists of four

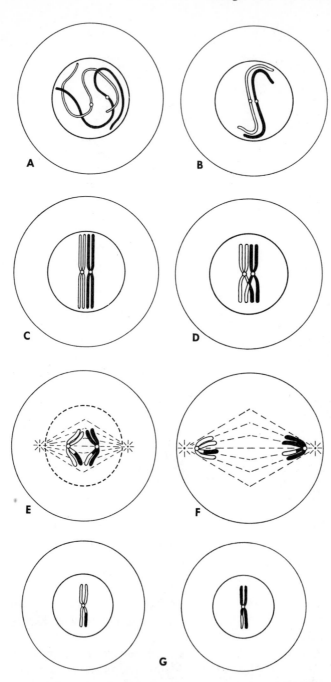

Figure 2–4 The first meiotic division. One of the 23 chromosome pairs is depicted. Chromosome from one parent is shown in outline, chromosome from the other parent in black. *A,* Leptotene; *B,* zygotene; *C,* pachytene; *D,* diplotene, showing one chiasma (several may be present, and two, three, or all four strands may be involved); *E,* metaphase; *F,* anaphase; and *G,* telophase. (From Thompson and Thompson: *Genetics in Medicine.* 1st Edition. Philadelphia, W. B. Saunders Co., 1966.)

strands, each two strands joined at the centromere. The centromere does not split during the first meiotic division; the daughter cells at the end of the first stage contain one of each of the homologous pairs. In the second meiotic division (Fig. 2–5), the centromere divides and single strands go to opposite poles. As cell division completes, there are now four cells, each with 23 chromosomes.

While both ovum and sperm

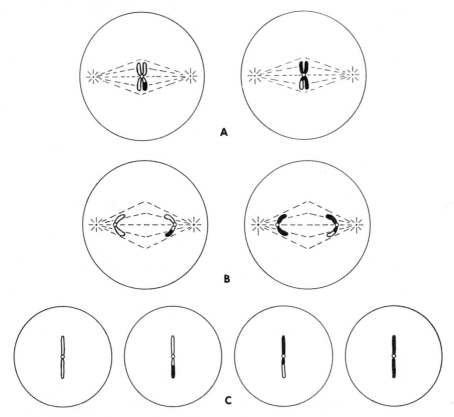

Figure 2–5 The second meiotic division. *A*, Metaphase; *B*, anaphase; and *C*, telophase. (From Thompson and Thompson: *Genetics in Medicine.* 1st Edition. Philadelphia, W. B. Saunders Co., 1966.)

undergo meiosis, there is a significant difference. In the male, the four resulting sperm are identical in size. In the female, however, the first meiotic division results in two cells that are identical as far as chromosomes are concerned but that differ greatly in size. Most of cellular material goes to one cell, the *secondary oocyte*. The other cell, the *first polar body*, contains the chromosomes but has only a very small amount of cellular material. The same process occurs at the second meiotic division, with the secondary oocyte producing the ovum and the *second polar body* (Figs. 2–6 and 2–7). The significance of this disparity in size is that should the ovum be fertilized, it contains all of the material of the original oocyte that will nourish the zygote prior to implantation in the uterine wall.

CHROMOSOMES

The rod-shaped chromosomes exist in a variety of lengths and shapes. Not only the chromosomal number but also the size and shape of the chromosomes are specific for each species. Humans have 46 chromosomes, which are paired: 22 pairs of *autosomes* and one pair of *sex chromosomes*. Autosomes are alike in both sexes. Females have two X sex chromosomes; males have one X chromosome and one Y chromosome. Both autosomes and sex chromosomes

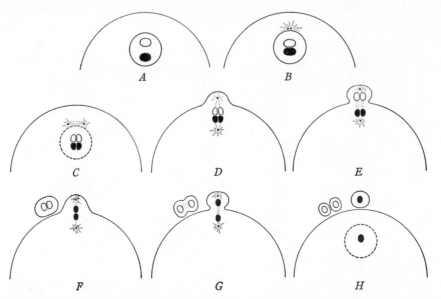

Figure 2–6   Diagrams of the maturation of the ovum in an animal with two chromosomes. *A–E,* Budding off of the first polar body. *F, G,* Formation of the second polar body and subdivision of the first. *H,* Mature egg with polar bodies. (From Arey: *Developmental Anatomy: A Textbook and Laboratory Manual of Embryology*. Revised 7th Edition. Philadelphia, W. B. Saunders Co., 1974.)

carry genes that govern traits, with the possible exception of the Y chromosome.

Human chromosomes have been classified on the basis of size and the position of the centromere. Since it is sometimes difficult to identify all 23 pairs of chromosomes in an individual sample, it has become an accepted practice to organize them into seven groups, identified by the letters A through G in order of decreasing length. A systematically arranged set of chromosomes is called a *karyotype* (Fig. 2–8). Cells used for karyotyping may be white blood

Figure 2–7   Living human ova, shown as photomicrographs (Shettles). × 150. *A,* Secondary oocyte, with first polar body (beginning to subdivide), lying within the space bounded externally by the dark zona pellucida; at the left, spermatozoa lie on the zona. *B,* Ripe egg, said to be artificially fertilized and showing all three polar bodies; unsuccessful spermatozoa are embedded in the locally elevated zona pellucida. (From Arey: *Developmental Anatomy: A Textbook and Laboratory Manual of Embryology*. Revised 7th Edition. Philadelphia, W. B. Saunders Co., 1974.)

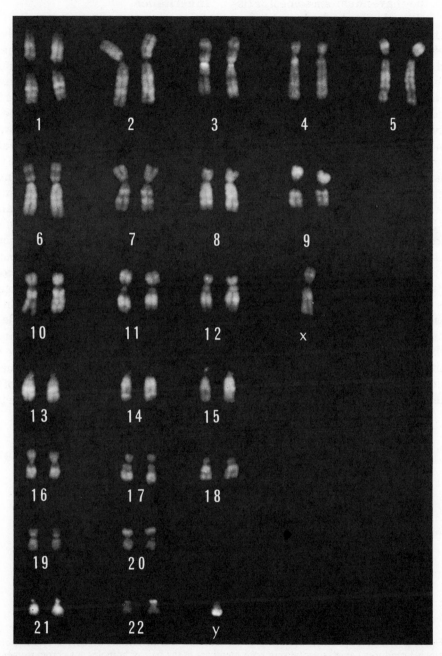

Figure 2–8   Normal human metaphase karyotype (from peripheral blood) stained with fluorescent quinacrine mustard, as described by Caspersson, Zech, Johansson, and Modest, *Chromosoma, 30*:215 (1970), and as published by Caspersson, Zech, and Johansson in *Experimental Cell Research, 62*:490 (1970). Magnification × 2500. (From Page, Villee, and Villee: *Human Reproduction: The Core Content of Obstetrics, Gynecology and Perinatal Medicine.* 2nd Edition. Philadelphia, W. B. Saunders Co., 1976.)

cells (since red blood cells have no nucleus, they have no chromosomes) or tissue cells obtained during biopsy. Epithelial cells from the lining of the cheek are frequently used. Amniotic fluid is used to study fetal chromosomes. The cells are cultured and treated chemically, and slides are prepared for examination and photography. Individual chromosomes are then cut from the photograph, matched in pairs, and mounted according to the standard classification, called the Denver Classification because of its adoption at a meeting in Denver, Colorado, in 1960.

Figure 2–4, *D* through *G*, illustrates another facet of chromosomal inheritance, a process called "crossing-over," in which two chromosomes of a pair may exchange certain sections and thus certain genetic traits at the same *locus* (i.e., at the same location on the chromosome). Note in Figure 2–5 that in the four daughter cells one of the "white" chromosomes has exchanged sections with one of the "black" chromosomes.

Variations in Chromosomal Inheritance

Mitosis and meiosis do not always occur normally. As a result, chromosomal abnormalities occur in a small percentage of infants. Because of the large number of genes located on each chromosome, it might be expected that any chromosomal change would produce not just one but a constellation of changes. It appears that it is the total effect of the imbalance of genetic material that is responsible for the changes.

Several types of chromosomal abnormalities can occur, involving either the autosomes or the sex chromosomes. The most common is *nondisjunction* (Fig. 2–9). If during the meiotic process a chromosome pair fails to separate normally, one gamete will contain two of a particular chromosome while the other will not have that chromosome at all. If the two-chromosome gamete then joins with a normal gamete to form a zygote, the zygote will have three of that particular chromosome, hence the term

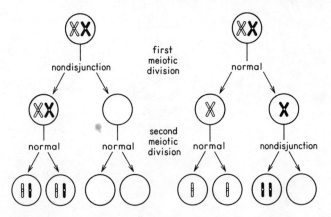

Figure 2–9 Nondisjunction occurring at the first and second meiotic divisions. Nondisjunction at meiosis I produces gametes containing both members of the pair of homologous chromosomes concerned, or neither member. Nondisjunction at meiosis II produces gametes containing (or lacking) two identical chromosomes both derived from the same member of the homologous pair. In experimental organisms and probably also in man, nondisjunction occurs much more frequently at meiosis I than at meiosis II. Gametes lacking a chromosome (other than the X) are usually apparently unable to form a viable zygote. (From Thompson and Thompson: *Genetics in Medicine.* 2nd Edition. Philadelphia, W. B. Saunders Co., 1973.)

Figure 2–10   Trisomy 21 karyotype. Note the three number 21 chromosomes. Compare this karyotype with Figure 2–8. (From Walker, Carr, Sergovich, Barr, and Soltan: *J. Mental Deficiency Research*, 7:150, 1963.)

trisomy (Fig. 2–10). The gamete with no autosome does not seem to be able to form a viable zygote. Nondisjunction can also occur during mitosis, after the zygote has been formed.

Down's syndrome (Fig. 2–11), which is related to trisomy of chromosome 21, is usually the result of nondisjunction. Occasionally, Down's syndrome is due to a second type of abnormality, *translocation*, in which a piece of one chromosome breaks off and subsequently attaches itself to another chromosome. In translocation Down's syndrome, the long arm of the twenty-first chromosome breaks off and subsequently attaches itself to either a chromosome of the D group (chromosomes 13 to 15) or another chromosome of the G group (chromosomes 21 to 22) (Fig. 2–11).

Such differentiation has value in genetic counseling. When the basis of Down's syndrome in an individual child can be determined (by obtaining a family history related to Down's syndrome, by karyotyping the baby, and sometimes by karyotyping the parents as well), the likelihood that the syndrome may be repeated in future children can be evaluated more accurately. The risk of Down's syndrome in a second child is much greater if the mother is a translocation carrier than if the cause is nondisjunction. Only about 5 per cent of children have Down's syndrome due to translocation rather than to trisomy 21; about 2 per cent of these babies have inherited the translocation from a parent. The mother of a baby with Down's syndrome due to translocation is usually of normal childbearing age; the risk of trisomy increases markedly in older mothers (Table 2–2).

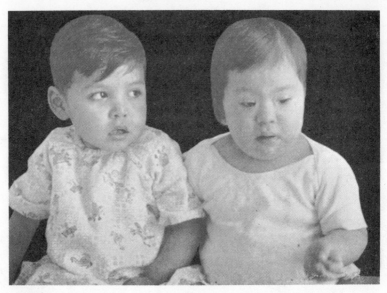

Figure 2–11   A three year old Canadian Indian girl with trisomy 21 (right) and a normal Canadian Indian boy of the same age. Canadian Indians are of Mongolian origin. Note that the trisomy 21 or "mongolism" phenotype is quite different from that of a normal Indian child. (From Thompson and Thompson: *Genetics in Medicine*. 1st Edition. Philadelphia, W. B. Saunders Co., 1966.)

In addition to trisomy 21, trisomy 18 (or trisomy E) and trisomy D also result from nondisjunction, the letters in both instances referring to the group of chromosomes involved. These babies usually have multiple and severe deformities and die in the first months after birth (Fig. 2–12).

Other chromosomal breaks include *deletion,* in which a piece of a chromosome breaks off and is lost; *duplication,* in which an extra piece of chromosome either is in the chromosome itself, is attached to another chromosome (translocation), or exists as a separate unit; the development of *isochromosomes* because of abnormal splitting; and chromosomal *mosaicism* in which an individual has at least two different groups of cells with different chromosome complements. Mosaicism always occurs after fertilization during the

Table 2–2   RISK OF DOWN'S SYNDROME*

| | Risk of Down's Syndrome in Child | |
Age of Mother	AT ANY PREGNANCY	AFTER THE BIRTH OF A MONGOL
–29	1 in 3000	1 in 1000
30–34	1 in 600	1 in 200
35–39	1 in 280	1 in 100
40–44	1 in 70	1 in 25
45–49	1 in 40	1 in 15
All mothers	1 in 665	1 in 200

*From Thompson and Thompson: *Genetics in Medicine*. 1st Edition. Philadelphia, W. B. Saunders Co., 1966. (After Motulsky, based upon the data of Carter and McCarthy.)

Figure 2–12 Infant with trisomy of a chromosome in group E, probably chromosome 18. Note the overlapping fingers, rocker-bottom feet, simplified patterns of the ear, and dorsiflexion of the big toe. (From Thompson and Thompson: *Genetics in Medicine.* 2nd Edition. Philadelphia, W. B. Saunders Co., 1973. Courtesy of D. H. Carr.)

process of mitosis, leaving cells with two different types of chromosomes to develop.

A number of anomalies are a result of sex chromosome alterations. Individuals may possess varying combinations of X and Y chromosomes. Klinefelter's syndrome (XXY), which occurs once in every 400 male births (Fig. 2–13), and Turner's syndrome (XO), which occurs once in every 3000 live births (Fig. 2–14), are two of the more common abnormal combinations.

In general, individuals with unusual combinations of chromosomes will be male if they have a Y chromosome (e.g., XXY) and female if they do not (e.g., XO). The higher the number of extra chromosomes, the greater the likelihood of abnormality in the visible characteristics.

The following example of nondisjunction in a single ovum illustrates how some unusual combinations may arise. Nondisjunction may take place in the sperm as well.

XX
(First meiotic division)

XX   O
(Second meiotic division)
XX   XX   O   O

The potential combinations following fertilization with a normal sperm (XY) would then be:

	XX	O
X	XXX	XO
Y	XXY	YO

We have already noted that XO represents Turner's syndrome and XXY Klinefelter's syndrome. YO would be nonviable. Females with the XXX pattern have frequently been found in surveys of hospitals for the mentally retarded and among women in infertility clinics. They may be relatively common in the general population as well.

When ambiguity of the genitalia makes it difficult to assign a sex to an infant, chromosome analysis can be helpful. An additional evaluation is the examination for a *Barr body* (*sex chromatin body, chromatin-positive body*) (Fig. 2–15). The Barr body is a chromatin mass derived from one of the X chromosomes, therefore the number of Barr bodies is one less than the number of X chromosomes. A normal male (XY) or a female with Turner's syndrome (XO) would have no Barr body. Both a normal female (XX) and a male with Klinefelter's syndrome

Figure 2–14   A girl with Turner's syndrome, XO karyotype. These girls are usually short and may have webbing of the neck, low set ears, poorly developed breasts with widely spaced nipples, and juvenile external genitalia. Note the absence of pubic hair. The ovary is usually only a streak of connective tissue. (From Barr: *American J. Human Genetics, 12*:118, 1960.)

(XXY) would have one. An XXX female would have two Barr bodies.

GENES

Genes exist in pairs because chromosomes are paired. The functions of genes at any specific point on each chromosome are the same for all chromosomes of that type. For example, a gene governing eye color is at a specific locus on a specific chromosome

Figure 2–13   A young man with Klinefelter's syndrome, XXY karyotype. These men are usually tall, with small testes and sparse pubic hair. Approximately 20 per cent of the time they have gynecomastia (female development of the breasts), as this man does. Many affected males are mentally retarded. (From Thompson and Thompson: *Genetics in Medicine.* 2nd Edition. Philadelphia, W. B. Saunders Co., 1973. Courtesy of M. L. Barr.)

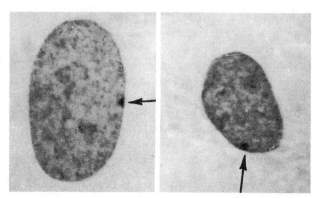

Figure 2–15   Sex chromatin or Barr bodies are indicated by the arrow. (Feulgen, magnification × 2200. Courtesy of Dr. Ursula Mittwoch, Galton Laboratory, University College, London. From Villee: *Biology.* 6th Edition. Philadelphia, W. B. Saunders Co., 1972.)

and at the same spot on every other chromosome that is identical to that chromosome. Geneticists are beginning to map the loci of some human genes; loci in some species, such as fruit flies, have already been mapped. In any pair of genes there are contrasting forms or states of the gene, known as *alleles.* Some genes have multiple alleles; there are three alleles for blood types A, B, and O. If an individual has the same alleles for a trait on each gene of a pair, he is said to be *homozygous* for that trait. A man with two alleles for A type blood, designated AA, is homozygous for A blood. When alleles differ, the individual is *heterozygous,* such as a man with AB blood. In heterozygous combinations one allele, the *dominant* allele, will manifest itself in the *phenotype* (visible characteristics). One cannot tell from the phenotype what the *genotype* (genetic characteristics) is, a matter of very practical concern in many instances.

Consider the father with blood that types Rh positive, who is married to an Rh negative mother. The capital letter D represents the positive allele, with a lower case d representing the negative allele. The positive father may be homozygous, with a genotype DD, or he may be heterozygous, with a genotype Dd. The only possible genotype for the negative mother is dd because recessive alleles are only expressed when no dominant alleles are present. Thus, recessive traits always represent a homozygous situation for that particular trait. The probability that this couple will have a child who is Rh positive will vary with the father's genotype. In the first example, the father is homozygous, i.e., DD (less frequently the case).

	D	D
d	Dd	Dd
d	Dd	Dd

As you can see, every child will have the genotype Dd, and the phenotype will be positive.

In the second example, the father has the genotype Dd.

	D	d
d	Dd	dd
d	Dd	dd

The probability is that 50 per cent of the children will have the genotype dd, and thus their phenotype will be negative.

It is very important to understand what this probability means. It does *not* mean that if this couple have two children with the genotype Dd the next child will be dd, nor does it mean the reverse. Because of the way in which genes segregate in meiosis and recombine at fertilization, each child born to a family has exactly the same probability of inheriting a specific condition as every other child of those two parents. (The obvious exception is the X-linked trait discussed below, in which the sex of the child is a factor.) The probability of a child's inheriting a specific trait is analogous to the toss of a coin. If a coin is tossed a great number of times, one expects an approximately equal number of heads and tails. But even if a person happens to toss "heads" 50 times in a row, the chance of tossing either "heads" or "tails" is still even on the fifty-first toss. Chance alone determines which alleles will be present in a particular zygote. Thus, in the case of Rh incompatibility, even if the father's genotype is Dd, it is perfectly possible that all of the children will be Dd (with a positive phenotype), and it is also possible that all will be dd (with a negative phenotype).

Both normal and pathologic traits are inherited through alleles of a gene that may be dominant, recessive, or X-linked. Many traits are controlled by more than one gene; this mode of inheritance is termed *polygenic*. Since genes are located on chromosomes and since each parent normally contributes 23 chromosomes to the zygote (see Chromosomes, above), inheritance from each parent is equal in terms of numbers. Genetically, there is no "chip off the old block" in the sense that no child can be just like either parent, nor is it likely that brothers and sisters (with the exception of monozygotic twins) will share identical genes. Two children of the same parents may resemble each other closely in genotype or in phenotype, or they may be very different, depending on the genes that they have received by chance and on the interaction of those genes with environment. The real surprise is not that some children fail to resemble either parent

very closely but that, considering the almost infinite number of possible combinations of the thousands upon thousands of genes involved, strong similarities are seen fairly often between people who are only distantly related. We need no more than a very simple understanding of genetics to realize that each child is truly different from other children and from his parents, a unique individual in his own right.

Twins may or may not have the same genotype. Dizygotic (fraternal) twins result when two separate ova are fertilized by two separate sperm. The genotype, including sex, is no more likely to resemble that of the twin than is the genotype of any other brother or sister. Monozygotic (identical) twins result when one egg and one sperm unite to form a single zygote and then split at an early stage of zygote development. Monozygotic twins do have the same genotype and must be of the same sex.

THE GENETIC INHERITANCE OF CHARACTERISTICS

Dominant Characteristics

For a *dominant* allele to be manifest in the phenotype, only one gene from one parent is necessary. The illustration of the Rh factor above shows dominant inheritance. The dominant gene (in this case D) must be present in one parent (genotype DD or Dd) and must be present in the child for the trait to be inherited. The chance, or *probability*, of a dominant trait's being inherited is 50 per cent if the parent contributing the gene is heterozygous, which is usually the case. There are nearly 800 pathologic traits caused by dominant genes, in addition to the many, many normal traits governed by them. Examples of the former include hyperphalangy of the thumb; one type of achondroplastic dwarfism; and Huntington's chorea, a degenerative disease of the central nervous system that usually affects young adults. For the individual who knows he or she carries a dominant gene for a condition such as Huntington's chorea, or who suspects the possibility, feelings about marriage and childbearing may be strongly influenced by this knowledge.

While dominant traits are commonly expressed whenever the gene is present, the term *lack of penetrance* is used to describe an individual who carries and transmits a gene for a dominant trait but who does not express the trait in his own phenotype. Environmental interaction may be one factor accounting for lack of penetrance, but it is probably not the only factor. As genetic knowledge increases, it is likely that more specific reasons will be found to explain variability within individual genes.

Recessive Characteristics

Recessive genes are expressed in the phenotype only when one recessive allele is inherited from *each* parent. All of us carry many recessive genes, transmitted through generation after generation, but unexpressed until they find a "mate," i.e., a second identical allele. Approximately 800 recessive diseases are known, most of them rare.

Cystic fibrosis is a condition inherited through recessive genes. For purposes of illustration, the normal dominant gene is designated "F" and the recessive gene for cystic fibrosis "f." An individual with the genotype FF neither has the disease nor is a carrier of the recessive gene. The genotype Ff denotes a carrier (one recessive gene), while ff is the genotype of the person with cystic fibrosis. The following diagrams illustrate the inheritance of a recessive trait. We would suggest to

nurses that it is much easier to construct this type of diagram than to try to remember probability figures. This can be done in an instant and clearly demonstrates possible combinations.

In this first example, neither parent has the disease nor is a carrier; thus, no child can have the condition or be a carrier.

	F	F
F	FF	FF
F	FF	FF

If only one parent is a carrier (Ff), there is a chance that 50 per cent of the children will be carriers (Ff), but no child will have cystic fibrosis. It is through such combinations that recessive genes may be carried for many generations, yet never expressed.

	F	f
F	FF	Ff
F	FF	Ff

If both parents carry the recessive gene (Ff), the mathematical probability is that 25 per cent of the children will have cystic fibrosis (ff), 50 per cent will be carriers (Ff), and 25 per cent will be neither (FF).

	F	f
F	FF	Ff
f	Ff	ff

Again, remember just what probability means (page 23). If this seems to be unduly emphasized, it is only because so many misunderstandings are encountered, both in the literature describing the experiences of others and in life.

Now that children born with many recessive disorders are not only surviving infancy but growing to adulthood and possible childbearing, three other possibilities occur, which were rare until recent years. The first is the combination of an individual with the condition (ff) and an individual who is neither a carrier nor has the disease (FF). As you can see, all of the children would be carriers, but none would have cystic fibrosis.

	f	f
F	Ff	Ff
F	Ff	Ff

If, however, an individual with cystic fibrosis should mate with a carrier (who, in all likelihood, would not know he was a carrier), the chance is that half of their children would have cystic fibrosis and the other half would be carriers.

	f	f
F	Ff	Ff
f	ff	ff

In the event that two individuals with cystic fibrosis should mate, every child would also have cystic fibrosis; there is no alternative.

	f	f
f	ff	ff
f	ff	ff

Sickle cell disease is another condition caused by recessive alleles. Persons who are carriers (Ss) have sickle cell trait; those individuals with two recessive genes (ss) have sickle cell anemia. Unlike most recessive traits whose presence is detected only after an affected child is born (such as the child with cystic fibrosis), carriers of the sickle cell gene can be identified. Since approximately 10 per cent of American blacks carry the sickle cell gene, sickle cell screening becomes an important factor for couples considering childbearing (see genetic counseling in Chapter 5). The prevalence of sickle cell trait is much higher in parts of Africa, where it apparently gives the individual an increased resistance to malaria.

X-linked Characteristics

The dominant and recessive genes discussed above are located on the 22 pairs of autosomal chromosomes. The remaining pair of chromosomes are sex chromosomes. Normal females have two X chromosomes; normal males have one X chromosome and one Y chromosome. For traits that are inherited through genes located on the autosomal chromosomes, it makes no difference whether a gene comes from the mother or the father. Virtually all of the characteristics known to be carried by the sex chromosomes, however, are located on the X chromosomes. They are recessive traits, expressed only when they are not masked by a normal X chromosome. Thus, females who have two X chromosomes may carry an X-linked trait, but it will not be expressed because of the presence of a normal X chromosome. Only if a female carries two affected chromosomes would the trait be expressed, a mathematical possibility but a rare occurrence (see the third example below).

In males, however, the recessive X chromosome will always be expressed when it is present, because there is no dominant allele on the Y chromosome to match it. Thus, males can never be carriers of X-linked traits; either they must express the trait, or it will be totally absent.

Hemophilia is possibly the best known example of an x-linked trait. Let X represent the normal X chromosome (which is dominant) and x the recessive gene for hemophilia. There are three possible combinations:

If the mother carries the hemophiliac allele (Xx) but the father does not (XY), the probability is that half of the daughters will be carriers (Xx) and half of the sons will have hemophilia (xY). The remaining half of the sons and daughters will receive the normal allele.

```
        X    x
 X     XX    Xx
 Y     XY    xY
```

If the mother carries no gene for hemophilia (XX) but the father is a hemophiliac (xY), all of the daughters will be carriers (xX), but the sons will neither have the disease nor be carriers.

```
        X    X
 x     xX    xX
 Y     XY    XY
```

Should a woman who is a carrier (xX) marry a man with hemophilia (xY), their daughters would all be either carriers or have hemophilia (xX or xx) (because they could inherit two recessive genes), while half of the sons would have the chance of having hemophilia (xY).

```
        x    X
 x     xx    xX
 Y     xY    XY
```

Some traits that are suspected to be X-linked are dominant rather than recessive. For example, in one type of oral-facial-digital syndrome (a disorder with a number of characteristics, including unusual facial appearance, absence of certain teeth, and a digital malformation such as syndactyly), transmission is from affected females to their daughters. Sons are rare in these families, but those who are born are unaffected. It is thought that the gene may be lethal to the male fetus. Thus, the sons who receive the particular gene die in utero, while those who receive the normal allele survive but do not inherit the trait.

Polygenetic Inheritance

If all traits were transmitted by single genes in one of the ways described above, our understanding of inheritance would be greatly simplified.

Many traits, however, are influenced by more than one gene and, hence, are termed *polygenetic*. Common problems that are believed to be polygenetic in origin include diabetes mellitus, spina bifida, anencephaly, cleft palate, gout, and allergic disorders. Interaction with the environment appears to be an important factor in the expression of a polygene. This would explain why these conditions tend to appear in families yet do not follow the classic patterns of inheritance.

REFERENCES

1. Arey, L.: *Developmental Anatomy: A Textbook and Laboratory Manual of Embryology*. Revised 7th Edition. Philadelphia, W. B. Saunders Co., 1974.
2. Asimov, I.: *The Genetic Code*. New York, The Orion Press, 1962.
3. Borek, E.: *The Code of Life*. New York, Columbia University Press, 1965.
4. Dobzhansky, T.: *Mankind Evolving*. New Haven, Yale University Press, 1962.
5. Eppink, H.: Genetic Causes of Abnormal Fetal Development and Inherited Disease. *JOGN Nursing* 6(5):14, 1977.
6. Horan, M.: Genetic Counseling: Helping the Family. *JOGN Nursing* 6(5):25, 1977.
7. Mellman, W. G.: The Genetic Basis for the Variability of Hereditable Disease. *Journal of Pediatrics*. 72:727, May 1968.
8. Page, E., Villee, C. A., and Villee, D. B.: *Human Reproduction: The Core Content of Obstetrics, Gynecology and Perinatal Medicine*. 2nd Edition. Philadelphia, W. B. Saunders Co., 1976.
9. Papazian, H. P.: *Modern Genetics*. New York, W. W. Norton and Co., Inc., 1967.
10. Smith, D. W.: Genetic Basis for Clinical Disorders. *Southern Medical Journal*. 64:Supplement #1, 4, Feb. 1971.
11. Thompson, C.: Legal Aspects of Genetic Screening. *JOGN Nursing* 6(5):34, 1977.
12. Thompson, J., and Thompson, M.: *Genetics in Medicine*. 2nd Edition. Philadelphia, W. B. Saunders Co., 1973.
13. Ursprung, H.: Developmental Genetics. *In* Cooke, R. E. (ed.): *The Biological Basis of Pediatric Practice*. New York, McGraw-Hill Book Co., 1968.
14. Wright, S. W.: Chromosomal Abnormalities in Man: The Autosomes. *In* Nelson, W. E., Vaughan, V. C., and McKay, R. J. (eds.): *Textbook of Pediatrics*. 9th Edition. Philadelphia, W. B. Saunders Co., 1969.

Chapter 3

BIOLOGIC READINESS FOR CHILDBEARING

The biologic functioning of the male and female reproductive systems is a complex and fascinating process. While this might be said of each body system, it is only in the reproductive systems that two distinct individuals must function in concert to achieve their biologic purpose.

Consider, for example, that the character of the mucus of the female cervix changes in consistency to facilitate the passage of sperm into the female reproductive tract at precisely the time that the ovum is ready for fertilization. Or consider that the zona pellucida, the area surrounding the cytoplasm of the ovary, admits a single sperm and then repels others.

In this chapter, we will examine the reproductive tracts from a biologic point of view; in the chapters that follow, we will consider more closely how social and psychologic factors interface with reproductive biology.

The reproductive system serves three functions, all closely interrelated. Satisfying sexual desires is the first; without a strong sexual drive the human race might never have survived the long course of history. The production of some very potent hormones is a second function. The third is procreation, beginning with the production of the ovum and sperm and continuing for several weeks following an infant's birth.

ANATOMY OF THE REPRODUCTIVE SYSTEM

In both males and females the reproductive system is divided into external and internal components. The major structures will be described here, and their functions will be discussed in greater detail later in the chapter.

MALE GENITALIA

The *penis* and *scrotum* are the external organs of the male reproductive system. Although the *testes* are found within the scrotum, they are generally considered internal structures.

Within the penis are three cylinders of spongy tissue: two *corpora cavernosa* and the *corpus spongiosum*. The urethra runs through the corpus spongiosum. A network of blood vessels and nerve endings crisscrosses the spongy tissue of each of these cavities; during sexual excitement they are engorged with blood, and the penis becomes characteristically stiff. The smooth, round head of the penis is the *glans penis,* a highly sensitive structure with many nerve endings. In an uncircumcised male, a retractable foreskin *(prepuce)* covers part of the glans; circumcision totally exposes the glans (Fig. 3–1).

The scrotal sac (Fig. 3–2) contains a testis and its *spermatic cord* in each of two separate compartments. Within the spermatic cord, from which the testis is suspended, are blood vessels, nerves, muscle fibers, and the *vas deferens* through which spermatozoa leave the testes. The spermatic cord enters the abdomen through the inguinal canal.

Internal reproductive organs in the male are the testes and the duct system. In the latter, spermatozoa are both stored and transported.

Within each testis are many seminiferous tubules in which spermatozoa are produced. The combined length of the seminiferous tubules of both testes measures several hundred yards, which allows the production and storage of hundreds of millions of sperm.

Each testis is enclosed in a tight fibrous sheath *(tunica albuginea).* If mumps occurs in an adult male, the virus may infect the testes. They will swell, but because the tunica albuginea is unyielding, the seminiferous tubules may be destroyed, and the man will then become sterile.

From the seminiferous tubules, sperm enter the *epididymis* and then the vas deferens. They pass from the vas through the *ejaculatory duct* into the urethra.

Figure 3–1 Male genitalia.

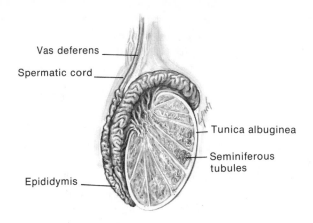

Vas deferens

Spermatic cord

Tunica albuginea

Seminiferous
tubules

Epididymis

Figure 3–2 Testis and epididymis.

Seminal Fluid

Seminal fluid, or semen, is produced by several glands, including the *prostate* and the *bulbourethral glands;* the epididymis; the vas deferens; and the *seminal vesicles.* In addition to containing spermatozoa, semen includes amino acids, certain amines that give it a characteristic odor, fructose, and *prostaglandins.* Prostaglandins are fatty acid derivatives secreted by the seminal vesicles that affect uterine muscle (see also Chapter 23).

Fluid from the seminal vesicles is believed to have a part in initiating sperm motility. The alkaline secretions of the bulbourethral gland may help to neutralize the acidic vaginal secretions that harm sperm. Some of this sticky fluid is secreted prior to ejaculation; because it may contain a few spermatozoa, pregnancy can result even when ejaculation does not occur (Chapter 5).

The Completion of Spermatogenesis

The initial development of an individual sperm during the process of mitosis has been described in Chapter 2. Before a sperm can become functional, i.e., capable of fertilization, it must complete its development. The nucleus shrinks, becoming the head of the sperm, and most of the cytoplasm is shed. A pointed acrosome forms at the front of the sperm, while a tail forms behind (see Fig. 2–2, page 12).

Biochemically, the sperm's energy is directed toward motility. Only motile sperm are capable of fertilization; sperm motility is one major factor evaluated during an infertility examination (Chapter 5). In the female reproductive tract, sperm may remain motile for as long as a week, although they are considered capable of fertilizing an ovum for only 48 to 72 hours.

The final step in sperm maturation is called *capacitation.* Probably because of some enzymatic difference, capacitation takes place only in the female reproductive tract; if a sperm is returned to the seminal fluid, the process is reversed *(decapacitation).* Just exactly what occurs during capacitation is unclear; probably the acrosome is detached.

Before mature sperm can be produced, there must be adequate production of follicle-stimulating hormone (FSH) (page 46) and of other hormones, particularly thyroid hormone. Because a temperature lower than body temperature is necessary for the production of mature spermatozoa, they cannot be produced when the testes are undescended.

EXTERNAL FEMALE GENITALIA

The female reproductive tract is also divided into external and internal structures. The external genitalia, collectively termed the *vulva* (covering), are the mons pubis (mons veneris), the labia majora, the labia minora, the clitoris, and the vaginal opening.

The *mons pubis* is composed of fatty tissue; it covers the bony pubic symphysis (page 37). Following puberty, it is covered with hair (Fig. 3–3).

The *labia majora* (labium majus is the singular form) are also composed of fatty tissue and contain nerves, blood vessels, and smooth muscle fibers. The covering skin of the labia majora contains hair follicles and sebaceous glands, but the inner surface is smooth and hairless. The labia majora are usually close together; the area between

them, visible only when the lips are parted, is the *pudendal cleft*.

The *labia minora* are thin, pink, and hairless. Posteriorly, the major lips merge with the minor lips. Anteriorly, the major and minor lips divide, with the upper portions forming the *prepuce* of the clitoris and the lower portions meeting beneath the clitoris to form the *frenulum*. The prepuce completely covers the clitoris in most women.

Between the labia minora is an area, the *vestibule* of the vagina, that contains the clitoris and the opening of the urethra and the vagina. The *clitoris* is homologous to the male penis; it consists of two *corpora cavernosa*, the tips of which are attached to the pubic bone. In function it is more like the glans of the penis, in that it contains many nerve endings and is highly sensitive. Like the penis, the clitoris becomes engorged

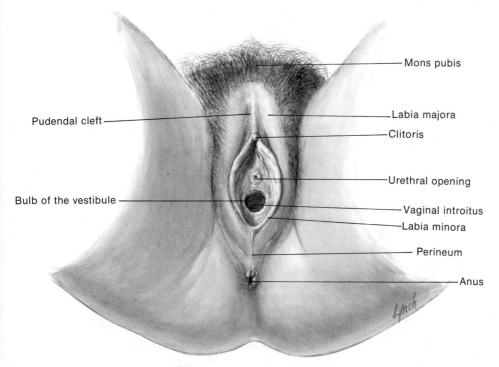

Pudendal cleft

Bulb of the vestibule

Mons pubis

Labia majora

Clitoris

Urethral opening

Vaginal introitus

Labia minora

Perineum

Anus

Figure 3–3   Female genitalia.

with blood during sexual excitement. However, because of its attachment, it does not become erect in the way that the penis does.

The introitus (or opening) of the vagina is an area highly sensitive both to pain and to sexual stimulation. The appearance of the opening tends to vary with the shape, or the absence, of the *hymen,* a pinkish membrane composed of elastic and collagenous tissue.

Traditionally, great social importance has been attached to the intact hymen as proof of virginity, but it is a very unreliable sort of evidence. Not only may the hymen be torn accidentally, but it may sometimes remain intact following intercourse. The rare imperforate hymen (i.e., the hymen with no opening at all) is corrected by surgical incision (hymenotomy).

Usually the virginal hymen will admit one fingertip, sometimes two, or a tampon. If the hymenal orifice is small, self-dilatation, either with the fingers or with a dilator, for 2 to 3 weeks prior to initial intercourse not only will make intercourse less difficult but may prevent a tearing of the hymen that predisposes to bladder infection, often called "honeymoon cystitis."

Provision of good preventive care would suggest that this information should be more widely disseminated. The anticipation and prevention of such problems are considered one value of a premarital examination. However, considering that many, probably most, women never have such an examination and that many women have initial sexual intercourse prior to marriage, some other way of educating both women and men should be found.

Alongside the vaginal opening are masses of erectile tissue, the *bulb of the vestibule,* and the muscular ring of the *bulbocavernous* muscle. These muscles allow for a certain amount of voluntary control over the size of the vaginal opening. Like the anal sphincter, the vaginal opening can be relaxed or tightened. The muscles can also be tightened through exercise. Such exercise should always be taught to mothers, preferably in the prenatal period (Chapter 9).

General body tenseness, anxiety, or physical pain communicates tenseness to the vaginal muscles. Such tenseness can make a vaginal examination much more difficult for a woman. It is a cycle in which anxiety and tenseness lead to pain, which, in turn, makes the woman more tense. The more a woman is able to relax, the less uncomfortable she will be, and the more she will relax.

The same cycle of tenseness—pain—tenseness may be a problem in sexual intercourse. *Vaginismus* is the term that describes such intense spasm of the muscles surrounding the vagina that the vagina itself cannot be penetrated.

Behind the vestibular bulbs are two small *Bartholin's glands* (greater vestibular glands), with ducts opening between the edge of the hymen and the labia minora. Bartholin's glands, homologous to the bulbourethral glands in the male, were once thought to play a major role in vaginal lubrication. Now that the vaginal walls themselves have been shown to be the chief source of lubrication, the function of these glands is unclear. Bartholin's glands may be infected by the gonococcus or by other organisms, with resultant abscesses or cysts. *Skene's ducts* (paraurethral ducts), which are found on each side of the urethral meatus, are also subject to infection. Between the vulva and the anus is the perineum, made up of skin, muscle, and fascia.

INTERNAL FEMALE GENITALIA

The internal organs of the female tract are a pair of ovaries and uterine

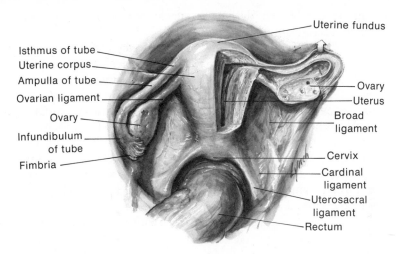

Figure 3–4   Female pelvis, posterior view.

(fallopian) tubes, the uterus, and the vagina (Figs. 3–4 and 3–5).

The Ovaries

Flanking the uterus and attached to it by the ovarian ligaments are the almond-shaped ovaries. Each ovary is approximately 1½ inches × 1 inch × ¾ inch (3.8 cm. × 2.5 cm. × 1.9 cm.) and weighs ½ ounce (15 grams). The periphery (cortex) of the ovary contains follicles in all stages of development (page 44), while the central medulla has many convoluted blood vessels. Each follicle contains one ovum (egg).

Figure 3–5   Internal female reproductive organs.

Unlike the testes, which deliver sperm through a duct system, there is no tube attached to the ovary through which the egg passes directly into the uterus. Instead, the follicle containing the egg must rupture (page 52), and the ovum must be "captured" by the end of the uterine tube. Thus, it is important that the ovarian capsule be thin.

Prior to puberty the ovary appears smooth and glistening, but as years go by, with a follicle rupturing each month, it becomes scarred.

The Uterine Tube

The uterine (fallopian) tube is about 4 inches (10.2 cm.) long. At the uterine end, it extends within the wall of the uterus and opens into it.

The tube itself contains four segments. Beginning at the ovarian end, they are:

1. The *infundibulum,* which is funnel-shaped (hence the name) and fringed by "finger-like" projections, the *fimbria.*

2. The *ampulla,* which accounts for half the length of the tube, and in which fertilization occurs.

3. The *isthmus,* a thin segment resembling a cord.

4. The *interstitial* segment, which passes through the myometrium of the uterus. The diameter of the tube becomes progressively smaller and is very small in this segment.

The motions of the fimbria that occur at the time of ovulation may attract the ovum into the tube in some way, probably by ciliary action, for if the fimbria are diseased or cut off, the result is relative infertility.

The tubes are lined with hairlike *cilia.* The sweeping action of these cilia, along with the peristalsis of the muscular tubal wall, propels the ovum through the tube. Unlike the motile sperm, the ovum has no innate mobility.

Patency of the tubes is very important. Surgical ligation of the uterine tubes is an effective means of sterilization. Gonorrhea can cause sterility because the purulent exudate that is produced fastens the mucosal surfaces of the lining of the tubes together, and often seals off the infundibulum as well. In countries where abortion by vacuum aspiration has been practiced for a number of years, subsequent sterility from collapse of the tubes has occurred in some women who have had repeated aspiration procedures.

Two methods for determining the patency of the tubes are:

1. The Rubin test, in which carbon dioxide gas is introduced into the uterus and the pressures measured.

2. Serial x-ray studies following the injection of a radiopaque fluid.

(See discussion of infertility in Chapter 5.)

The Uterus

The hollow, pear-shaped uterus is moored to the pelvis by eight ligaments (page 40) and attached to the pelvic floor through the vagina. Prior to any pregnancy, the uterus is approximately 3 to 3½ inches long (7 to 9 cm.) and 2 inches (5 cm.) wide at the top. Following the tremendous expansion of pregnancy, it returns almost, but not quite, to this original size. Normally, the uterus is tilted forward (anteverted, anteflexed) (Fig. 3-6).

The uterus consists of two parts, the corpus (body) and the cervix, but four areas may be described:

1. The fundus, which lies above the openings of the uterine tubes and is the uppermost part of the corpus.

2. The corpus.

3. The narrow isthmus where the corpus joins the cervix.

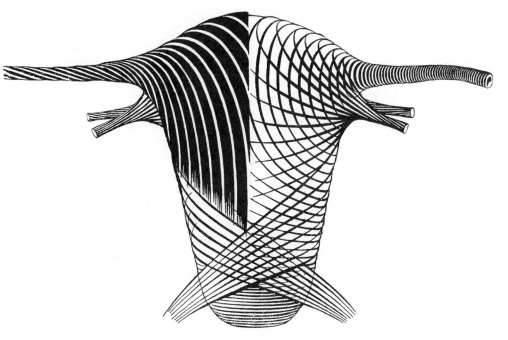

Figure 3–6   Highly schematized representation of the complex interlacing of the myometrial fibers, showing external longitudinal bands and internal circular arrangement. (From Bumm: *Grundriss zum Studium der Geburtschülfe*. 13th Edition. Wiesbaden, J. F. Bergmann, 1921.)

4. The cervix, or neck, which projects into the vagina.

The fundus is a landmark for obstetric care in every phase of pregnancy. For example, the height of the fundus is one indicator of the age of the normally developing fetus. That prolongation of the uterus into which the uterine tube spins is termed the *cornu* (horn).

During pregnancy, the isthmus forms the *lower uterine segment,* with the remainder of the corpus and fundus forming the *upper uterine segment.*

About half of the inch long (2.5 to 3 cm.) cervix protrudes into the vagina (Fig. 3–5) and is visible on vaginal examination with a speculum. The cervical canal expands somewhat between the *internal os,* where the cervix enters the isthmus, and the *external os,* which opens into the vagina. The external os, which is visible through the speculum,

appears round prior to first childbirth; subsequently, it is transverse with an *anterior lip* and a *posterior lip.*

Prior to pregnancy, the walls of the uterus are approximately 8 mm. thick and consist of three layers:

1. The perimetrium, a serous outer layer.

2. The myometrium, layers of intertwined smooth muscle.

3. The endometrium, a mucous membrane covered with ciliated columnar epithelium.

The perimetrium covers all of the uterus except the lower part of the anterior wall; at this point it turns upward to cover the bladder.

About 90 per cent of the upper uterus, including the fundus, consists of myometrium. By contrast, 10 per cent or less of the cervix is composed of myometrium, the cervix consisting chiefly of fibrous connective tissue. The transition area occurs in the lower 1 cm. of the isthmus. A change in muscle fibers during pregnancy allows for growth of the uterus.

The glands and blood vessels of the endometrium change constantly with the menstrual cycle. These changes are discussed in detail later in this chapter.

The Vagina

Above the hymen, the vagina serves as a repository for semen, a duct for uterine discharges (menstrual flow, for example), and a birth canal. The vagina tilts posteriorly from the vulva to the place at which it joins the cervix. Because of the angle of attachment to the cervix (almost a right angle), the anterior wall of the vagina is shorter than the posterior wall by about an inch. (The anterior wall is approximately 2.4 to 2.8 inches or 6 to 7 cm. in length; the posterior wall 3.2 to 3.6 inches or 8 to 9 cm.)

The projection of the cervix into the upper one-third of the vagina creates a blind vaginal pouch surrounding the cervix. Four fornices describe the upper segment of the vagina in relation to the cervix:

1. The posterior fornix, which lies behind the cervix.

2. The anterior fornix, which lies in front of the cervix.

3. Two lateral fornices, one on each side of the cervix.

Ordinarily a collapsed tube, the vagina is soft and so highly distensible that it will accommodate an infant's head at the time of delivery. Unlike the vaginal introitus, the walls of the vagina above the hymen are largely insensitive.

The vagina has a mucosal inner layer and a fibromuscular layer. Prior to a first delivery, the thick mucous membrane of the vagina appears in folds, called *rugae,* which are stretched to give the vagina a smooth appearance during delivery. Within the mucosa are layers of several types of cells: flat cells closest to the surface; parabasal and intermediate cells; and small, round basal cells. Beneath the vaginal mucosa is a fibromuscular layer that consists of predominantly smooth muscle in the upper layer and then changes to connective tissue cells at the deeper levels. This fibromuscular layer may become stretched or torn during childbirth.

Other Pelvic Organs

Because of their proximity, both the rectum and anus and the urethra and its meatus must be considered in relation to the genitalia. As Figure 3–5 demonstrates, the bladder is anterior to the uterus and the rectum posterior. This pelvic "geography" explains many of the minor problems of pregnancy and the postpartal period that are discussed throughout the text.

SUPPORTING STRUCTURES OF FEMALE GENITALIA

A variety of systems support the genital organs and structures. They include the bony pelvis, muscles, ligaments, and segments of the circulatory and nervous systems.

The Bony Pelvis

The pelvis consists of four bones: two innominate bones, the sacrum, and the coccyx. The innominate bone is divided into three areas that in childhood were distinct bones: the ilium, the ischium, and the pubis. Pelvic bones articulate at the two sacroiliac joints, the

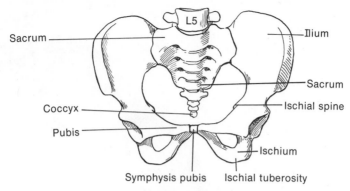

Figure 3–7 Female bony pelvis.

sacrococcygeal joint, and the symphysis pubis (Fig. 3–7). The fibrocartilage lining these joints becomes soft during pregnancy. This softening allows mobility of the pelvis during labor, but does not result in any change in pelvic size.

The size and shape of the bony pelvis are significant in determining whether a woman will be able to deliver her infant vaginally or whether a cesarean section may be necessary. Measurement of the pelvis is a part of the prenatal examination and is discussed in Chapter 8.

The *linea terminalis* divides the pelvis into two sections. The upper or *false* pelvis is of little obstetric interest; it does provide the general direction for the entry of the fetus into the true pelvis.

The lower or *true* pelvis determines the shape and direction of the birth canal and supports the muscles of the pelvic floor. The shape and size of the false pelvis give no indication of the shape and size of the true pelvis. The true pelvis has a basically cylindrical shape, which curves anteriorly much as a bent stovepipe (Fig. 3–8). Because of this curve, the canal is slightly less than 2 inches (4.5 cm.) anteriorly but is 5 inches (12.5 cm.) posteriorly.

Both the entrance and outlet of the true pelvis are smaller than the middle portion. The entrance is termed the *superior strait,* or plane of the inlet, and the outlet is the *inferior strait,* or plane of the outlet (Fig. 3–9). It is the shape of the superior strait that determines the type of pelvis. Figure 3–10 illustrates the four pelvic types:

a. Gynecoid, which is rounded and "roomy."

b. Android, which is heart-shaped and funnel-shaped, narrowing from top to bottom.

c. Anthropoid, an ellipse, which is elongated from front to back.

d. Platypelloid, a flattened ellipse.

In most women the shape of the pelvis is somewhat between these four types. When there is doubt, the shape of the anterior segment is the guide. Approximately 50 per cent of childbearing women have a gynecoid pelvis, considered the most favorable for normal delivery. The anthropoid pelvis is the next most common. Because the funnel-shaped android pelvis narrows from top to bottom, vaginal delivery is difficult. The flat platypelloid pelvis is relatively rare. Disease in early life that has caused contraction and distortion of the pelvic bones may present obstetric complications.

Pelvic inclination refers to the angle that the inlet makes with the horizon. When a woman is standing

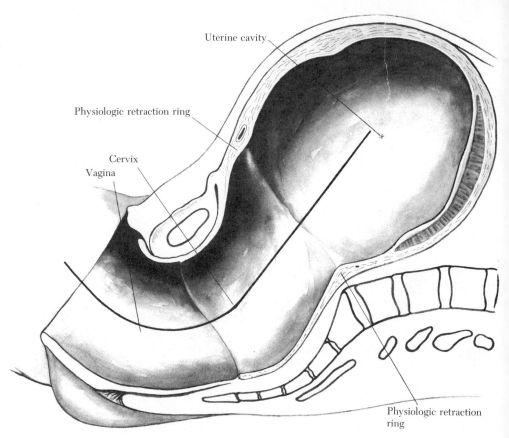

Uterine cavity

Physiologic retraction ring

Cervix
Vagina

Physiologic retraction
ring

Figure 3–8   The pelvis curves anteriorly, much as a bent stovepipe. The uterus, cervix, and vagina are diagrammed as if all the component parts were distended at one time. The axis is the central curved line. (From Greenhill and Friedman: *Biological Principles and Modern Practice of Obstetrics.* Philadelphia, W. B. Saunders Co., 1974.)

erect, pelvic inclination is about 55 to 60 degrees.

The *axis* of the pelvis is formed by drawing a line perpendicular to each of the pelvic planes (Fig. 3–8). In the gynecoid pelvis, the curve begins at about the level of the spine. The pelvic axis is another important consideration in delivery.

Muscles and Fascia of the Pelvic Floor

The pelvic floor, or pelvic diaphragm (Fig. 3–11), is made up of two identifiable muscular diaphragms: (1) the deeper, stronger muscles and (2) the superficial muscle structures that close and control the urethral, anal, and vaginal orifices. Internally, the pelvic diaphragm forms the base of the abdominal cavity and is covered with peritoneum. It serves to anchor the cervix, vagina, rectum, and bladder. The muscle layers are surrounded by connective tissue, fascia, adipose tissue, and skin.

The deeper levator ani muscles are composed of the pubococcygeal, the iliococcygeal, and the puborectal muscles. The vagina, rectum, and urethra actually pass through this muscular diaphragm, which forms a sling-like support for the birth canal. Each pelvic organ has a fascial sheath surrounding

Figure 3–9 The pelvic inlet and outlet. (From Greenhill: *Obstetrics.* 13th Edition. Philadelphia, W. B. Saunders Co., 1965.)

delivery. Persistent bowel and bladder problems may result from a weakening or tearing of these tissues.

The superficial layer of the pelvic floor is composed of the urogenital diaphragm, the perineal body, the vulva, and the glands of the vulva. The *urogenital diaphragm* is formed by the bulbocavernous muscle, the ischiocavernous muscle, and the superficial transverse perineal muscles. It surrounds the upper part of the urethra and the lower part of the vagina, which supports the upper portion of the urethra. When there is an increase in intra-abdominal

or embracing it that supports it and assists in maintaining its anatomic relationship to the other pelvic organs and the bony pelvis.

Four fascial layers arise from the deeper fascial covering of the levator ani muscles: (1) one layer extends in the front to the bladder and continues on to the pubic bone to form the pubovesical ligament; (2) another, the retrorectal layer, travels to the sacrum to form the uterosacral ligament; (3) two other layers, between the bladder and vagina and between the vagina and rectum, branch to each side to form the base of the broad ligament that attaches to the pelvic side wall and to each side of the uterus. It is the fascial layers surrounding the vagina with the bladder in front and the rectum in back that are most subject to tearing during the course of

Figure 3–10 Caldwell-Moloy classification of pelves. *A,* Gynecoid; *B,* android; *C,* anthropoid; and *D,* platypelloid.

Inferior fascia of
urogenital diaphragm

Bulbocavernosus m.

Ischiocavernosus m.

Deep transverse
perineal muscle

Superficial trans.
perineal muscle

Obturator m.

Levator ani

Ischial spine

External anal
sphincter

Ischiorectal fossa

Gluteus maximus

Figure 3–11 Topographic anatomy of the important perineal structures showing the interrelationships between bony, muscular, and visceral structures. (From Greenhill and Friedman: *Biological Principles and Modern Practice of Obstetrics.* Philadelphia, W. B. Saunders Co., 1974.)

pressure, the pressure is transmitted to the upper urethra as well as to the bladder, and urine does not escape. However, if the urogenital diaphragm has been torn or stretched during childbirth, the bladder neck and urethra may sag downward, allowing urine to escape when intra-abdominal pressure increases. This is called *stress incontinence*. Often nurses are the first to hear of the symptoms of stress incontinence; a woman may feel it is too small a problem to mention to a physician, even though it is very aggravating to her.

The pelvic floor muscles and fascia differ in strength and tonus from one mother to another. They tend to be weaker in the mother who has delivered babies previously than in the mother who is delivering for the first time. The

quality of pelvic floor support and the integrity of these tissues can be maintained or enhanced by an attentive birth attendant and by a knowledgeable care-agent during postdelivery recovery and adjustment.

Pelvic Ligaments

Four significant ligaments serve to bind the pelvic bones together and add strength to the pelvic structure: (1) the interpubic ligaments between the pubic bones strengthen the symphysis pubis, (2) the sacrotuberous ligaments between the sacrum and the ischial tuberosity, (3) the sacrospinous ligaments between the sacrum and the ischial spines, and (4) the sacroiliac ligaments between the sacroiliac joints and the inguinal ligaments between the anterior superior iliac spine and the pubic bone. The sacroiliac ligaments are probably the strongest in the entire body. The sacrotuberous and sacrospinous ligaments form the back portion of the pelvic outlet.

Other major ligaments supporting the pelvic organs are summarized in Table 3-1. Figure 3-4 illustrates several major ligaments.

Circulation

Three paired vessels form the main arterial blood supply of the uterus (Fig. 3-12). They are: (1) the uterine arteries, branches of the hypogastric arteries; (2) the ovarian arteries, branches of the aorta; and (3) the funicular arteries (not shown), branches from the vesical arteries that join the ovarian arteries at the fundus. As Figure 3-12 shows, all of these vessels are highly convoluted with frequent anastomoses.

Veins follow the same paths as the arteries. The uterine veins empty into plexuses in the broad ligaments. The blood then flows through veins in the broad ligaments to the hypogastric vein and then to the common iliac vein. The ovarian veins empty into the renal vein on the left and the vena cava on the right. Veins penetrate all the layers of the uterus and are especially plentiful in the myometrium. Like the arteries, they anastomose frequently.

The arteries and veins of the uterine wall are unique in that they

Table 3-1   LIGAMENTS SUPPORTING THE PELVIC ORGANS

Ligament	Location	Comments
Broad	From the lateral walls of the uterus to the lateral pelvic wall.	Upper two-thirds: two thin layers of peritoneum. Divides pelvic cavity into anterior and posterior segments. Folds contain uterine tubes, ovaries, round and cardinal ligaments, blood vessels, lymphatics, and nerves.
Cardinal	Lower one-third of broad ligament, from cervix to lateral pelvic wall.	Dense connective tissue. Main supporting structure of uterus (along with muscles of pelvic diaphragm and perineum). Contains uterine artery and vein.
Round	From the uterus, just anterior to the insertion of the uterine tubes, upward and outward through the inguinal canal to the labia majora.	Forms the upper margin of the broad ligaments.
Uterosacral	From the posterior upper cervix backward to the fascia of the second and third sacral vertebrae.	Exerts traction, which keeps the uterus in normal position.
Anterior	A peritoneal fold between the bladder and the uterus.	
Posterior	A peritoneal fold between the uterus and the rectum.	
Ovarian	Suspends ovary.	Short.
Infundibulopelvic	Ovarian hilum to the lateral pelvic wall.	Contains ovarian vein and artery.

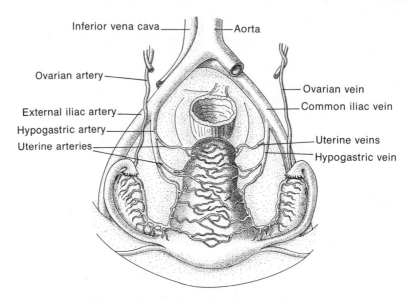

Inferior vena cava
Aorta
Ovarian artery
Ovarian vein
Common iliac vein
External iliac artery
Hypogastric artery
Uterine arteries
Uterine veins
Hypogastric vein

Figure 3–12   Blood supply of uterus and ovary.

have no outer coat and so lie directly on the muscular bundles, where they form large blood spaces called sinuses. Because of this, the ovarian and pelvic veins are able to dilate as blood volume increases during pregnancy. It is estimated that their capacity is increased by more than 60 times by the thirty-sixth week of pregnancy. A second apparent advantage of this property of the ovarian and pelvic veins is the neutralization of changes in systemic pressure that is afforded, such as the sudden high central pressure that occurs during acute straining.

The pelvic organs are also richly supplied by lymphatic vessels and lymph nodes. The lymphatic system follows the overall pattern of the major blood vessels.

Nerve Supply

Both motor and sensory fibers from the autonomic and central nervous systems supply the genitalia (Fig. 3–13). Parasympathetic motor fibers stimulate vasodilatation and cause the inhibition of muscular contraction; sympathetic motor fibers affect vasocon-striction and muscular contraction. The *hypogastric plexus* is a large plexus of motor fibers formed above the promontory of sacrum near the bifurcation of the aorta. Sensory fibers arise from the spinal cord through the sacral nerves.

A basic knowledge of neural function is valuable in understanding a number of clinical phenomena that will be discussed in greater detail in the chapters that follow. For example, because sympathetic motor fibers that stimulate muscular contraction originate in the ganglia at the level of the T-5 to T-10 vertebrae, spinal anesthesia to the level of T-5 will tend to abolish contractions of the uterine fundus. However, a transection of the spinal cord above the level of T-5 will not necessarily prevent labor and delivery.

The stimulus for pain in hollow viscera such as the uterus and tubes is either stretching or ischemia. Thus, a cervical biopsy is only mildly uncomfortable but dilatation (as for a dilatation and curettage) requires anesthesia. A twisting of the tube that interferes with blood supply will cause severe pain.

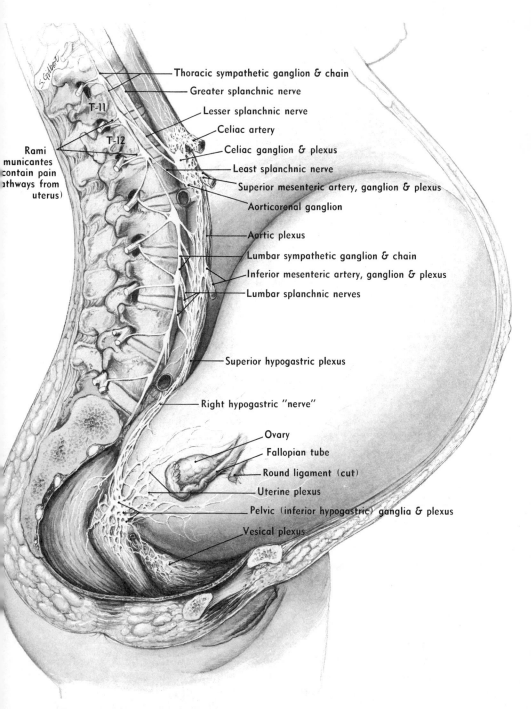

Figure 3–13   Schematic representation of uterine nerve supply showing nerve routes arising from the thoracic and lumbar spinal nerves and traversing through the lumbar sympathetic chain to the aortic plexus, superior hypogastric plexus, and pelvic plexus. (From Bonica: *Principles and Practice of Obstetrical Analgesia and Anesthesia.* Philadelphia, F. A. Davis Co., 1967.)

Figure 3–14 *Left,* Diagram of the breast as a "forest of trees." *A,* Alveolus; *B,* ductule; *C,* duct; *D,* lactiferous duct; *E,* lactiferous sinus; *F,* ampulla; *G,* nipple pore; *H,* areolar margin. With full development of the uterine-menstrual cycle, groups of gland secreting cells (alveoli) bud from the small ducts (ductules). The alveoli secrete milk under the influence of prolactin, a hormone of the pituitary gland. *Right,* Diagram of an alveolus. *A,* Uncontracted myoepithelial cell; *B,* contracted myoepithelial cell; *C,* gland secreting cell; *D,* ductule opening. Gland secreting cells are arranged in a circle about the ductule opening. About the alveolus is a contractile cell. When sucking begins, this cell, under the influence of oxytocin from the pituitary gland, contracts and squeezes the milk into the duct system. This reflex is called "let-down." (From Applebaum: *Pediatric Clinics of N. America, 17*:205, 1970.)

BREASTS

While the breasts are not genitalia, they are influenced by the same hormones and play an important role in both sexual and reproductive functions. Externally, the nipples and the darkened areolae are the most obvious areas of the breasts. The nipples contain many nerve fibers, which make them highly sensitive. While nipples normally protrude, they may be flat or inverted. Occasionally, a woman may have one or more accessory nipples and/or breasts. These are usually found along a "milk line" extending from the normally located nipple to the groin, as are multiple nipples in other species. The small papillae that appear on the surface of the nipples and the areolae are the *tubercles of Montgomery,* glands that secrete a lipoid substance that lubricates the nipples.

Internally, the breast is arranged in *lobes,* composed of about 15 to 20 *lobules* and *lactiferous ducts* (Fig. 3–14).

Lactiferous ducts from each lobe join to form the *ampulla* or *lactiferous sinus.* From each ampulla a milk duct opens into the nipple. Connective and fatty tissue support the lobes.

Breast changes during pregnancy are discussed in Chapter 6 and those of lactation in Chapter 19.

THE ENDOCRINE SYSTEM AND REPRODUCTION

Even during the embryonic and fetal period, hormones are necessary for the proper development of the reproductive organs. Hormonal influence continues to be significant throughout life, both in normal physiologic functioning and in pharmacologic intervention in a variety of circumstances.

The endocrine secretions that affect the reproductive system come from two sources: the anterior lobe of the pituitary gland and the ovaries or testes.

These hormones are, in turn, affected by the hypothalamus and the central nervous system.

Endocrine functioning involves both positive and negative feedback. For example, a steroid hormone such as estrogen can stimulate the release of a gonadotropin such as luteinizing hormone. This is positive feedback. Negative feedback occurs when a hormone, such as a large amount of progesterone, prevents the release of a gonadotropin. The concentration of a particular hormone in the blood determines whether the feedback will be positive or negative. Examples of both positive and negative feedback can be found in the discussion of hormonal action that follows.

Neural Control of the Endocrine System

At one time the anterior pituitary gland (the adenohypophysis) was considered the "master" of the endocrine system. It is known now that the "master" is itself influenced by the hypothalamus, which in turn can be stimulated by still higher nerve centers (Fig. 3–15).

Six factors have been isolated in the hypothalamus, each of which controls the release of one of the hormones of the anterior pituitary. Three factors affect reproductive hormones; together they are termed gonadotropin-releasing factors and include: (1) follicle-stimulating hormone releasing factor (FRF), (2) luteinizing hormone releasing factor (LRF), and (3) prolactin inhibitory factor (PIF).

The gonadotropin-releasing factors are carried to the anterior pituitary by way of the hypothalamic-hypophyseal portal system (Fig. 3–16).

Several brain centers modify the action of the gonadotropin-releasing factors. These centers are located mainly in the limbic system, a group of brain structures surrounding the hypothalamus and including the hypothalamus as one of its central elements. The centers are influenced by positive and negative feedback levels of steroid hormones (estrogen, progesterone, and testosterone) and probably by anterior pituitary hormones (follicle-stimulating hormone [FSH], luteinizing hormone [LH], and luteotropic hormone [LTH]). The limbic centers are also sensitive to emotional stimuli, such as stress, and to factors external to the individual, such as light.

Examples of central nervous system influence on gonadotropin excretion can be found in animals and in humans. In sheep, goats, and deer, for instance, changes in the weather and in the amount of light during the day elicit responses in the nervous system that, in turn, increase the quantity of gonadotropins during the mating season. This, in turn, allows birth during a season of the year when the chances of survival are greatest.

Although there is no directly analogous behavior in humans, stress, mediated through the central nervous system to the endocrine system, certainly affects fertility. Rose[17] found that levels of testosterone rose and fell in combat soldiers in response to the degrees of stress to which the men were exposed. A stressful emotional problem may suppress luteinizing-releasing factor (LRF) in a woman so that luteinizing hormone is not released, ovulation does not occur, and amenorrhea results. The emotional correlates of infertility are discussed in more detail in Chapter 5.

The Anterior Pituitary and the Reproductive System

The anterior pituitary secretes three gonadotropic hormones, i.e., hormones that act upon the gonads. These hormones are: (1) follicle-stimulating

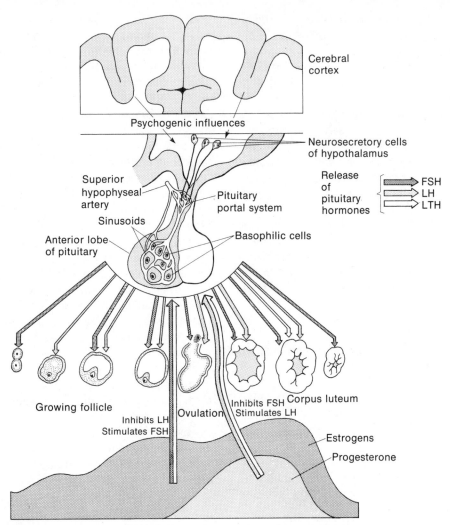

Figure 3–15 Diagram of the interaction between the nervous system, the endocrine system, and the ovarian cycle.

hormone (FSH); (2) luteinizing hormone (LH), usually called interstitial cell-stimulating hormone (ICSH) in the male; and (3) luteotropic hormone (LTH), also called lactogenic hormone or prolactin.

Follicle-Stimulating Hormone in the Male. FSH is essential for initiating the conversion of spermatogonia into sperm. In addition, it potentiates the effects of LH in promoting the production of testosterone.

Follicle-Stimulating Hormone in the Female. At the time of puberty, FSH stimulates the growth of the ovaries. From that time onward its primary function appears to be the initiation of the growth of the follicles. During each monthly cycle, 20 or more primordial follicles begin to develop under the influence of FSH. Ordinarily, one will outgrow the others and expel its ovum, i.e., ovulate. All of the others degenerate completely.

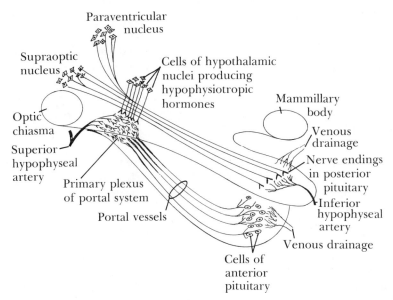

Figure 3–16 Diagram of hypothalamus and pituitary gland showing the portal system of the vasculature. (From Villee: *Human Endocrinology*. Philadelphia, W. B. Saunders Co., 1975.)

FSH is not secreted continuously; FSH output follows a cyclic pattern that is related to the output of estrogen. As estrogen production rises, the level of FSH falls (an example of negative feedback). Figure 3–15 shows this relationship during the menstrual cycle, discussed below. The level of FSH is high on day one, drops to its lowest point on day 14 when estrogen levels are peaking, and begins to rise again on about day 25 in preparation for the beginning of the next cycle.

Luteinizing Hormone (Interstitial Cell-Stimulating Hormone) in the Male. LH (ICSH) stimulates the production of testosterone by the interstitial cells of Leydig in the testes.

Luteinizing Hormone in the Female. Whereas FSH initiates follicular growth, LH, acting along with FSH synergistically, is necessary for final growth and for ovulation. Together they cause rapid swelling of the follicle shortly before ovulation, which probably contributes to the rupture of the fol-

licle. LH may also have a direct effect upon the breaking open of the follicle. It is known that an especially large amount of LH is secreted on the day immediately prior to ovulation, a condition termed the *ovulatory surge* (Fig. 3–15). Note also in Figure 3–15 that LH appears to be stimulated by estrogen (positive feedback).

LH is also responsible for the change of follicular cells into lutein cells following ovulation. (See discussion of the ovarian cycle, below.)

Luteotropic Hormone in the Male. At this time the role of LTH in the male is not considered significant.

Luteotropic Hormone in the Female. On the basis of animal experiments it is believed that LTH is responsible for the maturing of the corpus luteum and its secretion (see below). In animals LTH also stimulates the development of the mammary glands and milk production, hence the name prolactin. The name used for this hormone generally depends upon the function being described; remember that LTH and prolactin are one hormone with more than one action. LTH has not been proved to exist in humans.

HORMONES PRODUCED BY THE REPRODUCTIVE SYSTEM

Testosterone, secreted by the interstitial cells of the testes; estrogens, produced by the cells of the ovarian follicle and the corpus luteum; and progesterone, secreted by the corpus luteum, are the principal hormones produced by the male and female reproductive systems. During pregnancy the placenta also secretes both estrogens and progesterone (Chapter 6). (Small amounts of both estrogens and testosterone are also secreted by the adrenal cortex in both men and women.)

Testosterone

The production of testosterone begins in the second month of embryonic life. Testosterone is essential for the development of the penis, scrotum, prostate gland, seminal vesicles, and genital ducts. It is also essential for the descent of the testes. A deficiency of testosterone during this period of development may lead to male hermaphrodism, i.e., a male with ambiguous external genitalia.

The major production of testosterone begins between the ages of 11 and 13, dwindles after the age of 40, and by the age of 80 is only 20 per cent of the amount of peak years. It is testosterone production during adolescence that is responsible for the development of the distinguishing characteristics of the male body:

1. The penis, scrotum, and testes enlarge.

2. Male hair distribution is achieved.

3. Because of hypertrophy of the laryngeal mucosa and enlargement of the larynx, the voice changes; at first there is hoarseness, later a deepening of the voice.

4. Protein is increased in the body; muscles become stronger.

5. The quantity of the bone matrix increases; bones become thicker and have increased deposits of calcium salts.

6. The basic metabolic rate increases from 5 to 15 per cent.

7. Red blood cells are increased by 15 per cent.

8. There is slightly increased reabsorption of sodium in the distal renal tubules.

Testosterone is also necessary for the completion of spermatogenesis, i.e., the conversion of spermatogonia into sperm, a process begun by FSH (page 46). If the hypothalamus is functioning normally, testosterone acts as a feedback control system that inhibits the secretion of the gonadotropins (FSH, LH, and LTH). It is believed that testosterone does this by inhibiting the gonadotropin-releasing factors of the hypothalamus.

The Estrogens

There is no single substance, estrogen, but rather a group of estrogens. However only two, *β-estradiol* and *estrone,* are secreted in quantities large enough to be considered significant. Of these two, estradiol is considered the major compound. The singular word estrogen is commonly used for these substances.

Estriol is the oxidized end-product of estradiol and estrone; it is formed in the liver shortly after the estrogens are secreted, from that part of the estrogens that has not entered cells. Other substances conjugated from estrogens in the liver are glucuronides, sulfates, and estroproteins.

Small quantities of estrogens are secreted even in childhood, but it is at puberty that the production of estrogens, now 20 times greater, becomes such a major factor in female life. The estrogens:

1. Are responsible for the development of primary and secondary sexual characteristics.

2. Are essential to the hypothalamic-pituitary-ovarian cycle.

3. Influence the thickening of the uterine endometrium during the proliferative and secretory phase of the endometrial cycle.

4. Diversely affect reproductive function.

5. Appear to influence numerous body processes.

Estrogens in the Development of Female Characteristics. Just as testosterone is responsible for the distinguishing characteristics of males, the estrogens govern female traits. During puberty:

1. The uterus, vagina, uterine tubes, and external genitalia increase in size. Fat is deposited in the mons pubis and labia majora.

2. The cells of the vaginal epithelium change from cuboidal to stratified, which enhances their resistance to trauma and infection.

3. The cells and glands of the uterine endometrium increase in number, a preparation for possible pregnancies in the future. Similar changes occur in the lining of the tubes, where the increased number of ciliated cells aids the ovum in traveling toward the uterus.

4. Breasts grow and the milk-producing system begins to develop (to be completed under the influence of other hormones, progesterone and prolactin).

5. Bone growth is accelerated for several years. Because estrogens cause the epiphyses to unite with the shafts of long bones at an earlier age than does testosterone, the average woman does not become as tall as the average man.

6. Fat is deposited in the subcutaneous tissues, particularly in the breasts, buttocks, and thighs.

7. The basic metabolic rate is increased, but not to the extent of the increase caused by testosterone.

8. Female hair distribution occurs.

Estrogens stimulate motility in the uterine tubes, which brings the fimbriated end of the tube into contact with the ovum, aiding in its capture and propelling it into the end of the tube.

The effects of estrogens alone and of estrogens and progesterone combined on the ovarian and endometrial cycles are discussed more fully below. Following implantation, estrogens stimulate the development of both the myometrium of the uterus and the ductile system of the breasts.

Progesterone

In the woman who is not pregnant, progesterone, produced by the corpus luteum, governs all of the morphologic and biochemical changes of the endometrium during the second half of the menstrual cycle (see below) (Fig. 3–15). These changes prepare the body for pregnancy or gestation (thus they are progestational). Progesterone also maintains the endometrium during pregnancy, making continuation of pregnancy possible (Chapter 6).

Before progesterone can be effective, tissues must first be exposed to estrogens. This has practical value in diagnosis. If, for example, in the absence of pregnancy the endometrium fails to bleed after the administration of progesterone, a low level of estrogen is being secreted by the ovary.

Progesterone has a number of other functions, some of which will be discussed in greater detail later. Under the influence of progesterone, the endocervical glands secrete a thick mucus that will not form fern patterns and that impedes sperm migration, a factor important in the contraceptive effects of progestins (see page 61).

Progesterone reduces the excitability of the myometrium; contractions that normally recur in uterine muscle are reduced and become sustained and tetanic rather than clonic.

Alveolar development of the breasts and the preparation of the breasts for lactation require progesterone. Progesterone exerts a feedback mechanism on the releasing factors of the hypothalamus, which is demonstrated elsewhere in this chapter. The effect of progesterone on the elevation of basal body temperature is important in understanding basal temperature in relation to both contraception and infertility (Chapter 5). Progesterone also stimulates respiration, so that the CO_2 tension of the blood is decreased during the last half of the menstrual cycle and during pregnancy.

THE MENSTRUAL CYCLE

The interaction of the hypothalamic, pituitary, and gonadotropic hormones controls the cyclic changes that occur in a woman's body from the time of *menarche* (first menstruation) until *menopause* (the cessation of menstruation). These changes include the ovarian and endometrial cycles as well as variations in basal body temperature and changes in other areas of the genital tract. Although each cycle is closely interrelated with the others, each will be discussed separately.

Each cycle is discussed on the basis of an "idealized" 28 day cycle, in which the first day of the menstrual period is day one. Such numbering is convenient because the onset of menstruation is readily identified. Many normal cycles are either shorter or longer than 28 days; it is merely convenient in a textbook to discuss a 28 day period in which ovulation is presumed to occur on day 14.

THE OVARIAN CYCLE

Because the cyclic changes of the endometrium are dependent upon the cyclic changes in the ovary, the ovarian cycle must be understood first.

At the twentieth week of fetal life there are about 7 million *oogonia* (immature ova) in the human ovary, the largest number that there will ever be. By the time an infant girl is born, the oogonia have been reduced to approximately 1 million, have begun their first meiotic division (Chapter 2), and are called *primary oocytes*. They do not undergo further change until ovulation occurs. Their number at puberty is about 0.5 million. Approximately 450 primary oocytes will ovulate; consider how few will eventually be fertilized.

Figure 3–17 *A,* Follicle with early formation of oolemma or zona pellucida. (From Shettles: *Ovum Humanum.* New York, Hafner Publishing Co., 1960.) *B,* Follicle of a slightly later stage at the 18th day of the cycle showing *a,* ovum; *b,* oocyte nucleus; *c,* oolemma or zona pellucida; *d,* follicular epithelium with mitochondria; *e,* Call-Exner body or vacuole; *f,* theca folliculi with internal and external layers not yet differentiated; *g,* blood vessels containing erythrocytes; *h,* basement membrane; *i,* mitosis in follicular cell. (Magnification ×345.) (From Bloom and Fawcett: *A Textbook of Histology.* 9th Edition. Philadelphia, W. B. Saunders Co., 1968.)

A

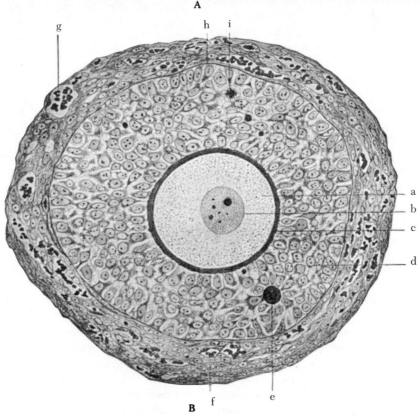

B

Figure 3–17 *See legend on the opposite page.*

The Follicular Phase

In the 2 weeks prior to ovulation, the primary oocyte undergoes the changes that prepare it for fertilization under the influence of the follicle-stimulating hormone (FSH). FSH output is very high at the beginning of the cycle (Fig. 3–15). The oocyte, along with the follicular (or granulosa) cells that surround it, is now called a follicle and is found in the periphery of the ovarian cortex (Fig. 3–17). The follicular cells are at first flattened, but they enlarge, become cuboidal in shape, and multiply in number. Follicular fluid, containing estrogen, develops between the follicular cells, accumulating in the center of the follicle to form a vesicle. Two layers of cells develop around the follicle, the outer *theca externa* and the inner *theca interna*. Theca interna cells play a part both in estrogen production and in the formation of the corpus luteum (see below). A mucoid membrane, the *zona pellucida,* develops between the primary oocyte and the follicular cells.

Thus developed, the immature primary follicle is now a *vesicular* or *graafian* follicle (having been first described by the anatomist de Graaf). During a normal cycle, several follicles will begin to develop, but usually only one will mature to the graafian follicle stage. The others degenerate and disappear. Should more than one follicle mature, rupture, and subsequently be fertilized, fraternal twins will develop. Identical twins, in contrast, develop from a single ovum.

As the graafian follicle matures, it moves to the surface of the ovary. Shortly before the follicle ruptures, it is approximately ½ inch in diameter (10 to 15 mm.) and could easily be observed if the ovary were to be removed for some reason.

Within the follicle the oocyte is also enlarging. Yolk granules are deposited in the cytoplasm for nourishment, should fertilization occur. Before the follicle ruptures, the first meiotic division is completed.

Changes continue to take place in the graafian follicle. At a late stage the ovum and the follicular cells bordering it (called the *corona radiata* because they appear as a radiating crown) may become detached from the wall of the follicle. Finally, on about the fourteenth day of the cycle, under the influence of FSH and LH, the follicle ruptures, and both the fluid *(liquor folliculi)* and the ovum and corona radiata are discharged from the ovary (Fig. 3–18).

The exact mechanism of ovulation itself is not well understood, but experimental evidence suggests that it is a slow process of extrusion, involving a gradual opening and oozing rather than an explosive event.

Variations in the overall number of days in the total cycle are usually variations in the length of the follicular phase.

The Luteal Phase

Following ovulation, the extruded ovum makes its way into the uterine tube. It may be fertilized in the outer one-third of the tube and subsequently makes it way to the uterus. Beginning shortly before ovulation and during the first 3 days following this (about days 14 to 17 of the cycle), capillaries invade the granulosa of the follicle, and both the granulosa and the theca interna become filled with a yellow material, hence the name *corpus luteum* (yellow body).

The corpus luteum produces progesterone and estrogen. Observe in Figure 3–15 that there is a slight dip in estrogen production following ovulation. This occurs because estrogen secretion by the graafian follicle has ceased, but the corpus luteum is as yet not fully formed and producing estrogen

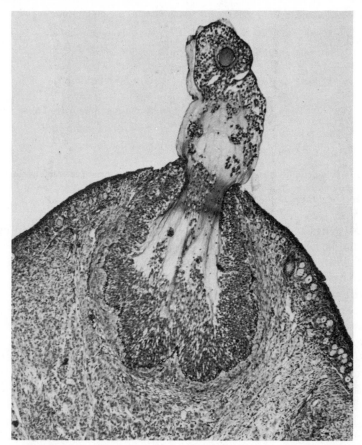

Figure 3–18 Photograph of a rabbit follicle taken at the moment of ovulation. (From Page, Villee, and Villee: *Human Reproduction: The Core Content of Obstetrics, Gynecology and Perinatal Medicine.* 2nd Edition. Philadelphia, W. B. Saunders Co., 1976.)

at peak level. Note, in Figure 3–15, that the rise in progesterone level begins before ovulation; this is because the cells of the corpus luteum are beginning to mature in the graafian follicle.

Peak development of the corpus luteum comes about a week after ovulation, or about day 21 of the cycle, the time at which implantation will occur if the ovum is fertilized. From that point in time its development depends upon fertilization. If there is no fertilization, degeneration of the corpus luteum (now called the corpus luteum of menstruation) occurs rapidly. It ceases to secrete

progesterone and estrogen, and the level of these hormones falls abruptly. Toward the end of the regressive phase, the corpus luteum is whitish in color and is called the *corpus albicans*. Following degeneration, it is replaced by connective tissue. The drop in hormone production leads to menstruation about a week later (see below).

Should the ovum be fertilized, the life of the corpus luteum (now termed the corpus luteum of pregnancy) is extended by chorionic gonadotropin, which is produced by the trophoblast that developed from the fertilized ovum

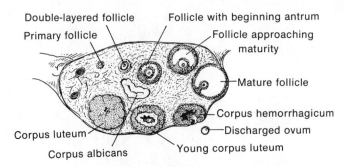

Figure 3–19 Schematic diagram of ovary, showing the sequence of events in origin, growth, and rupture of the ovarian follicle and the formation and retrogression of the corpus luteum. Follow clockwise around the ovary, beginning at the primary follicle.

(Chapter 6). It will then continue to enlarge and be active throughout the first 3 months of pregnancy, with peak production of hormones during the first 60 days. The placenta gradually replaces the corpus luteum as the producer of estrogens and progesterone during pregnancy.

The luteal phase lasts from 13 to 15 days, regardless of the overall duration of the menstrual cycle. A luteal phase of less than 12 days is considered abnormal; a luteal phase of more than 16 days is suggestive of pregnancy. The presence of pregnanediol, a breakdown product of progesterone, in the urine indicates that luteinization has taken place.

The complete ovarian cycle is diagrammed in Figure 3–19 and summarized in calendar form in Figure 3–20.

THE ENDOMETRIAL CYCLE

A second cycle, concurrent with and influenced by the ovarian cycle, prepares the endometrium for the implantation of the ovum should fertilization occur. The ovarian cycle involves the ovary; the endometrial cycle involves the uterus.

Before describing the phases of the endometrial cycle, the endometrium itself should be considered in somewhat

Figure 3–20 Calendar of ovarian cycle.

more detail. Although the line of demarcation between the three layers of the endometrium is not sharp, they are the (1) zona basalis, (2) zona spongiosa, and (3) zona compacta.

The thin zona basalis, which lies next to the myometrium, responds very little to hormonal changes. Portions of the zona spongiosa, in which the endometrial glands are located, respond to ovarian steroids and are shed during menstruation. The zona compacta forms about one-third of the endometrium during the fourteenth to twenty-eighth days of the menstrual cycle. It is totally shed during menstruation.

Like the ovarian cycle, the endometrial cycle is divided into phases. The major phases are the proliferative, which precedes ovulation, and the secretory, which follows it. The first 4 days of the idealized cycle are the menstrual phase; some authors consider the menstrual phase as an early part of the proliferative phase. Terminology varies somewhat from one text to another. Although the menstrual phase begins on day one of the cycle, in function it is a terminal activity and so will be discussed after the other phases.

The Proliferative Phase

The proliferative phase of the endometrial cycle corresponds to the follicular phase of the ovarian cycle. Estrogens produced by the developing follicles cause the initially thin endometrial epithelium to thicken; the epithelial cells increase in number through mitosis and become taller and columnar. The glands of the zona spongiosa hypertrophy and become more convoluted; blood vessels also grow. At the time of ovulation the endometrium is approximately 2 to 3 mm. thick (0.08 to 0.12 inch) (Fig. 3-21).

The Secretory Phase

Following ovulation, the endometrium continues to thicken in preparation for the fertilized ovum. The secretory phase of the endometrial cycle corresponds to the luteal phase of the ovarian cycle. Glands and blood vessels coil (Fig. 3-21). Progesterone, produced by the corpus luteum, is the principal hormone that influences the changes of the secretory phase. At full development, about a week after ovulation when the endometrium is prepared to receive the embryo, it contains thousands of microscopic blood vessels surrounded by soft, spongy tissue. At this time also (about day 21 of the cycle), the biochemical activities of the endometrium (oxygen consumption, lipid storage, glycogen storage, and so on) are at their maximum, again in readiness for the implantation of the fertilized egg.

As in the ovarian cycle, what happens next depends upon whether or not fertilization occurs. If within 24 to 48 hours of ovulation (days 14 to 16) fertilization does take place, the changes of the secretory phase will continue and intensify under the influence of progesterone from the corpus luteum. If there has been no conception, the corpus luteum regresses, as described previously, and levels of estrogen and progesterone drop. The endometrium becomes infiltrated by polymorphonuclear leukocytes. The last days of the secretory phase may be called the *ischemic phase* or phase of regression, as the endometrium prepares for menstruation.

The Menstrual Phase

Spiral arteries in the endometrium are the key to the occurrence of menstruation. These arteries are very sensitive to fluctuations in the ovarian

A

Figure 3–21 Appearance of the human endometrium at various phases of the menstrual cycle. *A*, (1) Midfollicular phase; (2) late follicular phase; and (3) early luteal stage.

B

Figure 3–21 *Continued   B,* (1) Midluteal stage; (2) late or premenstrual phase; and (3) menstrual phase. (From Papanicolaou, Traut, and Marchetti: *The Epithelia of Woman's Reproductive Organs.* Commonwealth Fund, 1948.)

Figure 3–22   Calendar of idealized endometrial cycle.

steroids. The fall of estrogen and progesterone levels causes the constriction of intermittent segments of the spiral arteries in the endometrium, cutting off the supply of blood to the zona compacta and part of the zona spongiosa.

The combination of vasospasm and loss of hormonal stimulation leads to necrosis in the endometrium, particularly necrosis of the blood vessels. During the 24 to 36 hours preceding the onset of menstruation, blood seeps into the deeper layers of the endometrium, forming hemorrhagic areas. It is at these hemorrhagic sites that the separation of the necrotic outer layers of the endometrium occurs. The desquamated tissue and the blood in the uterine cavity initiate uterine contractions that expel the uterine contents. About 30 to 50 ml. of blood and an additional ounce of serous fluid are expelled during menstruation. When blood loss exceeds 80 ml., iron supplementation is required to prevent anemia. Women who report consistently heavy menstrual periods should have their hemoglobin level checked. *Menorrhagia* is the term for an abnormally heavy menstrual flow.

Physical Symptoms During the Menstrual Phase

Understanding the hormonal and physiologic basis of menstruation is only a part of understanding menstruation as it occurs in the lives of women. Menstruation can be viewed in two interrelated aspects: the physical symptoms encountered and the meaning of menstruation for an individual woman.

Symptoms related to the menstrual cycle fall into the general classifications of premenstrual tension and edema and of dysmenorrhea (painful menstruation).

Premenstrual Tension and Edema. Premenstrual tension is an "umbrella" term that describes a variety of symptoms some women experience for 1 or 2 days, or longer, during the second half of the endometrial cycle. Because of the timing of premenstrual tension and because the symptoms usually do not occur during anovulatory cycles (although menstruation does), the symptoms are thought to be associated with the corpus luteum. Among the symptoms reported fairly commonly are irritability and nervousness, less purposeful activity, and increased appetite.

Edema is also fairly common in the days prior to menstruation. Edema may be associated with premenstrual tension in some manner. However, successful treatment of the edema has not been shown to relieve the symptoms of premenstrual tension with any more frequency than would treatment with a placebo.

Dysmenorrhea. Dysmenorrhea is classified as primary or secondary. Secondary dysmenorrhea is that condition in which a specific pathologic reason can be demonstrated as the basis for pain. For example, there may be a malformation of the uterus, inflammation, and so on. In primary dysmenorrhea, no specific pathologic cause is discernible.

Like premenstrual tension, primary dysmenorrhea appears to be related to the function of the corpus luteum in some manner; it is rare during anovulatory cycles. This explains why young girls infrequently experience dysmenorrhea with initial menstrual periods, which are usually anovulatory. Women using oral contraceptives that prevent ovulation (Chapter 5) also have little or no dysmenorrhea; these preparations are therefore sometimes used in the treatment of particularly disabling dysmenorrhea.

There is little doubt that dysmenorrhea is a medical problem for a significant number of women in American society. Fay,[7] in a study of 701 girls in grades seven through twelve in Minnesota, found that 279 students (42.5 per cent) reported some pain during their menstrual cycles and that 196 students (27.7 per cent) lost time from school. In the group that reported pain, 76.3 per cent said they required bed rest for relief, 32.2 per cent had consulted a physician, and 66.6 per cent curtailed some favorite activity. Almost all of the students reporting pain said that they took some type of medication for it, including aspirin, aspirin with codeine, sleeping pills, and tranquilizers.

In another study, Doster[6] found that 38 per cent of a group of 1410 senior high school girls reported dysmenorrhea. Two-thirds of the girls with dysmenorrhea reported that they sometimes missed school because of it, and nearly half (45 per cent) reported that they missed some school during every menstrual period. Eighty per cent said that they needed some degree of bed rest, and 73 per cent felt that their pain required medication. Doster used the same questionnaire to study 720 women employees in the Denver school system and summarized his data with women classified into two groups—one of teachers and clerical workers (white

Table 3–2   MENSTRUAL PAIN AMONG 25 SAMOAN GIRLS*

Amount of Discomfort	Number	Per Cent
None	2	8
Abdominal only	3	12
Back only	10	40
Abdominal and back	4	16
Extreme discomfort†	6	24

*From Mead, M.: *Coming of Age in Samoa.* New York, New American Library, 1949.

†Extreme discomfort was so characterized by the girls; in no instance were the girls so ill that they could not work.

collar workers) and the other of lunchroom workers. While a higher percentage of white collar workers reported having had dysmenorrhea at some time, more lunchroom workers said they had dysmenorrhea regularly. Other studies of the frequency of dysmenorrhea have been done by Golub and Goldenwasser.

Table 3–2 summarizes Mead's findings concerning menstrual pain in a group of 25 adolescent girls in three villages in Samoa.[14] Future studies that try to differentiate those women who have dysmenorrhea regularly from those who rarely do would seem very important, as this is a physical problem that involves so many women.

Cyclic Changes in the Endometrium

Endometrial Hyperplasia and the Endometrial Cycle. When ovulation does not occur, the endometrium continues to proliferate under the influence of estrogen. Eventually there will be marked endometrial hyperplasia (i.e., cell proliferation). When estrogen levels do fall, the endometrium will often be shed in a patchy fashion, with excessive and prolonged bleeding.

Endometriosis and the Endometrial Cycle. Endometriosis occurs when patches of endometrium are found outside the uterus, most often in the cul-de-sac, the uterine ligaments, the ovaries, or the serosa of the uterus and bowel. The mechanism causing this is believed to be the regurgitation of menstrual blood through the uterine tubes. When endometriosis occurs in the ovaries, cysts filled with old blood (chocolate cysts) are a classic finding (Fig. 3–23).

Endometriosis most commonly occurs in white women who have never

Figure 3–23 The gross appearance of endometriosis of the ovaries. Cross sections of ovaries show the hematomas (chocolate cysts). (From Sampson: *American J. Obstetrics and Gynecology*, 4:489, 1922.)

been pregnant; many have long-term infertility. Quite typically many are unmarried career women. This *may* be related to the production of progestins that occurs during pregnancy; progestins do cause endometriosis to regress and are one form of therapy. Surgery is also used in the treatment of some women.

Endometriosis may be quite painful, particularly during the menstrual phase (the endometrium outside the uterus responds to the hormonal cycle in the same way that the uterine lining does). On the other hand, some women have few symptoms.

Other Cyclic Changes in the Endometrium. As Figure 3–24 indicates, there are many additional changes in the endometrium that can be used to "date" the cells taken during an endometrial biopsy to determine what is happening during the cycle. Such studies are helpful in the evaluation of various gynecologic problems, particularly infertility.

Changes in the Cervical Mucus

The mucus secreted by the endocervical glands also changes with the levels of estrogen and progesterone. Immediately following menstruation, when the level of both hormones is low, secretion of mucus is slight and the mucus is quite sticky. As the level of estrogen rises, secretion of mucus increases and the mucus becomes more and more elastic. By day 13 of the idealized cycle, cervical mucus exhibits *spinnbarkeit* and *ferning*.

Spinnbarkeit (literally the ability to spin) refers to the property of cervical mucus to make a thread when it is placed between two glass slides. The length of the spinnbarkeit varies over a period of several days. It is longest immediately prior to ovulation (Fig. 3–25); at this time the cervical mucus resembles fresh egg white, both in appearance and viscosity.

Ferning describes the branching pattern that cervical mucus exhibits at the time just prior to ovulation when it is allowed to dry on a glass slide. Ferning is caused by the increased sodium and water content of the mucus at this time. The disappearance of spinnbarkeit and ferning indicates that ovulation has occurred (see discussion of infertility, Chapter 5).

As progesterone secretion rises during the second half of the cycle, endocervical glands secrete a thick mucus that impedes sperm migration. This property is an important factor in the contraceptive effect of progestins. As progesterone levels fall toward the end of the cycle, mucus again becomes scant.

Changes in the Vagina

Both the epithelial cells of the vagina and vaginal pH are influenced by the hormonal cycle. Cells exhibit different characteristics at different stages that may be identified by laboratory examination. The pH of the vagina is acid through much of the cycle (pH about 4.0 to 5.0). This is probably because of the activity of vaginal tract bacilli, which break down glycogen, producing lactic acid. The pH rises shortly before and during the menstrual phase because of alkaline cervical secretions and menstrual flow.

Changes in Basal Body Temperature

At approximately the time of ovulation or shortly afterward, basal body

DATING THE ENDOMETRIUM
APPROXIMATE RELATIONSHIP OF USEFUL MORPHOLOGICAL FACTORS

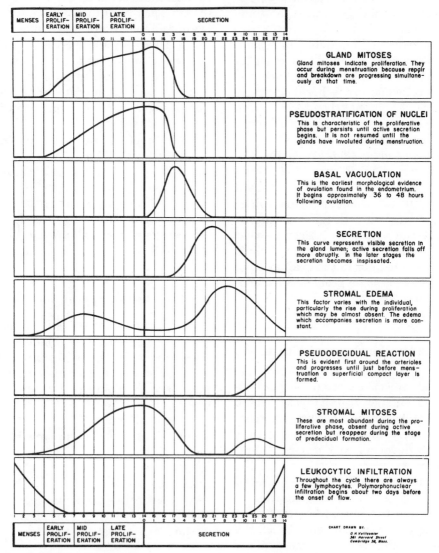

Figure 3–24   Criteria for dating the endometrium. Each curve represents the approximate quantitative change in each of eight factors considered most helpful. (From Noyes, Hertig, and Rock: *Fertility and Sterility*, 1:3, 1950.)

En la parte superior

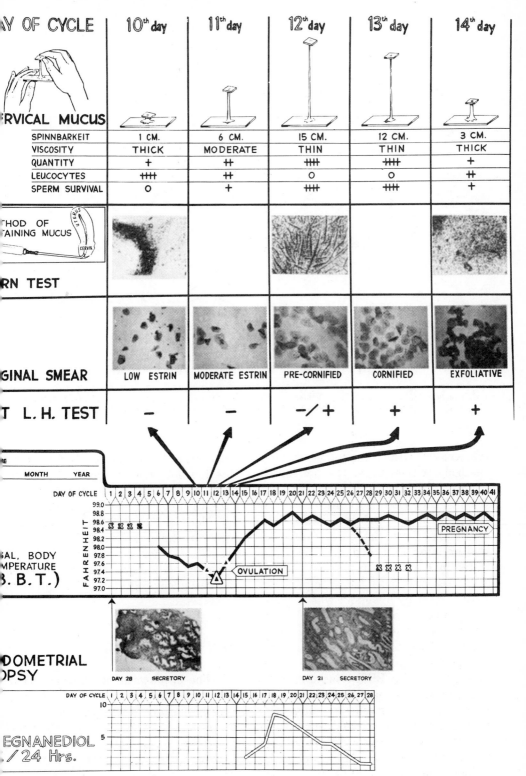

Figure 3–25 Clinical and laboratory changes at the time of ovulation. (From Cohen: Lying-in. *J. of Reproductive Medicine*, 1:182, 1968.)

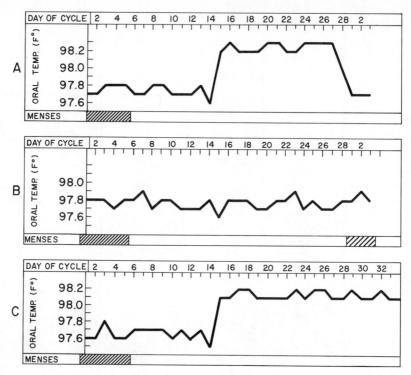

Figure 3–26 Typical oral basal body temperature curves in *A,* a normal cycle; *B,* an anovulatory cycle; and *C,* early pregnancy. (From Page, Villee, and Villee: *Human Reproduction: The Core Content of Obstetrics, Gynecology and Perinatal Medicine.* 2nd Edition. Philadelphia, W. B. Saunders Co., 1976.)

temperature (BBT), the temperature of the body at rest, rises. The increase is usually from 0.4 to 1.0 degree (Fig. 3-26). The rise is believed to be influenced by progesterone. Immediately prior to the temperature rise, there is often a marked drop, also illustrated by Figure 3–26.

A record of basal body temperature may be kept by a woman who is using the temperature-calendar method of contraception (Chapter 5) or by a woman with an infertility problem (Chapter 5). Special graphs are available for recording BBT. It is very important that any woman who is recording BBT, for whatever reason, understand that she must take her temperature each morning before she gets out of bed. The thermometer should be kept at the bedside and should even be shaken

down the night before. If she rises to get the thermometer or to go to the bathroom before she takes her temperature, the BBT will not be valid.

Note in Figure 3–26 the temperature variations during an anovulatory cycle and when pregnancy occurs. If pregnancy does occur, the BBT remains high because progesterone continues to be secreted.

THE CLIMACTERIC

The *climacteric* is that period of time, usually several years, during which ovarian function becomes less and less responsive to the stimulation of the gonadotropic hormones. Ovulation eventually ceases, and estrogen production slowly declines.

Menopause is the specific point in time at which menstruation ceases. (The word is often used incorrectly to refer to the climacteric.) The date of a woman's menopause can only be determined in retrospect. When she has not menstruated for a period of 6 months, the date of her last menstrual period is considered to mark her menopause.

While the body is in this process of disengagement from its cyclic preparation for pregnancy, pregnancy is possible and does occur during the climacteric. Since mothers of this age (commonly 45 to 55) are felt to be obstetrically at risk and the risk of a defective baby is greatly increased, contraception is usually advised for a year following the menopause.

The majority of the physiologic changes and symptoms of the climacteric (summarized in Table 3–3) are related to the decrease in estrogen production. No woman exhibits all of the symptoms noted; most will exhibit one or two, a few several. The difference is due in part to the fact that the amount of estrogen decrease varies from one woman to another. Estrogen is produced by the adrenal cortex as well as by the ovaries. In some women, estrogen production may be sufficiently adequate so that few or no symptoms occur. The cells of the vagina may continue to show the effects of estrogen for more than 10 years after the cessation of menstruation. Possibly emotional factors, such as a woman's feelings about her life and about her femininity also influence the severity of some symptoms of the climacteric (Chapter 4).

Although estrogen production declines, the gonadotropic hormones not only continue to be produced but are produced in excess. (Remember the feedback mechanism; as estrogen and progesterone levels rise, the levels of the gonadotropic hormones decrease.

During the climacteric, estrogen does not respond to the secretion of FSH and so more FSH is secreted.) Thus, the level of gonadotropins in the urine of the postmenopausal woman is high; this urine is the source of human gonadotropins used therapeutically to stimulate follicular growth.

Estrogen Replacement Therapy

It is readily apparent from scanning Table 3–3 that most of the changes that occur during the climacteric and in postmenopausal women are related to the decreased production of estrogen. Many physicians feel that this represents an endocrine deficiency and therefore feel that estrogen should be replaced for the remainder of life, just as other hormones are replaced when they are deficient. Other physicians use estrogen replacement only in specific individual instances. It is virtually always prescribed for women whose ovaries are diseased and/or removed before the age of 45. The dosage given to postmenopausal women is usually lower than that given to younger women for various gynecologic reasons.

There are certain disadvantages and contraindications to estrogen therapy, probably the chief reason why there is not universal agreement about its value. Episodes of uterine bleeding may occur, although this is often caused by a dose that is larger than necessary. Because estrogen appears to accelerate the growth of endometrial and breast cancers, it is contraindicated in women who have had any history of these malignancies within the preceding 5 years. Mainly as a precaution against the development of these malignancies, a regimen of 21 days of medication followed by 7 days of no medication is usually suggested.

Since the purpose of hormonal

Table 3–3 PHYSIOLOGIC CHANGES IN PERIMENOPAUSAL AND
POSTMENOPAUSAL WOMEN

	Symptoms	Physiologic Basis
SYSTEMIC CHANGES	Hot flashes: sudden sensations of heat. Night sweats. Flushes: sudden reddening of face. Cold hands and feet (decreased blood supply). Dizziness (episodic decreased blood supply to brain).	Withdrawal of estrogen after many years of exposure *may* cause instability in hypothalamic vasomotor centers. Blood vessels do not dilate and constrict as formerly. These are probably the most widely discussed symptoms of the climacteric, but occur in only 20 per cent of women.
MUSCLE CHANGES	Decline in general muscle tone: Supporting muscles of uterus, bladder, and rectum lose tone and strength; muscle strength declines in arms and legs; decline in smooth muscles of bladder wall.	Estrogens function in protein storage, needed for muscle development.
REPRODUCTIVE CHANGES	Menstrual irregularity. Atrophic changes in vagina: vagina shortens, becomes more narrow, less elastic, and more susceptible to inflammation, infection, irritation, itching, discharge. Lining of vagina becomes pale and thin; may be painful during intercourse (dyspareunia). Shrinking of uterus.	Withdrawal of estrogen.
SKELETAL CHANGES	Osteoporosis leads to: loss of body height increased incidence of fractures slow healing of bone weakening of spinal vertebrae with low back pain, bowed posture, "dowager hump." Changes in joint cartilage may lead to aching joints.	Estrogen aids bone to utilize calcium; in the absence of estrogen, bone demineralization is significantly accelerated.
SKIN CHANGES	Fat pads beneath skin absorbed. Elastic material within skin absorbed; wrinkling. Brown spots on skin. Loss of firmness of breasts.	
CORONARY ATHEROSCLEROSIS	Thickening of arteries appears to be hastened.	Estrogen deficiency appears to correlate with the development of arteriosclerosis; conclusive evidence lacking.
MISCELLANEOUS CHANGES	Burning on urination following intercourse.	Thinning of vaginal lining between vagina and bladder and urethra.

therapy prior to menopause is often to stimulate normal ovarian function, both estrogen and a progestin may be given. Following menopause or total hysterectomy, only estrogen is used.

Estrogen therapy, once started, should not be discontinued abruptly. Estrogen can be gradually discontinued, but sudden withdrawal may result in endocrine imbalance and serious mental distress. Arras[2] reports evaluating a patient who became withdrawn, confused, and semicomatose following a mitral commissurotomy. When several weeks of studies failed to reveal a reason for her mental symptoms, she was to be transferred to a mental institution. A nurse during a clinical conference asked why her estrogens had never been restarted (she had had a total hysterectomy 2 years before). In less than 24 hours after estrogen therapy was resumed, the patient began to communicate; within 8 days she was planning her discharge from the hospital and her return to work.

SEXUAL INTERCOURSE

The reproductive organs function not only in the production of hormones and of ova and spermatogonia, but also as the means of sexual intercourse. Intercourse is very much more than a physiologic phenomenon. Katchadourian states, "There is no denying the importance of knowing where the nerve centers are, but the current that feeds those centers is emotion."[12] In subsequent chapters we will look at the social and emotional factors in human sexuality during particular stages of life. Our purpose here is to examine the physiologic aspects of sexual intercourse as a foundation for understanding some of the concerns of couples during pregnancy and in the postpartal period and the interrelation between intercourse and fertilization, contraception, and infertility.

Physiologic Reactions to Sexual Stimuli

Sexual stimulation, whatever its source, activates the parasympathetic nervous system and inhibits the sympathetic system. An almost immediate reaction to parasympathetic stimulation is the relaxation of the arterial walls, which leads to *vasocongestion,* as more blood flows into an area than can be handled quickly by the veins. The most dramatic example of vasocongestion is the erection of the penis. Arterial blood under high pressure flows into the corpora cavernosa and spongiosum, the erectile tissue of the penis (see Fig. 3-1). Because venous flow is partially occluded and because the erectile tissue is surrounded by a strong fibrous coat, the pressure causes ballooning of the erectile tissue, and the penis becomes long and hard. The testes also increase in size because of vasocongestion.

Vasocongestion also occurs in the vaginal walls, which become darker in color. The congested walls of the lower vagina are called the *orgasmic platform* (Fig. 3-27). The clitoris, like its homologue the penis, also becomes erect from vasocongestion, although more slowly. The labia, uterus, and breasts are also affected and increase in size as well as change in color. In both men and women a flushing response of the skin, temperature change, and perspiration accompany sexual activity, again related to vasodilatation and congestion. Skin reactions are somewhat more common in women.

A second physiologic response is increased muscle tension. Muscle tone increases in both smooth and skeletal muscles; part of the increase is volun-

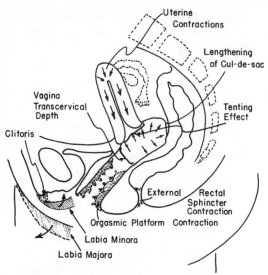

Figure 3–27 The female pelvis, orgasmic phase. (From Masters and Johnson: *Human Sexual Response.* Boston, Little, Brown & Co., 1966.)

tary, such as the flexing of muscles, and part involuntary, such as the muscular contractions of orgasm. The myometrium of the uterus also contracts, a consideration in planning care for some women who are pregnant.

Other physiologic responses include elevation of heart rate, blood pressure, and respiratory rate; hyperventilation; and increased secretion of saliva.

Secretion in the genital area (as well as of the sweat and salivary glands) is another correlate of sexual arousal. In males the genital secretion is limited. The bulbourethral (Cowper's) glands may secrete a small amount of alkaline mucus, which may neutralize the urethra (through which acidic urine has passed) and make it "safer" for sperm survival.

The vagina secretes a clear, alkaline fluid that may also neutralize the normally acid vaginal tract. The mechanism of vaginal secretion is unclear; it may be related to vasocongestion. The female bulbourethral (Bartholin's) glands and the cervix contribute limited secretions.

The Cycle of Sexual Response

In both men and women sexual response occurs in four phases: (1) the excitement phase, (2) the plateau phase, (3) the orgasmic phase, and (4) the resolution phase.

The *excitement* phase is the time of arousal. The couple become more aware of sexual excitement and less aware of other factors in their environment. Strong distractions, either internal or external, may inhibit sexual desire during the early part of the excitement phase. For example, a parent's concern about a new baby (internal) or the baby's cry (external) may be a barrier to sexual arousal.

The *plateau* phase precedes orgasm and is characterized by intense muscle tone throughout the body. Sensory perception of other stimuli is poor and becomes even less acute as *orgasm* is approached. Other changes already described—flushed skin, pounding heart, heavy breathing, and so on —also mark the plateau phase.

At the moment of orgasm, voluntary control is lost; the response not only is genital but also involves the entire body. Women are physiologically capable of multiple orgasms in rapid succession; men are not (see refractory period, below).

During the *resolution* phase, which follows orgasm, both genital organs and other body areas return to a prearousal state. Many persons feel pleasantly weary and go to sleep. Others may feel exhilarated, relaxed, hungry, or thirsty or may experience one of a wide variety of other possibilities.

While there is considerable individual variation, sexual responses are basically similar in both men and women. However, certain important differences do exist. Figure 3–28 diagrams male sexual response, based on the research of Masters and Johnson;

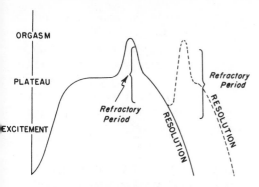

Figure 3–28 The male sexual response cycle. (From Masters and Johnson: *Human Sexual Response*. Boston, Little, Brown & Co., 1966.)

Figure 3–29 illustrates female response.[13] Note the presence of a refractory period in the male cycle. (The term *refractory period* refers to the time that must elapse, following stimulation, before a cell, tissue, or organ can respond again.) During the refractory period, a male cannot respond to sexual stimulation, no matter how intense it is. No such refractory period occurs in females, hence the potential for multiple orgasms. Note also in comparing Figures 3–28 and 3–29 that while there is

one basic pattern for male response, several variations in response are possible for females.

There is a great deal more that might be said about the physiology of sexual intercourse. Particularly helpful sources of information are Masters and Johnson[13] and Katchadourian and Lunde.[12]

Fertilization as Result of Sexual Intercourse

When sexual stimulus becomes intense, the reflex centers of the spinal cord send out rhythmic sympathetic impulses to initiate *emission*, the forerunner of ejaculation. Peristaltic contractions begin in the ducts of each testis, the epididymis, and the vas deferens, and spermatozoa enter the internal urethra.

Ejaculation follows when impulses sent from the spinal cord to the skeletal muscles encasing the base of the erectile tissue of the penis cause rhythmic increases in the pressure of the erectile tissue. Semen is thus expressed from the urethra to the exterior. The average

Figure 3–29 The female sexual response cycle. (From Masters and Johnson: *Human Sexual Response*. Boston, Little, Brown & Co., 1966.)

ejaculation contains approximately 100 million spermatozoa, some of which will be either immature or "senescent." Although only a single sperm will fertilize the ovum, the number of sperm is a significant factor in fertility (Chapter 5).

Spermatozoa are deposited at the mouth (os) of the cervix. Pregnancies have been reported from semen deposited on or near the vulva without intromission, a factor that is an important consideration in evaluating certain contraceptive practices, such as coitus interruptus (Chapter 5).

Throughout most of the cycle, viscid cervical mucus is a barrier to the ascent of the sperm from the cervix through the uterus to the uterine tube, where fertilization normally occurs. Sperm appear in the cervical mucus almost immediately after coitus; many never pass further. It has already been noted in the discussion of estrogen that at the time of ovulation the mucus increases in amount and becomes less viscid, making it more favorable for sperm penetration than at other times. Progesterone, on the other hand, makes the mucus unfavorable for sperm migration, so that very few reach the endometrial cavity either during the luteal phase of the menstrual cycle or when a woman is taking an oral contraceptive containing progestin.

Spermatozoa probably pass through the cervix by the movement of their tails. Upon reaching the uterus, they are apparently assisted in their passage to the tube by uterine contractions rather than by their own motility. Prostaglandins *may* be the agents that initiated the uterine contractions following coitus.

Probably only a few hundred to a few thousand of the original millions of sperm ever reach the ovum in the distal uterine tube. Those that do, however, do so in a few minutes. These few are very likely the healthiest and the most vigorous sperm. Other sperm remain in the cervix, in the junction between the uterus and the tube, and in the isthmus of the tube. Some pass out of the body; others enter the endometrium of the uterus or the peritoneal cavity.

ADDITIONAL FACTORS IN BIOLOGIC READINESS

Development of the reproductive tract is the most obvious factor in biologic readiness for pregnancy. However, a number of additional biologic factors interact to affect the body's readiness. Such factors should be a part of educational programs for young people prior to the time of first sexual intercourse and also for women during and after childbirth. They include: (1) parental age, (2) maternal nutrition, (3) maternal health (chronic conditions, infectious processes, and use of medication), (4) hereditary disorders, and (5) Rh incompatibility.

Each of these areas is discussed more fully in the chapters that follow.

REFERENCES

1. Applebaum, R. M.: The Modern Management of Successful Breast Feeding. *Pediatric Clinics of North America, 17*:203, 1970.
2. Arras, B.: Don't Underrate Those Clinical Conferences. *RN, 38*(7):41, 1975.
3. Davis, M. E.: Menopause and Estrogens. Chicago, Budlong Press, 1969.
4. Diekelmann, N., and Gallaway, K.: A Time of Change. *American Journal of Nursing, 75*:994, 1975.
5. Dienhart, C. M.: Basic Human Anatomy and Physiology. 2nd Edition. Philadelphia, W. B. Saunders Co., 1973.
6. Doster, M. E., McNuff, A., Lampe, J., and Corliss, L.: A Survey of Menstrual Function Among 1668 Secondary School Girls and 720 Women Employees of the Denver Public Schools. *American Journal of Public Health, 51*:1841, 1961.

7. Fay, A.: Dysmenorrhea, A School Nurse's Findings. *American Journal of Nursing,* *63*:77, 1963.

8. Greenhill, J. P.: *Obstetrics.* 13th Edition. Philadelphia, W. B. Saunders Co., 1965.

9. Greenhill, J. P., and Friedman, E. A.: *Biologic Principles and Modern Practice of Obstetrics.* Philadelphia, W. B. Saunders Co., 1974.

10. Guyton, A. C.: *Basic Human Physiology.* 2nd Edition. Philadelphia, W. B. Saunders Co., 1977.

11. *Introduction to Endocrinology.* Prepared by Educational Design, Inc. for Merrell-National Laboratories. Cincinnati, 1966.

12. Katchadourian, H. A., and Lunde, D. T.: *Fundamentals of Human Sexuality.* New York, Holt, Rinehart & Winston, 1972.

13. Masters, W. H., and Johnson, V. E.: *Human Sexual Response.* Boston, Little, Brown & Co., 1966.

14. Mead, M.: *Coming of Age in Samoa.* New York, New American Library, 1949.

15. Moore, K. L.: *The Developing Human.* 2nd Edition. Philadelphia, W. B. Saunders Co., 1977.

16. Page, E., Villee, C. A., and Villee, D. B.: *Human Reproduction.* 2nd Edition. Philadelphia, W. B. Saunders Co., 1976.

17. Rose, R. M.: Androgen Excretion in Stress. *In* Bourne, P. G. (ed.): *The Psychology and Physiology of Stress.* New York, Academic Press, 1969.

18. Ziegel, E., and Van Blarcom, C. C.: *Obstetric Nursing,* 6th Edition. New York, The Macmillan Co., 1972.

Chapter 4

THE SOCIAL AND CULTURAL CONTEXT OF CHILDBEARING

If the bearing and rearing of children were solely biologic, human lives would be far less complex—and far less satisfying and interesting. The word "culture" has been used by so many people in so many different ways that it seems important to define it in the way in which it is used here. An early anthropologist Edward Tylor described culture as " . . . that complex whole which includes knowledge, belief, art, morals, law, custom or any other capabilities and habits acquired by man as a member of society."[76] All of our behavior that is not instinctive (and very little human behavior is governed by instinct), all that we have learned, and all of our customary ways of doing things are a part of our culture.

Recognizing the influence of culture on childbearing is important for two fundamental reasons:

1. Culture influences how every man and woman experiences and deals with childbearing in his or her own life.

2. Culture affects the way in which *we* as nurses deal with and are affected by childbearing.

Individuals learn many of the values of a society from the families in which they grow to adulthood. These values are supplemented and modified by educational institutions, mass media, and a number of other forces in a technologic society such as our own. Nevertheless, families remain important, and in order to care for childbearing families in the best possible manner, we need to be aware of family characteristics and the ways in which we interact with families of varying lifestyles.

One way of looking at family lifestyles is in terms of social class. Over the past decades a number of similar but slightly varying class groupings have been developed, based on criteria such as income, education, and occupation. These classes have also been divided into subgroups, such as lower-middle, middle-middle, and upper-middle. The semantics of social class designation seem unfortunate. They appear to infer that upper is good and lower is bad. We intend no such judgment here; it is our belief that in each group there are strengths and weaknesses.

Another influence on family lifestyles is ethnicity. The forebears of American families have come from nearly every part of the world. For some families, America has been a "melting pot," and over several generations many cultures have blended. Other families have more distinctive ways of living, either because of their own choosing or because of barriers that have been raised to their entry into the "mainstream" of American life.

Some individuals and families have deliberately chosen alternate lifestyles. Families who participate in the counterculture are an example.

As we examine family lifestyles, even briefly, it is important to recognize other social factors that influence family life. Two interrelated factors that seem particularly relevant to childbearing families at this time are the women's movement and maternal employment.

The discussion in this chapter is necessarily brief. Just as we must continually increase our knowledge of other aspects of nursing practice, we must also grow in our understanding of the significance of culture as it influences families in every aspect of their lives.

SOCIAL CLASS

Families of the Affluent Society

Sociologists divide relatively or absolutely affluent families into three distinct social groups:

1. An upper-middle class of successful professional people, such as physicians, lawyers, and executives of large businesses.

2. A lower-upper class of families with considerable wealth, but wealth that is relatively recently acquired (the newly rich).

3. An upper-upper class, with both great wealth and a certain social prestige that no amount of money can purchase.

Because the number of sociologically defined upper class families is small (in a great many communities there are no people who would be considered upper class by these definitions) and because these families seem to share many characteristics in relation to childbearing, we are grouping them together here.

Both husbands and wives in affluent families are likely to be well educated. Some exceptions occur in the families of professional men who marry before their education is completed, with wives dropping out of school to support the family in the interim.

These families are aware of contraception and probably use it effectively, although other factors besides lack of knowledge (Chapter 5) may certainly influence the occurrence of conception. On the whole, these families are likely to have approximately the number of children they desire when they wish to have them.

Affluent mothers will usually seek good medical care early in pregnancy. Often the doctor will be a personal friend or a neighbor or a member of the same clubs (with the possible exception of families in very large cities). The doctor-patient relationship may be very different from that of the physician treating a blue collar mother, even if the latter is his private patient, or caring for a lower class mother in the outpatient department. Nevertheless, even upper class mothers may be subject to feelings of awe and/or fear toward their physician. Socialization to respond to the doctor as if the physician were on a pedestal is not always neutralized by social status or education.

Nurses and student nurses, who are usually from middle class families, sometimes feel threatened by mothers from families more affluent than their own. They may even keep their contacts to a minimum because of such feelings. In our own experience when students have selected a mother for care and study throughout pregnancy, they have avoided these mothers, saying, "There's nothing I can teach her" or "She already knows everything I can tell her." We believe that such an appraisal is as unfair as assuming that our efforts will be wasted on a lower class mother.

Mothers and fathers in these affluent social groups have a certain amount of flexibility in the extent of involvement that they have with their infants because helpers can be hired. Fathers will be less likely to be participants in routine care, such as diapering, feeding, and bathing the baby, partly because of the press of "business" and partly because it is not customary. For men in the upper levels of corporate business (and perhaps even more for the young, middle class man aspiring to those levels), family relationships are part of a triangle that involves the corporation, rather than "another woman," as the third angle. "Success here," said one official, "are guys who eat and sleep the company. If a man's first interest is his wife and family, more power to him—but we don't want him."[83] While such attitudes may have modified somewhat since that statement was made in 1951, partly because such a philosophy is less acceptable to many of today's young families, there is little question that similar attitudes are still present.

We caution against automatically interpreting this difference between upper and middle class norms of father participation, and our own expectations of a father's role, as a lack of caring. In our assessment of parental attitudes toward their baby (a significant part of nursing observation), social class differences should be borne in mind.

Mothers from affluent families may choose to delegate other responsibilities, such as house care, to hired helpers and thus have more time to spend with their babies, or they may allow helpers to assume most or all of infant care. The total abdication of responsibility for baby care—all of the feeding, bathing, and even holding— suggests a rejection of the baby, although it may also indicate a severe lack of self-confidence, fear of harming the baby, anxiety about not being a good mother, or some other factor. How such a lifestyle may affect the baby will be influenced, at least in part, by the relationship that the baby has with other important people in his life— caretakers, grandparents, and the like.

Because most upper and upper-middle class mothers and fathers are reasonably well educated, some may tend to super-intellectualize the experiences of childbirth and the care they plan for their babies. Such trust may be placed in "experts" and books that their own feelings and reactions may be ignored and denied. This is particularly true of first babies, when parents have had no experience of their own with which to temper the advice of "experts." Variations in this experience, or in their baby's characteristics and/or appearance, may be difficult to cope with. We wish we could say to them, "Relax. Enjoy your baby. He's fine." We may be able to help them accept the concept of "range of normal" behavior that will make them more comfortable with these variations.

Middle Class Families

Middle class families have been grouped in various ways. For our purpose of looking at families in relation to childbearing, we have included the "upper-middle class" as a category of the affluent family groups. Two large groups remain, which appear to differ in a number of ways: a lower-middle class and a middle-middle class.

LeMasters,[49] calls the lower-middle class the "most rapidly growing group of parents in the United States." At least one factor is the mobility of blue-collar workers, as the number of blue collar jobs shrinks and as greater numbers of blue collar children complete high school and at least some additional education.

Lower-middle class parents are usually high school graduates. They may have some college education and may even have graduated from one of the smaller colleges. By occupation they may be salesclerks in small businesses (shoe shops or hardware stores, for example), lower-paid municipal employees, and so on.

Incomes are often less than those of the best-paid blue collar workers, and often wife-mothers work to supplement earnings. While the mother's income is not usually necessary to provide basics such as food and clothing, as it often is in lower class families, her earnings can mean a home in a nicer neighborhood (which, in turn, can mean that her children go to a nicer school), better furniture, a vacation, and so on, all of which are important to these families who identify themselves more closely with the more affluent white collar workers. Credit is often used extensively. and indebtedness may be a chronic state, as the family tries to pattern their standard of living after that of the television family shows and the slick magazines.

Lower-middle class families are often caught in a "crunch" in relation to medical care, including, of course, obstetric care. Economically, they find it increasingly difficult to afford good private care. They may lack the comprehensive hospitalization insurance that gives security to the unionized blue collar worker. Usually they are ineligible for free care or for care at reduced cost through clinics because their incomes are too high. Moreover, even if they were eligible, their close identification with the middle class makes such care difficult for them to accept. They

may be embarrassed when the public health nurse comes to the door, associating her visit with that of the "welfare department." Medical costs can become a real burden if, for example, the mother has a longer period of hospitalization than was expected, or if their baby requires the very expensive care of an intensive care nursery (averaging $200 a day or more). These expenses are not covered by many hospitalization insurance policies, if the family is fortunate enough to have insurance at all.

Lower-middle class marriages tend to have more companionship and less sex-role segregation than do those of blue collar families. Both husband and wife share an interest in their home and in a hope for a better life for their children. Because these families are often upwardly mobile (both husband and wife may have grown up in blue collar families), there is less reliance on other family members (i.e., the extended family of parents, brothers and sisters, aunts and uncles) and more on one another (i.e., the nuclear family). This may limit the kind of support the young couple can count on in caring for the new baby and other young children.

Companionship and cooperation are the expectations of most husbands and wives in *middle class* marriages, even if these are not always found. Indeed, lack of companionship may be seen as a valid reason for divorce. Such cooperation involves not only the sharing of the work to be done, but also the sharing of ideas and experiences. Much of the impetus for husband-father participation in childbirth comes from this group—in part because of the value given to sharing and also because of an openness to new ideas and a lifestyle that includes participation in groups in which individuals and couples exchange ideas and feelings.

These couples fulfill the expectations that many nurses have of what parents "should" be like. They accept our advice and are interested in the emotional as well as the physical aspects of pregnancy and infant care, a value that we share. Many of our breast-feeding mothers come from these middle class families. In short, our cultural model of the "good mother" and the "good family" is closely related to their behavior. However, we need to be very careful that we don't judge other families by this middle class model, labeling them as less than adequate when they behave in a different way.

The high ideals that middle class parents have for their children can be disadvantageous when both parents feel so overwhelmed by their idea that the total responsibility for producing "the perfect infant" is theirs alone. As a result, they may feel anxious and inadequate.

We also find parents in this class who have a very clear vision (although not always a realistic one) of how they plan to relate to their child in an intellectual and emotional sphere, but a less clear comprehension of day-to-day physical care. The college professor mother who was unsure about how long she should boil her baby's drinking water is an example. One reason for this uncertainty is probably that both fathers and mothers were reared in small, middle class nuclear families themselves and never had much experience with, or even exposure to, small children. David Steinberg writes:

> I knew nothing about babies when Dylan was born. I'm an only child and have never spent any time at all with babies. My confidence in myself as a father was very shaky. I felt deeply afraid of Dylan, always fighting an urge to close my eyes and shove responsibility for him over to Susan . . . I got very depressed at my lack of baby sense.[73]

We find that many middle class mothers share the same kinds of uncertainty, especially with their first babies.

Blue Collar Families

The term "blue collar family" encompasses a large but somewhat diminishing number of Americans, as automation and social change decrease the number of blue collar jobs. Traditionally, these jobs have included factory work, repair work, truck driving, bricklaying, carpentry, and many similar occupations. Many blue collar workers belong to strong labor unions.

There is a considerable range of both income and job security in blue collar families. Incomes may exceed that of many white collar workers, with fringe benefits and seniority within the union system offering a high level of security. Other blue collar workers have incomes that barely meet their basic needs, and jobs that are far less secure.

Segregation of sex roles seems to be a common characteristic of the relationship of many, but not all, blue collar husbands and wives. Some recent observations suggest that this kind of role segregation may be a little less rigid than formerly, but it is often still apparent.

Role segregation is significant in obstetric care. Many of our prenatal classes and our changing patterns of admitting fathers to delivery rooms, to cite but two examples, are based on middle class values of the joint sharing of roles and responsibilities.

A corollary to the segregated sex roles is the more limited communication between men and women, including husbands and wives, than is often found in many middle class families. Lines of communication are strongest between members of the same sex, and especially between family members of the same sex. A woman may turn to her mother or sister for advice; her husband will consult his brother. A nurse or other professional from a middle class environment may wrongly interpret such communication as evidence of a poor family relationship rather than as representative of a cultural pattern.

Familes in Poverty

An estimated 9 million or more Americans, roughly 22 per cent of the population, have incomes that barely enable them to meet their daily needs. Sociologists call these families the lower-lower class.

The middle class stereotype of such families is one of unwed mother, non-whites, and often of people who neither try nor care. Like most stereotypes, it describes some families and misses the mark many times.

For example, while the percentage of families headed by women is certainly higher among the poor (approximately 25 per cent as compared with approximately 10 per cent in the population as a whole), three-quarters of lower class families are *not* headed by women. And although nonwhite families are overrepresented (only 10 per cent of all families but more than 20 per cent of poor families are nonwhite), it is obvious that the overwhelming number of poor families, nearly 80 per cent, are white.

A knowledge of families who live in poverty is crucially important to nurses who care for mothers and babies. Many will be high risk mothers and/or have babies with special needs and problems. Prenatal care is often sporadic or nonexistent. Family planning is ineffective in many instances. Nutrition is usually poor.

Who are these families? They are Spanish-speaking and black families in urban ghettos and Anglo-Saxons in Appalachia. They are black or white farm-ers in the rural South—some tenants, some with their own small bits of land. They are the migrant families who follow the harvests along the Atlantic Coast from Florida to New England, or from Texas to the mountain states or the Midwest or across the deep South, or along the Pacific Coast. They are displaced farm workers who unsuccessfully sought jobs in the urban North. They are miners displaced by automation. They are American Indians. They are probably the most diverse group of families in the United States.

Not all of the poor are unemployed. Unskilled workers, day laborers, and domestics may work harder on a given day than a middle class man or woman. But income is low and work is often sporadic and inconsistent. A 2 week rainy spell can mean no income for an outdoor laborer. Nor do these jobs carry the fringe benefits—medical insurance, vacations, sick leave, and the like—that offer security to the unionized blue collar worker and the upper-middle class family.

Lower class families are often characterized as being improvident for not planning ahead. The mother who comes to the hospital to deliver with no money set aside to pay her bill, no clothes for the baby, and no bed for him at home is easily labeled a "poor mother" by middle class standards. After all, it is reasoned (and sometimes said) she had 9 months in which to get ready. It is worth considering that each day's needs in that 9 months may have seemed so pressing at the moment that they consumed the limited funds available.

ETHNICITY

Black Families

For an increasing number of middle and working class black families, family organization is not unlike that of middle and working class white families. But for the poor black family, especially the family living in an inner city slum or at the end of a rural dirt road, family structure may vary considerably.

Many poor black families are headed by women, probably for a number of reasons. During the days of slavery, marriage between slaves was not recognized, and families were frequently broken up as members were sold to different masters. Black women, who could produce more slaves and who also often served as mistresses for their owners, were often accorded higher status than black men.

In the years that followed the abolition of slavery, job opportunities were often more available for women than for men, both in the rural South and in the North, where 10 million blacks migrated in the years between 1910 and 1960. Many fathers, unable to find employment, fled from their families.

Still another factor is our system of financial support for the poor in the United States (Aid to Families with Dependent Children—AFDC), which in many states does not allow payment if an unemployed father remains at home. Under such a system, families are financially better off if the father leaves than if he were to remain at home without a job. Since fathers with limited education and job skills are often the "last hired and the first fired" from their jobs, it is easy for a family to feel that consistent income from the government is more important than having a father at home.

Extended family organization is frequent in poor black families. In contrast to nuclear families that include only a father, mother, and their nonadult children, in an extended family other relatives live together. If we consider all of the world's families, the extended family system is far more prevalent than the nuclear family organization. There may be a grandmother living with her daughters, her granddaughters, and their children (her great-grandchildren). A teen-aged mother may turn her baby over to her own mother, or even to her grandmother, to care for while she continues her adolescent activities. Although this may seem an unusual pattern of infant care by American middle class standards, it is a common form of childrearing in many parts of the world.

Rainwater[62] observed that in Pruitt-Igoe, a low-cost housing project in St. Louis that he and his coworkers studied closely over a period of time, the babies seemed very secure in their homes. Quite a few people cared for them; they received considerable attention, being passed from mother to sister to grandmother and later toddling from person to person. Their care was regarded as routine. Normal development was greeted with neither anxiety nor undue interest.

If this description seems idyllic, remember that there are many problems as well. Incomes are low, with concomitant poor nutrition, inadequate housing, and marginal health care. Homes are adult-centered rather than child-centered; when children's needs conflict with adults' needs, those of the adults will often prevail. When new babies join the family, children of two years or older may easily be pushed into the background.

Understanding differences in behavior is specifically important for maintaining our relationship with patients from poor black families. For example, in conducting classes for mothers, a lack of interest on the part of the mothers in what a baby should be expected to do at a particular stage of development does not necessarily indicate a lack of interest in their babies, but merely that such indices are not as important to them as they are to us or to the middle class mother (who may be striving to have her baby compete with the baby next door).

In teaching a family about baby care, we need to try to discover just who is going to take care of the baby once he is home. If the mother is not to be the primary caretaker, some contact needs to be arranged with the person who will be.

Not only may the mother not be the primary caretaker, she may have limited authority as to what care is given. If her mother or grandmother believes that catnip is a constituent of baby formula (not an uncommon practice in the author's part of the country), it may be difficult for the mother to overrule the practice, even if we have convinced her that it is not such a good idea.

Much lower class black behavior seems to be in conflict with our middle class norms—views about the desirability of marriage, legitimacy of children, and sexual relations, for example.

But Rainwater summarizes the norms of the 10,000 residents of Pruitt-Igoe as being the same as those shared by most Americans: "Lifelong marriage is the only really desirable way of living." "Children should be born only in marriage relationships; to procreate outside marriage is to fall short of the way things ought to be." "Any kind of sexual relationship outside marriage is dangerous, although it is attractive."[62]

It would appear, then, that it is not the norms that differ dramatically, but the ability to achieve those norms. As one father said, "I want my kids to be respectable and presentable wherever they go . . . I got seven boys . . . and I sure would like for one or two of them to be somethin'. I know they can't all make it, but if only one or two of them could be somethin'. . . ."[62]

Interracial Marriage: Black and White. Marriage between a black person and a white person has been illegal in some states and socially unacceptable to many people. Nevertheless, interracial marriages are increasing, although the couples involved face many obstacles and will probably do so for years to come—obstacles such as finding a home and maintaining relationships with black and white families and friends. (See Wolf.)

Nurses who meet interracial couples during childbearing may be uncomfortable at first because they are dealing with an experience new to them. The couples may be alienated from their own families and from friends, although this will not necessarily be true, and therefore may be particularly in need of support. If we interact with them as people, as potential mothers and fathers, rather than as stereotypes, and if we examine the basis of our own feelings, we will find that interracial couples are no different from the other families we meet.

Spanish-American Families

Spanish-speaking Americans and Americans of Spanish heritage live in many areas of the United States. There are Mexican-Americans in Texas and California, Puerto Ricans in the Northeast, and Latin-Americans in Florida and Georgia. Some Spanish-American families have been in the United States for many generations; others are newcomers. Some of these families have adopted the lifestyle of "middle-America," but many others, because of language barriers, poverty, fear of or experience with discrimination, and loyalty to their own traditions have retained a cultural heritage that "Anglo" nurses and other professionals do not always understand.

Extended family relationships are very important to most Spanish-Americans. Although a young couple may live in a separate home, many relatives often live close by and will be seen very frequently. The advice and counsel of relatives is likely to be important in childbearing. There may be discussions among many family members before an important decision is made. The extended family, rather than the medical professional, may be regarded as the ultimate authority by the young couple (see below).

A second and equally important facet of Spanish-American life is the influence of *compadrazgo*. Compadres, or coparents, have social and economic obligations to one another beyond those that godparents have in most of American society. Compadres are expected to always be friends, no matter what happens; subsequently, there is a feeling of special obligation. The compadrazgo system offers each child a greater number of people upon whom he can depend for the necessities of life.

> ... A woman will not hesitate to leave her husband and children to go to the aid of a compadre who needs help. When Paula's compadre, who lives in Hayward (about twenty-five miles from San Jose), was expecting her last baby, Paula left her own family for two weeks to care for her compadre during her confinement."[19]

Sex role division and a *double standard of sexual behavior* are characteristic of the relationship between men and women. It is not unusual for a husband to be several years older than his wife, who often marries between the ages of 16 and 19, a fact that enhances male dominance. There is limited dating prior to marriage, with very little acceptance of premarital sexual activity for girls. Women are categorized as "good women" and "bad women." One girl who became pregnant "out of wed-

lock" reported that "her family would throw her out" but added that she still wished to have the baby.

Childbearing is seen as a privilege and an obligation of married women; to be barren or to have only one or two children often elicits the sympathy of the community. Large families are still desired by many couples.

Many Spanish-speaking families have specific ideas about health care, about how they should act in situations of health and illness, and about the way in which the curer—nurse, physician, or *curandera* (folk-healer)—should behave. Many Spanish-speaking people are hesitant to seek care from someone who does not understand their beliefs.

Consider a pregnant mother who (in our view) needs hospitalization at some point in her pregnancy for diabetic control, perhaps, or for hypertension. There may be discussion among family members, relatives, and neighbors as to the proper course of action. We can become very distressed that our opinion about the necessity of the proposed hospitalization is not accepted as final, but it is the family group that has the ultimate authority to make such decisions. In the eyes of the Spanish community, the role of the curer is to advise, not to dictate. Authoritarianism is likely to drive patients away. The woman will rarely be openly defiant; she will smile and answer "si." But unless family consensus confirms medical opinion, medical advice may be ignored.

How is a nurse expected to behave? Clark further describes the behavior of Paula, a curandera in California previously referred to, whose behavior typifies the expected role.

> Paula's manner is as warm and friendly as her kitchen-dispensary.
> She observes the requisite social amenities and always behaves in a manner which her clients regard as courteous. For

example, she is always careful to wait for an invitation to enter the house before she goes in. She knows that she is expected to sit down with the family, drink a cup of coffee, and make small talk before getting down to the business at hand. . . . After a decent interval, the illness can be mentioned and the patient seen.

Families from Asian and Middle Eastern Societies

In the United States live many families from Asia—from China, Japan, India, Korea, Vietnam, the Pacific Islands and many other Far and Middle Eastern nations. Some of these families have lived in the United States for several generations; others have only recently immigrated. Although families from Middle and Far Eastern cultures are not homogeneous, many share certain characteristics that are important for us to recognize if we are to help these families cope with and grow during childbearing.

The Importance of Family Support. When many of us think of family support during pregnancy, we think first of a nuclear family and the support that comes from the husband. For many Middle and Far Eastern women, however, the traditional support during pregnancy comes from women in the extended family—their mother, aunts, and sisters.

The Male Role. The traditional Asian husband will see pregnancy as "women's business"; his cultural values often tell him that it is not proper for him to be actively involved with his wife's pregnancy, labor or delivery. To judge his degree of participation by our Anglo-Saxon standards and to thereby label him as being uninterested is, at the very least, unfair.

Because men are not expected to care for women, many Asian and Near Eastern women prefer a female physician or midwife and are very uncomfortable with a male physician. If they live in a community where there is no woman available for total obstetric care, a nurse can help to some extent by protecting the mother's modesty with particular care and by reminding professional colleagues of this special concern.

Traditional Practices. Traditional practices associated with childbearing will vary with the society and with the individual family. Check with the woman about concerns such as the:

1. Foods she believes are important for pregnant and newly delivered mothers.
2. Foods she customarily eats (see also Chapter 9).
3. Activities that are considered appropriate for mothers during pregnancy and the postpartum period.

A prolonged convalescence is customary for many societies, with special proscriptions about diet, bathing, and avoiding the "outside" or "unclean" world. Although these customs may seem unusual to us, from the viewpoint of ancient societies such practices probably served the new mother well by protecting both mother and baby from infection when there was no way to treat infection.

Similarly, the prohibition against the father's entering the room of the new mother and baby, common to many traditional societies, may have served to protect the new mother from intercourse and possible pregnancy too soon after birth during century after century when abstinence was the only sure means of contraception.

American Indian Families

Indian. The label is ours, not his. He has been an Indian for only 500 years. For as many as twenty-five thousand years, he has been Ottawa, Dakota, Shoshone, Cherokee —or one of several hundred distinct people who controlled this continent.[16]

Nearly 800,000 men, women, and children of American Indian tribes constitute approximately 1 per cent of the population of the United States. More than half live on or near reservations. Approximately 350,000 Indians live in urban areas in the Midwest and West (Fig. 4–1).

Most of the students and nurses who read this book may never care for Indian families. Yet because their health and human needs are so great, it seems important for anyone interested in people and in their care to become aware of the problems that Indians face, in order to serve, whenever possible, as an advocate for better opportunities for them.

Most of the Indians of the United States live in poverty; in general they are the poorest of the poor. Median family income in 1970 was $5,832, compared with $6,864 for black families and $11,549 for white families. (Median income means that 50 per cent of families would have incomes below that level and 50 per cent would have higher incomes.) One-third of all Indian families were below the "poverty line" ($3,743 for a nonfarm family of four). Unemployment on the reservations ranges from 37 to 51 per cent.

Hunger, malnutrition, and poor health are constant facts of life. Even water, so taken for granted by most of us, must be hauled many miles on some reservations. Although neonatal mortality (death within the first 28 days of life) has declined as more Indian infants are born in hospitals, infant mortality (deaths in the first year) on reservations averaged 23.5 deaths per 1000 births in 1971 at a time when the figure for the United States was 19.2 deaths per 1000

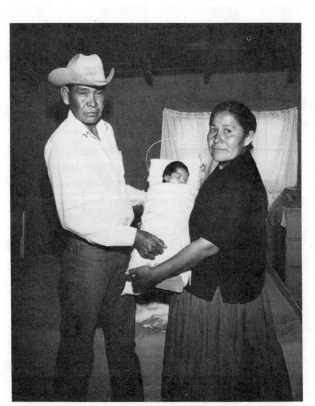

Figure 4–1 Navajo parents in Arizona with their new baby. Note the traditional cradle. (From the Office of Information Services, Indian Health Service, U.S. Public Health Service, Silver Spring, Md.)

births. These figures represent an improvement, however. The rate was 50.3 in 1960, 39.0 in 1965, and 24.8 in 1970. Indian infant deaths in Arizona were 108 per 1000 births in 1971 (the most recent figures available), twice as high as in the worst of the black ghettos and more than five times the white infant mortality rate in the United States (16.8 in 1971). This figure, too, represents improvement; the rate was 203 in 1966 and 120 in 1969.

Health care for Indians who live on reservations, other than the traditional care of the medicine man, is provided through the Division of Indian Health of the United States Public Health Service. Because of a shortage of personnel, it is largely crisis-oriented and overcrowded. An Indian may travel 90 miles to a clinic to find 200 to 300 persons ahead of him, with no hope of even being seen.

Transportation presents a major barrier to health care. Many families live miles from the nearest improved road. The *New York Times* (February 19, 1969) told of a Navajo woman who carried her sick baby 30 miles from her hogan (earth-covered dwelling) to the nearest traveled road. The *Times* noted that in the previous year 20 infants from the Pine Ridge Reservation in South Dakota were dead on arrival at medical stations. Eighteen of the deaths were attributed to delay in reaching medical aid.

Traditional beliefs about health care and the interrelatedness of health and other aspects of life, such as religion, are important in Indian culture. Today most medicine men and Indian families recognize that some conditions (appendicitis, for example) are best treated by the "white man's medicine" while others are more appropriately treated in traditional ways (such as the Navajo "sing" or through a combination of Western and Indian medicine).

For Indians living on reservations, much of life in general is dictated by the Bureau of Indian Affairs, and matters of health are controlled by the Public Health Service. Both of these services are agencies of the United States government. The history of governmental intervention in Indian affairs has not always been one of which we can be proud, nor is it ideal today—a discussion well beyond the scope of this book. But nurses with an understanding of and an appreciation for Indian cultural values can make a difference in Indian care.

RURAL FAMILIES

Approximately 57 million people live in rural America; of this number about 47 million are nonfarm families, living in small towns and villages scattered throughout the country.

Does life in rural areas differ from that in urban areas? In a time of mass media the differences are less distinct than formerly, but they remain. Recognizing some of these differences can be helpful as we care for childbearing families.

In contrast to the many impersonal relationships of people in urban areas, most relationships in rural communities are between people who know each other. The grocer is known by name and, in turn, knows his (or her) customers. Nurses and physicians will usually know the majority of their patients, unless they are serving unusually wide geographic areas. Families accustomed to this lifestyle can be tremendously overwhelmed by the apparent impersonality of a major medical center, where they must deal with a vast number of strangers in a single day. (The environment also intimidates the average urban resident, but they may have some skills for coping with impersonality.) Just knowing the name of their nurse, or their baby's nurse, and the name of their physician means a great deal to families.

Because "everyone knows everyone else" in a rural community, there is a great deal of pressure to conform to the community's norms and limited tolerance of those who deviate from these norms. For example, a single mother who wished to keep and raise her baby was forced to move to an urban community from her small hometown. "The people in my hometown would never accept me or my baby," she told us. "I was not even welcome in my church. My parents were suffering too."

The significance of family ties, such as she expressed, is seen as far more important in rural areas. The family is the central group for a rural man or woman; for urban dwellers the family may be but one of many groups with which an individual is associated. An urban woman may, for example, belong to a club or professional group for many years with little or no involvement by the rest of her family.

Still another difference is the attitude toward change. In rural communities life changes less from day to day and from year to year than in large cities where change may be an inevitable part of daily life. Social attitudes change more slowly, and one may expect conservative attitudes toward issues such as male and female roles, single parenthood, and abortion, for example.

One easily overlooked aspect of rural life is the frequency of poverty. While one person in fifteen in suburbia and one person in eight in the city, lives in poverty, one of every four persons in rural areas is poor. Among nonwhites living in rural communities, three of every five persons is poor. Poverty looms large in part of Appalachia, at the end of dirt roads throughout the South, on the

Indian reservations already described, and along the paths that migrant workers follow year after year.

Rural poverty is not just a rural problem. Families who can find no way to support themselves in small towns or on farms migrate to inner city ghettos where they are ill-prepared for urban life. Although this migration has slowed in recent years, as it has become obvious that cities are no longer the promised land, the effects will be felt for many years.

Medical care in many rural areas, including care for mothers and infants, is often limited. Hospitals with limited facilities, particularly for high risk care; a limited number of physicians, many of them on the verge of retirement; and an inadequate number of professional nurses contribute to high infant mortality and morbidity in many rural communities. A concentrated effort toward the regionalization of perinatal care in many states is being initiated in an attempt to overcome these difficulties over the next few years (Chapter 9).

Appalachian Mountain People

More than 24 million people live in Appalachia (Fig. 4–2); another 3.5 million Appalachians live in urban areas including Cleveland, Detroit, and Pittsburgh, where they have migrated in search of employment, in many instances with minimum success. The poor and working class people of Appalachia tend to share values that may not always be understood and may therefore be misinterpreted by health care professionals with middle class values. A few examples are cited below.[75]

Time Orientation. Middle class Americans are largely *future oriented*; they plan today for events that are going to happen at some future time;

Figure 4–2   Appalachia and Southern Appalachia. (From Tripp-Reimer and Friedl: *Nursing Clinics of N. America, 12*:41, 1977.)

Appalachians, like many of the world's peoples, are frequently *present oriented*. Prenatal care, which involves seeking medical care *now* to prepare for a *future* event may have low priority. Another aspect of their time orientation—a flexible attitude toward schedules—may lead to broken appointments. An appointment at 8:00 A.M. today may be kept "sometime today" or "sometime this week."

Relationship of Man and Nature. While middle class Americans tend to believe that man controls his own destiny to a large extent, Appalachians (again, like many of the world's peoples) believe that man has very limited control, if any, over the forces of nature. If one has no control over events—if "what will be will be"—then preventive health care such as prenatal and well baby care makes very little sense to that individual.

Importance of the Extended Family. The most important group influencing the Appalachian woman are her kinspeople, the members of her extended family. Their advice, especially about age-old matters such as pregnancy and birth, will often take precedence over the advice of professional strangers.

THE COUNTERCULTURE: ALTERNATIVE LIFESTYLES

Any family, any commune, is like a Rorschach test. What you see when you come here says more about who you are than what it is. Visitors . . . completely miss what's really going on because they don't see what these things mean to us. (Melville,[52] quoting a member of an Oregon commune.)

Our knowledge of the counterculture, those young men and women who have chosen to live in a style different from that considered "mainstream American," is important not only so that we may give care to those young people but also because some facets of their alternative lifestyles may be advance signals of changes that will later become a part of the society as a whole. This is already evident in matters such as hairstyle and dress, and I think we are seeing examples in facets of childbearing as well.

The decision to live apart from the mainstream is hardly unique to the twentieth century. The Old Testament Jews saw themselves as a people set apart; so did the early Christians. Convents and monasteries offered medieval women and men the opportunity for communal living. Nineteenth century America saw both successful communities (Shakers, Oneida, The Harmony Society, for example) and many brief, less successful attempts at communal life (Brook Farm, Oberlin, Utopia, and a long list of others). Nathaniel Hawthorne lived at Brook Farm for a time. Bronson Alcott, the father of Louisa May Alcott, was one of the founders of a small, short-lived group called Fruitlands.

What of the people who choose alternative lifestyles today? It is estimated that there are more than 2000 communal groups in the United States at present, and in addition many couples and individuals reside outside of the communes with similar ways of life. Many communes are rural, but they exist in urban apartments and homes as well. Communities are scattered throughout almost every region of the country, although they are rare in the Southeast and Midwest. California, northern New Mexico, Southern Colorado, Washington, Oregon, Vermont, and the Hudson River Valley are popular areas. Some communities are small, with eight to ten members; the larger groups usually number 20 to 40. Despite regional and individual differences, there are also similarities because there is migration from one communal group to another.

Philosophically, communal groups appear to be of two basic types: those whose members are, in a sense, retreating from contemporary lifestyles and those formed with a specific mission in mind. Examples of the former are Twin Oaks in Virginia and Morningstar Ranch in California. Personal fulfillment and a more viable lifestyle are major foci of the individuals who live in these groups.

Koinonia, founded near Americus, Georgia, in 1943 and Synanon, founded in California in 1958, are well-known examples of communities with a mission. Koinonia is an interracial community (consider what that meant in rural Georgia in the 1940's) formed for the purposes of demonstrating Christian ideals of community life and assisting local farmers by introducing scientific farming. Synanon, which began with an emphasis on group therapy for drug addicts, has grown into a community of over 1200 with 6 million dollars in property. Such wealth is very atypical of most communal groups.

Observers have noted with some interest that in many communal groups there is little talk of "women's liberation." In those communities that succeed, everyone works quite hard, with heavy field work done by the men and cooking, sewing, and childcare mainly done by the women. A major difference from the life of women in suburbia, however, is that these tasks are not done in isolation but in the company of other adults. Moreover, the entire community, fathers as well as mothers, sees childcare as important.

"Unmarried" married couples may live in communities or as individual couples. Their commitment to one another is usually longstanding, although it may not last, just as the commitment of the "legally" married may not. It is the *idea* that a document from the government makes the difference between being married and being single that is rejected. In much the same way, birth certificates may be scorned as "the fatal beginning of an official assembly line which leads to compulsory public education, military conscription, social security and taxation."[52]

A single mother who is part of the counterculture is more likely to be from a middle or upper class background and often is college educated. Unlike single mothers in the past, she may not share the guilt about an "out of wedlock" pregnancy, probably due in part to changing attitudes in mainstream society. These single mothers lead a life somewhat different from that of the lower class single mother, who often lives with her own mother or relatives in an extended family. The single mother of the counterculture is more likely to live in a community, with a group of other single mothers, or alone.

A detailed examination of the counterculture is obviously beyond the scope of this book. Our suggestions for further reading include the works of Kanter, Melville, and Hedgepeth listed in the chapter references.

Childbearing and the Counterculture

Many of the expressed values of the counterculture concerning childbearing and childrearing are not very different from the ideals expressed in this and other nursing texts. For example, there is emphasis on the role of the father during pregnancy, at the time of delivery, and in childrearing. Natural childbirth is common, although many of us would find it more difficult to accept delivery within the community with nonprofessionals serving as midwives. Breast-feeding is almost universal, as is close, intimate contact between mother and baby during infancy. In some groups the child is rarely left with anyone but the mother and father, while in others childrearing tasks may be shared, even to the point of exchanging breast-feeding infants among several lactating mothers.

There is considerable interest in nutrition, particularly in organic foods and herbs. One potential problem during pregnancy is that protein intake may be low. Diets with adequate protein can be planned within the framework of the dietary desires of most mothers, but some education and care in menu planning are necessary. For some mothers, the expense may be prohibitive.

The emphasis on naturalness and intimacy may put couples in conflict with the traditional medical world of hospitals and clinics—a world in which technology and bureaucracy often seem to be more important than people and relationships from the couples' point of view.

Bell* talks of this conflict and his

---

*Dr. Bell's book, *A Time to be Born,* one that we highly recommend to all nurses who care for mothers and babies, describes in very readable fashion the first days of four infants, three sick babies in a medical center hospital and Stephen Benson.

reaction to it in describing the birth of Stephen Benson.[10] At the time he wrote the book, Dr. Bell was a pediatric house officer in an intensive care unit of a medical center—practicing medicine in a way as foreign to life in the commune as the bloodletting of the eighteenth century is to cardiac pacemakers. Stephen's parents, Kristin and Peter, lived on a farm with 13 other people. Kristin had received prenatal care from an obstetrician who was unwilling to participate in a home delivery. She said of him, "I don't think he likes us very much," and added, "We want to do everything possible for our baby. We don't want it to be unsafe, but we feel that it would be better for the child to be born at home." The couple agreed that should complications occur, they would go immediately to the hospital, a 15 minute drive.

In describing the labor, Bell comments, "We were witnessing something we had never seen in a hospital, a child being born in an atmosphere of love and caring. I wondered if the baby would somehow recognize this and, as Kristin and Peter believed, to be a better, happier person because of it." A friend sang quiet songs during the long hours of labor. Kristin ate ice chips and sipped tea. At the time of Stephen's delivery, Bell records:

Finally, the vagina had stretched enough, and with a push the infant's head came out. Peter held the head and slowly guided out the shoulders and body of his son. The wet, warm, slippery body began to move, and after a cough, he began to cry . . . Peter and Kristin began crying, sobbing with joy as their son moved about, flexing his arms, opening his eyes, looking around for the first time.

. . . The door opened and the other house members came in, everyone laughing, crying, hugging each other, rejoicing, and welcoming the new child . . . Still overcome with joy, he (Peter) dried the baby, handing him carefully to Kristin, and they cried together for the joy of the new life they had produced.

Their son was not crying but moving about, carefully studying this strange new world in the arms of his loving parents.[10]

What kind of persons will Stephen and his contemporaries, the children of the counterculture, be as adults? Melville[52] quotes a father in Taos Pueblo, "The test of this whole thing . . . will be the next generation . . . the kids who grow up here, they're going to be really high people, absolutely out of sight."

Veysey,[77] in looking at the children of earlier generations who sought alternative lifestyles, found that most of the children "slipped back into more conventional beliefs and styles of living" and that at least some "were soon enthusiastically playing baseball." He comments, "In America it seems little easier for radicals to hold on to their children than it is for any other parents."

Nursing and the Counterculture

We have chosen to stress some of the positive aspects of the counterculture, recognizing that there are problems as well. Misuse of drugs, venereal disease, and other health and social problems of our general society can hardly bypass those who choose to live differently.

As with everyone whose values differ from our own, it is important to listen to his or her ideas attentively and seriously. Bancroft,[8] in describing her nursing practice within the counterculture, concludes that there was "no need for us to participate in the life style of our clients . . . As long as we did not try to impose our values on them, they did not impose theirs on us . . ." But, she adds, "It mattered a great deal that the staff were willing to work with hip clients."

THE SINGLE PARENT FAMILY

It is customary, and comfortable, for us to think of childbearing in terms of a husband-father and a wife-mother, married to one another. Much of our effort during the past decade has been devoted to breaking down barriers that have separated a husband from his wife and newborn child during significant phases of the birth of the child. While this continues to be an extremely important focus of our nursing practice, we must be just as interested in the needs of single parents.

In March, 1975, it was reported that 13 per cent of all American families were headed by single, separated, divorced, or widowed women—a total of 7.2 million families. About one of every seven children under 18 years of age in the United States lives in a home without a father. Not all of these children were legally fatherless at the time of birth, of course, but the single pregnant woman is by no means a rarity.

The exact number of single mothers bearing children is difficult to compute because a number of states do not record illegitimacy on birth certificates (a practice with much to commend it). Moreover, because of this, the poor, the black, and the very young mother are probably overrepresented in statistics. The mother with a higher income, frequently a white mother, may be able to travel to a state that will not record illegitimacy on her baby's birth certificate, and thus is probably underrepresented. Also unrepresented in statistics is the mother who is single at the time of conception and marries during, and perhaps largely because of, her pregnancy. For many couples, marriage under these circumstances may be short-lived, and the mother becomes a single parent at some future time.

Recognizing all of these limitations to the statistical data, we can still find some useful information about single mothers in the reported figures. Statistics are reported in terms of the total number of illegitimate births, the number of illicit births per 1000 live births, the number of illicit births per 1000 unmarried females, and the number of births to mothers who are white or nonwhite.

If we look at trends over a 36 year period (1938 to 1974), the number of births to single mothers has increased markedly (Table 4–1). Almost five times as many babies were born to unmarried mothers in 1974 as in 1938.

In looking at the age of the mothers (Table 4–2), the greatest number of babies are born to single mothers between the ages of 15 and 19. This was true in 1938, as well as in 1974. Two of every 100 unmarried girls in this age group and 3 of every 100 unmarried women between 20 and 29 years of age bear children, but absolute numbers are lower in the older age groups because so many women over 20 years of age are married. The rate, however, is dropping in every age group except the 15 to 19 category.

Table 4–1   BIRTHS TO SINGLE MOTHERS IN 1938, 1957, 1968, AND 1974, BY RACE OF THE MOTHER

	White		Nonwhite		
Year	Number	Per Cent	Number	Per Cent	Total
1938	41,200	47	46,700	53	87,900
1957	70,800	35	130,900	65	201,700
1968	155,200	46	183,900	54	339,100
1974	168,500	40	249,600	60	418,100

Table 4-2 NUMBER, RATIO, AND RATE OF BIRTHS TO SINGLE MOTHERS IN 1938, 1957, 1968, AND 1974, BY AGE OF THE MOTHER*

				Age of Mother			
Year	Under 15	15–19	20–24	25–29	30–34	35–39	40 and Over
			NUMBER OF BIRTHS TO SINGLE MOTHERS				
1938	2,000	40,400	26,400	10,000	5,000	3,100	1,000
1957	4,600	76,400	60,500	29,800	18,000	9,400	2,800
1968	7,700	158,000	107,900	35,200	17,200	9,700	3,300
1974	10,600	210,800	122,700	44,900	18,600	8,200	2,300
			ILLEGITIMACY RATIO (ILLICIT BIRTHS PER 1000 LIVE BIRTHS)				
1938	608.5	135.5	36.6	16.4	13.2	15.3	14.2
1957	660.9	138.9	44.4	26.1	24.9	25.7	29.1
1968	810.2	267.2	82.6	38.9	41.0	47.1	51.4
1974	653.1	202.3	110.7	48.6	49.9	69.4	77.7
			RATE OF ILLEGITIMACY (BIRTHS PER 1000 UNMARRIED FEMALES)				
1938	0.3	7.5	9.2	6.8	4.8	3.4	1.1
1957	0.6	15.6	36.5	37.6	26.1	12.7	3.3
1968	0.0	19.8	37.3	38.6	28.2	14.9	3.8
1974	0.0	23.2	30.9	28.4	18.6	10.0	2.6

*Adapted from the following sources: (1) Schacter, J. and McCarthy, M.: Illegitimate Births: United States, 1938–57. In *Vital Statistics–Special Reports, Selected Studies*, Vol. 47, No. 8. (Washington, D.C.: U.S. Government Printing Office, 1960); (2) *Trends in Illegitimacy: United States, 1940–1965.* (Washington, D.C.: U.S. Government Printing Office, 1968); (3) mimeographed reports for 1968 data from National Center for Health Statistics; and (4) *Monthly Vital Statistics Report*, Vol. 24, No. 11, Feb. 13, 1976.

In 1974, of all babies born to mothers between the ages of 15 and 19, approximately 20 per cent were born to single mothers. Of babies born to mothers under 15 years of age, 65 per cent of the mothers were unmarried at the time of birth. (This represents a decrease from over 80 per cent in 1968, probably due to the legalization of abortion.) Because of this, much of the emphasis, both in terms of care during and the prevention of the single pregnancy, has been directed toward the adolescent single mother. Special needs of adolescent mothers are discussed in Chapters 7 and 10.

Apart from the particular needs of the adolescent mother, what can we say about single mothers?

1. Single mothers represent a diverse group of people—diverse in terms of age, race, socioeconomic status, and individual characteristics. Reasons for pregnancy outside of marriage vary; they may be related to personality characteristics of the mother, such as low self-esteem; to cultural patterns in which successive generations of women in the same family have become single mothers; to ignorance of the physiology of conception and/or effective contraception; to the desire for a child; and to a variety of other reasons important to a particular mother.

2. Not every pregnancy is unwanted by an unmarried mother, nor is every pregnancy seen by the mother as a problem (any more than every preg-

nancy to a married mother is wanted, planned or without problems). Nurses and other professional workers tend to view single mothers from the perspective of their own values, values that are not necessarily shared, or shared with the same level of intensity, by the mother herself. A part of our role is to assess what the pregnancy means to an individual mother.

3. Pregnancies outside of marriage may fall into one of several categories. The couple may have no intention or desire to marry one another. Or one partner may desire marriage, but the other may feel uninterested or unready. Contrary to the popular myth, it is not always the woman who desires marriage. Fairly frequently we see instances in which the man is very willing to marry, but the woman states that she "is not ready to settle down." These couples may continue their relationship during their pregnancy and after the birth of the baby. Some couples, as noted in the discussion of the counterculture, may choose to live together without a legal ceremony but may have a real commitment to one another and to their children. Pregnancy may occur to a couple already planning marriage, or to a woman following divorce. Or pregnancy may be the result of rape or incest. Pregnancy due to extramarital intercourse may result in a situation in which the mother is married but her husband is not the father of the conceptus.

UNMARRIED FATHERS

Hundreds of studies, articles, and books have examined unwed mothers; very few have looked at the fathers of their babies. Why?

One reason is the double standard for sexual behavior in our society. Not only are men not condemned for sexual intercourse, but the adolescent boy receives many subtle (and some not so subtle) messages that sexual intercourse is expected. Society at large, and the medical world as well, places little blame on him when pregnancy occurs. Consider the following statements, part of a discussion following the presentation of a paper on the "Unwed Teen-age Mother" at the Pacific Coast Obstetrical and Gynecological Society:

There is no question of the increased frequency of this aberrant behavior of young women in our culture . . . If we are to discover the least common denominator of illegitimate pregnancy we must investigate wherein the unwed mother's own mother failed in programming her daughter with enough basic emotional control to restrain her instinctive procreative drive until she meets the conditions required by the cultural mores.[46]

. . . I will tell them, and in many instances I sense that they know it to be true, that if they indulge in teen-age sexual intercourse and pre-marital intercourse most of the time their sexual partner has no respect for them whatsoever, and if he ever did, he usually loses it very rapidly.[7]

A second reason for little emphasis on the unmarried father is that he is, in a sense, invisible, while the mother is not only highly visible but in many instances a problem to a society that must support her and her child.

Traditionally, we have not expected much from the father involved in an unwed pregnancy. Our laws, which require only the consent of the mother for such actions as adoption and abortion, do, in fact, discourage the father's participation. And certainly there are some fathers who choose not to be involved.

However, when mothers and the professional people working with them have included the father in planning, they have found that many fathers were far more interested than they expected. Many chose to act responsibly when they were given the opportunity.

Auerbach describes two different paternal reactions to out-of-wedlock pregnancy.

> The first woman had conceived due to contraceptive failure. The relationship with the father was shaky before the pregnancy and rapidly deteriorated after the announcement of expectant motherhood. Throughout her pregnancy her baby's father made no effort to help her in any way. She subsisted on a welfare check in an apartment house for singles only. After the baby was born she continued to live there with minimum financial support from her parents at the sufferance of the apartment house superintendent.
>
> The second woman chose to conceive. While the father served a brief prison term, she decorated their rented house with care and devotion to the needs of their baby. They attended childbirth preparation classes together and he accompanied her to the obstetrician's office for prenatal visits. The physician treated them as he did married couples. Six months after the delivery of their daughter, they were hoping to have another child within two years.[5]

Pannor and his associates report that "the relationships between unwed mothers and fathers are much more meaningful than popularly supposed, and that unwed fathers have more concern for their offspring than is generally realized."[60] They describe a sense of isolation, alienation, and feelings of being cut off and denied meaningful human contact as some of the fathers' emotions.

In some clinics and hospitals, male partners are included in planning and support to the extent that they and the mother wish them to be. Part of our nursing role is to accept and support these fathers.

DECISIONS THE SINGLE MOTHER AND FATHER MUST FACE

Unmarried parents must make one of four decisions: marriage, raising the child by a single parent, releasing the child for adoption, or abortion.

Marriage

Couples who are considering marriage because of pregnancy need to face their motives realistically. Does one, or both, of them feel guilty, if not for the act of coitus itself, for the pregnancy? Are sympathy or pity factors in their decision? In the months that follow such a decision, a bride may wonder, "Would he have married me if I were not pregnant?"

"Did she trick me into this?" may cross the mind of the groom. Such thoughts may be less important now than they will be in later years. Several of our patients have found that this kind of question becomes an issue during a subsequent pregnancy, when old feelings are rekindled.

Vincent[78] suggests that couples must face the reality that the question "Would he have married me if . . . ?" is unanswerable and is one form of a very universal problem. All couples, at some time during their marriages, drag events of the past into arguments, whether the issue be premarital pregnancy or some other circumstance of courting or early marriage. Thus, premarital pregnancy in itself does not constitute an absolute contraindication to marriage.

If marriage is chosen as the desired course, a wedding such as the couple would have had if there were no pregnancy may be a good idea. A hurried, secretive ceremony may be remembered longer by the couple themselves than the fact of a premature conception.

Often marriage, or at least marriage during the course of the pregnancy, is not desirable. No one can make this decision but the couple themselves, but the alternative of waiting until after the baby is born and perhaps placing the infant for temporary foster care before a marriage decision is made, might be suggested.

Keeping the Child Without Marriage: The Mother as a Single Parent

A mother's decision to keep her baby although she remains single is influenced by cultural norms and by individual circumstances. Women of lower socioeconomic classes are far more likely to feel that they should keep their babies than are the middle class mothers. Quite a few of these lower class mothers are themselves products of single parent families; perhaps their own survival makes the idea of bringing up a child alone less threatening or strange.

Support for her chosen course from her parents is another positive factor that increases the likelihood that a mother may keep her baby. Older women who are already maintaining their own households, women who continue to have a relationship with the putative father (and who may consider future marriage a possibility), and women who have had prior pregnancies that were not carried to term have also been found to be more ready to keep their child.[50]

A mother who is a single parent faces some pressing issues concerning her lifestyle, both before and after the baby is born. She must decide where she will live; how she will meet increasing financial needs; how she will obtain medical care, both for herself and later for the baby as well; and how she will begin or continue a job or further education.

Where Will She Live? The options available to her include: (1) living with her parents or other relatives, (2) living with her partner, (3) living with a friend, (4) living alone, (5) living in a maternity home, or (6) living in a foster home provided by some communities if she is under 18.

Each of these alternatives presents both advantages and problems that are highly individual. Living at home with genuinely supportive parents who accept their daughter and her pregnancy may be the best of all possible alternatives. However, in other instances constant friction between a young woman and her parents may make such a situation impossible. Still other parents totally reject an unmarried daughter. One of our patients, formerly married but now divorced and living at home, told us that her father would banish her when he discovered that she was pregnant. She was quite positive about this because he had already disowned her sister for the same reason.

Both in the past and somewhat more openly today, a woman may choose to live with her sexual partner, although marriage is not desired by one or both at the present time. Many nurses find this arrangement hard to accept; our feelings may affect our nursing relationship with this woman and this couple if we do not recognize and deal with them.

From a purely financial standpoint, living with a friend or living alone can present problems. At some point, income may cease; what will the woman do then? The problem is not unsolvable but needs realistic planning (see below).

Maternity homes, such as the Florence Crittenton homes, at one time played a significant role in the care of unmarried women during pregnancy. They are used far less today. A number have closed after many years of operation; others remain open but operate below capacity. The combination of legal therapeutic abortion and wider public acceptance of pregnancy outside of marriage is probably responsible for this decreased use. Those homes that do remain open offer the advantages of privacy and a protected environment, and often counseling and the chance for continued education are provided. Good medical care is usually assured. No good maternity home pressures the mother into placing the baby for adoption, as some mothers seem to fear.

A foster home is an individual home licensed by the state. Foster homes are more commonly used for infant and child care, including the care of an infant awaiting adoption, but a young pregnant girl may also qualify for placement.

How Will Financial Needs Be Met?
Most single mothers who deliver and keep their infants will have financial problems, regardless of socioeconomic status. The median family income for families headed by women was $6,400 in 1974, compared with a median income of $13,800 for husband-wife families. In our society even well-educated women rarely command the salaries of men with similar levels of education. With a high proportion of single mothers being teenagers and coming from nonwhite families, earning opportunities are even further restricted.

Each mother needs someone who will realistically help her balance the expenses of pregnancy and childrearing with the funds available to her. The economically poorest of patients may have a social caseworker who can help her assess her finances. For women with somewhat higher incomes, financial counsel may be more difficult to find. In some communities, home economists who are employed by the city or county government will help with budgeting.

Nurses can provide information about the costs of medical services and the resources available for meeting these and other needs. To those who would wonder if this is truly *nursing* care, we wonder how we can say it is not.

How, for example, can we encourage a diet adequate for good prenatal care and remain oblivious to the fact that the mother can afford only pinto beans and fatback?

Many hospitals and clinics have departments or social workers to whom mothers can be referred for financial advice and assistance, and this should be done whenever it is possible Referral, for many mothers, means not merely telling them to go to Room 31-C if they need help, but describing to them the service that is available and assisting them in whatever way seems individually appropriate. Although it is important for each mother to assume as much responsibility as possible in seeking help, women will vary in the amount of initiative they will be able to command, particularly when much of their coping strength is already channeled into dealing with the pregnancy itself.

Sources of financial assistance that may be available to an individual mother include: (1) employment, for at least part of the pregnancy; (2) help from the father of the child; (3 Medicaid; (4) food stamps; and (5) resources particular to the individual community.

Individual community resources may be services offered by an agency related to the National Foundation-March of Dimes, individual churches or groups of churches, women's clubs Jay-cettes, and the like. When there is a definite gap in community services nurses may be able to persuade such local groups to undertake unmet needs as projects. Such groups are not only helpful in securing clothes and food for mothers but in equipping hospital nurseries when a definite need is brought to their attention.

Support payments for the baby from the putative father that are or dered by the court may be a source of financial assistance *after* the infant is born, as may be public aid through Aid to Families with Dependent Children (AFDC). If the unmarried mother already has a child, she may be eligible for AFDC payments before delivery. Such eligibility is determined by the Department of Social Services of the AFDC. For some mothers the thought of any type of government assistance (which they translate as "welfare") is totally unacceptable. A nurse may be someone with whom they can share their feelings, explore alternatives, and eventually arrive at the best decision for themselves.

How Will She Obtain Medical Care? In the United States obtaining medical care is closely related to finances. At this point we would say that each nurse should be aware of the options for maternity care available in her own and neighboring communities and their relative costs in relation to other advantages and disadvantages, such as availability of transportation; length of waiting time; and, of paramount importance, the quality of care given.

Placing the Baby for Adoption

Mothers should know that the decision to place the baby for adoption is not final and irrevocable until after the infant is born. The length of time following birth in which a mother may change her mind varies with the laws of each state. Counsel and support should be available to each mother not only at the time that she struggles to make her initial decision but during the weeks and months that follow. She will need reassurance that a good home will be found for her baby as she questions, to herself and to others, "Am I really doing the right thing?"

Adoption may be handled directly or through a licensed agency. In direct adoption the baby is placed in a specific adoptive home by the mother or couple. Usually this is less desirable than placement through a licensed agency, which preserves the anonymity of both natural and adoptive parents and has experience in selecting an adoptive home and dealing with the legal requirements.

While it is common to think that the adoptive decision is made near the time of birth, a mother may initially decide to keep her baby and then find, as the infant becomes a toddler or a preschool child, that caring for him is more than she can manage. A door should be left open for a change of plans at any time.*

Abortion

Since the Supreme Court ruling of January 22, 1973, a woman may legally choose abortion of any fetus before the seventh month of pregnancy, the time defined as the legal age of viability. The wording of that ruling (Roe vs. Wade, Texas—41 LW 4213) declared that since physicians, philosophers, and theologians are unable to reach a consensus on the issue of when life begins, it was not appropriate for the courts to speculate about it. For the purposes of constitutional protection, the unborn child was not to be considered a person.

Almost all of the existing laws that limited abortion were declared unconstitutional because they were considered to invade the privacy of the pregnant woman. In the first trimester, abortion was judged to be strictly a medical decision between a woman and her doctor. From the beginning of the second trimester until the seventh month, individual states were allowed to enact

---

*This later change of plans is dramatized well in a film "I'm Seventeen, Pregnant, and I Don't Know What to Do." (Appendix I.)

laws to protect the health of the mother. But only after viability of the fetus was attained was the state permitted to limit abortion decisions to those instances in which the life or health of the mother was jeopardized.

In a second significant decision (Doe vs. Bolton, Georgia—41 LW 4233), a number of related laws were also declared invalid because they, too, were considered to violate the privacy of the pregnant woman. No longer could abortions be done only in accredited hospitals, only for residents of the state in which they were performed, or only when approved by a hospital abortion committee or the consensus of consulting physicians.

Abortion is discussed in Chapter 23.

THE WOMEN'S MOVEMENT

The women's movement is not a recent phenomenon. Because the status of women is so closely related to our nursing practice, we would urge nurses to broaden their own knowledge of the movement by reading the works of authors such as Friedan, de Beauvoir, Sanger, Rossi, and others.

How does the women's movement relate to health care for childbearing families? First, because the majority of professional nurses are women, nurses have traditionally had less power to affect care than physicians and hospital administrators, the majority of whom are men. Ashley[4] points out that "nurses were not the equals of physicians in political and economic spheres, and so nursing's continuing subjection to male dominance resulted. . . They sought approval from men, not liberation. As a result, from the first decade of the century onward, physicians and hospital administrators have remained in positions of dominance and control over nursing and health care."

As recently as 1976, the president of the American Medical Association, Dr. Max Parrott, characterized nursing as ancillary to medicine and dependent upon it.[69]

As women become stronger, politically and economically, nurses will also practice from a position of greater strength. We may become more outspoken concerning issues that deal with health care for childbearing families rather than deferring to others. We may seek to align public opinion on both national issues and problems within our own community, such as family life education in the school system, birth control information for all sexually active women (regardless of age or marital status), and family-centered care in maternity units, to name but three of many possible examples.

The status of women has also affected women's power in relation to their own health care, a large measure of which is obstetric and gynecologic care. As recently as the 1960's, obstetrician-gynecologists made decisions for women such as withholding birth control devices from unmarried women and deciding when a woman could be sterilized. The formula for sterilization (the woman's age times the number of children she had delivered had to equal or be greater than 120) was not dropped by the American College of Obstetric and Gynecology (ACOG) until 1969 and is still a "rule of thumb" in many hospitals. By this formula, a woman of 25 would have had to have delivered five children before she could elect to be sterilized; a woman with four children would have to wait until she was 30. Pity the poor family that chose to have only two children; nature would solve the mother's fertility problem before the age of 60, at which time the ACOG formula would permit sterilization! Even if overpopulation were not one of the most pressing of the world' problems, the failure to allow women to make such decisions seems almost unbelievable.

The foregoing is one illustration of why many women have felt that they have been unfairly treated by male physicians who have had so much control over their lives. In response, the women's movement has inspired a number of activities.

Learning to understand their own bodies and sharing their knowledge with other women has been one focus of the movement. *Our Bodies, Ourselves* is the result of such a study by one group, the Boston Women's Health Book Collective.[13] Originally published by the New England Free Press on newsprint and distributed to women's groups, the book is now available commercially. In a very frank and readable way, this volume discusses anatomy and physiology, female sexuality, venereal disease, birth control, abortion, and the many facets of pregnancy. *Vaginal Politics* by Ellen Frankfort[25] and *Free and Female* by Barbara Seaman[71] have similar goals. Frankfort warns (appropriately, we believe) that one danger of the health movement is that young women may become totally anti-doctor, as have some young couples at the time of pregnancy. The message is not total mistrust of physicians, she emphasizes, but understanding that doctors have areas of specialized information that can be utilized—"but not blindly."

The concerns of the women's movement for women's health parallel those of maternity nursing, although individual points of view certainly will differ. In relation to pregnancy, the emphasis is on making childbearing a fulfilling experience rather than a stressful one. Counseling for pregnant women who are experiencing difficulties, establishing pregnant couples groups, and placing heightened emphasis on dealing with the feelings as well as the physiologic facts of pregnancy are some suggested goals. The increased use of nurse-midwives for normal preg-

Some Relationships between the Status of Women
and the Health Needs of Women

Low Status of Women

↙ ↘

Women lack power to affect their own health and social needs

Nurses (because most nurses are women) lack power to affect health care of women

↘ ↙

Male dominance of health care for women, including childbearing

↓

Health care structured to suit male professionals

↓

Desires and needs of women often ignored

↓

Entire family (mother, father, children) shortchanged from generation to generation nancies, similar to the English model, is proposed, as well as the formation of organizations of visiting laywomen who would help with postnatal concerns. Maternity leave, not only for mothers but for fathers, so that the family can be together during the days following birth is already policy in Sweden. Providing daycare at every place of employment to enable the mother to return to work and to continue to breast-feed is a goal of some feminist groups.

Another area of concern to the women's movement has been the status of abortion in American society. Abortion is viewed by many women in "the movement" as a part of the right of a woman to control her own body. Obstruction to abortion, whether in the form of laws, hospital policy, high prices, physicians, adverse public opinion, or poor communication that keeps a woman from knowing what services are available, is a target for concern and for action of many women's groups (Chapter 23).

The Women's Movement and Changing Sex Roles

A second focus of the women's movement that seems particularly relevant to nursing care for childbearing families is the attempt to free both men and women from the stereotyping of sex roles. It has become obvious that the roles of women as wives and mothers cannot change to any great extent without changes in the roles of men as husbands and fathers.

What defines masculinity and femininity? Is it behavior such as bathing and diapering a baby or repairing an automobile engine? Is it a feeling, such as tenderness or sympathy? Is it a personality trait, such as aggressiveness or passivity? As people become parents, some are asking, "Can we raise children who will be free of sex stereotypes?"

To a large extent, sex roles are defined by cultural norms. There are societies in which sewing is the work of men rather than women, and even in our own country fine tailoring is frequently a man's occupation. In segments of our society the male dancer has been considered unmasculine (many little girls but few little boys go to dancing school); in other groups dancing is a male prerogative.

So, too, with the characteristics of personality. Mead[51] points out that among the Arapesh of New Guinea both men and women display traits that in our limited cultural perspective we might call maternal and feminine. They are "co-operative, unaggressive, responsive to the needs and demands of others." Among another tribe, the Mundugumor, in marked contrast, both men and women are ruthless, aggressive individuals with little that we would call maternal or feminine in their personalities. In a third group, the Tchambuli, women are the dominant, impersonal, managing persons while men are "less responsible" and emotionally dependent.

Mead concludes:

If those temperamental attitudes which we have traditionally regarded as feminine—such as passivity, responsiveness, and a willingness to cherish children—can so easily be set up as the masculine pattern in one tribe, and in another be outlawed for the majority of women as well as for the majority of men, we no longer have any basis for regarding such aspects of behavior as sex-linked. And this conclusion becomes even stronger when we consider the actual reversal in Tchambuli of the position of dominance of the two sexes, in spite of the existence of formal patrilineal institutions.[51] (Author's note—patrilineal institutions might be expected to support male dominance.)

There seems little doubt that sex roles are changing in our own society. Can anyone imagine, if television had existed in Victorian days, that Victorian fathers (or the actors portraying them) would have appeared discussing the relative merits of two brands of diapers. Even a few years ago, fathers were rare in prenatal classes and labor rooms and nurseries. It was an unusual father who had the opportunity to touch his baby before the day of discharge. While this kind of situation still exists in some hospitals, it is rapidly changing.

Now society has, in a sense, given its permission. "It's all right to help at home and care for your baby. It doesn't make you a sissy. You may even like it" is the nonverbal message of television and magazines and even cocktail party conversations. A few men have experimented with being "househusbands" while their wives are employed.

As nurses, our practice changes too. More and more we find ourselves relating to couples, rather than to mothers, two people instead of one.

Changes in sex roles are by no means evenly distributed throughout our society. Most social change begins in urban areas and among middle class families, and sex role changes follow similar patterns. As we have already noted in the discussion of social class, sex role differentiation is still characteristic of many blue collar families and upper class families.

In single parent families one parent cannot and should not attempt to assume both male and female roles, although some mothers may feel, and may even be told, that they must do so. Nurses can assure the single mother that she is only expected to fulfill a mother's role. Male role models may be assumed by relatives or friends or other males in the community.

FAMILIES IN WHICH THE MOTHER IS EMPLOYED OUTSIDE THE HOME

In spite of a popular myth that American families consist of fathers who are breadwinners and mothers who are homemakers (which the early sections of this chapter should have dispelled), a great number of American mothers have been employed outside the home for many years. In 1973, one out of evey three mothers of preschool children was gainfully employed. Six million children under the age of six have working mothers; 2.5 million working mothers have children under three years of age.

What is the effect of maternal employment on our society, and particularly on our families? In the general press and in popular discussion, mothers who are employed outside of their homes have often been treated as one homogeneous group. No real understanding of maternal employment is possible, however, without looking at the varied reasons why women seek employment.

Many mothers have no choice. They furnish all or most of the financial support for themselves and their children. In approximately 10 per cent of American households, a woman is the head of the family. Some of these women have never been married. Others are widowed, divorced, or separated from their husbands.

A second group of mothers work to supplement a family income that is, or seems to be, inadequate. Their husband may be unable to work because of physical or mental disability; even if he receives compensation of some sort, it is often insufficient for the family's financial needs. Unexpected expenses (frequently major medical expenses) may have overtaxed family resources. Two incomes may be necessary to meet basic needs or to provide the standard of living that would not be possible on one income. In nearly half of the families with two parents in which the mother works, the father's income is below $7,000.

For still other women, work offers

emotional satisfactions that are as compelling as, or even more important than, economic considerations. This group includes many educated professional women who have spent time and money preparing for a career. Mothers who find themselves lonely at home with little adult companionship may also choose to work for social and emotional rather than for monetary reasons. Being a mother does not, unfortunately, bring much prestige in American society.

These categories are by no means mutually exclusive. For many women the decision to seek employment outside of their homes is influenced by social, emotional, *and* monetary considerations.

Societal Attitudes toward Employed Mothers

Americans have some very contradictory attitudes about working mothers. The mother who works because she loves what she does or to provide income for "extras" (as opposed to basics such as food and shelter) is still largely regarded with ambivalence at best, and not infrequently with disapproval.

However, the lower class mother who accepts public assistance is often criticized for not putting her baby in a day care nursery and going to work to support herself and her child. Thus, we offer one standard to one group of mothers and a second to another group.

The effect of criticism on an individual working mother varies. In a neighborhood in which necessity dictates that all mothers be employed away from home or when a mother's friends are equally career-oriented, the problem of criticism from her peers may be minimal. It is the mother who is "bucking the trend" of behavior in her own neighborhood who may feel guilty because of the attitudes of her contem-

poraries. As some of the studies reviewed below indicate, this guilt, rather than her working per se, may in turn affect her family.

Family Attitudes toward Employed Mothers

A second source of comment and potential criticism comes from within the woman's own family. The mother's parents and relatives, or her husband's, may also create tension and anxiety by their comments. "When you (or your husband) were little, I stayed home and took care of you (him)," implies that the mother should do the same. The amount of stress that such comments can cause will depend on many factors: the support that a husband gives his wife's desire for employment and the couple's overall relationship with their parents are two such factors.

A major consideration in terms of family dynamics is the effect of the mother's employment on her relationship with her husband. If the mother gives her limited time at home to housework and baby care and if the father does not participate in these activities, when do the parents find time for one another? How resentful does the mother feel about the apparent unfairness of such a situation? On the other hand, if the father fully supports the mother's need or desire for employment and if homemaking and childcare tasks are shared, this is not only less likely to be a problem but can become a positive factor in the children's development, as they see both mother and father in more than one role.

A father's refusal to help his employed wife with tasks at home may be due to his own enculturation (men don't do women's work), or it may be a way of showing his unhappiness with his wife's employment. Lancaster[48] points out that it is not the husband who is unalterably opposed to his wife's job who creates the most difficult situation. Rather it is the husband who says, "It's O.K.," but then refuses to share in the other tasks and/or expects everything to be done as if the wife were home all day.

Howell[38] estimates that it takes 105 hours a week (that's 15 hours a day, 7 days a week) for a woman to hold a fulltime job and care for a home and family without help. Since some domestic chores are inevitable (cooking and dishwashing are hard to avoid, for example) it is easy to see that some important aspects of infant and child care, such as holding and singing and playing peek-a-boo, might be difficult to find time for, or that a mother with such a schedule might be too tired to play or even to talk if she must carry dual responsibilities alone.

One might hypothesize that if the mother's income is important to the family economically, the father would willingly share other tasks or, at the very least, be grateful for his wife's contribution. In some families, however, a wife's economic contribution may serve to make her husband feel that he has failed as a provider, and thus as a man, and thereby may increase family tension. Douvan[22] reports that in homes in which the mother's working suggests the father's inadequacy, sons chose the father as a role model less frequently, were generally less active, and often showed a rebellious response to adult authority.

New studies of mother and infant interaction that show that importance of parenting for attachment and development during the early months (Chapter 20) raise questions about what happens when the mother is employed during this time.

Studies of babies receiving care by someone other than their mother have shown these babies to behave somewhat differently. This difference could be re-lated to having received care from other people, or it could be related to a difference in the personality of their own mother (and thus the mothering they receive from her).

Moore[54] found that children receiving day care before one year of age showed more fears and more dependent attachments to their parents than those children who were not in day care until after they were three years old. Infants who had a succession of child care arrangements during the first year demonstrated marked attention seeking and dependent behavior. When Moore compared "home-reared" children with those receiving any other kind of care, the home-reared infants appeared less aggressive, more obedient, and more concerned with approval. Schwarz and associates report similar findings.[70]

Murray[56] also found differences in babies who received care from their own mother as opposed to those who received care from multiple sources, but suggests that the difference may be more related to the mother's personality. He found that the mothers who had sole responsibility for their baby's care (other than the care given by the father) when the baby was six months old were more self-confident and more personally involved with their baby than the mothers who shared care with one or more caretakers. At one year the babies who had been cared for by their mother alone had a more positive interaction with their mother, who, in turn, interacted more with her baby. We are impressed by the similarity of these findings with those of Klaus and associates[47] and Kennel and associates,[45] who found that mothers with early contact with their babies appeared more confident and interacted more frequently with them. Greenberg[31] reports similar findings for fathers (Chapter 20).

Long-term studies will be necessary to determine if the differences in mother-child interaction and infant personality during the first year are important as the child grows older. It seems obvious that such studies are vitally important to our society.

The effect of mothers' employment on older children has been investigated. Burchinal[15] found no apparent effect on personality, school-related characteristics, or social development in the school-aged children of 1100 families. The study included families in which the mother was employed during the first three years of the child's life, the second three years, and the first six years, as well as children of mothers who had never been employed. Some of the children who were tested were in the seventh grade; the remainder were eleventh graders.

Siegel reports similar findings.[72] She matched children for such factors as family size, age of siblings, and family income level, so that she could more closely estimate if the differences she found were related to the fact that the mother was employed. The matched pairs of children, one of an employed mother and one of a mother who was not employed, were observed during free play period in kindergarten for self-reliance, conformity, and aggression. Siegel found no major differences in the two groups of children.

In the case of mothers of adolescents, there is some evidence that part-time employment may have a positive effect by helping adolescents become more independent. This may be because the part-time job helps the mother make the transition from the nurturing, protecting role of the mother of young children to the "letting go" that is important in allowing adolescents to mature.

The Mother's Feelings About Employment

How a mother feels about employment may be as important as employment itself in its effect on her children. Because of the proscriptions of our society about a mother's job, guilt is probably the emotion most commonly shared by employed mothers. Guilt is intensified if the baby has an accident while his mother is at work, if an older child is doing poorly in school, or if an adolescent commits some act of delinquency. A mother who feels guilty forgets that children whose mothers are not employed also have accidents and school problems and have trouble with the law.

Guilt can lead to efforts to compensate for being away part of the day by giving children attention and affection when their mother is home (not necessarily bad) or to overcompensate by being unable to say "no," buying too many toys and "things," and so on (obviously harmful).

Employment may either enhance or lower a mother's self-esteem, and this, in turn, affects her children. If a mother feels good about herself because of success in her job, her positive feelings can be contagious. On the other hand, if her self-esteem is lowered by employment ("If I had married a different man who could care for me and my children more adequately, I would not have to work"), her negative feelings may affect her children. The effect of her employment on the father's feelings about himself is also significant (above).

Career or Job

One variable that has not been examined closely in formal studies is the effect of a "career" versus the effect of a "job" on infants and children. We use the term career to describe work that is not limited to hours at a place of employment, but that makes many additional demands on time if one is to be reasonably effective—time for continuing education, traveling to attend professional meetings, reading, and even preoccupation with a challenging problem during the time a parent is at home. We consider nursing practice to be a career in this sense. Women who are lawyers, physicians, business executives, artists, writers, and teachers are other examples. A "job," by contrast, demand's one's time and energy only during the hours actually worked; assembly line work in a factory is an example.

In past generations, the number of mothers of infants and young children with careers was rather limited. But the number increases each year, as women seek and find new opportunities.

It has been suggested that a career is one's own favorite child. This is an issue to be considered not only by mothers, but by fathers as well. The demands of a man's career can shortchange his family, if he allows them to, just as much as the demands of a career on a woman. Although problems are not inevitable, career-oriented families, both fathers and mothers, must consider what is important to them as they plan their families. Successful parenting cannot be fit into odd moments of leftover time.

Infant and Child Care for the Employed Mother

One of the biggest problems for mothers who must, or choose to, work is finding child care—care that is not merely safe but that will be a positive factor in their infant's and child's development. For the mother who knows she must return to work within a few weeks after her baby's birth, this can be a major concern during pregnancy.

Potential caretakers commonly include another family member, such as a grandmother living in the home or nearby; someone who is hired to come into the home; or an individual or day care center to which the baby is taken. In some families the husband and wife may arrange their employment so that one of them will always be with the baby. In a few families the husband may care for the baby while his wife is employed away from home, but this is still the exception in most American households. Communal living arrangements provide caretakers for a limited number of couples.

Although individual circumstances affect the decisions that a mother makes, social factors also appear important. Traditionally, few middle class mothers have chosen group care for small babies. This has been due, at least in the past, to the paucity of day care centers in middle class neighborhoods, but it also seems to be related to a reluctance to use such centers, even if they were present. Taking their baby to someone, either an older woman or perhaps a young mother with children of her own, is more acceptable to these mothers. An often preferred but more expensive alternative is hiring someone to come into the family's home to care for the child. Aside from the expense, finding a suitable person is difficult in many areas.

For mothers with more limited economic resources, day care may be the only alternative, unless they are living in an extended family. Currently there is licensed day care for about only 10 per cent of the children under six years of age whose mothers are employed. And only a small percentage of these facilities provide truly comprehensive services. Much day care is custodial, providing safety but little more. Some is neglectful.

What should parents look for in choosing a caretaker? For small infants and children, a one-to-one relationship between caretaker and child would appear to be best. Murray[56] wonders whether a caretaker with four infants can provide sufficient responsiveness and stimulation.

The individual should be a warm,

stimulating, nonrejecting person. Continuity is also important. A baby will need to form an attachment to his caretaker, just as he must to his parents, if he is to develop in an emotionally healthy way.

The caretaker's philosophy and rules of care must be similar to those of the parents; few small children can live by two sets of rules. Consider the confusion, for example, if parents encourage their eight month old baby to try to feed himself and to experiment with the textures in his food, but his caretaker slaps his hand if he puts it in his plate and roughly scrubs his face with a washcloth, frowning all the while, when food misses his mouth.

For the adolescent mother, married or unmarried, the caretaker is often her own mother, an aunt, or even a grandmother. Under these circumstances it is often difficult for the young mother to make suggestions about how she feels the baby should be cared for. Young mothers tell of their distress over some of their own mothers' practices (dressing the baby too warmly on a hot day, for instance), yet they feel unable to change the situation. Moreover, they may be unable, economically and/or emotionally, to care for the baby without that parent's help.

Unanswered Questions

The mother who is employed is an integral part of American life. Many of our childbearing women will return to work within a few weeks following delivery. It is necessary for us to be knowledgeable about the effect of maternal employment on children, both in order to help these women integrate their roles of wife, mother, and worker and to make a contribution to public planning for infant and child care for those families in which the mother is away from home.

There are no clear answers for the employed mother who is concerned about depriving her child, and almost all are concerned about this. Many more questions need to be explored. Does the age or sex or social class of the child make a difference? Is an unhappy mother at home better than a cheerful, hired caretaker? Is the effect of full-time work different from that of part-time work? Are fathers as effective as mothers in caring for infants and small children? The answers to these and similar questions are highly important to our society.

CULTURAL NORMS OF NURSES WHO CARE FOR CHILDBEARING FAMILIES

It is important that we recognize the cultural factors that influence the behavior of childbearing families. It may even be more important for us to understand how cultural factors influence our professional lives. In essence, nurses and other professional workers are influenced by two sets of norms—those of their own cultural heritage and those acquired in the process of becoming a professional person.

Norms of the Nurse as a Person

Cultural factors that influence families also influence nurses. We bring to nursing the norms of our social class, our religion, the community in which we live, and the many other facets of our own cultural heritage. In the preceding pages, we have already illustrated some of the ways in which our values may differ from those of our patients—in relation to families in poverty and to American Indian families, for example. Many additional illustrations will be found throughout this book.

The "middle class" values of many

nurses and other professionals can be a major barrier to providing health care for those who do not share them, if we do not consider these values in our planning. For instance, for many years the middle class assumption about unwed pregnant women has been that the pregnancy was an "accident," and the solution has been a hurried marriage or adoption. We now know that neither our assumption nor our solutions are necessarily correct, either for women who are not middle class or even for those who are.

Religious beliefs are another of our cultural norms that may conflict with patient values in many areas of nursing, and particularly in issues surrounding childbearing, such as family planning and abortion. The cardinal principle is that professionals, such as nurses, have no right to impose personal convictions or feelings on patients.

Norms of the Nurse as a Nurse

Values and norms of nurses can enhance good perinatal care, or they can be barriers to good care. Examples may be seen throughout this text and on any day on virtually every clinical unit.

One of the most pervasive cultural influences upon us is the "medical model" of childbearing. In sharp contrast is the view that for most mothers childbearing is a normal physiologic process. A basic question might be phrased, "Who runs the show?" Is childbearing a family function, supported and assisted by nurses and physicians? Or is childbearing within the purview of professionals, with compliance expected from families and those families who do not follow "orders" labeled as "bad"?

Although there have been some changes in recent years, the medical model of childbearing predominates in the United States. The medical model

has even been upheld in the courtroom (Fitzgerald vs. Porter Memorial Hospital, No. 75–1203). The issue: could physicians and administrators bar fathers from the delivery room? In a ruling of the Seventh Circuit Court of Appeals, written by Justice John Paul Stevens (now a Justice of the United States Supreme Court), it was stated that an obstetric procedure "is comparable to other serious hospital procedures" and thus maternity patients had no greater right to determine hospital procedure than did other hospital patients.

Is the medical model essential to good perinatal care? Is it a barrier? Or does it really matter? Many nurses question this view of childbearing; others support it in whole or in part. Practices that evolve from the medical model and are a part of the cultural context of childbearing include labor in bed, usually in a recumbent position; elective induction of labor when there is no clear medical indication for this; separation of the family during the majority of the intrapartum period; frequent use of anesthesia, forceps, and episiotomy, and so on.

A physiologic, family-centered "culture of childbearing" does not need to be antimedical, although frustration with the prevailing system has led some couples to reject the system altogether for varying reasons. Physiologic care will work in rhythm with the woman's body, often making many of the procedures described above unnecessary during normal labor and delivery. Family-centered care makes parents informed partners in decisions and allows them to be together throughout as much of childbearing as they choose to be.

Beds that permit labor and delivery without a hurried rush down the hall and rooms that allow the same (and do not necessarily resemble operating rooms) are examples of environmental changes related to the idea that childbearing is a physiologic, family-centered process. Experiments with early discharge, which may return the mother and her infant who have no complications to their home 12 hours following delivery, along with modifications in hospital care following delivery are additional examples of changes in our norms that will be discussed, along with other options, in appropriate sections of this book.

Few of us wish to return to nineteenth century obstetrics, but the opposite extreme, that of seeing childbearing totally in terms of a medical model that is a part of nursing subculture as well, seems no more desirable.

When the Values of Families Differ from the Values of Nurses

Families come to childbearing with many and varying cultural values. Nurses, too, meet these patients with their own set of values. How can nurses give the best of care to patients whose life experiences and values differ from their own? A number of suggestions have already been made in this chapter. They are summarized below, along with some additional principles.

1. Every family can be treated with dignity, as individuals rather than as cases, regardless of whatever makes them seem "different."

2. We can talk with every family using terms that are familiar to them. This may mean the use of another language, such as Spanish, or the use of idiomatic English. Often it will mean learning what terms a family or group uses that differ from those the nurse will ordinarily use.

3. We must understand the social organization of the families with whom we work, so that we will see why in some families the mother must defer decisions to the father and others in the extended family group, whereas in other situations the woman alone may make decisions about her plans.

4. We can involve the family in the planning of their care, so that plans are made in accordance with their priorities and needs.

5. We must understand the role expected of nurses by families with different cultural heritages and must work within these expectations as far as possible. This may involve slowing our pace (not an easy accomplishment) and observing social amenities that may seem time-wasting to us but are important to the families.

6. We can be willing to learn things that may differ from what we have previously experienced.

7. We must avoid making promises we cannot keep.

Knowing and working with families from a variety of cultural backgrounds add richness and depth to our nursing practice when we appreciate the significance of culture in the life of every individual.

REFERENCES

1. Abernethy, V.: Illegitimate Conception Among Teenagers. *Nursing Digest,* IV(3):8, 1976.
2. Adair, J., and Deuschle, K.: *The People's Health: Anthropology and Medicine in a Navajo Community.* New York, Appleton-Century Crofts, 1970.
3. Aichlmayr, R. H.: Cultural Understanding: A Key to Acceptance. *Nursing Outlook,* 17:20, 1969.
4. Ashley, J.: Nursing and Early Feminism. *American Journal of Nursing,* 75:1465, 1975.
5. Auerbach, K. G.: Behavior During Pregnancy: A Sociological Analysis. Unpublished doctoral dissertation, University of Minnesota, 1976.
6. Baldwin, B.: Problem Pregnancy Counseling: General Principles. *In* Wilson, R. (ed.): *Problem Pregnancy and Abortion Counseling.* Saluda, N.C., Family Life Publications, Inc., 1973.
7. Baldwin, G.: Discussion to paper by Von der Ahe. *American Journal of Obstetrics and Gynecology,* 104:286, 1969.

8. Bancroft, A.: Pregnancy and the Counterculture. *Nursing Clinics of North America,* 8:67, 1973.
9. Beauvoir, S.: *The Second Sex.* New York, Alfred A. Knopf, Inc., 1957.
10. Bell, D.: *A Time To Be Born.* New York, William Morrow and Co., Inc., 1975.
11. Bell, R. R.: *Marriage and Family Interaction.* Homewood, Ill., The Dorsey Press, 1971.
12. Benson, L.: *Fatherhood: A Sociological Perspective.* New York, Random House, Inc., 1968.
13. Boston Women's Health Book Collective: *Our Bodies, Ourselves.* New York, Simon & Schuster, Inc., 1973.
14. Brill, G.: *Indian and Free: A Contemporary Portrait of Life on a Chippewa Reservation.* Minneapolis, University of Minnesota Press, 1971.
15. Burchinal, L., and Rossman, J.: Personality Characteristics of Children. *Marriage and Family Living,* 23:334, 1961.
16. Cach, E., and Hearne, D. (eds.): *Our Brother's Keeper: The Indian in White America.* New York, New American Library, 1969.
17. Chesterman, H.: The Public Health Nurse and Family Planning. *Nursing Outlook,* 12:32 (September), 1964.
18. Chung, H.: Understanding the Oriental Maternity Patient. *Nursing Clinics of North America,* 12:67, 1977.
19. Clark, M.: *Health in the Mexican-American Culture.* Berkeley, Ca., University of California Press, 1959.
20. Curtis, G.: Retreat from Liberation. *Texas Monthly,* June, 1975, p. 58.
21. Deloria, V.: *Custer Died For Your Sins: An Indian Manifesto.* New York, The Macmillan Co., 1969.
22. Douvan, E.: Employment and the Adolescent. In Nye, F., and Hoffman, L. (eds.): *The Employed Mother in America.* Chicago, Rand McNally and Co., 1963.
23. Eiduson, B., Cohen, J., and Alexander. J.: Alternatives in Child Rearing in the 1970's. *American Journal of Orthopsychiatry,* 43:720, 1973.
24. Francoeur, R. T.: *Utopian Motherhood: New Trends in Human Reproduction.* New York, Doubleday & Co., Inc., 1970.
25. Frankfort, E.: *Vaginal Politics.* New York, Quadrangle Books, 1972.
26. Friedan, B.: *The Feminine Mystique.* New York, W. W. Norton & Co., Inc., 1963.
27. Gano, H. J.: *The Urban Villagers.* New York, The Free Press, 1962.
28. Gans, H. T.: *The Levittowners.* New York, Pantheon Books, 1967.
29. Goodwin, L.: Middle-Class Misperceptions of the High Life Aspirations and Strong Work Ethic Held by the Welfare Poor. *American Journal of Orthopsychiatry,* 43:554, 1973.
30. Gottlieb, D., and Heinsohn, A. L.: *America's Other Youth: Growing Up Poor.* Englewood Cliffs, N.J., Prentice-Hall, Inc., 1971.
31. Greenberg, M., and Morris, N.: Engrossment: The Newborn's Impact Upon the Father. *American Journal of Orthopsychiatry,* 44:520, 1974.
32. Greenberg, M., Rosenberg, I., and Lind, J.: First Mothers Rooming-In with their Newborns: Its Impact upon the Mother. *American Journal of Orthopsychiatry,* 43:783, 1973.
33. Haire, D.: *The Cultural Warping of Childbirth.* Milwaukee, Wisc., International Childbirth Education Association, 1972.
34. Halpern, F.: *Survival: Black/White.* Elmsford, N.Y., Pergamon Press, 1973.
35. Hedgepeth, W.: *The Alternative: Communal Life in New America.* New York, The Macmillan Co., 1970.
36. Hill, R.: *Families Under Stress.* New York, Harper & Bros., 1949.
37. Hoffman, L., and Nye, F.: *Working Mothers.* San Francisco, Josey-Bass, Inc., Publishers, 1974.
38. Howell, M.: Employed Mothers and Their Families: Part I. *Pediatrics,* 52:256, 1973.
39. *Indian Health Trends and Services.* Washington, D.C., U.S. Department of Health, Education and Welfare; Public Health Service, 1974.
40. Jorgensen, V.: The Gynecologist and the Sexually Liberated Woman. *Obstetrics and Gynecology,* 42:607, 1973.
41. Judd, J.: Nursing Implications. Comment on an article by Greenberg and Morris: Engrossment. *Nursing Digest.* IV(1):22, 1976.
42. Kaiser, B., and Kaiser, I.: The Challenge of the Women's Movement to American Gynecology. *American Journal of Obstetrics and Gynecology,* 120:652, 1974.
43. Kanter, R.: *Commitment and Community: Communes and Utopias in Sociological Perspective.* Cambridge, Harvard University Press, 1972.
44. Keyserling, M.: Our Children are our Future: Early Childhood Development and the Need for Services. *American Journal of Orthopsychiatry,* 43:4, 1973.
45. Kennell, J., et al.: Maternal Behavior One Year After Early and Extended Post Partum Contact. *Developmental Medicine and Child Neurology,* 16:172, 1974.
46. Kimball, C.: Discussion to paper by Von der Ahe. *American Journal of Obstetrics and Gynecology,* 104:285, 1969.
47. Klaus, M., et al.: Maternal Attachment: Importance of the First Post-partum Days. *New England Journal of Medicine,* 286:440, 1972.
48. Lancaster, J.: Coping Mechanisms for the Working Mother. *American Journal of Nursing,* 75:1332, 1975.

108 The Social and Cultural Context of Childbearing

49. LeMasters, E.: *Parents in Modern America: a Sociological Analysis.* Homewood, Ill., Dorsey Press, 1970.
50. McCoy, G. and Muth, F.: The Alternatives in Continuing the Pregnancy. *In* Wilson, R. (ed.) *Problem Pregnancy and Abortion Counseling.* Saluda, N.C., Family Life Publications, Inc., 1973.
51. Mead, M.: *Sex and Temperament in Three Primitive Societies.* New York, Dell Publishing Co., 1963.
52. Melville, K.: *Communes in the Counter Culture: Origins, Theories, Styles of Life.* New York, William Morrow and Co., Inc., 1972.
53. *Monthly Vital Statistics Report.* Vol. 24, No. 11, February 13, 1976, Table 11, page 11.
54. Moore, T.: Children of Working Mothers. *In* Yudkin, S. and Holme, W. (eds.): *Working Mothers and Their Children.* London, Sphere Books, 1969.
55. Moustafa, A., and Weiss, G.: Health Status and Practices of Mexican Americans. Los Angeles, School of Public Health, University of California, 1968.
56. Murray, A.: Maternal Employment Reconsidered: Effects on Infants. *American Journal of Orthopsychiatry, 45*:773, 1975.
57. Newson, J., and Newson, E.: *Infant Care in an Urban Community.* New York, International Universities Press, 1963.
58. Nye, F., and Hoffman, L.: *The Employed Mother in America.* Chicago, Rand McNally & Co., 1963.
59. Pannor, R.: The Unmarried Father—the Forgotten Man. *Nursing Outlook, 18*:36, (November), 1970.
60. Pannor, R., Massarek, F., and Evans, B.: *The Unmarried Father.* New York, Springer Publishing Co., Inc., 1971.
61. Primeaux, M.: American Indian Health Care Practices: A Cross-Cultural Perspective. *Nursing Clinics of North America, 12*:55, 1977.
62. Rainwater, L.: *Behind Ghetto Walls; Black Families in a Federal Slum.* Chicago, Aldine Publishing Co., 1970.
63. Ringler, N. M., et al.: Mother to Child Speech at 2 Years: Effects of Early Postnatal Contact. *Journal of Pediatrics, 86*:141, 1975.
64. Rossi, A.: Family Development in a Changing World. *American Journal of Psychiatry, 128*:47, 1972.
65. Rossi, A. (ed.): *The Feminist Papers: from Adams to de Beauvoir.* New York, Columbia University Press, 1973.
66. Roszak, B., and Roszak, T. (eds.): *Masculine/Feminine.* New York, Harper and Row, Publishers, 1969.
67. Sanger, M.: *My Fight for Birth Control.* New York, Farrar Rinehart, 1931.
68. Schacter, J., and McCarthy, M.: Illegitimate Births: United States, 1938–57. *Vital Statistics–Special Reports, Selected Studies,* Vol. 47, No. 8. Washington D.C., U.S. Government Printing Office 1960.
69. Schorr, T.: Current Shock. *American Journal of Nursing, 76*:911, 1976.
70. Schwarz, J. Strickland, R., and Krolick, G.. Infant Day Care: Behavioral Effects at Preschool Age. *Developmental Psychology, 10*:502, 1974.
71. Seaman, B.: *Free and Female.* New York Coward, McCann and Geoghegan, Inc. 1972.
72. Siegel, A., et al.: "Dependence and Independence in Children." *In* Nye, F., and Hoffman, L. (eds.): *The Employed Mother in America.* Chicago, Rand McNally & Co., 1963.
73. Steinberg, D.: Redefining Fatherhood: Notes After Six Months. *In* Howe, L. (ed.) *The Future of the Family.* New York, Simon & Schuster, Inc., 1972.
74. *Trends in Illegitimacy: United States, 1940–1965.* Washington, D.C., U.S. Government Printing Office, 1968.
75. Tripp-Reimer, T., and Friedl, M.: "Appalachians: A Neglected Minority." *Nursing Clinics of North America, 12*:41, 1977.
76. Tylor, E.: *Primitive Culture.* New York, Henry Holt and Co., 1883.
77. Veysey, L.: *The Communal Experience: Anarchist and Mystical Counter-Cultures in America.* New York, Harper and Row Publishers, Inc., 1973.
78. Vincent, C.: *Unmarried Mothers.* New York, The Free Press, 1961.
79. Vincent, C., Haney, C., and Cochrane, C.. Familial and Generational Patterns of Illegitimacy. *Journal of Marriage and the Family, 31*:659, November, 1969.
80. Von der Ahe, C.: The Unwed Teen-age Mother. *American Journal of Obstetrics and Gynecology, 104*:279, 1969.
81. Washburn, W.: The American Indian. *The Americana: 1974 Annual.* New York Grolier, Inc., 1974, p. 63.
82. Weissman, M., et al.: The Educated Housewife: Mild Depression and the Search for Work. *American Journal of Orthopsychiatry, 43*:565, 1973.
83. Whyte, W. H.: "The Corporation and the Wife." *Fortune,* November, 1951, p. 109

Chapter 5

FAMILY PLANNING

In our society the term family planning has often been used as a synonym for contraception, which is unfortunate. Although family planning without the means of controlling birth would be virtually impossible, the mechanics of such control is a beginning, not an end in itself.

Family planning means advice to the apparently infertile couple, genetic counseling for the family of a baby with a genetically transmitted defect, or help for the woman who feels she cannot cope with pregnancy. It means education to help individuals and couples determine when, and if, they are ready to be parents, and then assistance to help them achieve their goal. Family planning may include adoption or artificial insemination.

Although nurses think of family planning primarily in terms of individual women and couples, we cannot escape the implications of our work for groups of people. For example, in an area where infant morbidity and mortality are high, can we improve the health of mothers and infants and even of older children through excellent family counsel? If we believe we can, how can we reach out to these families?

As a beginning, we need to be aware of the reasons why people choose to limit (or not to limit) their families, their motives for pregnancy, and their fears, as well as the advantages and disadvantages of various contraceptive devices. A special facility in communication is important, because family planning involves human sexuality, a topic some people find difficult to discuss.

MOTIVATION FOR CHILDBEARING

Every minute of the day, in every part of the world, children are born. Some are greatly desired; some are accepted as "God's will," with little understanding of the biologic principles of procreation; still others are viewed as "accidents" and are scarcely welcomed.

The motivations for pregnancy are many. Because the motivation for having a child may affect the child's development and the total family, it is an important consideration. Often the motivation is not apparent to the parent.

To create a new human being and to guide that infant, then child, then adolescent in a way that allows him to develop his own best self are deeply satisfying experiences, and rightly so. However, many of the motives discussed

109

below have negative connotations. The pregnancy and the child may meet a need in the lives of the parents that is not necessarily in the best interests of the child.

Childbearing as a Steppingstone into the Adult World. In many traditional societies, clearly defined "rites of passage" mark the transition to adulthood. There may be rituals, attended by the entire community; changes in the manner of dress; and so on.

There are fewer clear-cut indications of adulthood in our own society. Frequently both adolescents and young adults see pregnancy as an affirmation of their competency as adults. "We can do *something;* we can produce a child, therefore we are now a part of the adult world."

Childbearing to Save a Relationship. For some couples, childbearing is an attempt to "save" a faltering marriage or to stabilize a fragile relationship outside of marriage. This attempt may be the idea of one partner or of both.

One or both may feel that a child will give them a common experience that they can share, so that they will grow closer together. A woman may hope that a child will cause her mate to "settle down" and become more responsible and to care more about home and about her.

All of the odds are against the success of such an attempt. Pregnancy and the adaptation to a new member of a family add strain to even a firm, stable union; the stress on a fragile union may cause further disintegration.

Moreover, the child conceived for this purpose who fails in his appointed task is often rejected for that failure.

Childbearing as a Substitute for a Relationship. When the relationship between a man and a woman is poor, the woman, especially, may see in her child an opportunity for the satisfying rela-

tionship that is lacking with her partner. It is not difficult to imagine the tremendous burden such desires place on her relationship with a child who, in his early months and years, is very much a receiver of warmth and affection rather than a giver.

The unmarried girl or woman who feels she is unloved may also see a baby as an answer to her needs. She may have no special relationship with the baby's father but desires a baby as a love-object upon whom she can shower her love and who will love her in return. When the dependent, demanding baby fails to meet her needs, she is likely to feel highly ambivalent and frequently hostile toward the baby.

Childbearing to Please Others. "We had not planned to have children for several years, but the pressure from our parents, who wanted to become grandparents, was so intense that we decided to go ahead and start our family."

A variation on the theme quoted above is, "All of our friends were having children, and we felt left out, so we decided to have a baby too."

In a similar way, adolescents may experience *peer pressure,* which is not principally directed toward childbearing but toward sexual behavior that may result in childbearing. The more insecure an adolescent is, the more likely he is to feel the need to gain approval by competing with other adolescents in becoming sexually active or to copy the behavior of a sexually active peer. The fact that these experiences are frequently unhappy because the emphasis is on the sexual act itself and not on the relationship between the persons involved compounds the adolescent's insecurity and may lead to still more attempts.

Childbearing to Produce an Heir or a Child of a Specific Sex. "My husband wants a son," said the mother of two daughters, "and we are going to keep on having babies until there is a Quincy Gotrocks III."

"I've always wanted a little girl, to dress in pretty dresses and teach to sew and play the piano," said another woman.

But there are no guarantees that the child will be of the desired sex or even that the child of the desired sex will fulfill the parents' fantasy. Very likely, he or she will not. The baby may indeed be a little girl, but one who grows to love climbing trees and Little League baseball more than dresses and dolls.

Childbearing to Replace a Lost Child. When a sibling has died, some parents hope that another child may fill the void that they are experiencing. It seems important to discuss this issue as part of the counseling of parents after a child's death. Moreover, if the initial assessment during pregnancy reveals the death of a sibling, we need to be aware of this possibility and alert to any indications of this motive for pregnancy.

Childbearing to Affirm Femininity or Masculinity. For the woman who has doubts about her femininity or for the man who feels a need to prove his masculinity, the ability to become pregnant or to impregnate may be a way of affirming sexuality. The woman may seek a large family to confirm her womanliness; for the man fathering many children may represent "machismo" or maleness.

Childbearing as an Escape. Pregnancy may be viewed as a means of escaping from an undesirable situation. For the adolescent this may be an unhappy home life, with little realization that life in a forced marriage or as a single mother will often be no improvement. Older women also may see pregnancy as a chance for escape—from a job they don't like or as an excuse for

avoiding other expected activities, for example.

Childbearing to Fill a Void. Women who express a feeling of "emptiness" may see in pregnancy a way to fill the psychic void within themselves. For such women, the desire may be not for the child but for pregnancy per se. One pregnancy may be followed by another.

Pseudocyesis, a condition that mimics the symptoms of pregnancy (often called false pregnancy), may occur in these women when the void is unfilled by an actual pregnancy.

Childbearing as Therapy for Physiologic Problems. Pregnancy may be undertaken as a cure for menstrual cramps, backache, migraine headache, and a variety of other ills. Here again it is the pregnancy that is desired; the child may almost be a by-product.

Childbearing for the Emotional Satisfaction of Producing a Perfect Child. Every parent-to-be, and every parent, feels that his or her child is special. But some parents approach parenthood with the expectation of producing a "perfect child." They postpone pregnancy until the "perfect" time. Each detail is carefully planned. They expect to gain their satisfaction from their ability to produce a perfect child.

After the baby's birth the attempt to have everything "just so" continues. Here too there is a feeling of disappointment in the child who does not fit their plan. The scholar they fantasized is a nice but average child. Their athlete, in spite of all they do (and sometimes because of all they do), is on the second string.

Childbearing as an Act of Rebellion or Hostility. Adolescents, particularly, may choose sexual intercourse as a way of rejecting parental values. The more rigid they view their parents' values to be or the more uncomfortable their parents seem to be about sexual matters, the more valuable their sexual behavior becomes as a weapon.

Cohen and Friedman[16] quote one teen-aged girl, who had told her mother she was pregnant, as saying with great satisfaction, "Seeing the look of horror on my mother's face made the whole thing worthwhile."

The motives described here are mostly individual in nature. Social factors affecting high and low fertility are discussed in the section on population growth that follows. Some possible reasons for unplanned pregnancies are discussed later in this chapter.

POPULATION GROWTH: THE WORLD IN WHICH WE PRACTICE

Nurses have traditionally viewed population growth at the level of the individual family. The number of children born to particular parents has been more important to us than the fertility and reproductive rates of the nation and of the world. But population, as a national and as a worldwide issue, does affect us both as individuals and as nurses. As individuals, we are all a part of the problems of the world in which we live. As nurses, we find that "official" attitudes toward reproduction can mean government funds for family planning clinics or, conversely, severe limitations on providing the family planning advice that we may feel is highly important to the physical and mental health of a particular family. Emphasis on zero population growth can mean that we fail to appreciate the concerns of an infertile couple.

Demographers have been concerned with population trends for many years, but population growth became an important social and political issue in the 1960's. Three terms are used by demographers to describe trends in births:

1. *Crude birth rate* (CBR) is the number of births per year per 1000 population.

2. *General fertility rate* (GFR) is the number of births per year per 1000 women ages 15 to 44 years.

3. *Total fertility rate* (TFR) is the sum of the fertility rates for women of different age groups in a given year.

Such distinctions may seem unimportant to the average person, but they assist demographers in more clearly understanding births. For example, if a large number of women between the ages of 20 and 30 were having babies, both the crude birth rate and the general fertility rate would rise; the total fertility rate would give an indication of the reason for the rise, i.e., an increase in the birth rate for women in a particular age group. Thus, although all three measures roughly follow the same pattern of ups and downs, each gives specific information that is valuable. In comparing birth rates of the world's nations, particularly the rates of underdeveloped nations, crude birth rate figures are often the most readily available.

DEMOGRAPHIC TRENDS IN THE UNITED STATES

Population in the United States, as well as in the rest of the world, began to grow not because birth rates increased but because death rates decreased. This growth was slow in the eighteenth century, accelerated in the nineteenth century, and became very, very rapid in the twentieth century (Fig. 5-1). Throughout this period of population growth, birth rates have been decreasing. In the United States there was a decrease in the white population from 7.0 births per woman in the year 1800 to 2.1 births per woman in 1936. Figures for nonwhite women have not been recorded over as long a period of time, but in general the

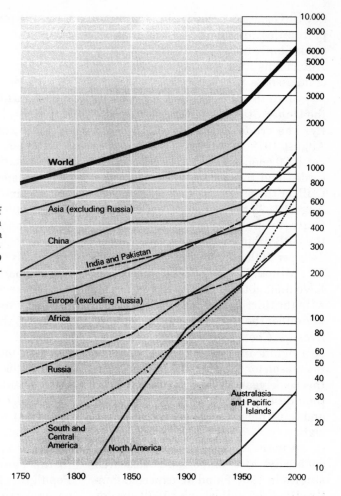

Figure 5–1 The growth of world population 1750–1950, with projections to 2000 (population in millions). (From Wrigley: *Population and History*. Copyright©1969 McGraw-Hill Inc. Used by permission of McGraw-Hill Book Co.)

downward trend has been the same, although the birth rate has been higher.

The fact that a level of 2.1 births per woman was achieved in the United States in 1936, considerably before the use of oral contraceptives and intrauterine devices (IUD's), suggests rather strongly that contraceptive technology is not the only factor in limiting births. Among the factors that apparently contributed to this low fertility rate were:

1. A higher proportion of women who never married.

2. A higher proportion of women who married at a later age.

3. A high level of unemployment and economic insecurity that motivated couples to postpone childbearing.

The downward trend of fertility in the United States reversed after World War II (the 1940's) with a tremendous rise occurring from 1946 through 1958. The "baby boom" came not from a rise in the number of large families but from a reduction in the number of childless couples and couples with only one child. The trends were the reverse of those of the depression years of the 1930's, as:

1. More women married.

2. Women married and had children at an earlier age.

3. Good job opportunities and opportunities for homes in the suburbs made family living the lifestyle of many Americans. Pregnancy was "in"; childlessness was suspect.

Since the 1957 peak, birth rates in the United States have decreased steadily. The crude birth rate (CBR) from August 1972 to August 1973 was 15.2 per 1000 population, the lowest ever recorded and 6 per cent lower than the CBR for the preceding 12 months. From August 1973 to August 1974 (the latest figures available at the time of writing) the CBR dropped another 3 per cent to 14.8 per 1000 population.

Although newer contraceptives have undoubtedly been a factor, again, as in the thirties, the decrease began before either the IUD or the oral contraceptives were being used widely enough to be a significant factor. Probably part of the reason for the drop is that couples in the peak years of the fifties achieved their desired family size rather quickly, and thus there were fewer births in the sixties.

A norm for smaller families is undoubtedly also important. Research studies in 1967 found an expected family size of 2.9 children; by 1972 similar studies found expected family size to be 2.1 children. Interrelating factors include a changing governmental policy toward family planning concepts (see below), an increase in the number of single women, the postponement of marriage and childbearing, and the desire or need of many women for jobs other than homemaking. The increased availability of abortion in the seventies has undoubtedly played some part. The rapidly rising cost of living may be related to postponement of marriage and childbearing and the need for women to work, much as economic factors in the depression years affected childbearing.

GOVERNMENT POLICY AND FAMILY PLANNING IN THE UNITED STATES

As early as the 1940's some political leaders had advocated federally supported family planning funds as part of maternal and child health programs for those states that wished them. But most Americans were not ready for such ideas, and there were many objections.

A major change in United States policy came in 1963, when Congress included the promotion of research on population growth in a foreign aid bill. Former President Eisenhower, who had previously blocked such legislation, now supported it as a means of helping nations keep fertility in check. But the program was slow in developing, and much of the hoped-for research into means of better fertility control was neither funded nor conducted.

In 1965 the Supreme Court of the United States ruled that laws prohibiting birth control were an invasion of "the right to privacy." Over the next 5 years congressional commitment to population problems grew, culminating in the Family Planning Services and Population Research Act of 1970, which encompassed support not only for research and family planning, but also for manpower training and preparation of informational materials, and created an Office of Population Affairs in the Department of Health, Education and Welfare with full authority for family planning programs in the United States.

It was during these same years that biologist Paul Ehrlich wrote *The Population Bomb,*[22] which brought widespread public attention to population growth and advocated immediate and forceful action to control population. In the early years of the seventies, however, population growth in the United

States dropped without the use of the strong measures suggested by Ehrlich.

DEMOGRAPHIC TRENDS IN THE REST OF THE WORLD

In 1900 the world's population was roughly 1.5 billion. By mid-1975 there were 4 billion people living on earth. Currently the world's population is increasing at the rate of approximately 2 per cent per year; in just 35 years, at this rate, the world will be expected to sustain twice the number of people as it does today.

As Table 5–1 indicates, population growth in most of the countries of Western Europe is as low as, and in many instances lower than, that of the United States. The decline in fertility began in many European countries in the 1870's and 1880's, not only before modern contraception but largely without the use of

Table 5–1   WORLD POPULATION GROWTH*

	Estimated Population (Mid-1973)	Birth Rate Per 1000 Population (CBR)	Death Rate Per 1000 Population	Per Cent Population Growth	Number of Years to Double Population at Current Growth Rate
World	3,860,000,000	33.0	13.0	2.0	35
West Germany	59,400,000	11.5	11.7	0.0	—
East Germany	16,300,000	11.7	13.7	−0.2	—
Finland	4,800,000	12.7	9.6	0.3	231
Sweden	8,200,000	13.8	10.4	0.3	231
Belgium	9,800,000	13.8	12.0	0.2	347
Austria	7,500,000	13.8	12.6	0.1	700
Hungary	10,400,000	14.7	11.4	0.3	231
United Kingdom	57,000,000	14.9	11.9	0.3	231
France	52,300,000	16.9	10.6	0.6	117
United States	210,300,000	15.6	9.4	0.8	87
Switzerland	6,500,000	14.4	8.7	1.0	70
Canada	22,500,000	15.6	7.3	1.2	58
Soviet Union	250,000,000	17.8	8.2	1.0	70
Japan	108,300,000	19.0	7.0	1.2	58
China (Mainland)	799,300,000	30.0	13.0	1.7	41
China (Taiwan)	15,000,000	27.0	5.0	2.2	32
Brazil	101,300,000	38.0	10.0	2.8	25
India	600,400,000	42.0	17.0	2.5	28
Bolivia	5,000,000	44.0	19.0	2.4	29
Nigeria	59,600,000	50.0	25.0	2.6	27
Venezuela	11,900,000	41.0	8.0	3.1	21
Phillipines	42,200,000	45.0	12.0	3.3	21
Thailand	39,900,000	43.0	10.0	3.3	21
Algeria	15,500,000	50.0	17.0	3.3	21
Morocco	17,400,000	50.0	16.0	3.4	21

*From data in *The Americana: 1974 Annual*. New York, Grolier, Inc., 1974. Source: Population Reference Bureau, Washington, D.C.

any mechanical devices, such as the condom. Coitus interruptus was probably the most commonly used method. Gardner[28] uses the phrase "the collapse of fertility" to describe this phenomenon in Western Europe, a situation that the countries themselves (though obviously not individual families) view with mixed emotions. In some countries governments have attempted to increase fertility by various programs, such as free obstetric and child care and the payment of subsidies to mothers. At present rates of growth, it would take 175 years for the population of Western Europe to double.

The population of the Soviet Union is growing at a far faster rate than that of the other nations in Europe (Table 5–1), although the birth rate is declining. During the 1960's the Soviets opposed any international efforts toward family planning. Since that time, however, there has been an acknowledgement that excessive population growth can hinder economic development. In 1973 a demographic center was created at Moscow University to study both Soviet and world population problems.

Outside of the United States and Western Europe, Japan has led the way in slowing population growth, with a 50 per cent drop in births from 1948 to 1960, perhaps the most rapid decrease in reproduction in the world's history. Three factors are considered significant in this decline:

1. A strong interest in fertility reduction by a majority of Japanese families that caused a downward trend in fertility beginning in the 1920's.

2. The very energetic role of the Japanese government in birth control practices, probably the most active of any government ever.

3. Widespread, legal, induced abortion (about 1 in every 20 pregnancies in the peak year 1955).

Even though other Asian nations, such as India, are beginning to realize that overpopulation is a serious problem, and some (Taiwan, for example) are achieving a modest degree of success in family planning programs, some observers fear that these steps may already be too little and too late.* For example, when compulsory vasectomy of men with three or more children was first under consideration in India, it was estimated that 100 surgeons or surgical technicians averaging 20 operations a day, 5 days a week, would take 8 years to cope with the existing candidates. In the meantime there would constantly be new candidates coming along. At today's rates the population of Asia will double in 30 years.

In the African nations, as death rates from diseases such as smallpox and malaria decline dramatically, governments vary in their feelings about population growth. Although some leaders are concerned about limiting fertility, others still consider their countries underpopulated and are suspicious of "outsiders" who advocate family planning. As Table 5–1 indicates, population increase is rapid in most African countries; the population of Africa will double in 28 years at current rates of increase.

Population growth in Latin America is the most rapid of all continents; continued growth at today's rates would mean a doubling of population in 25 years. Some governments support principles of family planning; in Venezuela the government appropriated a small amount of money for family planning programs in 1973 for the first time. Others are strongly opposed. There are approximately 80 million women o

*Note in Table 5–1 that Taiwan has a lower CBR than mainland China. However, because the death rate is also far lower, the rate of population growth is higher.

childbearing age in the Latin American nations; it is estimated that roughly 10 million middle class women use contraceptives. The remaining 70 million average six children each, although surveys indicate that many of these women desire only three children. A study in Puerto Rico more than 20 years ago showed a preference for small family size (Table 5–2).

THE PROBLEMS OF WORLD POPULATION GROWTH

How many people can the earth sustain? We really don't know the answer. One question, of course, is "sustain at what level—in the lifestyle of an Asian or African farmer or of a Western European or middle class American?" A range of from 8 to 15 billion people is the usual estimate, with 15 billion believed to be an absolute maximum at a very curtailed way of life. As we have already noted, the 8 billion mark will be reached within our own lifetime, just 35 years from now, if growth continues at current rates.

Some observers, such as Grant Cottam, a University of Wisconsin ecologist

Table 5–2   PUERTO RICAN ADULTS' VIEWS OF IDEAL FAMILY SIZE*

Ideal Family Size	Men (Per Cent)	Women (Per Cent)
0	0.3	0.1
1	2.2	2.4
2	45.7	50.5
3	27.0	26.7
4	12.5	10.9
5	4.7	3.8
6–8	4.2	3.2
9 plus	1.0	0.6
As God wills	2.3	1.9

*From Hatt: *Background of Human Fertility in Puerto Rico.* Princeton, N.J., Princeton University Press, 1952.

who was an official observer at the World Food Conference in Rome in 1974, feel that the world has possibly already reached its "carrying capacity" in terms of the number of people who can be fed using available resources. Only the food reserves of recent years have made survival possible, according to Cottam. Now that these reserves are gone to a large extent, he sees famine as inevitable *(Food and Population: Thinking the Unthinkable[25])*. In 1975 famine did occur in parts of central Africa and India and in Bangladesh.

Who is to feed the poor of the world is a major issue to be resolved throughout the remainder of this century. Not only will it probably become impossible to feed all of the world's hungry, but some people doubt the wisdom of even trying, feeling that food given to nations with no policy of population control will only lead to further population explosion and eventual disaster. Such ideas do not have universal acceptance. There are those who feel that technology, properly applied, can solve the world's food problems. Meanwhile the concept of triage, i.e., of cutting off food to groups of people who are starving, is unpleasant to everyone and unthinkable to a great many. Nevertheless, such triage already has occurred.

Starvation is not the only problem of unchecked population growth. The quality of life and economic standards of living are also adversely affected by rapid growth. For example, from 1945 to 1954 the gross domestic product of Latin America doubled, but rapid population growth kept the per capita increase far lower. Davis[17] says, "To put it in concrete terms, it is difficult to give a child the basic education he needs to become an engineer when he is one of eight children of an illiterate farmer who must support the family with the product of two acres of ground." Such problems are not limited to the developing nations. The cyclic dilemma of poverty leading to high fertility leading to poverty continues.

Another area sometimes overlooked in the concern for feeding the earth's people is the effect of high population density on life. Animal experiments (which can be applied to human populations only with great caution) indicate that when overcrowding exists, stress, rather than starvation, may be the major cause of death. Studies of chickens and of wild woodchucks have shown that caging too many animals together can cause a drastic increase in fatal heart attacks. Heart disease has also been found to increase in caged zoo animals (antelopes, deer, monkeys, and apes) when they are grouped together.

Calhoun[11] confined a population of Norwegian rats in a quarter acre enclosure and provided abundant food and protection from disease and predators. By the end of 27 months, the population could have expanded to 5000 animals, yet it stabilized at approximately 150. Although the adult rat mortality was unusually low, stress from the high level of social interaction led to such a disruption of maternal behavior that infant mortality was extremely high.

In other experiments Calhoun found that even moderate crowding affected rats by limiting their ability to carry pregnancy to term, to survive delivery, or to "mother" their litters. Males, too, showed behavioral disturbances.

SOLUTIONS: FAMILY PLANNING VERSUS POPULATION POLICY

What is to be done about world population growth? Certain writers such as Kingsley Davis[17] and Bernard Berelson[4] draw a sharp distinction between "family planning" and "population policy."

A basic tenet of the family planning concept is voluntary contraception. The goal of family planning is to help parents have the number of children they want, when they desire them. It is not inconsistent with family planning principles for a couple to have four or six or more children, if they so wish.

The aim of population control is to give society a feasible number of children. Although there are indications that many families, particularly poor families in many parts of the world, desire fewer children than they bear, just eliminating unwanted births would still leave a high birth rate in many societies.

No nation in the world has, as yet, developed what might be considered a population policy. Possible suggestions that might become part of such a policy include:

1. Payments to people for allowing themselves to be sterilized.

2. Compulsory sterilization after a given number of pregnancies.

3. Free abortion.

4. Required abortion for illegitimate pregnancies.

5. A system of taxation that gives economic advantages to single persons, such as taxation on marriage and on childbearing, elimination of tax exemptions for parents, and abandonment of tax policies that discriminate against couples when the wife works.

6. Creation of more opportunities for women to work outside the home, along with the assurance of equal education and equal pay for women.

7. Requiring a license to have children.

8. Temporary sterilization of all women by a technology not yet invented.

Although some of these suggestions are very much in conflict with our values (compulsory sterilization, for example), others, such as tax revision, may be politically unpopular but not totally unacceptable.

FAMILY PLANNING AND FAMILY HEALTH

Important as concerns about overpopulation are, they are not the only rationale for the planning of childbirth. Family health may also be affected in several ways:

1. The risk of stillbirth is relatively high for first births, low for second births, and increases thereafter, rising sharply after fifth and sixth births.[15]

2. The risk of infant and early childhood mortality increases steadily as the number of children in the family increases. (A second child has no advantage.) This has been found to be true in all social classes, although rates vary from one class to another.[1, 15, 29, 67]

3. Data on the relationship between family size and the frequency of specific diseases (respiratory infection, gastroenteritis, and so forth) are conflicting. Social class variation is probably one reason. The way in which data are gathered is important. If visits to a physician are the criteria for determining the frequency of illness, the mother of seven who is not overly concerned and does not seek treatment for a child's respiratory infection may appear to have a healthier family than the mother of two who does seek such assistance.

4. The risk of prematurity has been found to be higher when there is less than 12 months from the end of one pregnancy to the beginning of the next. Prematurity is the major cause of neonatal death (death within 28 days after birth) and a major cause of infant morbidity.

5. A number of studies show some decline in successful marital adjustment with increasing family size. One reason may be that success in controlling fertility may be a factor in marital satisfaction.[65]

6. Diminished maternal care has been found to be a correlate of some large families.[70] It is not difficult to understand the problems that a mother with several children under the age of six may have in meeting even the basic physical needs of each child individually.

7. Not only total family size but the spacing of pregnancy can affect family satisfaction. Before a subsequent child is born, a mother should feel both physically and emotionally ready. The father's feeling that he is ready is important too. When a previous child is 12 to 15 months old, he is still very demanding. It is hard for a mother to meet his still very strong needs for nurturing, as well as those of a new baby. By the time he is three years of age, the older child is less dependent. He is verbal enough to talk about the pregnancy and the new baby with his parents and to express his feelings about the baby.

A great volume of additional studies about the interrelation between family size and family health has been and is being conducted. One problem in studies of this type is determining what other variables are affecting the outcome. For example, malnutrition is often correlated with large family size, but is this because poor families are overrepresented in the large families of the study? One cannot compare the health of a middle class family with two children with that of a lower class family with six children. Future research should answer more of our questions.

SOCIAL FACTORS AFFECTING HIGH FERTILITY

Family planning programs presuppose, in principle at least, that access to information about and materials of contraception will decrease birth rates. Although this is obviously true up to a point, we have already seen that fertility rates in many nations fell, often sharply, before the advent of modern contraceptives.

Obviously other factors are important in influencing high fertility. At certain times, and in certain societies, both industrialized and agrarian, large families brought status to both man and woman, often enhancing their position in the community. A woman's chief claim to fame might be the numbers of her children and grandchildren. Fertility has been thus extolled, even in our own country, until relatively recently. Moreover, a large family was insurance against both high infant mortality and loneliness and lack of care in old age.

Religious Factors

Religious beliefs are related to high levels of fertility in various ways. In some predominantly Roman Catholic countries, such as some nations of Latin America, church opposition may influence governmental policy and may even make the use of birth control illegal, as it was in two states of the United States until the 1960's. Because of the large number of Roman Catholics and of families of other religions living in predominantly Roman Catholic countries, it is important for us to be aware of Catholic doctrine and practice in relation to birth control.

In July 1968 Pope Paul VI issued a 38 page encyclical *Humanae Vitae*, which defined Roman Catholic doctrine in relation to contraception, abortion, and sterilization. For contraception the rhythm method (and abstinence) is approved, and artificial means of birth control are rejected in these words:

If, then, there are serious motives to space out births, which derive from the physical or psychological conditions of husband and wife, or from external conditions, the church teaches that it is then licit to take into account the natural rhythms in the generative functions, for the use of marriage in the infecund periods only, and this way to regulate birth without offending the moral principles. . .

This encyclical was one more step in a long series of debates that have spanned the centuries of Christianity, influenced at various times by St. Augustine's condemnation of all contraception in the fourth century, Pope Gregory IX's decree in 1230 that contraception was to be considered the equivalent of murder, and St. Thomas Aquinas' views in the thirteenth century that the enjoyment of intercourse without the goal of procreation was not legitimate. By the mid-eighteenth century it was evident that in the Western world many couples, including Roman Catholic couples, were limiting their families. In 1930 Pope Pius XI issued *Casti Connubii*, reaffirming procreation as the primary goal of marriage and contraception as an "offense against the law of God and of nature, and those who indulge in such are branded with the guilt of a grave sin."

Not all Roman Catholics have agreed with these positions. One of the physicians chiefly responsible for the development of oral contraceptives, Dr. John Rock, a Roman Catholic, argues that the pill established a safe period similar to nature's safe period during pregnancy.

Following the encyclical of 1968, there was open disagreement in the Catholic press and among theologians about contraception. As Tables 5–3 and

Table 5-3   THE TREND OF CATHOLIC BIRTH CONTROL PRACTICE
BEFORE THE ENCYCLICAL*

	1955 (Per Cent)	1960 (Per Cent)	1965 (Per Cent)
Never used any method	43	30	22
Used rhythm only	27	31	25
Had used other methods	30	38	53

*From Westoff and Westoff: *From Now to Zero: Fertility, Contraception and Abortion in America.*
Boston, Little, Brown & Co., 1971.

5-4 indicate, women in the United States (and apparently in other parts of the world as well[72]) have been increasing their use of forms of contraception other than rhythm steadily over the last decades and have continued to do so following the *Humanae Vitae.*

In relation to our family planning practice, it seems evident that Roman Catholic families do not share a single set of beliefs about contraception. Individual wishes are our guide in counseling these families, as in any other family.

Black Fertility

When fertility statistics are tabulated by race, it is obvious that throughout the years black fertility rates are consistently higher. Further analysis of black fertility indicates that the reason lies in the higher number of blacks who are poor and who have had limited educations. Black women who are married to professional men or to men with college educations tend to have *lower* fertility rates than comparable groups of white women.

Black women interviewed in the 1965 National Fertility Study indicated a desire for the same number of fewer children (2.6 per woman) than the white women interviewed, but black women expected to have considerably more children (4.0 per woman). The chief difference between the black and the white women interviewed was therefore in the control of fertility rather than in the number of children desired. In this group of women only 8 per cent of the blacks and 28 per cent of the whites were completely successful in achieving both the number of children they desired and in timing the births as they desired. Although 58 per cent of the black couples and 60 per cent of the white couples were using some form of contraception, the methods of contraception used by black families were

Table 5-4   METHODS OF CONTRACEPTION USED MOST RECENTLY BEFORE
AND AFTER THE ENCYCLICAL BY CATHOLIC FECUND WOMEN UNDER 44,
MARRIED AT LEAST 4 YEARS*

	1965 (Per Cent)	1969 (Per Cent)
No method	7	4
Rhythm	35	32
Pill	14	37
Other methods	44	27

*From Westoff and Westoff: *From Now to Zero: Fertility, Contraception and Abortion in America.*
Boston, Little, Brown & Co., 1971.

often the least effective methods. For example, among black couples 30 to 44 years old, 25 per cent used the douche, probably the least effective of any method.

Another reason for high rates of fertility among black women may be the meaning of pregnancy for the unmarried, lower class, black adolescent. Having a baby may be the "rite of passage" that signifies that she is no longer an adolescent, just as marriage or college is in other segments of our society.

SOCIAL FACTORS AFFECTING LOW FERTILITY

In those nations in which fertility has been reduced, the principal factor appears to be industrialization, accompanied by increased job opportunities and education. Within nations, fertility is usually lowest among social classes in which women have the most education and opportunities for employment. The availability of skilled jobs lowers the economic value of children, makes it possible for more women to enter the work force, and raises the age of women at the time of marriage. No longer need the number of children she produces be the measure of a woman's status.

Postponement of marriage, coupled with social disapproval of premarital intercourse and out-of-wedlock pregnancy, was probably a factor in the longstanding low fertility rates of many European nations. Easily available abortion is also important; the very low fertility rates of the Eastern European nations and the sharp drop in the Japanese birth rate are undoubtedly related to the widespread availability of abortion in these nations.

CONTRACEPTIVE COUNSELING

A major role of nurses in a total program of family planning is that of counseling individuals and couples about the use of contraceptives. In order to do this we need knowledge of:

1. The contraceptives available today—the way in which each prevents conception and the advantages and disadvantages of each.

2. Effective ways of introducing contraceptive information, both to women or couples who have never used contraceptives and to those who have been unsuccessful or dissatisfied with a method they had been using previously.

3. The reasons why people avoid contraceptives or fail to use them effectively.

CONTRACEPTIVES IN CURRENT USE

Oral Contraceptives

Observation that the discharge of an egg from the ovary does not occur during pregnancy raised the initial questions about the possibility of using hormones to prevent pregnancy. Experiments followed that demonstrated the role of the corpus luteum, and in 1934 progesterone was isolated as the active chemical of the corpus luteum. But although the injection of progesterone prevented pregnancy, contraception by injection was not a practical solution.

As early as 1942 it had been discovered that oral estrogens would readily inhibit ovulation, but because long term use of estrogen without progesterone often leads to endometrial hyperplasia with irregular bleeding and prolonged hypermenorrhea, estrogen was not considered as a possible contraceptive.

In 1954 synthetic progestin steroids were developed that had the properties of progesterone but that were both more powerful and also active by the oral route. Human field trials followed in Puerto Rico in 1956, using a "pill" with a small amount of estrogen and one of the synthetic progestins. In May of 1960 oral contraceptives were first introduced for regular use; by 1965 they were the single most popular contraceptive in the United States.

There are a large number of estrogen-progestin combinations available. Because the various products differ from one another in amount and type of estrogen and progestin, some women are able to tolerate one preparation far better than another. It is important to reassure a woman that because she is having difficulty with one "pill" does not mean that she will be unable to use any form of oral contraception.

Action. The basic action of oral contraceptives is the prevention of ovulation. The hypothalamus is prevented from sending follicle-releasing factor (FRF) and luteinizing-releasing factor (LRF) to the anterior pituitary, thus blocking the release of follicle-stimulating hormone (FSH) and luteinizing hormone (LH), which, in turn, are necessary for ovulation (see Chapter 3). Remember that the formation of the follicle and its subsequent rupture are determined by FSH and LH. The cells of the ruptured follicle form the corpus luteum, which secretes progesterone. A metabolite of progesterone, *pregnanediol,* is found in the urine, evidence of the level of progesterone in the body.

In women taking oral contraceptives, direct examination of the ovaries does not reveal any newly formed corpora lutea. In addition, urinary levels of pregnanediol are about one-tenth the usual level during the postovulatory period (0.5 mg. rather than the usual 5.0 mg.).

Progestins have additional antifertility actions. Under ordinary circumstances, as was said previously, the mucus of the cervix becomes thin and watery midway during the menstrual cycle, making it less difficult for sperm to ascend into the cervical canal (Chapter 3). However, under the influence of oral contraceptives the mucus remains thick and sticky throughout the cycle and thus is hostile to sperm. Also, the endometrium matures more rapidly and thus becomes out of phase with the ovulatory cycle, making implantation less likely if fertilization should occur.

Regimens. An oral contraceptive containing both estrogen and progestin is taken for 20 days of each cycle. The first pill is taken on the fifth day of the menstrual period, regardless of the length of the period (and thus it is important when teaching a woman to always say fifth day and not last day). If there is no menstrual period, the second cycle of pill-taking begins on the seventh day after the completion of the 20 day course.

July

X ② ③ ④
⑤ ⑥ ⑦ ⑧ ⑨ ⑩ ⑪
⑫ ⑬ ⑭ ⑮ ⑯ ⑰ ⑱
⑲ ⑳ ㉑ 22 23 24 25

X = menstrual days

O = estrogen-progestin combination

When oral contraceptives fail, it is frequently because the user forgets to take her pill. Because of this, two regimens have been introduced to simplify pill-taking. In the 28 day regimen seven of the pills are placebos. The woman begins the pill on the *first* day of her menstrual period and takes one each day for 28 days. The active hormone is in the pills taken on days 5 through 26. She begins another package of pills immediately upon finishing one package.

In the 21 day regimen pills are taken during a complete 3 week period of the cycle; no pills are taken during the fourth week. However, the pill-taking cycle always begins on the same day of the week, again, an aid to remembering.

Side Effects. Among the most common of the side effects of oral contraceptives are those resembling some of the symptoms of pregnancy, such as nausea, weight gain, chloasma (yellowish-brown skin discoloration),

headache, leg cramps, and breast enlargement and tenderness. These side effects are more often a nuisance than a serious medical problem, but they are of great importance to the individual woman. Some women find that nausea is lessened if they take their pill in the evening rather than in the morning, a change that does not affect the effectiveness of the contraceptive. After the first or second cycle of pill-taking, these side effects disappear in the large majority of women. If not, changing to a product with a lower estrogen content may help.

Metrorrhagia (bleeding during the intermenstrual period) is also fairly frequent and is a symptom related to the amount of estrogen in the particular product in use.

Acne may become worse; here a product with increased estrogen may help. Vaginal infections are more common in women using the pill; preexisting conditions may become more difficult to treat when oral contraception is started.

Depression has been reported in about 5 to 10 per cent of women using oral contraceptives. Approximately the same number of women become depressed following tubal ligation or the insertion of an intrauterine device, suggesting at least the possibility that psychologic rather than hormonal factors may be responsible. Possible emotional factors might be religious conflicts about the avoidance of pregnancy, a subconscious desire for children, or ambivalent feelings about the woman's own sexuality.

Considerable attention has been focused on the increase of thromboembolism in women who use oral contraceptives. Laboratory data show an increase in certain coagulation accelerator factors (Factors VII, VIII, IX, and X) both in the pill user and in women who are pregnant. The mortality rate from thromboembolitic disease has been found to be as much as eight times as great among women using the pill, and the risk of thromboembolism is from five to ten times higher. Statistics on both counts vary from one study to another.

The rate of thromboembolism is considered to be related to the quantity of estrogen contained in the product used. Sequential preparations and those combined preparations containing 0.1 mg. of estrogen are associated with a risk of embolism that is two to three times greater than that of preparations containing only 0.05 mg. Products with still lower doses of estrogen and preparations containing only progestin are currently being evaluated. Theoretically, the absence of estrogen should reduce the incidence of blood-clotting, but this has not yet been demonstrated in studies.

As already mentioned, the possibility of pregnancy appears to increase very slightly with low estrogen products, but it nearly triples when pills containing no estrogen at all are used. Although the exact mechanism of progestin contraception is unknown, cervical mucus thickening (which affects the passage of sperm) and endometrial changes (which affect implantation) are two possibilities. Breakthrough bleeding, which at times is heavy, and failure of menstruation may also occur in some women and account for the higher drop-out rates among women using contraceptives with low or no estrogen.

Two recent British studies, one of 63 women and the other of 153 women, have found the risk of heart attack to be more than four times greater among women who use oral contraceptives than among nonusers. The risk is compounded if the woman has other risk factors known to be associated with heart disease: cigarette smoking, diabetes, high blood pressure, obesity, or high serum cholesterol levels. The effect is suspected to be synergistic (i.e., the action of one factor potentiates the action of another). A 4.2 per cent increase in the risk of heart attack was found with one other risk factor being present; a 10.5 per cent increase with two other factors; and a 78.4 per cent increased risk with three or more additional factors.[66]

Still another area of concern has been the possible effect of oral contraceptives on subsequent pregnancy. When Peterson[61] compared 442 women who had become pregnant after they ceased to use the pill with 699 women who used other forms of contraception or none at all, he found that the incidence of abortion and infant death or illness within the first month after birth was similar in both groups. Premature births and congenital anomalies were less frequent in the group using oral contraceptives than in the control group. Peterson also found that long-term pill usage failed to result in either increased or decreased fertility.

For the breast-feeding mother, oral contraceptives appear to decrease milk production. In those parts of the world where infant nutrition is still highly dependent on successful breast-feeding, this is a major factor to be considered in family planning programs.

Sometimes the side effects that women report come from improper usage. For example, women will tell us that they take their pills "every once in a while" and that they tend to have irregular episodes of bleeding. The bleeding makes them feel that the pill is harming them in some way, and so they discontinue its use. History-taking in family planning involves finding out not only what is used for contraception but how it is used.

Effect on Sexual Enjoyment. The real or perceived effect of any contraceptive on sexual enjoyment will be an important factor in its continued use. For many couples the pill enhances sexual pleasure because:

1. It is taken at a time other than the moment of intercourse, so that remembering to use a contraceptive does not intrude.

2. It is highly effective in preventing pregnancy, so that the fear of pregnancy is removed from intercourse. For many couples this fear interferes considerably with sexual enjoyment.

For a woman who is experiencing some of the more unpleasant side effects of oral contraceptives, sexual intercourse may seem unpleasant while the other symptoms last.

Masters and Johnson[50] report an additional relationship between sexual desire and oral contraceptives in some women. These women begin to lose interest in sex after using the pill for from 18 months to 3 to 4 years. In about 90 per cent of affected women, 3 to 6 months of using some other form of contraception resulted in an improvement in sexual desire. To date no studies have examined this association, but it seems worth our awareness.

Contraindications to Oral Contraceptives. Because there are several physical conditions that are considered a definite contraindication to oral contraception, a thorough history and physical examination are mandatory before the pill is initially prescribed and at regular intervals during the entire course of its use. An annual check-up is a minimum precaution; many physicians prefer to see women once every 6 months.

Because of the increase of clotting factors discussed above, no woman with a *past history of thrombotic episodes* (pulmonary embolism or thrombophlebitis, for example) or with an *existing thrombotic condition* should use oral contraceptives at any time. The *development of migraine* after a regimen of oral contraceptives is started is also considered an indication for discontinuance because the incidence of cerebral thrombosis may be higher in these women.

Any woman with a *history of liver disease* or with *existing liver disease* (such as hepatitis or cirrhosis) should not take oral contraceptives, as they have been shown to produce subclinical changes in liver function tests. These changes are not felt to be significant for women with a normal liver and no past history of liver disease.

Malignancies of the breast or reproductive tract, either past or presently existing, are also contraindications. Although estrogen has never been shown to cause such malignancies, it may cause exacerbations.

Vaginal bleeding for which a cause cannot be ascertained is a definite contraindication.

Since glucose tolerance is decreased, women with *diabetes* or with a *strong family history of diabetes* are advised to use other forms of contraception.

As previously mentioned, recent studies involving the risk of *heart disease* suggest that another form of contraception should be considered if more than one additional risk factor is present, even though the two limited studies done are not sufficient to prove a definite relationship.

Risks Versus Benefits in Oral Contraception. After becoming aware of the possible risks of oral contraception, it is not unusual to wonder if this is a safe means of prevention. One does not have to practice very long to discover that some women, and their husbands, are afraid of the pill. Some of these fearful women have limited educations and are strongly influenced by "granny tales," but well-educated women are also sometimes hesitant.

Current medical consensus recognizes that although there is some risk, there is also a risk factor in pregnancy. It is felt that if the appropriate contraindications are observed, the advantages of oral contraception in terms of effectiveness (p. 138), ease of administration, and acceptability by the woman and her mate far outweigh the risks. The ideal contraceptive, 100 per cent effective with no risks and no side effects, has yet to be discovered.

Intrauterine Devices

The idea that an object placed in the uterus could prevent conception is centuries old; Arab camel drivers placed stones in the uteri of their animals for that purpose many centuries ago. In modern times intrauterine devices (IUD's), usually of silkworm gut or gold or silver, were apparently first used to prevent pregnancy in Europe in the early twentieth century. However, IUD's came to be regarded as a possible cause of pelvic infection, and because of this and the occasional accompanying abnormal vaginal bleeding and/or perforation of the abdominal wall, their use fell into disrepute. It was not until new plastic materials became available that the potential of IUD's was again seriously considered.

The chief advantage of an intrauterine device is that, once inserted, very little thought need be given to contraception. This convenience is equally important to continued use and to sexual enjoyment. Once a week women are advised to make sure that the device is in place by checking for the presence of the thread that protrudes from the vagina. At the time of insertion we should be sure that each patient can "check for the string" effectively. She can do this by inserting her index finger in her vagina until the thread is felt. Obviously, if it is not felt, she should contact her physician or clinic right away.

A second important advantage of the IUD is its comparatively low cost, an important factor in family planning programs not only in underdeveloped nations but in our own country as well.

As a postpartal contraceptive, the IUD has one distinct advantage over the pill; it does not affect lactation. Although in the United States this may be a very important consideration for individual mothers, in those areas of the world where breast-feeding is still the only safe means of nourishing an infant, this is tremendously important.

Types of Intrauterine Devices. There are a number of different types of intrauterine devices; their advantages and disadvantages vary. Major characteristics of several IUD's are seen in Figure 5–2 and in Table 5–5. It is important to recognize that IUD's differ. Problems with one type of device do not necessarily mean that a woman will not be able to tolerate another type of IUD. Patient teaching also varies from one device to another. For example, women should be told that the copper Cu-7 should be removed 2 years after insertion. Because of the continuing changes in IUD's, nurses must constantly update their own information in order to answer women's questions correctly and to teach effectively.

Limitations and Side Effects. Intrauterine devices have five basic limitations:

1. They may be expelled by the uterus.

2. They often cause uterine bleeding and/or cramping.

3. They may perforate the uterus.

4. They may fail to prevent pregnancy, even though they remain in place.

5. They may cause infection.

The extent of each of these limitations varies with the type of IUD (Table 5–5). Exact comparisons between various types are difficult because the number of each type that has been inserted is unknown. Moreover, because a product must be in circulation for approximately 2 years before data on side effects begin to accumulate, comparison between devices available for a number of years and newly marketed products is also difficult. Experience with the Dalkon shield illustrates the problem of ascertaining limitations.

The Dalkon shield was first introduced in 1970. It had the advantage of a lower rate of expulsion than the other devices then in use; by 1973 it was reported that approximately 40 per cent of all IUD users had the shield. Early in

Lippes Loop

Saf-T-Coil

Cu-7

Dalkon Shield

Ypsilon

Figure 5–2 Intrauterine devices.

Table 5–5   INTRAUTERINE DEVICES

Device	Advantages	Disadvantages	Status, 1975
Lippes Loop	Proved relatively safe following several years of use	Expulsion or bleeding sufficient to cause removal in approximately 25% of patients	In use
Saf-T-Coil	Proved relatively safe following several years of use	Expulsion or bleeding sufficient to cause removal in approximately 27% of patients	In use
Cu-7	Causes less bleeding than inert IUD's; smaller size; ease of insertion	Leaches small amount of copper into system. Should be removed after 3 years of use	In use
Dalkon Shield	Lower rate of expulsion	Difficulties in insertion and removal; multifilament tail conveys bacteria to uterus	Original shield withdrawn from market; new design being developed
Ypsilon	Shape believed to lower rate of expulsion	Currently being tested	

1972, however, it became evident that there were some difficulties with the shield. Because of its shape and because it was the largest of all the IUD's, it was the most difficult to insert. It did not show up on x-ray. The tail sometimes came off during insertion. But most significant was the finding in 1974 that the multifilament tail, which differed from the tails of the other devices, could convey bacteria to the uterus. If the woman were to become pregnant, the chances of infection and septic abortion (Chapter 10) were high. In 1974 Dalkon shield-related infected abortions accounted for 88 per cent of all such infections in IUD wearers. Subsequently, the Dalkon shield was withdrawn from the market and has been redesigned.

Continuing research into new shapes and materials is being conducted in an attempt to deal with the varying limitations of the different products. The design of the Majzlin spring, for example, was created in an effort to lower the rate of expulsion; however, this device was so difficult to remove that the Food and Drug Administration forced its withdrawal from the market in 1974. A small percentage of women are unable to retain any IUD currently available.

Cramping at the time of insertion and an unusually heavy menstrual flow in the period following insertion are almost universal. Other complaints are of cramps and backache, spotting, and bleeding between periods, although these problems do not occur in all women. Anticipating these side effects and explaining that in most instances they last for only a few weeks may help many women tolerate them. The newer copper-containing devices appear to reduce the incidence of bleeding.

The International Planned Parenthood Federation estimates that about 2 per cent of women with IUD's can be expected to develop pelvic inflammatory disease within the first year of use. As noted in the example of the Dalkon shield, infection appears to be much higher with some devices than with others.

Current Research. Several additional types of IUD's are currently being tested. Tatum's Copper TCu-220C is a second copper-containing device. Because of a different type of design, developer Howard Tatum says the copper sleeves should last up to 75 years before being leached away.

The Ypsilon is a Y-shaped stainless steel and silicone device designed to prevent expulsion. The plastic T-shaped Alza device has a hollow vertical stem that releases progesterone into the uterine cavity for a year. Preliminary research indicates that use of the Alza device eases cramping on insertion and heavy menstrual flow.

At the time of this writing, IUD's are not regulated by the Food and Drug Administration (FDA), with the exception of the Cu-7 (because it leaches a small amount of copper into the wearer's uterus). However, because of the difficulties with some devices, the FDA and manufacturers have started a voluntary registry. Physicians will register each patient at the time of insertion and keep records of each woman's experience, with manufacturers reporting to the FDA every 6 months. Such paperwork seems important for the realistic evaluation of these devices, an evaluation significant to the safety of women and the embryo-fetus, should pregnancy occur. It must also necessarily add to the cost of each IUD.

Spermicidal Preparations

Spermicidal preparations come in various forms—jelly, foam, or cream. Foams are more recent innovations than jellies or creams; they are less messy and spread more readily over the cervix. Originally used in combination with a diaphragm (see below), these contraceptives are now also used alone. Although they are somewhat less effective alone, they are readily available at most drugstores without a prescription, and this can be a decided advantage.

The preparation itself consists of a chemical that immobilizes and kills sperm and a base that mechanically blocks the cervical os.

Many women who purchase spermicidal contraceptives receive no instruction in their use. But we can, if we have the opportunity, teach their most effective application. The preparation should be inserted into the vagina within an hour prior to coitus. The applicator is filled and inserted while the woman is lying on her back. If the applicator is inserted as far as possible into the vagina and then withdrawn one-half inch, it will be at the mouth of the cervix, where its contents should be deposited. The movement of the penis during coitus will distribute the foam (cream, jelly) throughout the vagina and over the cervix. If the woman gets out of bed prior to intercourse, she should insert a second applicator of spermicide. Getting out of bed following intercourse is not contraindicated, however.

The immobilization and killing of sperm take place in the 6 to 8 hours following coitus. There should be no douching during that time, since douching will either remove the spermicide or dilute it to the point of being ineffective, although it will not remove all of the sperm. Should the couple desire intercourse within the 6 to 8 hour period, reapplication of the spermicide is necessary. This is because vaginal secretions will dilute the spermicide and also because a certain amount of the preparation will leak from the vagina during and following coitus.

One disadvantage, apart from the necessity of applying the preparation shortly prior to intercourse, is that some women experience chemical irritation from the preparation itself. This is a relatively rare occurrence that may be an allergic reaction.

Diaphragm Plus Spermicide

A diaphragm is a dome-shaped device made of rubber with a metal spring contained within the rim. The spring fits the diaphragm to the walls of the vagina.

Diaphragms are always used in conjuction with a spermicidal preparation (see above). The diaphragm gives the additional advantage of a second mechanical barrier.

Diaphragms must be fitted by a physician or a nurse with specialized training. They come in a variety of sizes, with diameters ranging from 60 to 90 mm., and with several types of springs. Both the size and contour of the vagina influence the type and size of diaphragm for an individual woman. A diaphragm that is too small may not cover the cervix adequately; too large a diaphragm would, at best, be uncomfortable.

Most physicians and clinics prefer not to fit a virgin with a diaphragm, for once intercourse has stretched the vagina, the device must be refitted. Fit must also be checked: (1) following childbirth; (2) following therapeutic abortion or miscarriage; (3) following

any surgery; (4) any time there is a weight change of 10 or more pounds, either gain or loss; and (5) every 2 years.

Displacement of the uterus will influence the type of diaphragm that can be used. If displacement is severe or if adjacent organs are displaced (e.g., caused by a pronounced cystocele), use of a diaphragm may not be possible.

Once the diaphragm is fitted, the woman must learn how to position it properly. She needs the opportunity to practice insertion before she takes the device home with her.

The diaphragm is prepared for insertion by covering the dome and the rim with a spermicidal preparation.* With the woman lying on her back, or squatting, or with one leg flexed (Fig. 5-3), she squeezes the opposite rims of the diaphragm together and inserts it deep into the vagina. She needs to be able to feel that it is over the cervix and behind the pubic bone. Some women may prefer to use plastic or metal inserters.

The diaphragm should be inserted no more than 2 hours prior to intercourse and should remain in place from 6 to 8 hours following coitus. As with spermicides used alone, there should be no douching during this period. If intercourse is desired again more than 2 hours after the initial coitus or if more than 2 hours has elapsed after insertion but before coitus, additional spermicide should be inserted with an applicator, without disturbing the diaphragm. The diaphragm is removed by inserting a finger or the inserter over the front rim and pulling down and out. The device is then washed in soap and water, dried, and stored in a cool place. It should be

---

*Some recent reports have suggested that spermicide on the rim increases the possibility of dislodgment during coitus.

Figure 5–3 *A,* Finger recognizes cervix. Forms and sizes of cervix shown in upper left corner. *B,* Finger makes sure cervix is covered. *C,* "Front rim" test of fit. If finger cannot get by, neither can penis. (From Calderone: *Manual of Family Planning and Contraceptive Practice.* 2nd Edition. Baltimore, The Williams & Wilkins Co., 1970. Copyright © 1970 The Williams & Wilkins Co.)

checked for any holes each time it is used.

Disadvantages of diaphragms are mechanical and, for some women, personal. The mechanical difficulty is that even properly fitted diaphragms may slip out of place. Expansion of the vaginal canal during intercourse and frequent insertions of the penis are two common reasons for this. Dislodgment may be more likely when the female is above the male during coitus.

Use of a diaphragm will be difficult for a woman who feels she should not touch her genital area. She must be able to check the placement of the diaphragm, even if she uses an inserter to place it.

And, of course, the diaphragm, like the condom and spermicidal preparations used alone, requires forethought and action in the period immediately prior to intercourse.

Natural Family Planning

Nurses and physicians have in recent decades been less than enthusiastic about *natural family planning,* i.e., methods that are based on abstinence from intercourse during the time the woman is fertile. However, an increasing number of couples are indicating an interest in natural family planning. Some are concerned abut the side effects of other methods of contraception. Some prefer "naturalness" in many aspects of their life (natural food, for example). Some have theological reasons.

In response to this interest, the Health Revenue Sharing and Health Services Bill of 1975 requires that agencies receiving federal funds for family planning provide information and counseling about natural family planning.

The Rhythm Method. The rhythm method is based on the concept of abstinence from intercourse during the period in which the woman is fertile (i.e., the period in which there is a recently expelled viable ovum capable of fertilization by a viable sperm in the upper portion of the reproductive tract). The ovum is capable of being fertilized no longer than 48 hours after ovulation (and probably only 12 to 24 hours), but since sperm remain viable for at least 48 hours and possibly for as long as 96 hours, intercourse must be avoided from 4 days prior to until 3 days following ovulation. Estimation of the time of the "fertile period" may be done by means of a calendar method or by a calendar-temperature method.

THE CALENDAR METHOD.   The fertile period (and the corresponding safe period) is estimated in the following way by the calendar method. Consider a woman who has menstrual cycles that vary over a period of several months from 27 to 30 days in length.

1. Subtract 18 days from the shortest cycle duration (14 days for ovulation plus 4 days for sperm viability) to obtain the beginning of the period of abstinence:

$$27 - 18 = 9$$

Abstinence must begin on day 9 of the menstrual cycle.

2. Subtract 11 days from the longest cycle duration (14 days for ovulation minus 3 days for ovum viability) to obtain the day on which the period of abstinence may safely end:

$$30 - 11 = 19$$

Abstinence may end on day 19.

The best way to demonstrate this to a woman (and ideally to her mate) is by the use of a calendar. The example described above is shown on the following calendar:

```
        X  X  X  X  X   6
   7   8  ⑨ ⑩ ⑪ ⑫ ⑬
  ⑭ ⑮ ⑯ ⑰ ⑱ ⑲  20
  21  22  23  24  25  26  27
  28  29  30   X  X  X  X
```

X = menstrual period

O = fertile period

Note that the number of days in the menstrual period is not significant; the day is determined from the first day of the period.

Ovulation has been found to occur as early as day 8, meaning that the fertile period could begin as early as day 5 (and very rarely even earlier). The length of time between ovulation and menstruation appears to be more constant than the timing of the early part of the cycle, as we noted in Chapter 3.

THE CALENDAR-TEMPERATURE METHOD. A method using the calendar alone is based on the presumption that in a 28 day cycle ovulation occurs on the fourteenth day. However, there is fairly wide variation in the day of the cycle on which ovulation occurs in an individual woman. Several physiologic criteria are useful in aiding the estimation of the exact time of ovulation: cervical mucus may be analyzed, an endometrial biopsy may be performed, and so on. The most practical method is by the determination of basal body temperature.

As discussed in Chapter 3, basal body temperature drops before ovulation and then, because of the influence of progesterone, rises from 1 to 3 days following ovulation and remains slightly elevated throughout the remainder of the cycle. The period during which the drop occurs is brief; the rise is considered the best indicator of ovulation. Because of ovum and sperm survival, pregnancy can occur within 72 hours following the rise in temperature. Thus the fertile period is considered to extend 3 days beyond the time at which the temperature rises.

The temperature rise does not indicate the beginning of the fertile period, only the end. Thus it is used in conjunction with the calendar method.

Consider now the woman described above with the same menstrual cycle of 27 to 30 days.

1. The beginning of the fertile period is estimated as in the calendar method, i.e., the shortest cycle duration minus 18 days:

$$27 - 18 = 9$$

2. The end of the fertile period is the day of the temperature rise plus 3 days. If the temperature rise occurs on day 15, day 18 would be considered the last day of the fertile period.

It seems obvious that the rhythm method requires a high level of motivation on the part of both the woman and her mate and a certain amount of intelligent understanding as well. Even if periods are always totally regular and of 28 days' duration, abstinence is necessary from day 10 to 17.

Rhythm will be ineffective for women who ovulate irregularly and thus have cycles of widely varying durations. Basal temperature can be helpful, but factors other than ovulation can cause a rise in temperature.

The Ovulation Method. Some of the disadvantages of the rhythm method are overcome by the ovulation method. In 1952 two Australian physicians, John and Evelyn Billings, began to work with couples who were "rhythm failures." They postulated that certain physiologic concepts that were being used to help couples achieve pregnancy might also be useful in avoiding pregnancy. Along with Professor James B. Brown of the Royal Women's Hospital in Melbourne, Australia, they developed a body of knowledge that has come to be known as the ovulation method of family planning.

Basic changes in cervical mucus prior to ovulation have been described in Chapter 3. Successful use of the ovulation method requires a woman's awareness of these changes in herself. As her awareness develops, she begins to perceive, during the days following ovulation, at first an absence of mucus. These are the "dry days." As the ovum begins to prepare for ovulation, a small amount of yellow or white mucus is present; it is opaque and sticky. As levels of blood estrogen reach a critical point, the fertile mucus appears. At first cloudy but not sticky, the mucus becomes clear and resembles raw egg white. The woman perceives a feeling of wetness. This slippery mucus usually appears about 3 days before ovulation.

Following ovulation, progesterone causes the abrupt cessation of the clear, fertile mucus. Mucus again becomes sticky.

It is possible for more than one estrogen peak to occur during the cycle. For example, if the woman has a high temperature, the growth of the ovum may be temporarily halted and then resume.

Women using the ovulation method keep a chart noting changes in the mucus; a system of colored stamps is frequently used. Red stamps are for the days of the menstrual period; white stamps (with the outline of a baby on them—thus white "baby stamps") are for the fertile or unsafe days. Unsafe days are those from the appearance of the slippery, fertile mucus until 72 hours after the change to progesterone mucus.

Following ovulation, light green "baby stamps" are used for 4 days. Green stamps designate safe days. The chart, stamps, and instructions are included in Billings' book *Natural Family Planning: The Ovulation Method.*[5]

The ovulation method requires awareness of one's body and a high level of motivation. In order to become acquainted with her own mucus pattern, the woman must abstain from intercourse for one complete cycle and thereafter every other day in subsequent cycles to detect fertile mucus. And, of course, she must abstain (or use some form of contraception) on the days in which she is fertile.

An advantage of the ovulation method, for women who chose it, is that it is effective for women with irregular cycles (for whom the rhythm method frequently is not satisfactory) and can be used by lactating and premenopausal women (in whom a menstrual period may not occur) to indicate fertility.

Billings suggests that the method be taught to each woman by a woman. Men have no personal experience with the feelings and sensations accompanying the changes in mucus and thus cannot communicate in the way that a woman can.

The Symptothermal Method. The symptothermal method utilizes observations of basal temperature, cervical mucus changes, and secondary signs such as increased libido and mittelshmerz to help couples recognize the period of fertility.

A lay group, the Couple to Couple League (CCL) (see Appendix J) suggests that the female partner identify the signs and symptoms and the male partner keep the records. Together the couple interprets the record and thus each shares in the responsibility for pregnancy prevention. During the period of abstinence couples are encouraged to display affection through avenues other than intercourse, such as touch.

CCL also suggests that this method is best taught by one couple to another.

Condoms

Nearly one billion condoms are sold in the United States and Canada each year, making them the most widely used mechanical contraceptive in these countries. Most condoms are made of latex (hence the colloquial term "rubber") and may be purchased in lubricated or nonlubricated form. Condoms made from animal membranes are more expensive, but some men feel they interfere less with sensation.

Rarely does one see instructions abut the use of a condom. It is assumed that all men are familiar with this technique, but experience gained from working in the kind of contraceptive clinics to which men feel free to come (below) shows that this is not necessarily so.

Condoms must be used throughout coitus, including foreplay if the penis is inserted into the vagina, since urethral secretions can also contain sperm. Most condoms come already rolled; if not, they should be rolled just before they are used. In either instance approximately 1/2 inch should remain unrolled at the tip to collect semen if the condom does not have a specialized ending for that purpose. As the condom is unrolled over the erect penis, this end space should be squeezed so that air does not collect in it. At the time that the penis is inserted in the vagina, it is important to avoid catching the extended end against the walls of the vagina, as the condom might break.

If the condom is not prelubricated, spermicidal jelly or surgical jelly makes insertion easier. Spermicidal jelly also gives additional protection, of course. The lubricant is applied to the outside of the condom after it is on the penis.

Condoms can be used more than one time if they are properly cared for. As they cost approximately 50 cents each, some men find reuse economically necessary, although condoms are available at considerably lower cost through many family planning centers. If a condom is to be reused, it should be placed in a glass or jar filled with water im-

mediately after removal from the penis. As soon as possible, it should be carefully washed in warm, soapy water, dried, and powdered with cornstarch. (Skin condoms are kept in a mild boric acid solution.) Condoms being reused should be tested for leaks before each use by filling them with water. Condoms are best stored in the containers in which they are sold. They will deteriorate from heat and moisture if carried in wallets or pockets or kept in other than a cool, dry place.

Disadvantages. One danger in the use of the condom is that it will slip off following ejaculation because of the loss of erection or that semen will leak from the open end. In withdrawing, the man should hold the upper part of the condom tightly against the base of the penis. If the condom has slipped off the penis, it should be removed from the vagina immediately, with the open end held tightly closed. Sperm deposited on the external genitalia can cause pregnancy.

Tearing or rupture of the condom is quite rare. If this should happen, the woman should insert an applicator of spermicidal jelly into her vagina, if a spermicide is available. Many physicians and clinics urge that condoms always be used along with spermicidal preparations and/or a diaphragm in case of condom failure.

The prevention of the spread of venereal disease is frequently cited as one advantage of condom contraception, and this is a real benefit. But because of this, some couples associate condoms with prostitution and other practices that they consider unacceptable and therefore find condoms undesirable as contraceptives for themselves.

Some couples feel that the condom itself is a barrier to sexual pleasure; both men and women may express this sentiment. But others, by incorporating the placing of the condom into sexual foreplay, find no such disadvantage.

Coitus Interruptus

Coitus interruptus is one of the oldest methods of conception control. It is believed to have been responsible for the drop in birth rates in Western Europe late in the eighteenth century. Also called *withdrawal,* the method consists of the withdrawal of the penis from the vagina prior to ejaculation. It is free of cost and always available.

However, there are a number of important disadvantages. Sperm must not only avoid the vagina but must not be deposited anywhere on the external genitalia because of their mobility. This is true even if the hymen is intact. Since sperm are present in urethral secretions as well as in the ejaculate, pregnancy can occur even if withdrawal is successful.

And successful withdrawal is not easily achieved. The time at which ejaculation occurs may be as early as 2 minutes after intercourse begins or as long as 20 minutes. Not every man is aware of the time at which ejaculation is imminent. Moreover, not every man has total ejaculation in a single emission; sometimes small amounts of semen are "leaked" prior to the ejaculation of which the man is aware. As the time of ejaculation approaches, coital movements become less voluntary, and withdrawal becomes more difficult.

Although there are no physical side effects, as once supposed, there are psychologic drawbacks for both men and women. The constant anxiety that withdrawal will not take place in time and that pregnancy will occur is a major disadvantage, as are ungratified sexual needs, particularly for the woman, who must often face interruption before orgasm.

So although withdrawal is probably better than nothing in an emergency situation, it is hardly a method of choice, considering the many other forms of contraception available today.

CONTRACEPTIVE EFFECTIVENESS

How effective are the various types of contraceptives? *Theoretical effectiveness* describes how effectively a contraceptive prevents pregnancy under ideal conditions. Although there is no direct measure of theoretical effectiveness, it is estimated from the findings in the most successful groups of users.

Use effectiveness is determined by the actual number of pregnancies that occur in field trials when a method is offered to 100 women and is expressed in terms of pregnancies per 100 woman years.* There may be, and often is, a wide variation between the theoretical effectiveness of a product and its use effectiveness because of such factors as poor motivation on the part of the user and inconsistent usage. Studies of oral contraceptive failure demonstrate this principle quite well. Although theoretically there should be less than 1 pregnancy per 100 woman years with oral contraceptives, in reality some studies show failure rates as high as 25 pregnancies per 100 woman years.[74] As emphasized earlier, product improvement of oral contraceptives is directed not only toward achieving the optimum balance of estrogen and progestin but

---

$$*R = \frac{\text{Total number of conceptions} \times 1200}{\text{Total months of exposure}}$$

R = rate of failure
1200 = 100 women × 12 months

From the denominator are subtracted 10 months for each pregnancy and 4 months for each abortion.

also toward trying to make the pill "unforgettable."

If no contraception is used at all, the pregnancy rate is approximately 80 to 85 per 100 woman years. With *any* type of contraception, even with relatively inadequate ones such as douching and withdrawal, pregnancy rates are more than halved. The two most effective methods are those that do not rely on some activity at the time of coitus, i.e., oral contraceptives and the IUD.

The theoretical failure rate of oral contraceptives is approximately 1.0 pregnancy per 100 woman years for sequential products and 0.5 pregnancy for combined products (for reasons already discussed), making both better than 99 per cent effective. The average use failure rate is about 5 pregnancies per 100 woman years, although it may be decidedly higher in some populations.

Pregnancy rates with the IUD average 2 to 3 per 100 woman years, making the method slightly more than 97 per cent effective. One reason for such a high rate of effectiveness is that the most common reason for the failure of many types of contraceptives is patient failure, i.e., the failure of the couple to use the method properly. The IUD is the only type of contraceptive that is virtually immune to patient failure. It requires only a single decision rather than sustained motivation.

When pregnancy does occur, it may be because the device has been expelled without the woman's knowledge; hence the need to check for the string. Spontaneous expulsion is more likely in women who have never been pregnant.

Approximately 1 per cent of women with IUD's become pregnant with the device in place. Should this occur, the device is left in the uterus and is delivered along with the baby. The device itself does not seem to present any problem to the developing embryo-fetus, but the spontaneous abortion rate is approximately 40 per cent, which is not really surprising in view of the suspected modes of action.

The theoretical effectiveness of the methods that necessitate some activity at the time of intercourse is lower than that of either the pill or the IUD, yet in several instances not much lower. Failure rates are approximately 2 to 3 pregnancies per 100 woman years for the diaphragm (about the same as for the IUD), 3 to 4 for the spermicidal preparations such as "foam," and 2 to 5 for the male condom. Use effectiveness, however, is not nearly as high. Failure to use these devices prior to every act of intercourse and improper insertion of the diaphragm or foam probably cause most failures from these methods. Failures from the condom method result most commonly from carelessness during removal after intercourse. The penis must be allowed to return to normal size before withdrawal, and the rim of the condom must be held during withdrawal, so that it will not slip off and spill its contents. If a fresh condom is used at each sexual act, breakage is quite rare.

The rhythm method averages 14 pregnancies per 100 woman years. Failure is most likely in women with irregular menstrual cycles, such as adolescents, postpartal women, and premenopausal women.

Coitus interruptus and douching are the least effective methods of contraception among those commonly practiced in the United States today. Even the theoretical effectiveness is about 15 to 20 pregnancies per 100 woman years; use effectiveness is estimated at approximately 30 to 35. Thus one woman in three using these methods will probably become pregnant.

POSTCOITAL CONTRACEPTION: DIETHYLSTILBESTROL

From time to time newspaper and magazine articles express an interest in the idea of a "morning-after" contraceptive. Diethylstilbestrol (DES), given within 72 hours after coitus, is such a medication. In one study of 100 women, no pregnancies resulted when 25 mg. of DES was given orally twice daily for 5 days, beginning within the 72 hour time frame.[44] It is believed that DES acts at the implantation site and thus the need to begin its use before the time of implantation. The medication may also increase the speed of ovum transport through the genital tract.

Currently, DES is most commonly given to rape victims. It may also be given after a known failure of contraception (rupture of a condom, for example) or when no contraceptive is used. But in all instances it is considered an emergency treatment only; good contraceptive counseling should be a part of follow-up care.

Nausea is the most frequently mentioned side effect, affecting 34 per cent of the patients in Kuchera's study.[44] About 16 per cent of the women experience both nausea and vomiting. Other side effects, all relatively rare, include headache, vaginal spotting, dizziness, diarrhea, and fluid retention. No serious side effects were noted, and 45 per cent of Kuchera's population reported no side effects at all.

A correlation between DES taken during the first trimester of pregnancy and vaginal cancer in the daughters of the mothers who had taken it has been reported. In each instance (all of which occurred in the 1940's and 1950's) DES was given to mothers with a history of miscarriages. The drug was often given throughout the first 3 months of pregnancy to prevent the possibility of another miscarriage.

Should DES fail as a contraceptive and pregnancy result, the question of the effect on the fetus would arise. There is no evidence, currently, that a 5 day dose of DES will cause these subsequent cancers. However, those few women who find themselves pregnant may elect abortion.

NATURAL CHILD SPACING: IS BREAST-FEEDING A FORM OF CONTRACEPTION?

The term "natural child spacing" is heard with some frequency in these days when natural foods and natural cosmetics are very much in vogue. *Complete* breast-feeding, *without offering solids or supplements,* usually postpones the resumption of ovulation and menstruation for 7 to 15 months. Thus the minimum number of months between children, if all were to go according to schedule, would be about 16. Proponents suggest that this is the norm for the human species and is ideal for the child who is by this time a complete toddler.

However, breast-feeding carries *no* absolute *guarantees.* Although studies have shown that less than 1 per cent of women who completely breast-feed ovulate before their first menstrual period, it is fairly unusual for American women to offer neither solids nor supplements. Once menstruation has occurred, even though there is the possibility that the first period of a nursing mother is anovulatory, some other form of contraception should be used. Most of us would urge using other forms of contraception from the outset, although for the adamant believer in natural spacing our urging is likely to fall on deaf ears.

GRANNY TALES

The very fact that folk beliefs and "granny tales" abound with contraceptive advice shows a depth of concern that has been present in many different groups of people for a long time. Unfortunately, a large number of these beliefs are without foundation.

The idea that sperm can be washed away by douching seems the most pervasive of these beliefs about ineffective methods. Products advertised for feminine hygiene are frequent ingredients for these douching solutions. Shaking a cola beverage and then spraying it into the vagina is also popular.

Women have told us that pregnancy may be prevented by having intercourse while standing, jumping up and down following intercourse, and voiding or taking a hot bath afterward. Postpartum women have stated that the reproductive organs cannot function until 6 weeks after delivery, and thus they are "immune" during that time and need no contraception.

A list such as this could be very long. Our purpose here is to call attention to the existence of many erroneous beliefs and to raise the question, "How can we deal with them?" The answer is rather carefully, to say the least. Our objective is to substitute a more effective means of contraception without belittling the woman who has been using these other measures.

SURGICAL STERILIZATION

Twenty-nine per cent of couples in the United States who had reached their desired family size by 1973 had already undergone contraceptive sterilization, according to the National Survey of Family Growth in a study conducted for the National Center for Health Statistics. An additional 14 per cent said they intended to be sterilized. In 1970, 18 per cent of couples chose sterilization when they had completed their families; in 1965 the figure was 12 per cent. The same study found sterilizations to be almost evenly divided between male and female procedures.

Vasectomy is the operation for male sterilization. Perhaps the outstanding advantage of vasectomy is that it can be performed in a clinic or an office under local anesthesia. Small incisions are made on each side of the scrotum; the vas deferens is then cut and tied, blocking the passage of sperm (Fig. 5–4). Vasectomy does not diminish sexual drive or affect sexual performance. The man continues to have erection, orgasm, and ejaculation. Spermatozoa continue to be formed in the testes; they are absorbed by the body. Following vasectomy, the couple should continue to use some other form of contraception until examination of semen shows no sperm present, usually a period of 8 to 10 weeks.

Tubal ligation is the most common sterilization procedure for women. A segment of each uterine tube is tied with sutures and then cut to block the

Figure 5–4 Vasectomy.

passage of the egg to the uterus. Tubal ligation in no way interferes with the menstrual cycle. The egg, however, does not reach the uterus; it is absorbed. Until the 1970's tubal ligations were most conveniently performed within 2 to 3 days following delivery, when the uterine tubes were more readily accessible. However, with the development of a procedure for tubal ligation using a laparoscope, the operation may be done quite easily at any time.

In a laparoscope tubal ligation, the laparoscope is inserted through a small incision in or just below the umbilicus, enabling the surgeon to visualize the abdominal cavity. Carbon dioxide gas is injected into the cavity so that the organs are separated and easily identified. An electric cautery is introduced through a second incision, about an inch long, below the first. The tubes are then severed and cauterized. Some surgeons perform the procedure through a single incision. Although some women report no discomfort afterward, others feel the need of rest for a day or two and/or experience abdominal pain that is the equivalent of menstrual cramps.

Since general anesthesia is used, the operation is usually performed in a hospital. However, a woman may be discharged once she recovers from the anesthesia or within a day after surgery. By contrast, 4 to 6 days of convalescence are usually required following traditional abdominal tubal ligation. A still simpler tubal ligation, which requires only local anesthesia and thus rarely an overnight stay in the hospital, is currently being tested at Johns Hopkins University and in some Asian countries. Through a small abdominal incision, the tubes are drawn into a loop that is then held by a silicone-rubber ring.

Neither men nor women should be sterilized with the hope of reversing the procedure. Although this is occasionally possible, it is never assured for a particular individual. However, research is currently being directed toward the development of a reversible vasectomy procedure. Many physicians and some state laws require that both husband and wife sign the permission form for sterilization. Both should understand the document they are signing.

When middle class couples seek sterilization, they have usually made a decision before they contact their doctor. With lower class families, it is often the professional personnel who first introduce the idea of sterilization. It is easy for us to see both medical and economic value in sterilization for low income families with many closely spaced children and to be eager for these families to share our views. But there is quite a difference between informing a patient about sterilization as an option that he or she may wish to consider and answering questions concerning the relationship of sterilization to sexuality and general health, on the one hand, and pressuring or coercing them to make a decision, on the other hand. Yet even in this area there is disagreement, as the example below indicates.

In 1974 the South Carolina Medical Association adopted a resolution declaring that a physician has a "moral and legal right to insist on sterilization permission before accepting a patient if it is done on the initial visit." The resolution was in support of a South Carolina physician who was being sued because of his policy that women on welfare with as many as three children *must* consent to sterilization before he would care for them. In response, a law professor at the University of South Carolina stated that such compelled sterilizations deprive women of their right to make personal decisions regarding their bodies, in violation of the First, Fourth, Fifth, Sixth, Eighth, Ninth, Thirteenth, and Fourteenth Amendments to the Constitution. In the trial, in which the American Civil Liberties Union sued the physician on behalf of two black women in 1975, the court found for the women, but awarded only token damages. The South Carolina Department of Social Services terminated the Medicaid contract of the physician.

UNPLANNED PREGNANCIES: WHY?

It is obvious that not every woman who becomes pregnant does so by choice. Many women, however, accept the pregnancy and welcome the baby by the time of birth. An unplanned child is not necessarily an unwanted child. Others choose abortion or adoption or resign themselves to an unwanted pregnancy and baby. A few, while denying that the pregnancy is desired, appear subconsciously to wish for the baby.

The immediate cause of unplanned pregnancies falls primarily into one of three categories: (1) failure to use any method of contraception, (2) irregular or improper use of effective methods, and (3) use of ineffective methods.

Since no contraceptive is even theoretically 100 per cent effective, *contraceptive failure* is another possible reason for an unplanned pregnancy.

Inadequate knowledge may be a factor in unplanned pregnancies, as suggested earlier in this chapter. At the most basic level, some patients do not appear to be aware of the biologic facts of conception. For others, including some women with a high level of formal education, such as college students, there is the obviously erroneous but rather prevalent belief that conception cannot occur from a single act of intercourse, or even from several acts. "I

didn't do it very often; how could I be pregnant?" they ask. There may also be inadequate information about the efficacy of various contraceptive devices and practices, with reliance on inadequate practices such as withdrawal and douching.

For some unmarried patients, particularly girls still living at home with their parents, the *need to hide* pills or contraceptive devices in order to keep their coital activities secret makes use difficult.

And even in the "sexually-liberated" seventies many women apparently feel that sexual activity outside of marriage is permissible only if it is spontaneous, an "act of passion." The use of contraceptives makes the act "premeditated" and therefore unacceptable.

INTRODUCING CONTRACEPTIVE INFORMATION

Individual women and couples are motivated toward contraception for a variety of reasons. What seems to be an excellent rationale for limiting family size to one couple may have absolutely no appeal to another. Consider the concept of world population growth, discussed earlier in this chapter. To the family of a college professor—a sociologist or an ecologist, perhaps—world concerns may very well be the chief reason for a small family. But to the rural mother who cannot even see another house from her kitchen window, such an issue has no real or personal meaning. Providing for the children she already has or concern for her own health will probably be more valid for her. Stressing social issues to this mother may backfire. She may feel that we are more interested in the social issues than we are in her as a person. Or she may wonder if we want to limit the number of "her kind of people." Certain black leaders have expressed the feeling in recent years that whites want to control black power by limiting the birth of black infants.

Some of the patients who come to us are already highly motivated and basically desire specific information. Others have doubts, fears, and misconceptions that we may be able to resolve by facts.

There are other patients who never come to us; we seek them out because *we* feel they need contraceptive advice for reasons that seem very valid to us—a number of closely spaced pregnancies, for example. Although many women in this last group may welcome our interest and advice, others are plainly hostile. Overenthusiasm about either specific birth control methods or about the subject of contraception itself can make these women less, rather than more, accepting of what we have to say. To cite one of my own experiences as an example:

A few years ago I was sitting in a clinic waiting-room with a friend who was a patient. There was no way in which anyone could identify me as a nurse. A public health nurse walked through and spoke to a woman nearby, saying, "I'll be out to see you next week." When she left, the woman said aloud to all of us sitting there, "I know what she wants. She don't want me to have no more babies. I really hate that woman!"

It nevertheless seems worthwhile to continue to try to reach out to such families. When 165 black urban mothers in Baltimore were asked if physicians or nurses should initiate family planning discussions or should wait until they were asked, 92 per cent said the nurse should not wait. The women said that many mothers were too shy or lacked adequate knowledge to ask. They added that teaching family planning was a medical and nursing responsibility.[21]

How, then, can we talk with these various patients? The initial statement during a contraceptive interview might be something like, "I'm glad to see you this morning. How can I help you today?"

After talking with the woman during these first few minutes, you can assess her feelings about contraception and her level of motivation. Is she there because someone told her to come— perhaps her social worker, or her mother, boyfriend, or husband? Is she doubtful? Curious? Does she really think you have something to offer her?

What about her mate? If she is married, her husband's feelings about contraception are particularly important. If her sexual partner is constant, a single woman may also be strongly influenced by her mate's opinion. We need to give her the chance to talk about his feelings as well as her own. It would be even better if he were able to be present.

"Do you know how a woman gets pregnant?" may be the next logical question. Mitchell[52] suggests that for some women, anxious to discuss various methods, this question, which leads to a discussion of anatomy and physiology, gets in the way of her chief interest and is best deferred until later in the interview. For others, however, it may be the necessary door opener to an understanding of what contraception is all about. A pelvic model is very helpful in answering questions at this point. Lacking this, excellent illustrations are available in several pamphlets. Then, as various methods are discussed, they can be demonstrated in relation to the model or the drawings.

The woman or couple should decide what method is desired (and should feel free to reject any method if that is their wish). For a majority of patients, their own wishes can be the determinant of the methods they will use. For a few, there will be contraindications to specific methods, so it is always important to be sure that the woman understands that the final choice is dependent upon her physical examination and medical history. If an IUD is to be inserted or a diaphragm fitted, the process should be described to the woman before she sees the physician.

Once a method is chosen and, if necessary, approved by a physician, the woman must be taught very carefully and thoroughly the most effective use of the contraceptive of her choice. She needs ample time to tell us what she has learned in her own words and to practice the chosen method when that is appropriate, such as inserting a diaphragm or an applicator, or checking for the string or beads of an IUD.

There are also a number of practical questions that can be anticipated. "How much will I need? Where will I keep my supplies? How far in advance of intercourse should I use a particular product?" Estimated usage is aided if we can tell her how many applications are in a container of foam, for example. And although supplies should be kept out of the reach of small children, who have been known to eat oral contraceptives as well as nonoral products, coitally-related supplies have to be convenient or they will not be used. The kitchen shelf isn't much help if the bedroom is on the second floor or at the back of the house.

FAMILY PLANNING PROGRAMS: INCENTIVES AND BARRIERS

No family planning program ever achieves total success in the sense that it enables every family to eliminate all unwanted pregnancies (and enables families to have those children that they do desire). Some types of programs do seem particularly effective in helping "hard-to-reach" couples, however.

Stycos,[72] during field experiments in Puerto Rico, found that before a couple would use contraceptives effectively, they must first see that family size was a salient issue for them, usually in terms of the pressure of children on the resources of the family. The experiments found that for families who had never used any form of birth control, pamphlets that made the issues relevant and offered information were more successful than group meetings when initiating contraceptive use. As many as 50 per cent of the nonusers became users in this way. However, when trying to help families who had already used birth control methods become more consistent and systematic users, group meetings were found superior to pamphlets because of the opportunity offered for reinforcement and commitment.

Another factor in helping the hard-to-reach family has been the use of "peer counselors," i.e., members of the couple's own community. One New York City program employed women from the communities served by the hospital who could relate to patients in their own language and at their own level. The women who became counselors were prepared by taking 7 weeks of specialized family planning classes, which included training in communication skills as well as in providing contraceptive information and facts about anatomy, physiology, and human behavior. One important outcome of this project was the finding that at first many professional nurses seemed to feel that the counselors were infringing on their practice.

Hardin cites the following as an example of the need for involving peer counselors in family planning:

I recall one instance where a Mexican woman had an unwanted pregnancy. She went to the Planned Parenthood group to find out if she could get an abortion, and the counselor told her that she could, but she would first have to see a psychiatrist. The Mexican woman interpreted this as an accusation that she was insane. Poor Mexicans in this community don't use psychiatrists just to pass an otherwise boring afternoon. To them, the psychiatrist is the last stop on the way to the insane asylum. The Mexican woman in this case was scared speechless, would not see the psychiatrist and tried to abort herself—all because of the frightening word "psychiatrist." Now, had the counselor been a Mexican, she would have known how to explain the situation to the patient, get her to a psychiatrist and a safe medical abortion. This kind of thing also is involved in making birth control services truly available.[33]

The importance of the feelings of each woman's sexual partner has already been mentioned. Yet traditionally, family planning clinics have been almost totally woman-centered, probably because they have been associated with equally woman-centered obstetric clinics. Men have felt very much out of place in these surroundings, which is unfortunate for both partners. Women report that one reason for contraceptive failure is the objection of their mate to their choice of contraceptive. Some males may not only object to contraceptives that might interfere with sexual pleasure because they must be used at the time of intercourse, but may also object to the pill and the IUD because of a belief that such use might encourage their partner to engage in sexual activity with other men.

One attempt to remedy this has been the availability of contraceptive centers staffed by nonmedical personnel, located in convenient neighborhoods, and open during evening hours on a walk-in, no appointment basis. Such a unit offers clients their choice of condoms, foam, or jelly and instructs them in the use of these methods, often on a free basis. Although all of these devices are available at the local drugstore (if one has the money and is motivated to spend it in that way), contraception education is not.

It has been a rather significant discovery that male clients in these walk-in units have been very responsive to the chance not only to learn more about contraception but to ask about conception and the development and birth of the baby as well. (In one such clinic more than 90 per cent of the new patients and 98 per cent of the returning patients were male.) Even when the counselors are female, because these women are seen as professionals, they do not appear to be a threat to masculinity. It has been found, however, that separate group discussions for males and females are more effective; in the presence of females of their own peer group young males do not like to show an ignorance of any subject related to sex.[30]

Questions about contraceptives asked by young men in these clinics cover such basics as how to put on a condom and how foam is used. When they are encouraged to use a combination of condom and foam for maximum effectiveness, many request both methods.

Other programs have been aimed at males visiting maternity wards and in clubs and prisons.

"Modesty" is sometimes a reason for women to avoid family planning programs. Contrary to middle class myths, women from lower income families are often more reluctant to undress for examinations than women from higher income groups. They may also be more reluctant to discuss subjects such as sexual intercourse. Modesty is an even greater barrier in some other areas of the world. Encouraging participation in family planning programs may therefore involve assurance that modesty is preserved and that a conscientious program to assure privacy and adequate protection in the clinic itself is maintained.

Many patients in family planning clinics have a low tolerance for barriers. Yet we continue to erect them: inconvenient locations and times, which necessitate long and/or costly travel, and long, frustrating waiting periods once the clinic is reached. Hardin describes one such program that is, unfortunately, not unique.

When the clinic was established with private funds it was located conveniently to where the poor lived; they could walk to the clinic and walk home. Finally, the county was persuaded that birth control was a legitimate public health function, and it took over the clinic. But after about a year the county supervisors decided that it was too expensive to maintain this separate medical facility. They decided to amalgamate it with the county hospital to save the tax-payers' money and to be more efficient. The only difficulty was that the hospital was 10 miles out of town. Now, California has been built on the assumption that man was born with an automobile between his legs. But many poor people either don't have automobiles or they have only one and the man of the house needs that to drive to work. How is his wife going to travel 10 miles to the birth control clinic? There is a bus which leaves every hour, but it sometimes skips. If she does get to the hospital, the woman will have to wait two or three hours for service because it is necessary to make "efficient" use of the doctor's time, and to hell with the patient. If she is lucky, a woman may leave her house at eight o'clock in the morning and get back home at two in the afternoon. For a poor woman who may already have several children to care for this can be a nearly impossible situation. So it has proved to be. Once afflicted by "efficiency," the whole system so discouraged patients that use dropped drastically. Thus, it isn't enough to establish birth control facilities; they must be located conveniently to where poor people live.

Similarly, to make birth control fully available to the poor we have to involve the poor in the delivery of services. There is a chain of people involved in any organized birth control effort, and direct communication must finally be with a staff person who can speak as a peer.[33]

What can we do about such problems? Relocation is one possible answer; a different way of scheduling appointments is another. While we attempt to unravel some of the red tape, we can at least acknowledge some of the frustration with comments such as "I know how hard waiting must be for you" or "You must be tired after your long trip. We will see you as soon as possible."

FAMILY PLANNING DROP-OUTS

Once started, contraception is not necessarily continued. Table 5–6 summarizes some of the studies on the drop-out rates of family planning clinics. Why this failure to continue? Major reasons cited in a variety of studies include:

1. Diminished need for contraception, including pregnancy.
2. Difficulty in getting to the clinic.
3. Poor service.
4. Feelings of sexual partner.
5. Side effects of the contraceptive method (physical and psychologic).

Individuals who are more likely to drop out include those who are not currently married, the teenager, the woman near the end of her childbearing years, and the woman with two children or less.

INFERTILITY: THE OVERLOOKED SIDE OF FAMILY PLANNING

In a society concerned with limiting population, with developing newer modes of contraception, and with the issues of abortion, it is easy to forget that more than 15 per cent of all married couples are not childless by their own choice. Some of these couples are unable to conceive; in other instances the woman is unable to carry the pregnancy to term.

A couple is considered infertile when conception does not occur within a year during which intercourse is frequent and contraception is not used. *Primary infertility* means that the couple has never achieved a pregnancy. If one or more pregnancies have been established at some time but the couple is now unable to achieve pregnancy, the term *secondary infertility* is used.

Determinants of Fertility

Basic factors affecting the fertility of any couple are the ages of both husband and wife, the frequency of intercourse, and the length of exposure.

Both male and female fertility is at its highest at approximately 24 to 25 years of age. About 75 per cent of couples in whom both partners are approaching their mid-20's will conceive within 9 months. Female fertility declines fairly rapidly after age 30. When the man is over 40, only 22 per cent of couples become pregnant.[48]

Frequency of intercourse enhances fertility, not only because of the increased exposure but also because frequent ejaculation is a factor in sperm motility. Intercourse at least four times a week is advised for couples desiring pregnancy.

Length of exposure refers to the number of months of intercourse without the use of contraceptives. Eighty per cent of couples will conceive within a year; 90 per cent within 18 months. For those who do not, a fertility evaluation will attempt to pinpoint the reason. In all but 5 to 10 per cent of couples a cause may be found.

Physical Causes of Infertility

The reason for infertility in an individual couple may be physiologic or psychologic. In 30 to 40 per cent of couples the male partner is either completely or partially responsible.

Male infertility is usually due to sperm that are inadequate, either in number or in motility (Chapter 3). Impotence can also be a reason. Social factors such as motorcycle riding (because of heat in the scrotal area) and working in an environment that is too hot may affect fertility.

Common causes of female infertility involve the uterine tubes, the endocrine system, and the cervix. Tubal causes account for the largest proportion of female infertility and have been found more often in women of lower socioeconomic groups. Pelvic inflammatory disease, of either gonococcal or enterococcal origin, and postabortal sepsis are major causes of tubal closure. Data from Eastern European countries, where abortion by suction curettage has been performed for a number of years, suggest that repeated suction abortion may affect tubal patency.

Failure of ovulation accounts for approximately 15 per cent of all infertility. Possible reasons why a woman may not ovulate include low levels of pituitary gonadotropin, absent or damaged ovaries, absence of ova, and endocrine system dysfunction.

Cervical and uterine causes of infertility result in inability to carry a pregnancy to term, rather than a failure to conceive.

Emotional Factors in Infertility

A number of the biologic changes that are causes of infertility may have a psychologic basis in an individual man or woman.

In women these conditions include

Table 5–6 DROP-OUTS FROM FAMILY PLANNING PROGRAMS*

Study	Country Studied	Observation Period	Definition of Drop-out	Contraceptive Method Used	Sample Size for New Admissions	Drop-out Rate (as % of New Admissions†)
Dubrow and Kuder	U.S.A. (New York City)	2 years	"Failure to return for further follow-up"	Jelly, cream, diaphragm	2046	44.5
Creedy and Polgar	U.S.A.	1 year	Did not return 3 months before due date or 6 months after it	All	21917	51.47
Population Council	Korea (Koyang)	1 year	Not actively registered at end of observation period	Diaphragm, condom, foam	490	About one-third
Population Council	Pakistan (Comilla)	2 years	Unspecified	Condom, foam	129	Fewer than 10%
Population Council	Pakistan (Lulliani)	1 year	IUD not in situ at end of observation period	IUD	134	36.5
Population Council	Taiwan	14 months	IUD not in situ at time of interview	IUD	2000	33.0
Population Council	Taiwan	6 months	Unspecified	Pill IUD	1017 Not applicable	"Almost 1 in 2" "About 1 of 4"
Population Council	India	1 year	IUD not in situ at end of observation period	IUD	20000	33.0

Author	Location	Observation period	Reason for drop-out	Method	N	Drop-out rate
Hall	U.S.A. (Baltimore)	1 year	Pill would have run out if correctly used—did not return to clinic, IUD removed/expelled, accidentally pregnant	Pill IUD	12092	46.0 37.0
Kanagaratnam and Kim	Singapore	1 year	Not using pill 4 months after end of observation period	Pill	2992	45.5
Beasely et al.	U.S.A. (New Orleans)	1 year	Failed to comply with revisit schedule during observation period	All	9210	13.6
Reynolds	Trinidad and Tobago	2 months	Patient not returned to clinic 3+ months since missing last scheduled appointment	All	680	19.1
Gordis et al.	U.S.A. (Baltimore)	1 year	"Terminated relation with program"	Pill	100 sexually active nulliparous adolescents	Nearly 50%
Takeshita et al.	West Malaysia	1 year	Not using given contraceptive at time of interview	Pill (91%)	2609	35.3
Keeny and Cernada	Taiwan	1 year	IUD not in situ at interview (after end of observation period), pill not being used at end of observation period	IUD Pill	4820 2217	33.3 68.0

*From Bracken: *American Journal of Public Health*, 63:262, 1973.

†In reviewing the literature it was sometimes necessary to calculate the clinic drop-out rates from other data presented in the paper. In all cases the drop-out rate reflects the magnitude of dropping out for all reasons.

tubal spasm, failure to ovulate, rapid expulsion of spermatic fluid, and vaginismus (painful vaginal spasm). An additional cause may be an unconscious avoidance of coitus at the time of ovulation.

Women with psychogenic infertility appear to share certain characteristics. Although they express, and appear to believe that they have, a strong desire to become pregnant, after counseling sessions such conflicting emotions as intense ambivalent feelings toward their own mothers and a variety of fears become apparent. These fears may be of the pregnancy itself (will it make me unattractive to my husband?), of labor (will I or my child die?), or of becoming a mother (can I possibly be a good mother?). Many women with psychogenic infertility find it difficult to express hostility and feel very guilty about their angry feelings. When therapy has helped them to express hostility without guilt, they become more free to develop warm relationships with others, including their own husbands, and in many instances conception occurs.

In men, erectile impotence (impotentia coeundi) and ejaculatory impotence (ejaculatio retardata) are the principal causes of psychogenic infertility. In addition, men, as well as women, may unconsciously avoid coitus. *Primary impotence* is used to describe the condition in which there has always been impotence. *Secondary impotence*, which occurs at some time after normal sexual potency has been established, may be a major problem or a very transitory one. Any normal male may experience periods of transitory impotence. There is agreement that a high percentage of male impotence is psychologic in origin. Not only is this felt to be true of younger men, but some investigators feel that it is an important factor in male impotence of old age.

Early psychic trauma, feeding problems, illness in childhood, and overprotection and overindulgence by their mothers are some of the characteristics seen in many men with the complex problem of psychogenic infertility. In general these men appear unaggressive and often view their sexual relationships with women as aggressive, hostile behavior. Since the sexual problem is a part of a more extensive personality disorder, particularly if it is long-standing, success in treatment may be limited. Psychologic care, combined with re-education and retraining, is the principal treatment.

Evaluation of Fertility

The first step in helping an individual couple deal with infertility is to determine the reason. A thorough history is taken from both husband and wife. Significant information from the husband includes:

1. Occupation, past and present.
2. History of endocrine disorders.
3. Childhood diseases, especially if contracted during adulthood.
4. Genitourinary problems and/or surgery.
5. Excessive consumption of alcohol or use of tobacco.
6. Frequency of sexual activity.
7. Positions in coitus.
8. Impotence.

The wife will be asked about:

1. Occupation, past and present.
2. History of endocrine disorders.
3. Pelvic disease and treatment, and/or pelvic surgery.
4. Any previous pregnancies and their outcome.
5. Menstrual history.
6. Douching.
7. Coital technique.
8. Timing of coitus in relation to ovulation.

Occupation is important because hazards such as radiation and heavy metal poisoning affect fertility. Any disorder of the endocrine system, such as diabetes or thyroid disease, may be related to ovulatory failure. The contraction of a childhood disease during adult life, particularly of mumps, may lead to sterility (Chapter 3). Research has demonstrated that chronic alcoholism, nicotine intoxication, and habitual use of marijuana affect sperm production.

A complete physical examination follows the initial interviews. Specific fertility studies include the analysis of seminal fluid, the determination of ovulation, postcoital testing, and the determination of tubal patency.

Analysis of Seminal Fluid. Evaluation of seminal fluid for sperm count is a part of the initial evaluation of infertility. The specimen is obtained by masturbating directly into a clean bottle. The man should abstain from intercourse for 3 days before the sample is obtained. The specimen needs to be examined within 2 hours after collection.

In order to be considered "probably fertile" a specimen of seminal fluid should have greater than 20 million spermatozoa per ml., with more than 50 million sperm in the total specimen. The average ejaculation contains from 120 to 200 million sperm per ml. Counts between 20 million and 40 million may be considered subfertile, and some specific instructions may be given to the man about frequency of intercourse.

Sperm motility is also significant. Only motile sperm are able to reach the distal segment of the uterine tube, where fertilization takes place. Greater than 50 per cent of the sperm in a specimen of seminal fluid should be mobile, and more than 25 per cent should move forward. In addition, more than 70 per cent of the sperm in the sample should be of normal shape.

Failure to meet any of these five criteria in two or more samples suggests that male infertility is a very strong possibility, although only the total absence of motile sperm is considered absolute evidence of sterility.

Determination of Ovulation. The single most important tool in the determination of ovulation is the record of basal body temperature (Fig. 5–5). This is the same record that is kept by the woman who is employing the rhythm method of contraception. Again, we emphasize the importance of thorough patient teaching about the accurate taking and recording of basal body temperature. Ovulation is confirmed by endometrial biopsy.

Postcoital   Testing. Cervical mucus undergoes characteristic changes a few days prior to ovulation (Chapter 3). The Sims-Huhner postcoital test examines both the quality of the cervical mucus and sperm survival. The woman is asked to anticipate ovulation from her record of basal body temperature and to have intercourse with her husband from 4 to 8 hours before the test.* In the clinic or the physician's office, a specimen of mucus is taken from the cervical area with forceps. The physical characteristics of the mucus are first examined. Near the time of ovulation the mucus resembles fresh egg white and "can be pulled from the slide in a long thread which will then retract to its original globule."[57] When placed on a slide at room temperature, the mucus forms a delicate fern pattern that is observable under a microscope (ferning). The number of viable and nonviable sperm and the motility and active forward progression of viable sperm are also noted under the microscope.

If the results of the Sims-Huhner

---

*This length of time varies from one clinic to another. Page and associates suggest 4 to 18 hours.[57]

Figure 5–5 The use of a basal body temperature graph in infertility. (From Hamblen: *Southern Medical J.*, 38:339, 1945.)

test are less than optimal, the test is usually repeated, either during the same or the next cycle. Some clinics defer seminal fluid analysis until after examination of the sperm in a postcoital test.

   Determination of Tubal Patency. When semen analysis indicates that the husband is probably fertile, a Rubin test determines the patency of the uterine tubes by means of the insufflation of CO_2. CO_2 flows through the tubes into the abdominal cavity, irritates the subdiaphragmatic area as it rises when the patient sits erect, and causes a transient, referred pain in the shoulder.

Medications Used in the Treatment of Infertility

   When the only apparent reason for infertility is failure to ovulate, clomiphene citrate (Clomid) may be a useful treatment. Clomiphene appears to stimulate the release of gonadotropins (FSH and LH) by the anterior pituitary, which, in turn, stimulates the growth of the follicle and subsequent ovulation (Chapter 3).

   For clomiphene therapy to be successful, the pituitary must be capable of function and the ovary capable of response. Patients are screened to determine ovarian dysfunction (but not ovarian failure) and to rule out other types of reproductive tract problems, as well as untreated diabetes, or thyroid or adrenal disease that may be related to ovarian dysfunction. Any abnormal uterine bleeding must be evaluated. Patients with liver disease are not given clomiphene because it is metabolized in the liver. In women over 35 years old an endometrial biopsy to check for possible carcinoma is considered essential. The presence of some estrogen in the body, indicated by cervical mucus, biopsy of the endometrium, urine tests, or the administration of progestational agents suggests that a woman may be a good candidate for clomiphene therapy. Recognizing these constraints is important because of the widespread publicity given "fertility drugs" in the general press. Every infertile couple wonders, "Why can't I take these pills and solve my problem?"

A pelvic examination precedes each month's therapy. Following oral administration of clomiphene for 5 days, the woman is instructed to check basal body temperature to determine if ovulation has occurred. Endometrial biopsy and a rise in the urinary excretion of pregnanediol (a breakdown product of progesterone) are additional indications of ovulation.

Therapy is discontinued if:

1. The woman becomes pregnant.

2. The woman develops either visual symptoms (such as blurring of vision) or enlargement of an ovary.

3. After three cycles she has failed to ovulate.

4. After three ovulatory cycles she has failed to become pregnant.

The risk of multiple pregnancy is higher with clomiphene therapy (1:13) than in the general population (1:29), a fact that each couple should understand before the drug is given. Clomiphene has also been used experimentally to induce spermatogenesis, and in combination with human chorionic gonadotropin, given at midcycle, to enhance ovulation.[21]

ADOPTION

Adoption is one alternative for infertile couples who wish to become parents. Nurses who work chiefly with maternity patients are more likely to come to know mothers who give up their infants for adoption (Chapter 4) than couples who seek to become adoptive parents. Yet the same basic counsel is important for both groups: deal with a recognized adoption agency. In many communities departments of social services are an excellent source of information about recognized agencies.

Adoption is governed by state law (rather than by federal law), and thus regulations vary from one state to another. Although some privately arranged adoptions are probably successful, others have led to heartache. The mother who gives her infant for adoption, the adoptive couple, and the infant or child need the safeguards that recognized agencies afford.

The most frequently sought adoptive child is a white infant, newly born or a few weeks old. Relatively few such infants are available today. Most unwed mothers who feel they will not be able to care for a baby choose early abortion. Many homes for unwed mothers, once crowded, have closed their doors. A shortage of adoptive infants has led to some questionable practices, including the buying and selling of babies (often couched in more subtle terms) in some instances. At the same time older children, nonwhite children, and children with anomalies (even such minor ones as missing fingers) are often overlooked as adoptive possibilities.

Adoption by a single parent has become a possibility in some areas of the country, but with infants in very short supply, single parent adoption represents only a tiny fraction of adoptions.

Couples considering adoption have a great many questions, most of which are best answered by specially trained counselors in adoption agencies. Ideas about adoption are changing. For example, there have been some questions in recent years about whether the identity of the biologic parents should always remain a secret, a tenet of adoption practice for many years. Nurses serve families best when these questions arise by referring couples to those who are qualified to answer their questions, usually the social workers and counselors of recognized agencies.

ARTIFICIAL INSEMINATION

As an alternative to adoption, artificial insemination was rather rarely suggested to infertile couples; it was usually considered only if the couple themselves pursued the subject. But as widespread elective abortion has diminished the number of infants available for adoption, more attention has turned to the possibility of artificial insemination as an alternative.

Although infertility is the most common reason for artificial insemination, it is not the only one. For example, when a mother has previously delivered an erythroblastotic infant, and when her husband is homozygous Rh positive (Chapter 2), the couple may choose artificial insemination from an Rh negative donor. Following genetic counseling (below) that indicates that the husband carries a serious genetic defect or that the husband and wife share a recessive gene for a major disease, a couple may again choose artificial insemination.

Either donor semen or the husband's own sperm may be used for artificial insemination, the choice being governed by individual circumstances.

Husband Insemination. Malformations of the male or female reproductive tract that make it difficult or impossible to deposit semen in the posterior vaginal fornix are a major indication for insemination using the husband's semen. One of the earliest of all reasons for artificial insemination was penile hypospadias.

An adequate sperm count combined with low ejaculate volume or a low normal sperm count combined with a normal volume of ejaculate may suggest that the husband's semen be used for a number of inseminations before donor sperm is tried.

Donor Insemination. When the sperm count is very low or totally absent following medical therapy and when insemination using the husband's semen has not achieved pregnancy, donor semen may be used. Donor semen is also used when such factors as Rh incompatibility or genetic disease are the reasons for the insemination procedure.

Donors of semen often come from the university or medical community. They are paid for their semen, and they must agree both to the unrestricted use of their semen and to make no effort to discover the identity of the couples involved. Donors should not, to their knowledge, have any hereditary disease. Blood type, Rh factor, and serology are checked; ideally only compatible blood types are used. Matching the donor to the husband in relation to coloring and body type is not always possible, but physical characteristics serve as general guidelines. For example, semen from a tall, blond man would not be given to a Jewish or Italian couple who were short and olive-skinned.

Semen may be either fresh or frozen. Fresh semen must be delivered to the office or clinic shortly before the insemination procedure, which can be a disadvantage. On the other hand, freezing decreases sperm motility by about 40 per cent, and structural changes apparently take place in the individual sperm, lowering the conception rate.

The Insemination Procedure. Temperature charts for at least one cycle, and usually for several months, are reviewed. The initial day for insemination is then selected, about 1 to 2 days prior to basal temperature rise. Semen, obtained by masturbation into a clean cup (or a frozen specimen), is drawn into a syringe with a small length of polyethylene tubing attached. Or a metal cannula may be introduced into the cervix. A small amount (0.1 to 0.5 cc.) of semen is then inserted into the endocervical canal. The remainder of the semen is placed in a cervical cap—a small plastic cup that is held against the cervix by suction. After resting on the examining table for 15 minutes, the woman is ready to go home. She will remove the cervical cap about 6 hours later by pulling on the attached string.

Some physicians allow and encourage the husband to actively assist in the insemination procedure, believing that psychologically this is quite important. It is the husband who holds the syringe and deposits the semen. He is also instructed in the removal of the cervical cap. It is suggested that the couple have intercourse following the removal of the cap.

Two to three inseminations are done during each menstrual cycle, usually on alternate days, the last being performed on the day that the temperature drops just prior to ovulation.

When a woman's menstrual cycles are highly irregular, so that the time of ovulation is difficult to predict, she may be given clomiphene citrate, which is used to stimulate and control ovulation, or human chorionic gonadotropin, which will induce ovulation within 24 hours after administration if the follicle is ready.

Effectiveness of Artificial Insemination. An analysis of 630 couples who had artificial insemination with donor semen showed a success rate of from 55 to 78 per cent. Between 31 and 46 per cent of these successful couples achieved pregnancy in the first month. In six months 90 per cent of those who will become pregnant have already done so; rarely will there be success if pregnancy has not occurred within a year.[6]

Success with the husband's semen is as low as 15 per cent. The best results with frozen semen are no greater than 50 per cent.

GENETIC COUNSELING

The concept of genetic counseling is not new. The Babylonian *Talmud* noted many centuries ago that there were families in which blood did not clot. A case is described in which the sons of three sisters died during circumcision. A rabbi advised a fourth sister not to have her son circumcised.

Today, with nearly 1200 conditions identified as genetic in origin, it has been estimated that 25 per cent of medical problems in the United States can be traced in part to genetic factors. Genetic counseling has thus become an important medical specialty and a vital part of family planning counseling.

Goals

The birth of a child with a defect is one major circumstance that brings families for genetic counseling. A second is the knowledge that someone in the family—a cousin, a sister, or perhaps an uncle—has some abnormality. "Could the same thing happen to my child? Or could it happen to another of my children?" parents wonder. A young man, newly married, has just learned that his second sister has diabetes mellitus. "What are the chances that my children might have diabetes?" he asks. Thus one goal of counseling is to help determine the risks of occurrence of a particular trait.

For those conditions that are governed by a single gene, these risks are relatively easy to determine and explain. For disorders that are polygenic or appear to be influenced by familial factors, such as diabetes or cleft lip and palate, only empiric risk figures are available, i.e., calculations based on the occurrence of the particular disorder in a large number of births.

If a genetic condition already exists in one or more children in a family, an important goal of counseling is to help the family recognize their feelings about the child and accept those feelings. It is normal to feel sad about giving birth to a child with a serious mental or physical handicap. (See Chapter 22.)

In a number of conditions, genetic counseling can help to assure prompt medical attention for a child in utero who may have an inherited condition. For example, phenylketonuria (PKU) is an inborn error in metabolism that can be treated by a diet low in phenylalanine but if untreated leads to severe mental retardation. If one child in a family has PKU, counselors can alert both the family and the medical personnel who care for them to the need for prompt evaluation and early treatment at any subsequent delivery.

Other disorders can be diagnosed prenatally by amniocentesis and the cultivation and analysis of amniotic fluid cells. At least one condition, adrenogenital syndrome, is currently being treated in utero.

The importance of genetic counseling in ultimately reducing the number of abnormal genes in the population is the goal of some counselors, although this is not as significant in everyday practice as are the other goals that basically aim at helping individual families. Abnormal genes will never be totally eliminated because new ones arise by mutation in each generation, in addition to those that are carried undiscovered as recessive genes through many generations. However, because improved medical care now allows individuals to reach maturity and therefore to reproduce, when formerly they did not (children with cystic fibrosis, for example), there is concern that without attention to the population aspects of counseling the number of persons with genetic diseases will increase.

It is important to remember that every one of us carries recessive genes for three to eight "diseases" or conditions. The vast majority of these conditions will never be expressed in our own phenotype or in the phenotypes of our children, their children, or the children for many generations. For example, in the United States about four persons in every 100 are estimated to carry the gene for cystic fibrosis, yet only four in 10,000 suffer from the disease. One of 160 individuals carries the gene for galactosemia (an inborn error in metabolism), yet only one in 100,000 inherits the condition. Thus it is evident that most deleterious genes are carried, unrecognized, by apparently healthy people rather than by individuals with the disease. Even if someone with a particular condition marries a carrier, the odds of producing a child with the condition are two out of four, compared with one out of four if carriers marry.

The number of people with some genetically related traits is certainly increasing. For example, since the advent of insulin, individuals with juvenile diabetes mellitus no longer die at an early age. Many reproduce successfully. The possibility that their children will develop diabetes at some time in their lives is greater than for children who have no family history of diabetes. Yet diabetes is controllable and will probably be even more easily controlled in the future than it is today. Is the number of persons with diabetes a serious problem for society?

The Process of Genetic Counseling

A proper diagnosis is the foundation of genetic counseling. When a newborn shows signs of an abnormality (often first recognized by an observant nurse), possible causes are carefully evaluated (such as maternal rubella, kernicterus, and so on) before the disorder is accepted as genetic in origin.

Data from the extended family provide the basis for construction of a pedigree chart. Possible kinship between family members, the ages and causes of death of as many members as possible, exact diagnoses of any apparent familial disease, and the occurrence of spontaneous abortion and/or stillbirth are significant parts of the family history that are incorporated in the pedigree chart. Chromosomal studies are made of family members, when this is appropriate, as well as laboratory evaluations for carriers, when such persons can be determined.

It is only at this point that a discussion of risks is feasible. Counseling then attempts to help parents deal with the myriad of financial, medical, and social realities of their baby's condition. These questions are raised not just in relation to the affected baby but to the parents' considerations of future pregnancies.

What will the cost of care possibly be? What alternatives for care should be considered (as, for example, in the case of a child with a severely handicapping condition)? Will special medical treatment be needed (such as for the child with cystic fibrosis)? What is the eventual prognosis? How able is the family to cope with the emotional and financial demands of the condition? What resources are available to help them cope? Many of these are not questions that counseling can answer, other than to inform families about what a particular community has to offer. But by raising questions, parents can be helped to consider these issues, particularly when they are trying to decide to have another child, which is so frequently why such counseling is sought.

Alternatives to future childbearing may also be considered in the genetic counseling process. Some families choose sterilization as a means of preventing future pregnancies. Others seek information about highly reliable contraception. Adoption is an alternative that some of these couples choose.

Adoption, however, is by no means the right answer for every couple. For parents whose only child is defective, Macintyre[47] states, "there is a deep personal need to prove that they are capable of producing a normal child of their own." Macintyre uses the analogy of a baseball game to describe his perception of how parents feel when their infant, particularly a firstborn infant, is defective.

It's like being up to bat in a very important ball game where everything depends on you, and striking out; and the whole stadium boos, the whole of society boos, or you think it does. . . . For the individual who has struck out in that important ball game, there is a real need to offset society's criticism by hitting a home run the next time at bat. Adopting a child is like getting to first base on a "walk." It is no proof of your batting ability.[47]

Every couple will not feel this way, but the possibility that some will is certainly worth considering.

When the disorder in question is caused by a dominant gene carried by the father, artificial insemination may be an alternative for some families. With other conditions, pregnancy may be attempted with subsequent diagnosis in utero by the use of amniocentesis (Chapter 10) and possible therapeutic abortion. For example, when the disorder is X-linked recessive, thus affecting only male children, the knowledge that the fetus is a girl can make pregnancy far less stressful for both mother and father.

Abnormal fetal karyotypes may also be detected during the prenatal months. In a study reported by Nadler[53] at the 1969 International Congress on Congenital Malformations, 14 of 150 women undergoing amniocentesis in the fourteenth or fifteenth week of pregnancy were found to have fetuses with chromosomal abnormalities. Thirteen of the mothers were aborted at their request; in every instance the fetus was abnormal. The fourteenth mother decided against abortion and delivered an infant with Down's syndrome. The remaining 136 mothers delivered normal, healthy infants with no indications of abnormality.

Not every study using amniocentesis has resulted in such accurate predictions. Nadler suggests that the timing of the test at the fourteenth to fifteenth week, a period during which 90 per cent of the amniotic fluid cells can be successfully grown in culture, may be a factor in the extremely accurate predictions of this particular study. Nevertheless, 99 per cent success in the cultivation of amniotic fluid cells is becoming the rule rather than the exception.

Cultured cells from amniotic fluid are also being used to detect the presence or absence of some enzymes that lead to the diagnosis of certain biochemical disorders, such as galactosemia.

A single example of prenatal monitoring for detection of an inherited defect may illustrate its value.

A three and a half year old child was referred to us for chromosomal analysis. The youngster had several external congenital malformations and was suffering from bilateral renal dysplasia, severe growth retardation (she weighed only 8 pounds), and severe mental retardation. She has two phenotypically normal sisters. Results of the chromosome analysis indicated that the defective child's karyotype was genetically unbalanced, and analyses were performed on both parents. The father's karyotype was normal, but that of the mother indicated that she is a carrier of a balanced reciprocal translocation. . . .

The mother was pregnant at the time she was ascertained as having the genetic problem, and when she and her husband were informed that the risk of producing a second badly defective child might be as high as 50% both parents requested that the pregnancy be interrupted. They both desired more children, but neither could tolerate the thought of having another deformed one. We discussed the possibility of performing a prenatal chromosomal analysis on the developing fetus, and it was agreed that an attempt at such an analysis should be made. Amniocentesis was performed in the sixteenth week following the last menstrual period, and cultures were established from fetal cells in the amniotic fluid. By the eighteenth week the analysis was complete, and the fetal chromosome karyotype was obtained. It was obvious that the fetus carried the same translocation as the mother. . . . Since the karyotype represented that of a balanced carrier, we were able to predict that the child would develop normally. Furthermore, the parents were hoping for a boy and we were able to predict that their desires would be fulfilled in this regard also. In due time, at full term, the mother was delivered of a beautiful eight and a half pound, healthy son. The parents were ecstatic. . . .

Our ability to perform the prenatal chromosome analysis in this case literally saved the life of that youngster, for he would have been destroyed by therapeutic abortion on the basis of the high genetic risk involved, had we not been able to perform the prenatal evaluation.[47]

Genetic counseling is becoming one additional resource for families in their childbearing years. Like all counseling, it must never press solutions on families but rather should inform them of alternatives from which they can choose the best possible course for themselves.

REFERENCES

1. Baird, D., Walker, J., and Thompson, A. M.: Causes and Prevention of Stillbirths and First Week Deaths, *Journal of Obstetrics and Gynaecology of the British Empire,* 61:433, 1954.
2. Beasley, J. D., Harter, C. L., and Fisher, A.: Attitudes and Knowledge Relevant to Family Planning Among New Orleans Negro Women, *American Journal of Public Health,* 56:1847, 1966.
3. Beasley, J. D., and Harter, C. L.: Introducing Family Planning Clinics to Louisiana, *Children,* 14:188, September-October, 1967.
4. Berelson, B.: Beyond Family Planning, *Science,* 160:533, 1969.
5. Billings, J.: *Natural Family Planning: The Ovulation Method.* 3rd Edition. Collegeville, Minn., The Liturgical Press, 1975.
6. Board, J. A.: Artificial Insemination in the Human, *MCV Quarterly,* 8:13, 1972.
7. Bracken, M.B.: Factors Associated with Dropping Out of Family Planning Clinics in Jamaica, *American Journal of Public Health,* 63:262, 1973.
8. Bradbury, B.: Preventing the "Diaphragm Baby Syndrome": A Matter of Technique, Teaching, and Time, *JOGN Nursing,* 4(2):24, 1975.
9. Britt, S.: Fertility Awareness: Four Methods of Natural Family Planning, *JOGN Nursing,* 6(2):9, 1977.
10. Calderone, M. (ed.): Manual of Family Planning and Contraceptive Practice. 2nd Edition. Baltimore, The Williams and Wilkins Co., 1970.
11. Calhoun, J. B.: Population Density and Social Pathology, *Scientific American,* 206:139, February, 1962.
12. Campbell, A. A.: Design and Scope of the 1960 Study of Growth of American Families. *In* Kiser, C. V. (ed.): *Research in Family Planning.* Princeton, Princeton University Press, 1962.
13. Campbell, A. A.: Family Planning and the Five Million, *Family Planning Perspectives,* 1:2, October, 1969.
14. Carrighar, S.: Nature's Balance, The Teetering See-Saw. *In* Young, L. B. (ed.): *Population in Perspective.* New York, Oxford University Press, 1968.
15. Chase, H. B.: *The Relationship of Certain Biologic and Socioeconomic Factors to Fetal, Infant and Early Childhood Mortality.* Albany, N.Y., State Dept. of Health, 1961 and 1962.
16. Cohen, M., and Friedman, S.: Nonsexual Motivation of Adolescent Sexuality, *Medical Aspects of Human Sexuality,* 9:9, 1975.
17. Davis, K.: Population, *Scientific American,* 209:62, September, 1963.
18. Davis, K.: Population Policy: Will Current Programs Succeed? *Science, 158*:730, 1967.
19. DiPalma, J.: The Pill, Pro and Con, *RN, 34*:61, January, 1971.
20. Edmands, E. M.: A Study of Contraceptive Practices in a Selected Group of Urban, Negro Mothers in Baltimore, *American Journal of Public Health,* 58:263, 1968.
21. Edwards, R. G.: Studies in Human Conception, *American Journal of Obstetrics & Gynecology, 117*:587, 1973.
22. Ehrlich, P. R.: *The Population Bomb,* New York, Ballantine Books, 1968.
23. Finley, S. C.: Genetic Counseling, *Southern Medical Journal, 64*(Suppl. #1):101, 1971.
24. Flapan, M.: A Paradigm for the Analysis of Childbearing Motivations of Married Women Prior to Birth of the First Child, *American Journal of Orthopsychiatry, 39*:402, 1969.
25. Food and Population: Thinking the Unthinkable, *Science News, 106*:340, November 30, 1974.
26. Frank, R., and Tietze, C.: Acceptance of an Oral Contraceptive Program in a Large Metropolitan Area, *American Journal of Obstetrics and Gynecology, 93*:122, September 1, 1965.
27. Freedman, R.: Norms for Family Size in Underdeveloped Areas, *Proceedings of the Royal Society,* B, *159*:220, 1963.
28. Gardner, R. N.: *The United Nations and the Population Problem: Planning for the 1974 World Population Conference.* Rensselaerville, N.Y., The Institute on Man and Science, 1973.
29. Gilson, J. R., and McKeown, T.: Observations on All Births (23,970) in Birmingham, 1947. Effect of Changing Family Size on Infant Mortality, *British Journal of Social Medicine, 6*:183, July, 1952.
30. Gobble, F. L., Vincent, C. E., Cochrane, C. M., et al: A Nonmedical Approach to Fertility Reduction, *Obstetrics and Gynecology, 34*:888, 1969.
31. Greene, W.: Triage: Who Shall Be Fed? Who Shall Starve? *N.Y. Times Magazine,* January 5, 1975, 9.
32. Hamblen, E. C.: Minimal Standards for Sterility Surveys, *Southern Medical Journal, 38*:339, 1945.
33. Hardin, G.: Multiple Paths to Population Control, *Family Planning Perspectives,* 2:24, June, 1970.
34. Hatt, P. K.: *Background of Human Fertility in Puerto Rico.* Princeton, Princeton University Press, 1952.
35. Hellman, L. M.: Choices and Challenges for the Federal Family Planning Program, *American Journal of Obstetrics and Gynecology, 117*:782, 1973.
36. Hopkins, P., and Clyne, M.: Management of

the Home Confinement. *In* Howells, J. (ed.): *Modern Perspectives in Psycho-Obstetrics.* New York, Brunner/Mazel, 1972.

37. Inman, W. H., and Vessey, M. P.: Investigation of Deaths from Pulmonary, Coronary, and Cerebral Thrombosis and Embolism in Women of Childbearing Age, *British Medical Journal, 2*:193, 1968.

38. Jaffe, F.: A Strategy for Implementing Family Planning Services in the United States, *American Journal of Public Health, 58*:713, 1968.

39. Jekel, J., Klerman, L., and Bancroft, D.: Factors Associated with Rapid Subsequent Pregnancies Among School-Age Mothers, *American Journal of Public Health, 63*:770, 1973.

40. Kennedy, R. E., Jr.: Population, *The Americana Annual,* 1974, *The Americana Annual,* 1975.

41. Kilby-Kelberg, S.: Why Some Won't Try the Diaphragm Method—Why Others Try and Fail, *JOGN Nursing, 4*(2):24, 1975.

42. Kippley, J., and Kippley, S.: *The Art of Natural Family Planning.* Cincinnati, The Couple to Couple League International, Inc., 1975.

43. Kistner, R. W.: The Infertile Woman, *American Journal of Nursing, 73*:1937, 1973.

44. Kuchera, L. K.: Postcoital Contraception with Diethylstilbestrol, *Journal of the American Medical Association, 218*:562, 1971.

45. Legans, J.: Artificial Insemination: Hope for Childless Couples, *JOGN Nursing, 3*(4):25, 1974.

46. Lynch, H. T., Krush, T. P., Krush, A. J., et al.: Psychodynamics of Early Hereditary Deaths, *American Journal of Diseases of Children, 108*:605, 1964.

47. Macintyre, M. N.: Prenatal Chromosome Analysis—A Lifesaving Procedure, *Southern Medical Journal, 64*(Suppl. #1):85, February, 1971.

48. MacLeon, J., and Gold, R. Z.: Male Factor in Fertility and Infertility, *Fertility Sterility, 4*:10, January-February, 1953.

49. Markash, R. E., and Seigel, D. G.: Oral Contraceptives and Mortality Trends in Thromboembolism in the United States, *American Journal of Public Health, 59*:418, 1969.

50. Masters, W. H., and Johnson, V. G.: Contraception and Sexual Pleasure, *Redbook,* May, 1975, 42.

51. McCalister, D., and Thiessen, V.: Prediction in Family Planning, *American Journal of Public Health, 60*:1372, 1970.

52. Mitchell, H. D.: How Do I Talk—Family Planning? *American Journal of Public Health, 56*:738, 1966.

53. Nadler, H. L.: Prenatal Detection of Inborn Errors of Metabolism, *Southern Medical Journal, 64*(Suppl. #1):92, February, 1971.

54. Notestein, F.: Zero Population Growth: What Is It? *Family Planning Perspectives, 2*:20, June, 1970.

55. Omran, A. R.: *The Health Theme in Family Planning.* Chapel Hill, N.C., Carolina Population Center, University of North Carolina, 1970.

56. Osborn, F.: Attitudes and Practices Affecting Fertility, *In* Young, L. B. (ed.): *Population in Perspective.* New York, Oxford University Press, 1968.

57. Page, E., Villee, C. A., and Villee, D. B.: *Human Reproduction.* 2nd Edition. Philadelphia, W. B. Saunders Co., 1972.

58. Peer-level Counselors Play Key Role in Success of N.Y.C. Family Planning, *Hospital Topics,* January, 1971, 85.

59. Pendleton, D.: IUD's: Intrauterine Danger? *Science News, 107*:226, April 5, 1975.

60. Perspectives in Genetic Counseling, *Pediatric Currents, 20*:9, February, 1971.

61. Peterson, W. F.: Pregnancy Following Oral Contraceptive Therapy, *Obstetrics and Gynecology, 34*:363, 1969.

62. Rainwater, L.: *And the Poor Get Children.* Chicago, Quadrangle Books, 1960.

63. Ratner, H.: Child Spacing II, Nature's Subtleties, *Child and Family, 9*:2, 1970.

64. Ratner, H.: Child Spacing III. Nature's Prescription, *Child and Family, 9*:99, 1970.

65. Reed, R. B.: Social and Psychological Factors Affecting Fertility: The Interrelationship of Marital Adjustment, Fertility Control, and Size of Family, *Milbank Memorial Fund Quarterly, 25*:383, 1947.

66. Shapiro, S.: Oral Contraceptives and Myocardial Infarction, *New England Journal of Medicine, 293*(4):195, July 24, 1975.

67. Siegel, E., Scurletis, T. D., Abernathy, J. R., et al: Postneonatal Deaths in North Carolina, 1959–1963, *North Carolina Medical Journal, 27*:366, 1966.

68. Siegel, E., Thomas, D., Coulter, E., et al.: Continuation of Contraception by Low Income Women: A One Year Follow-Up, *American Journal of Public Health, 61*: 1886, 1971.

69. Siegel, E., Thomas, D., and Coulter, E.: Family Planning—Changes in Attitudes and Practices Among Low Income Women Between 1967 and 1970–1971, *American Journal of Public Health, 63*:256, 1973.

70. Spence, J., et al: *A Thousand Families in Newcastle Upon Tyne: An Approach to the Study of Health and Illness in Children.* London, Oxford University Press, 1954.

71. Sterilization on the Rise, *Science News, 108*:58, July 26, 1975.

72. Stycos, J. M., and Back, K. W.: *The Family and Population Control.* Chapel Hill, N.C., The University of North Carolina Press, 1959.

73. Tabah, L., and Raul, S.: Preliminary Findings of a Survey on Fertility and Attitudes Toward Family Formation in Santiago, Chile, *In* Kiser, C. V. (ed.): *Research in Family Planning.* Princeton, Princeton University Press, 1962.

74. Tietze, C., and Lewis, S.: The IUD and Pill: Extended Use—Effectiveness, *Family Planning Perspectives, 3*:53, 1971.

75. Timby, B.: Ovulation Method of Birth Control, *American Journal of Nursing, 76*:928, 1976.

76. Tips, R. L., Smith, G. S., Lynch, H. T., et al: The "Whole Family" Concept in Clinical Genetics, *American Journal of Diseases of Children, 107*:67, 1964.

77. Tyler, C. W., Tillack, W. S., Smith, J. C., et al: Assessment of a Family Planning Program: Contraceptive Services and Fertility in Atlanta, Georgia, *Family Planning Perspectives, 2*:25, March, 1970.

78. Westoff, L. A., and Westoff, C. F.: *From Now to Zero: Fertility, Contraception and Abortion in America.* Boston, Little, Brown and Co., 1971.

79. Wishik, S. M.: The Use of Client Characteristics as Predictors of Utilization of Family Planning Service, *American Journal of Public Health, 60*:1394, 1970.

80. Wolf, S. R., and Ferguson, E. L.: The Physician's Influence on the Nonacceptance of Birth Control, *American Journal of Obstetrics and Gynecology, 104*:752, 1969.

81. *The Womanly Art of Breastfeeding.* Franklin Park, Ill., La Leche League International, 1958.

82. Wrigley, E. A.: *Population and History.* New York, World University Library, 1969.

83. Wynne-Edwards, V. C.: Population Control in Animals, *Scientific American,* August, 1964.

84. Zatvchni, G. E.: *Post-partum Family Planning: A Report on the International Program.* New York, McGraw-Hill Book Co., 1970.

Chapter 6

PHYSIOLOGIC CHANGE FOLLOWING CONCEPTION: MOTHER AND CONCEPTUS

From the moment an ovum is fertilized by a sperm, a pattern of development begins that will result, if all goes well, in the delivery of a healthy infant approximately 266 days later. From the fertilized ovum, or zygote, not only the infant but also the umbilical cord, the fetal membranes, the amniotic fluid, and the fetal portion of the placenta must develop. These products are jointly termed the *conceptus*. Concurrently, changes are taking place in the mother's body to accommodate and support this growing life.

Nurses who care for childbearing families must be aware of both embryologic development and maternal changes. Without an understanding of basic embryology, it is impossible to understand the capabilities and limitations of the term and preterm newborn, the reasons for many congenital malformations, and the rationale for certain practices in maternal care. A knowledge of the development of the conceptus in utero provides answers to questions such as, "I took an airplane trip

when I was 6 months pregnant. Is this why my baby has a congenital heart defect?" We can understand why a viral disease such as rubella will have devastating effects on the first months of pregnancy but may cause only minor problems or no malformation at all late in pregnancy.

A knowledge of the basic concepts of embryologic development and maternal change is also important for nurses who choose other fields of practice—nurses who may be giving medications to women who are pregnant, nurses in venereal disease clinics, nurses who work with adolescent girls who have heart defects, industrial nurses and public health nurses with special concerns for environmental health, and nurses whose friends, neighbors, and relatives will be pregnant.

The period of time during which the baby develops in utero is divided into three divisions, called *trimesters*. The developing conceptus is called an *embryo* until the end of the seventh or eighth week (embryologists vary in their designation) and a *fetus* from that time until birth. Some embryologists designate the first 1 or 2 weeks following conception as the period of the ovum.

The mean length of human pregnancy is 266 days, or 38 weeks, from the time of conception. Approximately 70 per cent of all mothers deliver within 12 days of this period, plus or minus several days (i.e., from 254 to 278 days after conception). Because the exact date of conception usually is not known, the duration of pregnancy is usually calculated from the date of onset of the last menstrual period, the total period being considered as 280 days, or 40 weeks.

The *embryologic age* of the embryo-fetus is dated from the time of conception. *Gestational age* is dated from the time of onset of the last menstrual period. Thus 2 weeks after conception the embryo is 2 weeks old in terms of embryologic age, but the gestational age is 1 month. In the pages that follow the embryo is described in terms of embryologic age. After the period of viability, gestational age may be determined by adding 2 weeks to embryologic age. This aids in understanding the characteristics of the preterm newborn who is the same gestational age.

A common method for estimating the date of delivery, or estimated date of confinement (EDC), is Nägele's rule, in which one counts back 3 months from the *first* day of the last menstrual period and adds 1 year and 7 days. Thus if the last menstrual period (LMP) is March 10, the EDC will be December 17. In the review of the menstrual cycle in Chapter 3 it was noted that there is considerable variation in the length of the proliferative phase of the menstural cycle, one major reason that the EDC is rarely exact.

PRINCIPLES OF GROWTH AND DEVELOPMENT

Growth and development follow very specific patterns in an orderly sequence. Both are part of a continuum that begins at the time of conception and continues for many years after birth.

The development of the embryo-fetus is dependent upon: (1) cell proliferation, (2) growth, (3) differentiation, and (4) integration.

The single fertilized ovum (zygote) divides by mitosis, as do the daughter cells, until trillions of cells are produced. The process of producing two cells from every one cell is so efficient that doubling the number of cells 45 times would result in all the cells needed for a complete individual.

Cell division, per se, does not result in growth. Growth is a result of: (1) the synthesis of protoplasm from amino acids, (2) the intake of water by the cells, and (3) the deposit of nonliving substances, such as fibers and parts of cartilage and bone.

Differentiation includes *morphogenesis,* by which the organs of the body and the body itself take shape, and *histogenesis,* by which the specification of tissues occurs. Changes in form are due to the fact that various regions of the body grow at different rates, both prenatally and postnatally. (See, for example, cephalocaudal development below.) Different structures result as cells migrate to various areas of the body and aggregate, and the resultant tissues fuse, split, fold, and bend.

Induction is the process by which one tissue transmits a stimulus that leads to the development of neighboring tissues. *Competence* is the process by which the adjacent tissue responds to the stimulus. If induction fails, either because of inadequate stimulus or because the tissue to be acted upon does not react properly, an organ may fail to appear *(agenesis)*, may be smaller than normal *(hypoplasia)*, or may be incompletely differentiated. Irregularities in induction can also lead to organ duplication, such as a double kidney, or to abnormal positioning of an organ.

Cells first become specialized and later develop into specialized tissues. In the early stage of differentiation the suffix-*blast* often designates a developing cell (e.g., neuroblast) which will develop into a particular type of cell (such as a nerve cell).

The final stage of development is *integration*, during which organ systems become able to function in a coordinated way. The endocrine glands and the nervous system are the mechanisms for integration.

DEVELOPMENTAL TRENDS

Both embryo-fetal development and development after birth are *cephalocaudal*, that is, they proceed from head to tail. The embryo's head develops more rapidly than the remainder of his body. Development of function, as well as of size, proceeds in a cephalocaudal direction. Thus a baby will raise his head and "reach out" with his eyes before he is able to use his arms and, still later, his legs.

Growth also proceeds from the *medial* aspect of the body to the *lateral* aspects. Thus the trunk develops before the arms and legs, which, in turn, precede the fingers and toes. As with cephalocaudal development, function following birth will also proceed in the same medial-lateral direction. Arms will be used before hands, and it will be many years before a child will be able to use his fingers for activities that require a high degree of precision.

General structures (i.e., arm buds and then arms) precede specific structures (i.e., hands and fingers). Postnatally, as noted, these general structures will be used before the more specific structures. Toys and activities for younger children should be planned with this principle in mind; a large soccer-sized ball is more appropriate for a preschool child than a baseball.

THE FIRST WEEK

Conceptus

Zygote undergoes cleavage as it traverses the uterine tube.

Forms morula, which reaches the uterine cavity in 3 to 4 days, undergoes further change to blastocyst stage.

Zona pellucida disappears about day 6 to 7.

Blastocyst attaches to endometrium, (beginning of implantation), day 6 to 7.

Mother

Vascular changes influenced by progesterone prepare the endometrium for implantation.

Decidual reaction.

The First Week

The ovum is fertilized in the distal third of the uterine tube. During the next 3 to 4 days, it travels to the uterus, probably as a result of muscular peristaltic movement of the tube. The corona radiata disappears, so that the fertilized ovum can pass through the narrow infundibulum of the tube, but the zona pellucida remains until after the ovum reaches the uterine cavity.

During transport, cleavage (mitotic division) begins. The cells that result, called *blastomeres*, first form a ball called a *morula* (Fig. 6–1*A*). After reaching the uterine cavity, the morula begins to change its structure; a cavity filled with fluid forms in the center. The morula is now a *blastocyst* (Fig. 6–1*B*) with two types of cells: larger cells (the inner cell mass) that will form the embryo and smaller trophoblasts from which will develop the fetal portion of the placenta, the amnion and the chorion (see below), and the umbilical cord.

Meanwhile, the endometrium, under the influence of progesterone from the corpus luteum, becomes highly vascular and stores glycogen in preparation for implantation.

On approximately the sixth day the zona pellucida disappears and implantation takes place, that is, the blastocyst attaches itself to the endometrium, commonly at the midposterior or midanterior portion of the fundus, and almost always close to a maternal capillary. Following the attachment of the blastocyst, the *decidual reaction* takes place, i.e., the endometrial stromal cells become large and pale. *Decidua* is the term used to describe the endometrium during pregnancy.

THE SECOND WEEK

Conceptus

Inner cell mass (embryo)—Embryo is a two-layered disc of ectoderm and entoderm, lying between a primitive amniotic cavity and the cavity of the yolk sac.

Trophoblast—Implantation continues; completed about 12. Trophoblast differentiates into *syncytiotrophoblast* (outer layer) and *cytotrophoblast* (Langhans' cells).

Advancing Langhans' cells tap venules and capillaries of endometrium, forming *lacunae* filled with maternal blood, the predecessors of the intervillous spaces, at about 9 to 11 days.

Chorionic gonadotropin produced by syncytiotrophoblast.

Mesoblastic (mesodermal) cells formed from the trophoblast at 11 days, give rise to the *amnion*.

The primary yolk sac develops.

Mother

Decidua engulfs blastocyst.

Chorionic gonadotropin acts on the corpus luteum of pregnancy to main-

A.   Morula

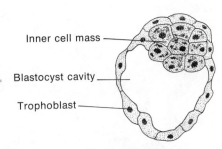

Inner cell mass

Blastocyst cavity

Trophoblast

B.   Blastocyst

Figure 6–1 *A*, The morula is a mass of cells; it resembles a mulberry in shape and contains blastomeres and trophoblast-producing cells. *B*, The blastocyst at approximately 5 days after conception, showing the inner cell mass (larger cells that will form the embryo) and prospective trophoblasts (smaller cells from which the fetal placenta, membranes, and cord will develop).

tain production of estrogen and progesterone and thus prevents the changes that would lead to menstruation.

Human chorionic gonadotropin found in the mother's serum and urine at 10 days; basis of pregnancy tests 2 to 4 weeks after conception.

The Second Week

The endometrium erodes at the point at which the blastocyst has attached itself, and the point of entry is covered by maternal endometrial cells. The area beneath the implanting blastocyst is called the *decidua basalis;* the *decidua capsularis* covers the implanting blastocyst. *Decidua vera* is the term used to describe the remainder of the uterine lining. Once the decidua has engulfed the blastocyst, the blastocyst is no longer in the uterine cavity. The

trophoblastic cells further differentiate and invade the decidua, as noted above and in Figure 6–2.

During the process of implantation, the future embryo has become a two-layered disc, consisting of ectoderm and entoderm. Table 6–1 indicates some of the major systems developing from each of these layers.

The *yolk sac,* which will further develop in the third week, does not store yolk in the human embryo, as it does in some species. Part of the digestive tract will develop from the entodermal roof of the yolk sac. A part of the sac, the proximal end of the yolk stalk, may persist to adulthood as an intestinal pouch (Meckel's diverticulum of the ileum). Some blood cells will be formed in the yolk sac during the third week.

The production of human chorionic gonadotropin by the syncytiotrophoblast is the basis of pregnancy testing.

Figure 6–2 Stages of implantation. *A,* The blastocyst approaches the endometrium; *B,* begins to erode the epithelium; and *C* and *D,* is progressively buried within the decidua.

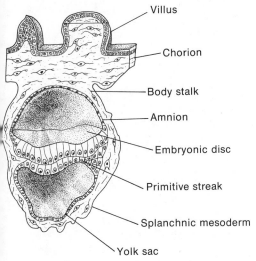

Villus

Chorion

Body stalk

Amnion

Embryonic disc

Primitive streak

Splanchnic mesoderm

Yolk sac

Figure 6–3   The right half of a human embryo of 14 days.

THE THIRD WEEK

Embryo

Embryonic disc becomes pear-shaped and then slipper-shaped (Fig. 6–4).
Primitive streak and primitive node (head process) develop.
Mesoderm develops between ectoderm and entoderm.
Cloacal membrane formed at caudal end of primitive streak.
Neural plate, neural groove, and foregut develop.
Supporting structures:
Amnion continues to develop.
Body stalk connects caudal end of embryo with the chorion.
Primary and secondary villi, and then tertiary villi, form.
Umbilical vessels forming in body stalk; blood vessels in villi, chorion, and yolk sac.
Circulation established between embryo and developing placenta.

Mother

Menstruation would have occurred during this week.

The Third Week

The embryo now has three layers of cells (ectoderm, entoderm, and mesoderm) and is divided precisely into right and left halves by the *primitive streak*. The ground work for the developing organ systems is thus established because from these three germ layers all of the systems will develop (Table 6–1). During the early stages of development, each germ layer has the potential for a variety of types of development. Cells differentiate first chemically and then physically by means of induction and competence, as already described.

The chorionic villi begin to resemble branching trees. At the placental site the chorion is called the *chorion frondosum* (i.e., leafy) and becomes the fetal component of the placenta (Fig. 6–5). As the developing embryo grows, the remainder of the chorion, which becomes the outer layer of the fetal membranes, is pushed against the wall of the uterus and its villi atrophy by the seventh week; it is then called the *chorion laeve* (smooth).

The missed menstrual period during this week is the sign that women most frequently associate with pregnancy. Because a single delayed or apparently missed menstrual period may be associated with a number of other circumstances, it is regarded as a presumptive factor. For example, amenorrhea may be caused by anemia, a debilitating disease such as tuberculosis, an endocrine disorder, strong emotional influences including a fear of pregnancy, and even by changes in climate or environment that a woman might encounter on vacation. Menstrual disturbances and other signs of pregnancy, such as breast changes, also occur in pseudocyesis, a condition in which a woman believes she is pregnant even though she is not. Pseudo-

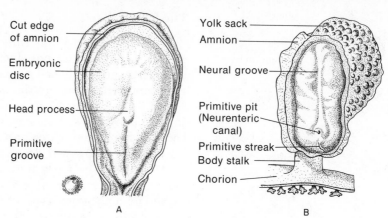

Figure 6–4 Human embryo viewed from above; *A,* at 18 days and *B,* at 19 days. (After Arey: *Developmental Anatomy: A Textbook and Laboratory Manual of Embryology.* Philadelphia, W. B. Saunders Co., 1974.)

pregnancy is usually the result of either an intense desire to be pregnant or an intense fear of pregnancy. When pseudocyesis is diagnosed, the woman should receive emotional counseling as well as physical care.

Another reason that cessation of menstruation is not considered a positive sign of pregnancy is the fact that vaginal bleeding, difficult to distinguish from menstruation, may occur following conception. Three of the many possible causes are cervical erosion, polyps, and threatened abortion. One of the reasons for difficulty in establishing the EDC is postconception bleeding.

Pregnancy may also occur in a woman with amenorrhea. The breast-feeding mother, for example, may conceive before she has her first menstrual period following delivery. Perimenopausal women may have amenorrhea for several months and therefore suspect that they have

Table 6–1 THE GERM-LAYER ORIGIN OF HUMAN TISSUES*

Ectoderm	Mesoderm (including mesenchyme)	Entoderm
1. Epidermis, including: Cutaneous glands. Hair; nails; lens. 2. Epithelium of: Sense organs. Nasal cavity; sinuses. Mouth, including: Oral glands; enamel. Anal canal. 3. Nervous tissue, including: Hypophysis. Chromaffin tissue.	1. Muscle (all types). 2. Connective tissue; cartilage; bone; notochord. 3. Blood; bone marrow. 4. Lymphoid tissue. Epithelium of: 5. Blood vessels; lymphatics. 6. Body cavities. 7. Kidney; ureter. 8. Gonads; genital ducts. 9. Suprarenal cortex. 10. Joint cavities, etc.	Epithelium of: 1. Pharynx, including: Root of tongue. Auditory tube, etc. Tonsils; thyroid. Parathyroids; thymus. 2. Larynx; trachea; lungs. 3. Digestive tube, including: Associated glands. 4. Bladder. 5. Vagina (all?); vestibule. 6. Urethra, including: Associated glands.

*From Arey: *Developmental Anatomy.* Revised 7th Edition. Philadelphia, W. B. Saunders Co., 1974.

Chorionic villus

Chorion frondosum

Chorion laeve

A   B

Figure 6–5 *A*, Human chorionic vesicle at 9 weeks, showing the chorion leave (smooth chorion) and the chorion frondosum, which will become the fetal component of the placenta. *B* shows a single chorionic villus. (After Arey: *Developmental Anatomy: A Textbook and Laboratory Manual of Embryology*. Philadelphia, W. B. Saunders Co., 1974.)

reached menopause—only to find themselves pregnant. Some healthy women have such irregular menstrual periods throughout their lives that it is difficult for them to know when a period is missed.

THE FOURTH WEEK

Embryo

Grows from 2 mm. (0.08 inch) in length (crown to rump) at beginning of week to 5 mm. (0.2 inch) at end of week.
Body becomes cylindrical, flexed, and C-shaped.
Organs develop rapidly:
Heart tube fuses at 22 days and begins to beat at 24 days; blood circulates through fetus and chorionic villi.
Anterior end of neural tube closes to form brain; posterior end closes to form spinal cord.
Pronephros (forekidney) and mesonephros (midkidney) develop.
Esophagotracheal septum has begun to divide esophagus and trachea.

Sense organs indicated.
Limb buds present.
Primitive jaws present (as branchial arches).
Somites develop
Yolk sac begins to diminish in size.
Supporting structures:
Chorionic villi develop into an early placenta.
Chorionic sac is 20 mm. (0.8 inch) or slightly larger in diameter.

Mother

Early breast changes may be noticed.

The Fourth Week

The fourth week has been called the period of the embryo with *somites*. Somites are primitive segments that lie in pairs next to the spinal cord. The three somites that are present at 21 days become a total of 42 during the fourth week. A muscle mass, supplied by a spinal nerve, primitive kidney tubules, and blood vessels that arise from the aorta, develops in relation to each somite. Each pair of somites will collaborate to produce a vertebra. Somites first appear in the region of the head, consistent with the principle of cephalocaudal development.

The fourth week is tremendously significant in the embryo's development. During these 7 days he changes from a relatively simple disc to a complex organism (Fig. 6–6). The body becomes curved because the neural tube grows more rapidly than the ventral surface.

The potential for several anomalies dates to this week. If the anterior end of the neural tube fails to close, *anencephaly* (absence of cranial vault) results. If the posterior end fails to close, meningocele develops. Should the esophagotracheal septum fail to develop properly, the baby will have a *tracheoesophageal fistula.*

Aside from the missed menstrual period, the first physical changes that the mother may notice during the fourth week are in her breasts, which may be sensitive as they begin to enlarge. In subsequent weeks nipples also will enlarge and become erectile, and the areolar area will darken. The sebaceous glands of the areola, called Montgomery's follicles, hypertrophy. Beneath the skin of the breasts, bluish veins may be traced. Breast changes are most obvious during first pregnancies.

FIFTH THROUGH SEVENTH WEEKS

Embryo

Crown-rump length 8 mm. (0.3 inch) at 5 weeks; 12 mm. (0.5 inch) at 6 weeks, 18 mm. (0.75 inch) at 7 weeks.
Five regions develop in brain.
Five main bronchi develop in lung.
Diaphragm separates abdominal and thoracic cavities.

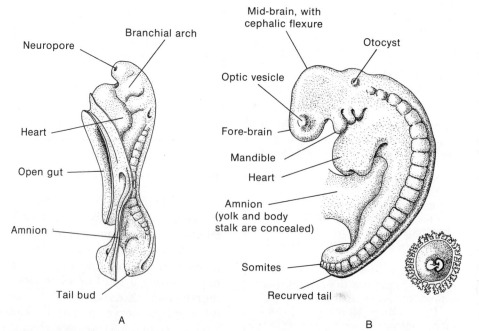

A

B

Figure 6–6 *A,* The human embryo at 24 days. *B,* The human embryo at 26 days. The heart begins beating on the 24th day. (After Arey: *Developmental Anatomy: A Textbook and Laboratory Manual of Embryology.* Philadelphia, W. B. Saunders Co., 1974.)

Hepatic buds and ducts form.

Exterior heart formation essentially same as at birth; valves and septa form in the seventh week.

A portion of the intestinal loop enters the cavity of the umbilical cord.

Metanephros (hindkidney) begins to develop.

Urorectal septum and anal canal develop.

Wrist and elbow develop at 32 to 34 days.

Face develops: definite eye and nostril; pigment in eye at 34 to 36 days.

Palate developing; upper lip formed.

External genitalia appear, but sex cannot be determined from their appearance. Internal gonads begin to differentiate.

Supporting structures:

Umbilical cord organizes.

Trophoblast invades spiral arteries; cotyledons form; beginnings of maternal-placental circulation.

Human placental lactogen can be detected.

Mother

Hegar's sign.

Goodell's sign.

Nausea present in some women.

Mucous plug.

Corpus luteum may begin to regress.

Fifth Through Seventh Weeks

These weeks complete the period of the embryo. By the seventh week the beginnings of all the essential external and internal structures are present. Most major structural abnormalities will have occurred, although it is only 6 weeks after the first missed menstrual period (Fig. 6–7). Note that a portion of the intestines is outside the abdominal cavity, which is too small at this stage to contain the rapidly growing intestinal tract. Normally the intestines will return to the abdomen in the tenth week. Should they continue to remain outside, the baby may be born with an *oom-phalocele* (a defect in the abdominal wall) or *gastroschisis* (a defect at the base of the umbilical stalk).

Deformities such as cleft lip and cleft palate occur during these weeks. Most congenital anomalies of the heart will have occurred before the end of the seventh week. If the diaphragm does not form correctly, the baby will have a *diaphragmatic hernia.*

The third and permanent kidney begins to develop early in the fifth week. Urine is first formed about the seventh to eighth week and from that time on throughout fetal life. Urine mixes with amniotic fluid, which the fetus drinks. Thus in the absence of fetal kidneys (renal agenesis) or in certain other abnormalities of the fetal urinary tract, the mother may have a decreased amount of amniotic fluid (oligohydramnios). However, since the placenta assumes the function of the fetal kidney during pregnancy, it is only during the perinatal period that the baby with a kidney abnormality experiences difficulty.

Imperforate anus, related to abnormal development of the urorectal septum, dates to the sixth or seventh week.

During the sixth week, the placenta is developing to the stage at which maternal placental circulation can take place. Each mainstem villus of the chorion develops into a lobule, called a *cotyledon,* divided from other cotyledons by *septa* (sheets of tissue) (Fig. 6–8). Within each cotyledon are blood vessels. At this time there are from 15 to 30 cotyledons; the mature placenta will contain about 200. The chorionic membrane in the placental area is called the *chorionic plate.*

Surrounding the cotyledons is the intervillous space, filled with maternal blood that comes from about 200 arterioles in the decidua basalis. The intervillous space is drained by collecting

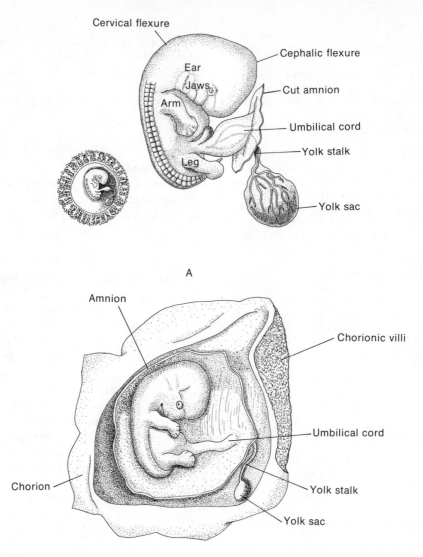

Figure 6–7 The human embryo. *A,* At 6 weeks and *B,* at 7 weeks. (After Arey: *Developmental Anatomy: A Textbook and Laboratory Manual of Embryology.* Philadelphia, W. B. Saunders Co., 1974.)

veins. Maternal blood flow at this stage is sluggish.

The umbilical cord is usually inserted near the middle of the fetal aspect of the placenta. The cord contains two umbilical arteries, which carry wastes from the fetus to the placenta, and one umbilical vein, which carries nourishment from the placenta to the fetus. When the cord is inspected at the time of birth, it may contain a single artery rather than two. The baby should then be inspected carefully, since there is a higher risk of anomalies in infants with a single umbilical artery.

Production of human placental lactogen is evident by the sixth week and continues to rise throughout pregnancy (Table 6–2).

As the placenta continues to de-

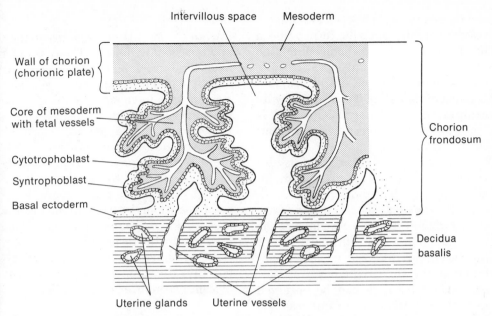

Figure 6–8 Cross section (diagram) of the human placenta. (After Arey: *Developmental Anatomy: A Textbook and Laboratory Manual of Embryology.* Philadelphia, W. B. Saunders Co., 1974.)

velop, maternal blood supply to the pelvis increases. This results in two changes that may be observed about the sixth week.

Hegar's sign is considered the most reliable sign of pregnancy during the first trimester. The isthmus of the lower uterine segment becomes softened and

Table 6–2   SUMMARY OF PLACENTAL FUNCTION

Function	Substances Involved	Comment
I. Nutrition	Oxygen Glucose Protein Fat Water Vitamins and minerals Electrolytes	
II. Elimination of waste	Breakdown products of fetal metabolism → mother's kidneys and lungs	
III. Antibody transfer	Immunoglobulin-G (IgG) transferred from mother to fetus	Fetus immune only to IgG organisms to which mother is immune
IV. Hormone production	Human chorionic gonadotropin	Early maintenance of corpus luteum
	Estrogens and progestins	Placenta major source of estrogens and progestins after second month
	Human placental lactogen (human chorionic somatomammotropin)	Promotes growth
	Human chorionic thyrotropin	

can be compressed between two fingers inserted in the anterior fornix and a hand placed on the abdomen behind the uterus (Fig. 6–9). In multiparas Hegar's sign appears about the sixth week; it is noted approximately 8 weeks following conception in primagravidas and is most fully developed in all women about the tenth week.

Softening of the cervix, along with succulence of the vagina and an increase of leukorrheal discharge, is called *Goodell's sign.* Goodell stated that if the cervix felt like the cartilage of the nose, pregnancy was unlikely, but if the cervix felt like the mucous membrane of the lip, pregnancy was possible. Goodell's sign can be observed as early as 6 weeks in primiparas and even earlier in some multiparas. Thick mucus fills the cervical canal, becoming a *mucous plug,* which will remain in place until the time of labor.

Because other conditions can result in findings similar to those of Hegar and Goodell, they are considered probable signs of pregnancy but not positive signs.

Some women experience nausea, either in the morning or at some other time during the day, from about the fifth to the twelfth week of pregnancy, and occasionally longer. The reason for nausea is uncertain, but by no means is every pregnant woman nauseated. Some women will have nausea during one pregnancy and not at all during another. In some societies apparently no pregnant women have nausea.

The *corpus luteum* may begin to regress as early as the sixth week, although well-developed corpora lutea have been found at term. During the first weeks of pregnancy progesterone produced by the corpus luteum is essential for the maintenance of pregnancy, but this function is assumed by the placenta soon after implantation.

EIGHTH THROUGH TWELFTH WEEKS

Fetus

At twelve weeks weighs 14 grams (1/2 ounce) and is 7 cm. (2.75 inches crown to heel).
Head 1/3 of total length.
Fetal movements begin at about 8 weeks.

Figure 6–9 Detecting Hegar's sign. The softened isthmus of the uterus is easily compressed between the hand placed on the abdomen and the fingers inserted in the vagina anterior to the cervix.

Thin skin develops.

Bones developing.

External genitalia become distinctively male or female in third month.

Eyelids develop and fuse.

Fingers and toes begin nail growth.

Liver becomes major producer of red blood cells.

Intestine returns to abdomen.

Supporting structures:

Placenta continues to grow; high maternal blood pressure (40 to 60 mm. Hg) in central intervillous spaces.

Amnion fills the chorionic cavity.

Chorion almost fills the uterine cavity.

Amnion and chorion remain in contact for the remainder of pregnancy.

Mother

Chadwick's sign.

Cardiovascular changes.

Basal metabolism falls.

Blood sugar low.

Increased salivation; mouth secretions acid.

Ureters and renal pelves begin to dilate about tenth week.

Enlarging anteflexed uterus rises above pelvic brim.

Fetal heart tones heard by ultrasound by 10 to 12 weeks (Chapter 10).

Weight gain for first trimester: 2 pounds (1 kg.).

Eighth Through Twelfth Weeks

Beginning in the eighth week the embryo is considered a fetus. He is now a recognizable human being (Fig. 6–10). In contrast to the embryonic period in which new structures are continually developing, the fetal period is primarily a time of growth and maturation. Because of this the fetus is less at risk than the embryo to many teratogens (below).

The crown-rump length more than doubles between the eighth and twelfth weeks, but head growth slows down, so that at twelve weeks the head represents only one-third of the total body length, rather than half.

The greatest noticeable change in the fetus is in the external genitalia. Until the end of the ninth week, the external reproductive organs of both males and females, which develop from analogous structures (Fig. 6–11), appear similar. Distinctive external genitalia are not present until the twelfth week.

In the mother enlarged blood vessels increase the blood supply of the vagina, which results in *Chadwick's sign,* a deep red-to-purple coloration of the vaginal mucosa. Other vaginal changes that are preparatory for vaginal distention at the time of delivery include muscle hypertrophy, mucosal thickening, and a loosening of connective tissue. Vaginal discharge becomes thicker and more profuse and is usually white to yellowish in color and crumbly in consistency. Because of an increased lactic acid content, this secretion is believed to help resist pathogens; douching will interfere with this protection. A douche should only be used during pregnancy when it it specifically prescribed.

During the third month the uterus rises out of the pelvis to become an abdominal organ. Note how the anteflexed uterus compresses the bladder (Fig. 6–12). The fundus is about midway between the symphysis pubis and the umbilicus at the end of the third month of gestation (Chapter 8).

Early dilatation of the ureters and the renal pelves is probably caused by hormones, although changes later in pregnancy are undoubtedly influenced by mechanical factors as well, since late dilatation is greater on the right, the side to which the uterus rotates late in pregnancy. Because of this dilatation, from three to four times more urine is contained in the "dead space" of the ureters and pelves than normally, re-

Figure 6-10 Eight week old embryo. (From Moore: *The Developing Human: Clinically Oriented Embryology*. 1st Edition. Philadelphia, W. B. Saunders Co., 1973.)

sulting in delayed flow and an increased susceptibility to urinary tract infection.

THIRTEENTH THROUGH
SIXTEENTH WEEKS

Fetus

A period of very rapid growth; at 16 weeks weighs 120 grams (4 ounces) and length is approximately 15 cm. (6 inches).

Period of rapid growth in the number of neurons in the brain.

Ossification widespread; evident on X-ray by 16 weeks.

Meconium present in intestines.

Lanugo growing on body; hair growing on head.

Fetus can suck thumb, swallow, make respiratory movements, protrude upper lip on stimulation, and has grasp reflex.

Mother

Desirable weight gain: 3/4 to 1 pound per week (0.34 to 0.45 kg.).

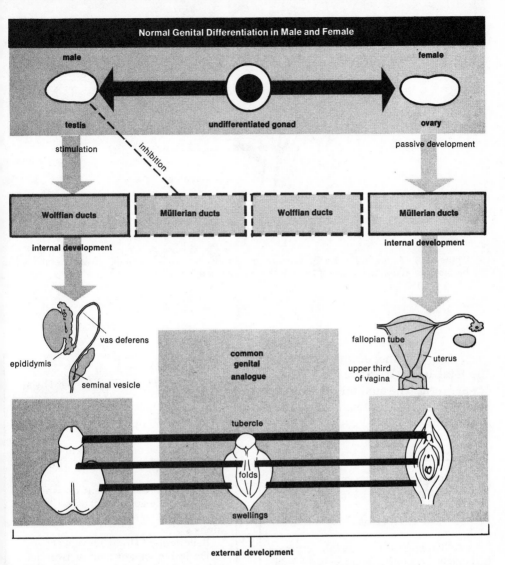

Figure 6–11 Normal genital differentiation in male and female. (From Hill: *AJN*, *9*:811, 1977. Copyright May, 1977, The American Journal of Nursing Co. Reproduced with permission from the *American Journal of Nursing*, Vol. 77, No. 5.)

Thirteenth Through Sixteenth Weeks

In relation to the individual's future potential, the period of the thirteenth to sixteenth week is highly significant, for it is the time when the number of neurons is increasing most rapidly. Insults during this period (rubella, for example) would limit neuronal development and hence intellectual capacity.

Meconium begins to be present in the intestines, where it will remain, under ordinary circumstances, until birth when it forms the first stools (Chapter 16). Meconium in the amniotic fluid is a sign of fetal distress.

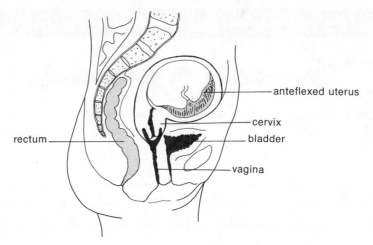

Figure 6–12 At the end of the third month, the corpus of the enlarged uterus rises out of the pelvis and becomes an abdominal organ. Note the sharp anteflexion of the uterus.

Lanugo, a fine, downy hair, covers the fetal body. It gradually decreases toward term. The amount of lanugo present at birth is one useful measure of gestational age.

SEVENTEENTH THROUGH
TWENTIETH WEEKS

Fetus

At 20 weeks the fetus weighs approximately 460 grams (8 ounces) and is 25 cm. (10 inches) long.

Lower limbs reach final relative proportions.

Bone marrow becomes increasingly important in blood formation.

Iron deposits begin to be stored.

Vernix caseosa begins to form.

More frequent and stronger movements.

Enamel and dentine for teeth deposited.

Eyelashes and eyebrows forming.

Brown fat begins to be formed.

Myelinization of the spinal cord begins.

Mother

Fetal heart tones may be heard by an examiner.

Fetal movements may be felt by an examiner and by the mother (quickening).

Fundus reaches the level of the umbilicus at approximately the fifth month.

Lower uterine segment drawn into body; anteflexion disappears.

Skin changes (see following sections).

Ballottement (16 to 32 weeks).

Desirable weight gain at twentieth week: approximately 8 pounds (3.75 kg.).

Seventeenth Through Twentieth Weeks

In the fetus the storage of iron during pregnancy is important for the subsequent well-being of the baby. Since most iron storage occurs after the twentieth week, it is not difficult to understand that the baby of low gestational age will have limited iron stores and a high risk of developing iron deficiency anemia. Preterm babies usually receive supplemental iron at some time during the first year. Another factor limiting iron stores is maternal intake, which usually must be supplemented during the second half of pregnancy (Chapter 9).

Vernix caseosa is a material that looks a little like white cheese. It is formed from the fatty secretions of the fetal sebaceous glands and dead epidermal cells. Vernix caseosa covers much of the skin during the second half of pregnancy and is thought to have a protective function. It can be seen on the baby at the time of birth (Chapter 16).

Brown fat is fatty tissue found principally on the back of the neck, behind the sternum, and around the kidneys, the subclavian area, and the carotids. Brown fat plays a role in newborn heat production (Chapter 15).

For the mother this period, approximately the midpoint of pregnancy, is the time during which pregnancy may be positively confirmed by the fetal heart tones heard and fetal movements felt by the examiner. Mothers are also becoming aware of fetal movement, a phenomenon called *quickening,* a term dating from the time when the word "quick" meant living. Thus the pregnancy, nearly halfway complete, is now confirmed both by others and by the mother herself.

Fetal heart tones are heard by the nonamplified stethoscope between 16 and 20 weeks of pregnancy. With ultrasonic auscultation, sounds may be heard as early as 10 to 12 weeks. Fetal heart sounds have been described as resembling the rapid "tick-tock of a watch heard through a pillow."[4] The "tick," representing systole of the fetal heart, is followed by a short pause and then by the "tock," which is the sound of the

closure of the valves in the fetal heart. The normal range of the fetal heart rate is from 120 to 160 beats per minute. If the rate heard is considerably lower, it may be the maternal heart rate instead; this can be ascertained by simultaneously checking the maternal pulse. Although rates outside of this range may indicate fetal distress, increased rates may also be related to fetal movement, palpation of the fetus, maternal fever, or to no specific cause. Pressure on the fetal skull leads to a decreased rate, a fact that becomes important during labor.

The best site for hearing fetal heart tones in the sixteenth to twentieth weeks is at the midline on the edge of the pubic hair. As the fetus becomes larger and his outline is palpable, heart sounds are heard best through the fetal back. Many nurses prefer to use a fetoscope (Fig. 6–13) because the sound of fingers holding the traditional stethoscope is eliminated.

Two sounds other than fetal heart rate and maternal heart rate may be heard: fetal (funic) souffle and uterine souffle. The fetal souffle is caused by the

Figure 6–13   The fetoscope allows the examiner to hear fetal heart tones through air and bone conduction while eliminating the noise of the examiner's finger holding a stethoscope.

rush of blood through the umbilical arteries and is synchronous with *fetal* heart sounds. Uterine souffle is a soft, blowing sound, synchronous with the *maternal* pulse, caused by blood flowing through the large arteries at the sides of the uterus. If the uterine souffle is sufficiently loud, it may be difficult to hear fetal heart tones. Other obstacles to auscultation are excessive amniotic fluid, external noise, and the location of the placenta on the anterior wall of the uterus.

The shape of the uterus continues to change during the fifth month. By the twentieth week anteflexion disappears, relieving the pressure on the bladder and thereby relieving urinary frequency for the next months. (Frequency returns late in pregnancy, as the large uterus again encroaches on the bladder space.)

Ballottement is a sign elicited when the examiner places two fingers in the mother's vagina and gives the fetus a gentle push (Fig. 6–14). The fetus is felt leaving and returning to the examiner's fingers; he bounces in the amniotic fluid like a beach ball in a swimming pool. Prior to 16 weeks the fetus is too small for ballottement; after 32 weeks he is too large in relation to the amount of amniotic fluid.

TWENTY-FIRST THROUGH TWENTY-FOURTH WEEKS

Fetus

At 24 weeks, weight is 720 to 960 grams (1½ to 2 pounds); length is 30 cm. (12 inches).

Alveolar cells beginning to make surfactant at about 24 weeks.

Skin pink to red because of visibility of blood in capillaries.

Primordia of permanent teeth begin to develop.

Nostrils reopen.

IgG levels rise, reaching maternal values at about 24 weeks.

Mother

Desirable weight gain: from 1/2 to 3/4 pound per week (0.24 to 0.34 kg.).

Twenty-first Through Twenty-fourth Weeks

The fetus' lungs come closer to the point at which survival following birth will be a possibility with the beginning of surfactant production (see section below).

Levels of IgG, the only immuno-

Figure 6–14 Eliciting ballottement. The fetal head or breech is pushed gently; it is felt moving away and quickly returning to the fingers. In short, the fetus "bounces."

globulin produced by the fetus under normal conditions, will protect the fetus and newborn from those diseases for which his mother has immunity. Included are most blood-borne viruses, bacteria, parasites, and fungi. The IgM molecule is too large to cross the placenta; when IgM is found in the newborn, it is considered to be the response of the fetus to intrauterine infection.

TWENTY-FIFTH THROUGH THIRTY-SECOND WEEKS

Fetus

Approximately 35 cm. (14 inches) and 1200 grams (2½ pounds) at 28 weeks; 40 cm. (16 inches) and 1900 grams (4 pounds) at 32 weeks.

Bone marrow becomes a major site of blood formation (28 weeks).

Subcutaneous fat minimal.

Moro's reflex at 30 weeks.

Alveoli appear in lungs; capillaries proliferate around alveoli; gas exchange possible at about 28 weeks.

If born, one in ten fetuses viable at 28 weeks gestational age; one in three viable at 32 weeks gestational age.

Glial cell formation and myelinization of brain.

Mother

Desirable weight gain: from 1/2 to 3/4 pound per week (0.24 to 0.34 kg.)

Fundus halfway between umbilicus and ensiform process at 7 months gestational age; three-fourths of the way at 8 months gestational age.

Striae gravidarum may develop.

Increased pigmentation may develop.

Twenty-fifth Through Thirty-second Weeks

The exchange of gases (oxygen and carbon dioxide) is not possible until: (1)

alveoli develop and (2) capillaries develop around the alveoli. This occurs at approximately 28 weeks, although it may be accelerated by stress, or delayed, as in the infant of a diabetic mother (Chapter 18).

A second stage of brain development, beginning about the twenty-eighth week and lasting into the year following birth, involves glial cell formation and myelinization. Poor nutrition, either prenatally or following delivery, during this period may result in learning disabilities, poor hand-eye coordination, and similar problems.

Mothers may note several skin changes in the third trimester. Red, slightly depressed streak marks on the abdomen and occasionally on the breasts, called *striae gravidarum,* occur in approximately half of all pregnant women. Within a few months following delivery, the marks will become silvery in color, but they will not entirely disappear.

Increased pigmentation also occurs along the *linea alba,* which is then termed the *linea nigra;* the vulva; and the face (the latter termed *chloasma,* the mask of pregnancy). Chloasma, usually most pronounced in Caucasian brunettes, is often aggravated by exposure to the sun. Protecting the face from the sun may make it less noticeable. A change of cosmetics will also be helpful, as will the assurance that changes in facial pigmentation will not persist after delivery.

THIRTY-THIRD THROUGH THIRTY-EIGHTH WEEKS

Fetus

Approximately 45 cm. (18 inches) and 2900 grams (6 pounds) at 36 weeks; 50 cm. (20 inches) and 3350 grams (7 pounds) at 38 weeks.

Viable.

Flexed limbs; well-developed muscle tone.

Testes descend at 36 weeks.

Lanugo mostly disappearing.

Pulmonary branching about two-thirds complete.

Placenta:

Cellular growth ceases at about 34 weeks.

Placenta at term weighs about 500 grams (approximately 1 pound); is 1/6 weight of fetus.

Mother

Fundus reaches level of ensiform process at about 32 weeks gestational age.

Lightening may occur about 36 weeks after conception (38 weeks gestational age).

Desirable weight gain: from 1/2 to 3/4 pound per week (0.24 to 0.34 kg.).

Thirty-third Through Thirty-eighth Weeks

Babies born during these weeks are potentially viable, although development continues for many years. Newborn characteristics and the significance of these characteristics in assessing gestational age are described in Chapter 15.

Lightening describes the descent of the uterus when the baby's presenting part (i.e., the part that will deliver first, most frequently the head) becomes fixed in the pelvis. Because lightening is more frequent in women who have good abdominal muscle tone, it is more likely to occur in primiparas, usually 1 to 2 weeks before labor begins. Many multiparas and some primiparas never experience lightening until after labor begins. Following lightening, the fundus

is approximately at the height it reached during the eighth month, about three-quarters of the distance between the umbilicus and the ensiform process. Abdominal contour changes, with the lower abdomen becoming more prominent. A mother finds that she breathes more easily, a welcomed sign, but pressure can cause frequent voiding and leg cramps. Walking may be more difficult.

Figure 6–15 summarizes the development of the embryo-fetus and Table 6–3 summarizes the signs of pregnancy.

HAZARDS TO THE DEVELOPING EMBRYO-FETUS

Developing within the mother's uterus, the embryo-fetus is not in safe and secure isolation, as was once supposed. He is, in fact, subject to a variety of hazards. Some are a result of conditions within his mother; maternal diabetes is an example. Some are a result of substances taken into his mother's body and subsequently transferred to his own, such as certain medications. Still others are a part of his mother's own external environment—a virus that she may have contracted or a chemical that may be present in the air she breathes or in her water supply.

Some of these hazards, such as radiation and the ingestion of certain drugs, can be controlled to a large degree. Others, such as some maternal infections, may pass unnoticed during pregnancy and be recognized only in retrospect, following the birth of a child who is not normal.

Teratogen is the term used to describe any environmental factor, chemical or physical, that affects the embryo-fetus adversely. Either too

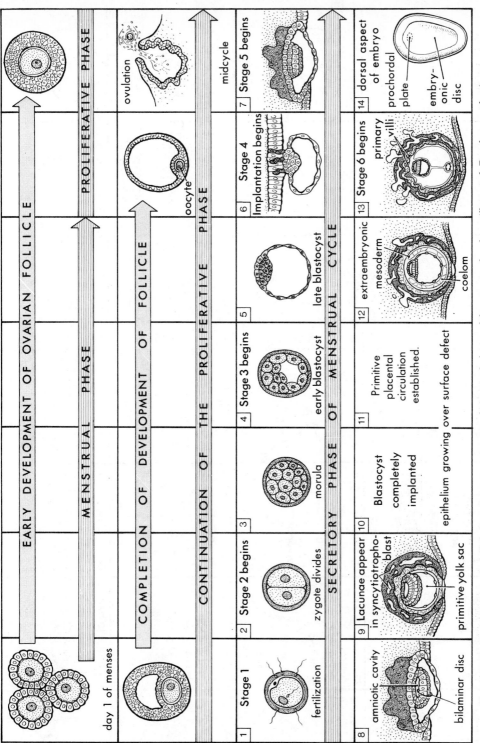

Figure 6–15 Development of a follicle containing an oocyte, ovulation, and phases of the menstrual cycle are illustrated. Development begins at fertilization, about 14 days after the onset of the last menstruation. Cleavage of the zygote in the uterine tube, implantation of the blastocyst, and early development of the embryo are also shown. The main features of the developmental stages in human embryos are illustrated. (From Moore: *The Developing Human: Clinically Oriented Embryology*. 2nd Edition. Philadelphia, W. B. Saunders Co., 1977.)

TIMETABLE OF HUMAN PRENATAL DEVELOPMENT
1 to 6 weeks

3

15 first missed menstrual period	16 Stage 7 begins	17 intra-embryonic mesoderm	18 Stage 8 begins	19	20 Stage 9 begins	21
primitive streak	notochordal process	trilaminar embryo	neural plate / primitive streak	neural fold / notochord / embryonic coelom	brain / neural groove / somite	neural groove / somite
			length: 1.5 mm		Thyroid begins to develop.	Heart tubes begin to fuse.

4

22 Stage 10 begins	23	24 Stage 11 begins	25	26 Stage 12 begins	27	28 Stage 13 begins
Heart begins to beat	rostral neuropore / primordia of eye and ear present. / caudal neuropore	heart bulge / rostral neuropore closes	otic pit / 3 pairs of branchial arches	arm bud	4 pairs of branchial arches, arm & leg buds present.	CR: 4.0 mm
Neural folds fusing.		2 pairs of branchial arches		indicates actual size	CR = crown-rump length.	

5

| 29 | 30 | 31 | 32 Stage 14 | 33 Stage 15 begins | 34 | 35 |
| CR: 5.0 mm | Lens pits, optic cups, nasal pits forming. | developing eye / nasal pit / primitive mouth | Hand plates (paddle-shaped) / Lens pits and optic cups formed. | hand plate / CR: 7.0 mm | Head much larger relative to trunk. / cerebral vesicles distinct / leg buds (paddle-shaped) | CR: 8.0 mm |

6

| 36 | 37 Stage 16 begins | 38 | 39 | 40 | 41 Stage 17 begins | 42 |
| Oral & nasal cavities confluent | foot plate | Upper lip formed. | CR: 10.0 mm | Arms bent at elbow. / Finger rays and auricular hillocks distinct / Palate developing. | finger rays | |

184

Figure 6–15 *Continued.*

Table 6–3 SIGNS OF PREGNANCY

Sign	When Appears	Basis	Other Possible Causes
	PRESUMPTIVE SIGNS		
Amenorrhea	Approximately 2 weeks after conception	Endometrium retained	Hormonal imbalance, emotional factors; Physical disease
Breast changes	As early as fourth week	Development of duct system; hormonal	Hormonal; not as valuable in multiparas
Nausea	Second and third months, primarily	Uncertain. Related factors may be reverse peristalsis, decreased gastrointestinal motility, decreased carbohydrate levels, psychosocial influences	
Quickening	16 to 20 weeks	Movements of fetus	Intestinal activity may stimulate fetal movement, especially in nulliparous women very desirous of child
Chadwick's sign	8 to 12 weeks	Increased vascularity of pelvic organs	Any cause of pelvic congestion
Urinary frequency	6 to 12 weeks	Enlarging uterus	Urinary tract infection; emotional factors
Sleepiness, fatigue	First trimester		Many possible reasons

much or too little of almost any physical or chemical agent can have a teratogenic effect on mammals of some species. However, not every agent that affects one species or even one subspecies will necessarily affect a different species in the same way or even in a way that is harmful. This means that there are limits to what we can learn about the effects of teratogens on humans from animal research. A substance may prove teratogenic in some animal studies but be safe for humans. Perhaps even more important, a substance may appear safe in animal studies yet prove deleterious to human embryos. An example of the latter is the drug thalidomide, which did not harm embryos in animal studies but produced phocomelia (malformed limbs) in human infants (Fig. 6–16). On the other hand dilantin has caused cleft palate in mice, and cortisone has caused both cleft palate and cardiac defects in mice and rabbits, but no human association has been demonstrated.

Timing is important in the way in which a teratogen may affect the embryo. A teratogen that comes in contact with the embryo during the third to eighth week of development, the period during which major organ systems are

Table 6–3   SIGNS OF PREGNANCY (*Continued*)

Sign	When Appears	Basis	Other Possible Causes
PROBABLE SIGNS			
Enlarged uterus		Growing fetus	Tumor; ascites
Hegar's sign		Hyperemia of pelvis	
Braxton Hicks contractions	From as early as 8 weeks throughout pregnancy	Normal uterine contractions	Hematomas; myomas
Ballottement	From 16 to 32 weeks	Fetus in amniotic fluid	
Palpation of fetal outline			Myomas, occasionally
Laboratory tests	7 to 14 days	Presence of human chorionic gonadotropin	
Goodell's sign	By the sixth week; may be earlier in multigravida	Pelvic congestion	Other causes of pelvic congestion
POSITIVE SIGNS			
Fetal movement felt by examiner	About 20 weeks		
Fetal heart heard by examiner	Doppler: 10 to 12 weeks; stethoscope: 16 to 20 weeks		
Fetal outline seen on X-ray or sonography			

being formed, will usually have a more devastating effect than the same substance introduced in the third trimester (Fig. 6–17). However, certain teratogens can affect the fetus even late in pregnancy; syphilis is an example of a disease that can cause late malformations in previously normally developed organs.

Certain teratogens appear to have a predilection for specific organs or systems, while others are more general in their action. Thalidomide, already mentioned, affected the limbs. Other agents may affect a broad range of systems.

Fetal tissues may respond to teratogens in several ways. They may atrophy or hypertrophy. Structures may fuse, or they may split. There may be a general inhibition of normal growth and development because of failure of induction or failure of competence.

In order to provide care for the pregnant woman and her developing child, nurses must be specifically aware of teratogens, which include infectious organisms, certain medications and other ingested substances, and radiation. Maternal conditions that may also affect the fetus adversely are discussed in Chapter 10.

Infectious Organisms as Teratogens

The most important organisms known to be teratogens are those of the TORCH group (Table 6–4):

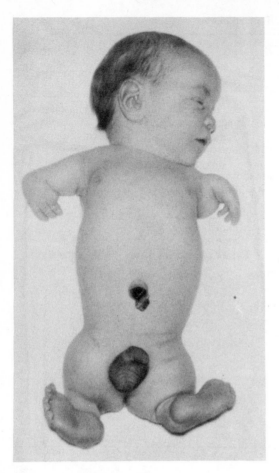

Figure 6–16   Newborn male infant showing typically malformed limbs (phocomelia) caused by thalidomide. (From Moore: *Manit. Med. Rev.*, *43*:306, 1963.)

T for toxoplasmosis
O for other (syphilis)
R for rubella
C for cytomegalovirus
H for herpes simplex

In many instances the fact that the mother has been exposed to the organism may not be evident until after the baby is born, because the disease is nonsymptomatic in the mother.

Toxoplasmosis, a disease caused by a protozoan, is nearly always unrecognized in the mother until the baby is born. All mothers should be cautioned about eating undercooked meat and about caring for cat litter, two principal sources of known contamination.

Serologic tests for *syphilis* should be a part of prenatal care for every woman, and in many states these are required by law. However, not all mothers receive prenatal care, and some may acquire syphilis following testing or may reacquire the disease after initial treatment. Moreover, because of the characteristics of the test, it will not become positive until 4 to 6 weeks after the initial infection. And because the mean length of time between treatment and a negative serologic reaction is 245 days, the test may remain positive following delivery, even though the mother has been treated and is no longer infected. Thus,

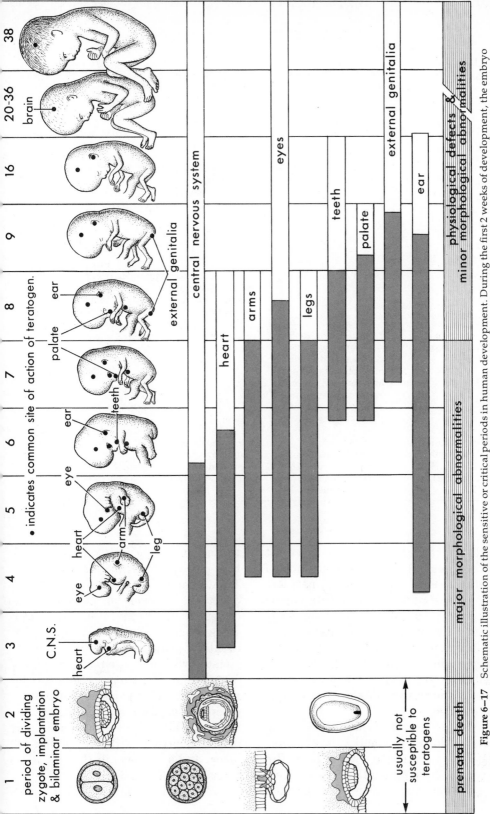

Figure 6-17 Schematic illustration of the sensitive or critical periods in human development. During the first 2 weeks of development, the embryo is usually not susceptible to teratogens. During these predifferentiation stages, a substance either damages all or most of the cells of the embryo, resulting in its death, or it damages only a few cells, allowing the embryo to recover without developing defects. The left side of the bars denotes highly sensitive periods; the right sides indicate stages that are less sensitive to teratogens. (From Moore: *The Developing Human: Clinically Oriented Embryology.* 2nd Edition. Philadelphia, W. B. Saunders, 1977.)

189

Table 6–4   THE TORCH DISEASES

Infectious Disease	Principal Sources	Transmission	Symptoms and Related Signs
Toxoplasmosis	Eating undercooked meats; cat litter; warm, moist soil	Transplacental passage; mother's infection may be unnoticed	Small for gestational age (SGA); central nervous system (CNS) damage; triad: chorioretinitis, hydrocephaly, cerebral calcification
Syphilis	Sexual activity of mother	Transplacental passage; contact with active maternal genital lesions	Premature labor; purulent nasal discharge (snuffles); skin eruptions: symmetrical rash— oral, anogenital, palms of hands and soles of feet; osteochondritis on X-ray; no signs may be present
Rubella	Infection of mother	Transplacental passage particularly during first 8 weeks following conception	Many organ systems may be affected: microcephaly, congenital heart disease, cataracts, deafness, etc.
Cytomegalic inclusion disease (CID)	Person-to-person contact —respiratory and venereal routes: virus probably persists in host tissues indefinitely; virus is worldwide —most adults have CMV at some time in life	Transplacental	SGA; petechiae (blueberry muffin baby); microcephaly; deafness; blindness
Herpes simplex— Type I (oropharynx), Type II (genital) (HSV)	Genital herpes in mother; transmission in nursery from other infected infants or nursery personnel	At or immediately preceding birth from exposure to infected genital secretions	May be asymptomatic at first; fever; vomiting; lethargy; meningoencephalitis

important as serologic testing is, it must be supplemented by the education of mothers and their sexual partners about the significance of syphilis during pregnancy and by the development of trust between nurses and patients, so that patients will tell us if they suspect they might have become infected. If initial tests are negative, repeat testing during the third trimester is often recommended.

Regardless of when syphilis is discovered during pregnancy, it is treated. Effective treatment with penicillin prior to the eighteenth week of pregnancy prevents fetal infection because the organism apparently does not cross the placenta until after that time. Treatment after 18 weeks is also highly effective, however, as penicillin also crosses the placenta to reach the fetus quickly and in adequate amounts. Fortunately, penicillin has never been associated with teratogenicity in spite of frequent use during pregnancy for many years. For patients sensitive to penicillin, erythromycin or tetracycline is used. Failure to treat syphilis may lead to abortion, stillbirth, premature labor, and symptoms in the infant, as described in Table 6–4.

Rubella is certainly the best known

Table 6–4   THE TORCH DISEASES (*Continued*)

Treatment	Possible Outcome	Special Points
No satisfactory treatment	CNS damage (76 to 100% if infant has disease symptoms); visual impairment	Instruct pregnant women about sources of disease
Treat mother with penicillin if diagnosed prior to delivery; treat baby with penicillin if diagnosed after delivery	CNS damage; hearing loss; mortality 10 to 30% if untreated	Serology determination for all women early in pregnancy important in prevention
Treatment of sequelae when possible	Severity and systems involved depend on time of disease; most serious in first 8 weeks after conception; less serious after 20 weeks	Infant may shed virus for a year or more following birth; nurses should know their rubella titer
No effective treatment	75% of infants will have CNS damage	Pregnant nurses should not care for these babies; virus excreted in saliva and urine of baby
Isolate baby	CNS damage; untreated mortality: 75 to 80%	Delivery by cesarean section when genital herpes diagnosed; personnel with herpes infections should not work in nursery

of the teratogenic viral infections; it is the one that first alerted researchers to the concept that there could be an environmental source of congenital deformity. The discovery followed rubella epidemics in Australia in 1939 and 1940. Because there had been no major rubella outbreak in Australia in the previous 17 years, the vast majority of young, pregnant women had no immunity and contracted rubella in large numbers, with a high incidence of what are now recognized as the classic sequelae in their newborn infants: cardiac defects (particularly patent ductus arteriosus and pulmonary stenosis), cataracts, deafness, mental and motor retardation, dental and facial defects, retarded intrauterine growth, and several others.

Through what mechanism the rubella virus affects development remains a mystery. It is known that the virus enters the fetus through the placenta and that it may persist in the newborn for as long as 4 years. Thus a newborn with evidence of congenital rubella may himself be a source of infection to susceptible individuals.

In 1970 a massive campaign was undertaken in the United States to vaccinate children under the age of 12 against rubella in order to curtail the spread of the virus to pregnant women. Since the rubella vaccine may be teratogenic to the fetus, it is important that no one be vaccinated who might be pregnant. Following vaccination, contraception should be used for 3 months to guard against pregnancy. Nurses need to be aware of their own rubella titers and should receive vaccine if they are not immune, both for the future health of their own families and so they will not unwittingly transmit the virus to patients if they should acquire an asymptomatic infection.

Cytomegalovirus (CMV) rarely produces symptoms, yet it is apparently fairly common. The effects of CMV are summarized in Table 6–4.

Herpes virus is classified as either Type I, causing disease above the waist, or Type II, causing disease below the waist. Herpes infection in newborns results in overwhelming systemic infection and often in death. It is believed that most newborn herpes infection is acquired from the mother's vaginal tract during delivery (and therefore is Type II). In recent years genital herpes has become the second most prevalent

Table 6–5   DRUGS THAT ARE HARMFUL TO THE HUMAN FETUS

Drug	Consequence	Comments
Alcohol	Fetal changes associated with chronic alcoholism	(See page 194)
Aminopterin Amethopterin	Gross deformity or death	
Chloramphenicol	Used near term may result in gray-baby syndrome; i.e., sudden collapse and death	
Cyclizine Diphenidol Thiethylperazine	Anticonvulsants whose use is not recommended in pregnancy	
Ethacrynic acid	Fetal and neonatal jaundice; thrombocytopenia	
LSD	Evidence for teratogenicity not conclusive but grounds for caution	
Mineral oil	Regular use may lead to reduced absorption of fat-soluble vitamins A, D, E, and K; reduced absorption of vitamin K may cause hypoprothrombinemia	
Morphine	Addiction in utero; withdrawal symptoms following birth; severe respiratory depression	
Nicotine	May affect fetal growth	Mothers who smoke heavily have babies with lower birth weight
Novobiocin	Near delivery associated with thrombocytopenia and hyperbilirubinemia	
Potassium iodide Radioactive iodine Prophylthiouracil	Congenital goiter, with possible respiratory distress from pressure of enlarged thyroid on trachea	Iodides may be found in "over-the-counter" cough medicines

venereal disease among young Americans.[7] It is therefore most important to identify the presence of this infection, especially late in pregnancy. When herpes is identified prior to delivery, this is an indication for cesarean section. Herpes is also the cause of common fever blisters (Type I), and therefore no one should be allowed in the nursery or in the mother's room who has such a blister.

Drugs and Hormones as Teratogens

No individual should practice self-medication at any time, but it is essential that a pregnant woman take no medication unless specifically prescribed by a physician who knows she is pregnant. Even then, it is a good idea for the woman to double check with the physician or nurse who is responsible for her maternity care. Moreover, women who might be pregnant must also be careful of the medicine they ingest because of the rapid embryologic development during the first weeks.

Table 6–5 lists medications that have been associated with problems in the human fetus or in the infant after birth. Some of these drugs, such as thalidomide and aminopterin, are proved to be teratogenic in humans. Some, such as morphine, do not cause

Table 6–5 DRUGS THAT ARE HARMFUL TO THE HUMAN FETUS (*Continued*)

Drug	Consequences	Comments
Reserpine	Nasal discharge, respiratory distress, lethargy, anorexia in newborn	
Salicylates	Neonatal bleeding in high doses; possible salicylate intoxication in high doses	
Streptomycin Dihydrostreptomycin Chloroquine	May affect inner ear of fetus	
Sulfonamides	Avoid during last trimester; possible hyperbilirubinemia, thrombocytopenia, kernicterus if given near term	
Testosterone Synthetic progestins (e.g., ethisterone, norethisterone)	Masculinization of the female fetus	At one time given to prevent spontaneous abortion
Tetracycline and derivatives	Inhibition of bone growth; discoloration of teeth	
Thalidomide	Phocomelia (seal-like limbs), amelia (absence of limbs), and other deformities	
Thiazides	Long-term use may lead to hyponatremia; diabetogenic effect on mother may have an effect on infant	
Trimethadione (Tridione) Paramethadione (Paradione)	A variety of defects may occur including facial defects, cardiac defects, cleft palate, and intrauterine growth retardation	

malformation but may present serious problems for the newborn at the time of birth. If the baby's system contains medications such as chloramphenicol or a sulfonamide at the time of birth, he may have the same problems he would have if given these drugs postnatally.

The Fetus of an Alcoholic Mother

When the mother has chronic alcoholism prior to her pregnancy, her child may develop abnormally. Jones and associates[5] report similar patterns of craniofacial, limb, and cardiovascular defects in eight unrelated children of three different ethnic groups born to mothers who had been alcoholics for an average of 9 years. The babies were small for their gestational age at the time of their birth and failed to "catch up" after birth. None of the children performed normally on developmental tests done from 3 months to nearly 5 years after birth, regardless of whether they were raised by their own mother or in a foster home.

What causes this pattern? It may be a direct result of alcohol toxicity or of toxicity from alcohol breakdown products or some other substances in the beverages consumed. It may also be related to the malnutrition that is common in chronic alcoholism. Further research may suggest additional possibilities.

Nutrition and the Developing Embryo-Fetus

Animal experimentation has produced a variety of malformations related to nutritional deficiency of such elements as vitamin A, riboflavin, zinc, and manganese. The only proven congenital malformation related to a specific dietary deficiency in humans is cretinism, which is related to a lack of iodine in the diet. Cretinism and adult iodine deficiency are prevalent in several areas of the world where soil and water do not contain sufficient iodine. Recently there have been reports that goiter is increasing in some parts of the United States because of a decrease in the use of iodized salt. Since mountainous and inland areas are most likely to be affected, pregnant women in these sections of the country should use iodized salt.

A general level of malnutrition has been correlated with low birth weight in babies; these babies are less likely to thrive after birth and have a higher incidence of infant mortality. Fetal malnutrition may be due to malnourishment in the mother or to failure of transport of necessary nutrients across the placenta. Maternal nutrition is discussed in detail in Chapter 9.

Radiation as a Teratogen

For many years it has been obvious that radiation is a direct cause of a number of congenital malformations. The specific organs affected depend upon the stage of fetal development at the time of exposure. The chance of defect is associated with the dose, but the range of safety is not known. Therefore, it is recommended that fertile women be exposed to X-ray only during the first 10 days following the onset of menstruation, except in an emergency.

Stewart and Kneale[12] suggest that X-ray during pregnancy may increase the risk of cancer in children under the age of ten. After an analysis of 15,000 children, they felt that "among one million children exposed shortly before birth to one rad of ionizing radiation, there would be an extra 300 to 800 deaths before the age of ten due to radiation induced cancer." A number of X-rays that might once have been felt necessary may now be avoided by the use of sonography, which has not been found harmful to the fetus. One example would be the confirmation of a twin pregnancy.

SUMMARY

The 38 weeks of pregnancy are a dynamic, constantly changing period for mother and conceptus. This chapter has examined physiologic changes. The next chapter will look at emotional and social changes that are equally a part of every pregnancy.

REFERENCES

1. Arey, L.: *Developmental Anatomy*. 7th Edition. Philadelphia, W. B. Saunders Co., 1965.
2. Blattner, R. J.: German Measles. *In* Vaughan, V. C. III, and McKay, R. J. (eds.): *Nelson Textbook of Pediatrics*. 10th Edition. Philadelphia, W. B. Saunders Co., 1975.
3. Giacoia, G., and Yaffe, S.: Drugs and the Perinatal Patient. *In* Avery, G. (ed.): *Neonatology*. Philadelphia, J. B. Lippincott Co., 1975.
4. Greenhill, J., and Friedman, F.: *Biological Principles and Modern Practice of Obstetrics*. Philadelphia, W. B. Saunders Co., 1974.
5. Jones, K., Smith, D., Ulleland, C., et al.: Pattern of Malformation in Offspring of Chronic Alcoholic Mothers. *Lancet, 1*: 7815, 1973.
6. Moore, K.: *The Developing Human: Clinically Oriented Embryology*. 2nd Ed. Philadelphia, W. B. Saunders Co., 1977.
7. Neeson, J. D.: Herpesvirus Genitalis: A Nursing Perspective. Nursing Clinics of North America, *10*:599, 1975.
8. Page, E., Villee, C., and Villee, D.: *Human Reproduction*. 2nd Edition. Philadelphia, W. B. Saunders Co., 1976.
9. Radioreceptorassay—A New Pregnancy Test. American Journal of Nursing, *76*:1281, 1976.
10. Reynolds, D., Stagno, S., and Alford, C.: Chronic Congenital and Perinatal Infection. *In* Avery, G. (ed.): *Neonatology*. Philadelphia, J. B. Lippincott Co., 1975.
11. Saxena, B., and Landesman, R.: The Use of a Radioreceptorassay of Human Chorionic Gonadotropin for the Diagnosis and Management of Ectopic Pregnancy. *Fertility and Sterility, 26*:397, 1975.
12. Stewart, A., and Kneale, G.: Radiation Dose Effects in Relation to Obstetric X-Rays and Childhood Cancers. *Lancet, 272*: 1006, 1957.
13. Ziegel, E., and Van Blarcom, C.: *Obstetric Nursing*. 6th edition. New York, The Macmillan Co., 1972.

Chapter 7

PSYCHOSOCIAL CHANGE FOLLOWING CONCEPTION: THE BEGINNINGS OF TRANSITION TO PARENTING

Just as the mother's body undergoes physiologic change to meet the demands of the growing embryo-fetus, so too do the lives of parents change as they prepare for new responsibilities. This is true not only for a first pregnancy but for every pregnancy. Psychosocial change involves work; the work of becoming parents has been labeled a crisis by some investigators. The more knowledgeable we are about the social and emotional work of men and women during the months of pregnancy, the more helpful we can be in assisting them as they make their plans for parenting.

In this chapter we will explore psychosocial changes, including the beginnings of attachment and the changes that occur in roles and relationships, as well as some of the ways in which culture interfaces with and affects these changes.

PREGNANCY AS A CRISIS

Many authors have described pregnancy as a crisis in the lives of the woman and man who are to become parents of a child. Crisis, in this sense, is defined as a turning point in the life of the individual.[4] Hill describes a crisis as "any sharp or decisive change for which previous patterns are inadequate."[18] Koos[20a] refers to "situations which block usual patterns of action and call for new ones." Loesch and Greenberg describe "acute disequilibria which under favorable conditions result in specific maturational steps toward new functions."[24] Each of these definitions can give us, as nurses, insight into the psychologic meaning of pregnancy for women and men about to become parents.

Pregnancy does represent a point from which there is no turning back. (Even if the decision is made to end the pregnancy in abortion, the fact of having become pregnant remains.) New patterns of action, i.e., behavior, will be necessary. Marital routines will change. The mother's employment outside the home will in some ways be affected, even if she continues to be employed. If this is a second or subsequent pregnancy for a couple, adjustments

196

must be made for other family members.

At each of the crises of life (for example, going to school for the first time, going away to college, marriage), successfully dealing with the crises leads to a more mature level of behavior. As the six or seven year old child successfully adapts to school, many "baby ways" are left behind. One need only compare first graders with second graders on the first day of school in September to observe such maturation.

The ability to cope with the crisis of pregnancy will also lead to maturation, which enables one to become a successful parent of either a first or a subsequent child. However, not every pregnancy leads to maturation. Factors that affect the developmental processes in pregnancy include:

1. The meaning of the pregnancy for the individual.

2. The individual's stage of development, i.e., readiness for pregnancy.

3. The acceptance or denial of the pregnancy.

4. The resources that the individual has to deal with the pregnancy.

PREGNANCY AS A DEVELOPMENTAL PROCESS

A number of professionals in the fields of nursing, medicine, and the behavioral sciences have considered pregnancy from a developmental perspective and have identified developmental *tasks*.

A developmental task is defined as "a task which arises at or about a certain period in the life of an individual, successful achievement of which leads to happiness and success with later tasks, while failure leads to unhappiness in the individual, disapproval by the society, and difficulty with later tasks."[16] Through the successful accomplishment of developmental tasks, women both prepare for parenthood and mature personally.

Rubin[37] identifies the following as maternal tasks during pregnancy: (1) "seeking safe passage for herself and her child through pregnancy, labor and delivery," (2) "ensuring acceptance of her child by significant persons in her family," (3) "bending-in to her unknown child," and (4) "learning to give of herself."

Klaus and Kennell have looked at tasks within the context of attachment.[20] They define attachment as "a unique emotional relationship between two individuals which is specific and endures through time." They have identified the tasks important to attachment as: (1) planning the pregnancy, (2) confirming the pregnancy, (3) accepting the pregnancy, (4) perceiving fetal movements, (5) accepting the fetus as an individual, (6) birth, (7) seeing the baby, (8) touching the baby, and (9) giving care to the baby.

Task number one, planning the pregnancy, is completed prior to pregnancy. Tasks six through nine follow birth and are discussed in Chapters 15 and 20.

Caplan[6] identified two tasks: (1) acceptance of the pregnancy and (2) perception of the fetus as a separate individual.

Confirming and Accepting the Pregnancy

Confirmation of the fact of pregnancy begins the developmental process for those couples who did not plan the pregnancy beforehand.

Acceptance of the pregnancy, and ultimately of the baby, is multifaceted. First the "idea" of being pregnant must be accepted, and then the fetus must be seen and accepted as an individual, separate and apart from the mother. The perception and acceptance of the fetus as a separate individual usually does not occur until fetal movements are perceived (quickening) after the twentieth week of pregnancy.

Acceptance not only by the mother but by other people significant to her is necessary. These "significant others" include her husband, her baby's father if not married, and her own mother. This acceptance means that there will be a reorientation of basic roles and relationships—a major aspect of the psychologic work of pregnancy.

Accepting New Roles and Reorienting Basic Relationships

The role of father or mother is added to that of husband or wife during the couple's first pregnancy. Subsequent pregnancies also bring role change—from the parent of one child to the parent of two, and so on. Both single and married parents also have additional roles, son or daughter, occupational roles, roles in the community, and so on. Although more attention has been focused on the transition to wife-mother and husband-father, other role transitions are important as well. The couple's relationship with their own parents assumes new dimensions as those parents become grandparents of their child. The changing relationship of an unmarried mother to her own mother can affect the way in which the child grows.

The process of assuming a new role involves grief, fantasy, observation, and role playing.

Grief is felt for the role left behind. No matter how desirous a couple is for a child, there is still the knowledge of the irrevocability of the occasion, as mentioned previously. This is true not only during the first pregnancy but as each new baby is anticipated. Grief may be for loss of independence, financial loss, loss of the relationship with the previous child who will no longer be the baby, or other factors important to a particular mother. Perception of this grief in herself may make an expectant mother feel guilty; this isn't the way she thinks she is supposed to feel. Knowing that these feelings are both common and "normal" can be reassuring.

Fantasy involves trying on the new role in one's mind. A mother imagines herself holding the baby, rocking him, and singing to him. Perhaps she pictures teaching a daughter to cook or sew. The father may fantasize playing ball with his son and taking him hunting or seeing his daughter in a school play. It is not unusual for the fantasy to involve not a newborn infant but a much older child. Both parents are trying to feel what it is like to be a mother or a father. During second and subsequent pregnancies both parents and siblings fantasize what life will be like with the expected baby.

In addition to fantasies of their own roles, parents also fantasize the roles of one another. The prospective father may imagine behavior by his wife that plays no part in her idea of her role, and vice versa. He may, for example, see her as breast-feeding their baby because that is traditional in his family, only to find that the idea has no appeal to her. She may have visions of his playing football with their son while she prepares dinner; she knows that he is highly unathletic now, but she imagines that having a son will change this. Both mother and father need to share their fantasies with each other.

The *observation* of other mothers and fathers is also a significant part of the development of parental role behavior. It is not unusual for couples, and particularly for mothers, to find that they are more interested in parents who are pregnant or who have recently had a baby. Old interests are changing; new values and ideas are being considered.

The opportunity to *play the role* of parents, with the infants of friends and relatives, is more difficult to arrange in nuclear families than in extended family living, in which infants are almost always present and many chances to care for them exist.

The period of preparation for childbearing is an ideal time for helping individuals and couples think about the way in which they view the roles of mother and father. Roles are a conglomeration of perceptions. We all have idealized, stereotyped ideas of what it means to be a mother or a father. Stereotypes have always existed, but television, viewed almost constantly since childhood by the current generation of parents, has probably affected our perception of what a father or a mother "ought to be" to an even greater extent. Role behavior is a result of reality impinging upon these stereotypes.

As roles change, basic relationships are altered. Consider the following example:

Prior to the birth of their first child, the end of the working day had been a time for Jan and Tom to share happenings—good and bad—with each other. A few weeks following the baby's delivery, Tom came home to find Jan too tired from the demands of mothering to give him the attention he had once received. He had hoped dinner would be ready so that he could make an evening business meeting. Not only had dinner not been started but Jan felt that (1) it was unfair of him to expect her to have dinner ready when the baby had been fussy all afternoon and (2) it was also unfair of him to leave her at home with the baby while he went out for an evening, even if it were business.

Jan wondered, "Doesn't my role as mother (caring for her fussy infant) come before my role as wife (having dinner ready)? After all, he's an adult; he should understand." She would also like him to assume the role of father (as she views that role) and help care for the baby now that he is home, but he may see his business meeting as even more significant to his father role, because for Tom a father's primary role is that of breadwinner.

Two basic problems are illustrated: differing perceptions of appropriate role behavior (e.g., how Tom and Jan perceive the priorities of the role of being a father) and conflict between the former role (wife) and the new role (wife-mother). If we can bring up these issues before they become problems, i.e., in the period before birth, and say, "This is a situation that all couples must deal with," some of these conflicts may be minimized.

Siblings and the Coming of a New Baby

The coming of each newborn affects the relationship of parents and every other child in the family. The changes that a new baby brings to the total family structure inevitably affect other children, as well as parents. There are changes in space, such as sharing a room or changing rooms. Possessions may change hands—the crib may be painted for the baby. A mother may be too tired during certain stages of pregnancy to participate in some formerly shared activities.

Siblings at every age, from the small baby to the adolescent, are affected. Very small children may not however perceive changes during the prenatal phase, unless their own activities change, as when a baby is weaned from the breast fairly rapidly.

Seeking Safe Passage

Rubin suggests that as a mother accepts the idea of her pregnancy, she also plans a safe passage for herself and her fetus.[37] As she becomes increasingly protective of the fetus, she becomes careful in her actions. She often tries hard to eat the foods suggested as being appropriate. She may avoid activities that she believes to be dangerous.

Seeking care that she believes to be competent and questioning even practices that formerly were taken for granted (riding in a car, hanging clothes) are further manifestations of her concern.

Learning to Give of Herself

The concept that during pregnancy the mother must learn to give of herself is also a contribution of Rubin's. Rubin sees giving in four contexts:

1. The fetus as a gift to the mother.
2. The mother's giving to the fetus in utero.
3. The mother's giving of the fetus in utero as a gift from herself to others.
4. The mother's exacting of gifts from the father and from friends as symbols of their concern.[37]

The theme of giving is evident in accounts of pregnancies in other cultures. Obeyesekere describes a craving, termed *dola-duka,* in Ceylon, which is a craving for specific types of food.[29] To deny the mother what she desires is considered a sin sufficiently grave to damage one's chances of rebirth. More immediately, it is believed that the ears of the fetus will rot if the woman's cravings are not satisfied.

Within the context of giving and receiving, perhaps the demands for gifts are preparatory to being able to give of oneself. We then need to question whether the mother who does not perceive of herself as being cared for, who is not "given gifts," may then have difficulty in meeting the many demands for giving that are placed upon a new mother.

Variables that Influence Achieving Developmental Tasks During Pregnancy

A number of factors may enhance or impede the achievement of the developmental tasks of pregnancy and ultimately of the tasks of parenting.

Success or Failure in Achieving Prior Developmental Tasks. A major block to the successful achievement of the developmental tasks of pregnancy is the failure to achieve prior tasks. For the individual or couple who has not yet resolved the tasks of adolescence and early adulthood, the intrusion of parenthood on uncompleted tasks may bring resentment of the pregnancy and rejection of the child.

Care by and Relationship to the Mother's and Father's Own Parents. From our own parents and our relationship with them, all of us develop, consciously and unconsciously, our understanding of what it means to be a parent and strategies for parental behavior. The fact that most parents who abuse their children were themselves abused as children points to this concept rather emphatically.

Expectations of Family and Society. The expectations of family and friends that developmental tasks will be achieved enhance their achievement. Conversely, the young mother or father who is told, or to whom it is implied, that for one reason or another she or he is not ready for pregnancy (too young, too immature, and so on) faces an added barrier.

When family and societal expectations become social pressures to become pregnant (the desire of the couple's own parents for grandchildren, pregnancy because one's peers are pregnant, and so forth) or when the pregnancy results in social disapproval (unwed pregnancy, pregnancies too closely spaced, too many children, for example) the achievement of tasks may be hindered.

The Relationship Between the Mother and Father. The relationship between the mother and father may also enhance or hinder the achievement of developmental tasks. If the father is supportive of the mother; if she, in turn, recognizes that he also has concerns and needs during the pregnancy (see below); and if their communication is effective most of the time; their relationship is likely to be a positive factor in achieving the developmental tasks of pregnancy. When serious problems exist in this relationship, however, it is not only more difficult to cope with the pregnancy, but the pregnancy is likely to put a further strain on the relationship. Parenthood is sometimes undertaken to strengthen a shaky relationship; however, the desired result is almost never achieved (see also motivation for pregnancy, Chapter 5).

Some couples do find themselves closer as a result of parenthood, but these are nearly always couples who have had a good relationship and good interpersonal communication prior to the pregnancy. Other couples begin to coexist, each in his or her separate world, as a result of pregnancy and parenthood—the mother becoming more absorbed in the world of her child or children while the father becomes absorbed in affairs outside of the home.

Feelings about Femininity and Masculinity. The mother who is ambivalent about or unsure of her own femininity may have difficulty accepting motherhood. Equally, the man who is unsure of his masculinity may find the idea of fatherhood threatening.

High Risk Pregnancy. When the mother has some condition, such as diabetes mellitus or previous difficult preg-

nancies, that puts the outcome of the pregnancy at risk, there may be major problems in achieving developmental tasks. This issue is discussed in Chapter 10.

EMOTIONAL REACTIONS TO PREGNANCY

Culture and the Emotional Changes of Pregnancy

Before we examine the emotional changes that have been observed in both men and women in our society, we must recognize that we do not really know whether they apply to prospective mothers and fathers everywhere or whether they are part of Western society. We do not even know if they apply to everyone in our own society. They may indeed be applicable, but systematic studies have not been done to confirm this.

The recognition of this fact has very practical significance. We cannot assess the emotional reactions of individuals of one cultural group by using norms for another group, just as in many instances we cannot judge the physiologic status of one group by norms established for another.

For example, in some societies or subsocieties it is expected that the father will become involved in pregnancy far more than in others. The middle class American father may thus attend prenatal classes with his wife; because the Chinese-American father does not behave in the same way does not mean that he does not care for his wife or child-to-be. Many examples of the role of culture have been given in Chapter 4 and elsewhere, and will be encountered in your practice.

Changes Occur in Both Mothers and Fathers

When researchers and caretakers first became interested in the emotional changes that accompany pregnancy, attention was focused almost exclusively on the expectant mother. Several cultural factors are undoubtedly related to this bias, including the idea that pregnancy is "women's business" and a longstanding concept that men in our society are not supposed to react to events in an emotional way, but solely in an intellectual manner. Thus only recently have the reactions and needs of fathers received much attention.

If we examine the evidence that is now accumulating, it is interesting to observe that many characteristics exhibited by women during pregnancy are directly or inversely related to characteristics in their mates. The mother's attitude about pregnancy will influence the father's attitude and vice versa. It is in this context that we will examine some of the major emotional components of pregnancy.

The extent to which these reactions are experienced by an individual man or woman will depend upon many factors, including the individual's age and level of maturity (not necessarily equal), the relationship of each with his or her own parents and particularly with the parent of the same sex, the couple's relationship to one another, the meaning of the pregnancy for each of them, their desire for the baby, and the reason for that desire.

Ambivalence

The popular belief that each mother and father is overjoyed when she or he learns about the pregnancy is not supported by investigation. This is true for married couples as well as for couples who are not married. There is no one reaction typical of expectant parents. Yet a degree of ambivalence seems very prominent in our society, and perhaps in all societies as we come to know more about them.

Sears[38] reported that as high as 25 per cent of women were ambivalent or displeased when they first discovered they were pregnant; Caplan[6] found as many as 80 per cent of the women in his group were at first unhappy when they found themselves pregnant.

Ambivalent feelings may be present even when the child has been planned and is desired. The mother (and father) may feel, "Oh yes, we want this baby, but maybe not quite yet." The feeling is similar to that experienced at any major change of lifestyle — graduation from school, or marriage, for example. We count the days until the Big Day finally arrives, and then we feel, "No, not quite yet." This is because once the change occurs, nothing will be quite the same. It may be better; it may be worse, but it will never be the same and that is frightening. We know how to cope with the known; will we be able to cope with the unknown? And so the couple feels as they face parenthood that nothing will ever be quite as it was before. Most couples expect their lives to be even better, but there are no guarantees.

Guilt about Ambivalence. Feelings of ambivalence are often unacceptable to men and women who are expectant parents, and because of this, such emotions may lead to feelings of guilt. Our myths tell us that, except in unusual circumstances, one should be delighted about the child who has been conceived. Because our ambivalent feelings are unacceptable to us, they are frequently not shared—even between the prospective mother and the prospective father. Each feels the other would think her (him) silly.

Helping Couples Cope with Ambivalence. For most couples all that is necessary is to communicate that: (1) feelings of ambivalence are common and very normal reactions, for reasons described above, and (2) feelings of ambivalence usually disappear as pregnancy progresses. One has time to become accustomed to thoughts of a new lifestyle and to make specific plans in terms of finances, housing, and all the multiple logistical details that accompany parenthood—not just at the time of the first pregnancy but at each succeeding pregnancy.

Concern for Change in Body Image

The concern of the pregnant woman about her changing body image is often paralleled by the reaction in her mate to her change in form. The changing shape is very tangible evidence for both men and women of the occurrence of sexual intercourse, and therefore feelings about intercourse and sexuality can be related to feelings about body image during pregnancy. If intercourse is felt in some way to be shameful, then the announcement to the world that intercourse has occurred may pose some difficulties, even when the child is desired.

Some mothers appear to deny their changing body. Adolescents, particularly, may continue to wear their regular clothes long past the time when they fit properly, as if to continue their identification with their nonpregnant peers. (Before concluding that denial is always the reason for this behavior, however, we need to determine whether there is a financial problem in acquiring maternity clothes.)

For many mothers the changing body image is confirmation that the pregnancy does indeed exist. Preparations for the coming baby, which may have seemed foolish and unnecessary when the pregnancy was first suspected, now become important. If the mother-to-be is employed outside of her home, the visible evidence of her pregnancy forces her to make plans with her employer for a leave of absence, perhaps, or for a "retirement," either temporary or permanent.

Men may react in varying ways to the changing shape of their mate. Some men find great satisfaction in this evidence of pregnancy, while others appear to be very uneasy around women who are pregnant, including their own wives. Husbands who are uncomfortable about their wives' changing anatomy may avoid prenatal classes in which anatomy is discussed and films of delivery and breast-feeding are shown. They may resist being, or be very uncomfortable as, participants in labor and delivery. Rarely is there an opportunity for them to discuss their concerns; most men will find it difficult to confide to either their mate or their buddies that they don't like the appearance of their pregnant mate.

Physical Symptoms as Emotional Reactions

Surprisingly similar physical symptoms can occur in both men and women during pregnancy, including nausea and vomiting, heartburn, indigestion, loss of appetite, and abdominal pain. We have been able to explain many of a mother's symptoms on a physiologic basis. Yet it appears that these symptoms have a social and/or emotional component as well, in that they vary markedly from one society to another, from one woman to another, and even from one pregnancy to another in an individual woman.

The "Sick Role." In 1951 sociologist Talcott Parsons[30] suggested that being sick involved not just physical symptoms but also circumstances in which certain behaviors were expected or permitted. If one were defined as "sick," one was then (1) exempt from normal social role responsibilities, relative to the nature and severity of the illness; (2) not expected to get well by an act of decision or will; (3) obliged to want to get well; and (4) obliged to seek technically competent help in relation to the severity of the illness.

These concepts are familiar to all of us. We say, "I can't go to work today because I'm sick" (exemption from normal responsibilities). "I wish I were well and could work" (obligation to want to get well and recognition that one does not get well by just wishing it were so). Someone may then say to us, "If you're sick, why don't you see the nurse or doctor?" (obligation to seek competent help).

Rosengren, in 1962, suggested a "sick role in pregnancy."[34] He postulated that a woman who had no organic illness during pregnancy but who considered herself ill:

1. Expected to be exempt from her usual social obligations and responsibilities.

2. Regarded pregnancy as a condition of abnormality that one should get over and return to the "normal round of life."

3. Expressed worry and concern about body changes during pregnancy and possible organic complications.

4. Considered that pain and suffering were anticipated corollaries of "being ill" and of "getting better."

5. Expected to act in the subordinate role vis-a-vis her attending physician.[35]

In a study of 76 pregnant women (44 clinic patients and 32 private patients), none of whom had any pathologic disorder, Rosengren reports

the following: "Women of comparatively low social status tended to regard themselves as more 'sick' during pregnancy than did women of higher social class standing."[34]

Rosengren had hypothesized that this would be so, in that he considered low social status an index of greater social disturbance than high social status. There was one exception to this:

Women who were or who had been employed in higher status occupation tended to regard themselves as more "sick" than those who held lower status jobs . . . Those women with higher educational level than their husbands had significantl higher sick role scores than those with similar or lower educational levels.[34]

One might speculate that in both of these instances pregnancy would be more disruptive of a specific way of life.

In the same article Rosengren also reported that there appeared to be an inverse relationship between social aspirations and sick role expectations. "Women who defined pregnancy as illness tended to express many negative social aspirations and many aspirations for material acquisition."

He further postulated that high sick role expectations would be found among the downwardly mobile while correspondingly lower sick role expectations would be found among the upwardly mobile. However, no significant difference was found between the upwardly and downwardly mobile. Nevertheless, when those women who were mobile in either direction were compared with those who were stable those who were stable had a lower tendency to take the sick role. The disruption of life, rather than the direction of the mobility, seemed to be the significant factor.

Brown[5] found that there were a number of differences when he compared 148 consecutive primiparas who had a high number of bodily symptoms with those who had few or no physical symptoms during pregnancy. All of the women were from working and lower class backgrounds. In general, the mothers with a high number of symptoms:

1. Had had different experiences with their own mothers and fathers, with frequent inadequacy and social disorganization during their "growing-up" years.

2. Reported more problems in interpersonal relationships, particularly with their husbands and close relatives.

3. Appeared socially isolated.

4. Were more dependent upon and insecure about their husbands.

5. Were more anxious and less able to cope with their anxiety.

6. Had a less favorable reaction to their pregnancy.

7. Had a greater incidence of sexual malfunctioning and difficult menstrual periods.

Brown concluded that in the women with many physical symptoms during pregnancy, a difficult pregnancy appeared to be a further incident in a troubled life.

The studies reported above examine social/cultural correlates of physical symptoms during pregnancy. Individual emotional correlates are more difficult to document. For example, how important is the role of the mother's feelings about her pregnancy in causing nausea and vomiting during pregnancy, and particularly in producing the prolonged vomiting called *hyperemesis gravidarum*? Are these physical symptoms a coping mechanism?

Physical Symptoms in Fathers. Trethowan suggests that one in five expectant fathers has one or more physical symptoms during his wife's pregnancy.[42] Curtis found that 65 per cent (42 men) of his study group of fathers, all of whom were considered to be psychologically normal, demonstrated physical symptoms.[8]

Nausea and vomiting have been reported as beginning at about 6 to 8 weeks, even in men whose wives did not complain of nausea. Loss of appetite is fairly common for some men, while other expectant fathers increase their food intake and may gain from 10 to 20 pounds during pregnancy. Some men change their diet patterns, such as increasing their milk intake "for the baby." An interesting parallel is found in many traditional societies in which it is felt that the father, as well as the mother, is personally responsible for the growth of the fetus and that his actions during pregnancy will affect the unborn child's normal development. In some of these societies diet restrictions are applied to both the father and the mother.

Restlessness, anxiety, and sleeplessness, especially as the time of labor approaches, are not uncommon in expectant fathers. Films and television situation comedies that frequently picture the distraught father and the calm mother are a reflection of the recognition of this situation in our society. As nurses working with couples in the last weeks of pregnancy and in labor and delivery rooms, we need to be conscious of the potentially high level of paternal anxiety at a time when everyone is expecting the father to be supportive of the mother. (See the father's supportive role below.)

Here again many traditional societies have provided for this anxiety by the practice of *couvade* (French, couver, to hatch, and Latin, cubare, to lie down). The couvade ritual takes various forms, all of which provide for male participation in childbirth. Among the Mohave Indians, transvestites mimic childbirth by being ceremonially delivered of stones. The Arapesh father shares his wife's childbirth bed. In other societies men may go to bed and enact the birth process in a ritualistic way. In our own society until relatively recently, twentieth century fathers have not been permitted a role in pregnancy and birth (other than conception).

Lacking a ritual and/or a role, many men responded to approaching delivery with physical symptoms. Trethowan found that it was not uncommon for either soldiers in the British army or civilians to experience abdominal cramps at the time of their wife's confinement.

Heightened Sense of Dependency

Both men and women commonly exhibit an increased need for dependency, a "desire to be mothered," during some phase of pregnancy.

Benedek[2] theorizes that the mother's heightened sense of dependence, her need to feel loved, enables her, in turn, to transfer love to the fetus and thus paves the way for the development of motherly feelings.

What happens, then, if the mother's dependency needs are not fulfilled? If she herself feels unloved, it may be very difficult for her to love her fetus, or her child after birth. If her husband is unable to meet her needs for dependency, she is likely to be disappointed in him, and their relationship can become strained.

If there is no husband, if the husband is not supportive, or if there is no extended family or other group, nurses may find women very emotionally dependent upon them, as these mothers struggle to cope with their need for security.

As the woman turns to her husband or mate to fulfill her dependency needs,

he may also be looking for "mothering," frequently from his wife but also from his own mother. Liebenberg[23] found that during pregnancy a number of husbands expressed a wish to be home on Mother's Day and wrote or called their own parents more frequently. This desire for mothering may make both husband and wife feel neglected. His need may coincide with a period during which his wife may not only be doing less for him because of her own decreased energy and self-absorption, but may also be making increased demands upon him to meet her own dependency needs. In our society in which many young couples may live far from parents, relatives, and long-time friends, the husband may be the only source of support (other than professional) available to his wife. And although he may feel neglected and angry, he may also feel guilty because he feels (and society indicates to him) that he should be supportive of his wife since she is the one who is pregnant. If these feelings go unresolved during pregnancy, they may be heightened after the baby is born, as the demands of the baby further interfere with the attention that the father formerly received and still desires from his baby's mother.

"Turning Inward"

Closely related to dependency needs is a "turning inward," described by Benedek as a "vegetative calmness." Even the busy extrovert usually finds herself "slowing down." One mother said, "I found myself quite content to sit and wash dishes, a job I've always hated. But now I'm not in a hurry to get on to other things. It gives me time to think about what it will be like when the baby comes."

For the mother who is busy completing her education or who has a career of her own, passivity may be distressing, particularly if she does not understand that her changing feelings are part of the normal process of pregnancy.

There does not appear to be a similar passivity in fathers. Often, in our society at least, he turns outward, becoming more concerned with his job or career as he feels increased financial responsibility, In Wapner's study of 128 first-time middle class fathers, the men's concern was not about income, per se, but about their ability to feel comfortable with the added responsibility.[45] We would suspect that for many fathers income itself might be a source of concern.

This apparent tendency for mothers and fathers to "go in different directions" can be stressful to a marriage. Maternal passivity, when not understood, may also be interpreted by the father as a rejection of him.

Anxiety

Few women experience pregnancy without some degree of anxiety at some stage. This appears to be true whether the pregnancy is planned or unplanned and whether the baby is wanted or unwanted.

Normal defense mechanisms seem to be relaxed, bringing old, unsettled conflicts closer to the surface. This is a useful function that enables the mother to resolve old conflicts in order to prepare for a new stage in her psychologic development.

Some fears will be old fears, fear of the dark, for example. Others will be related to the pregnancy itself. Will the baby be normal? Will delivery hurt? How will I behave if it hurts? Will I die? Fears about adequacy as a parent are a part of pregnancy for some mothers; for others this concern may not be important until after the birth of the baby.

Fears may appear during dreams. Mothers find it frightening to dream that their baby is born deformed or dead. They are usually relieved when they learn that many other prospective mothers have similar dreams.

If these anxieties are ridiculed rather than accepted, they are likely to be suppressed and to appear as physical or emotional symptoms.

Some mothers never mention fears or anxieties to nurses during the prenatal period. If they do not, the issue should be raised with a statement such as, "Most mothers find themselves worried at some time during their pregnancy about their health or the health of their baby," assuring them that such worries are quite common. This kind of permission to talk about concerns will often lead to a sharing of feelings.

The anxieties of fathers are less well documented but center primarily on their ability to provide financially, already discussed, and their ability to be a "father," i.e., to fulfill their image of the role of a father.

SEXUAL NEEDS DURING PREGNANCY

Physiologic and psychologic factors interface in human sexual relationships; this is as true during pregnancy as it is at other times.

Physiologic Changes

The research of Masters and Johnson[26] has increased our understanding of the physiologic changes in sexual response that occur during pregnancy. Thorough anatomic and physiologic evaluation of six women and interviews with 111 women and 79 of their husbands during the second, sixth, and eighth months of their pregnancy and again 3 months after delivery were the basis of their findings.

As already noted in Chapter 6, during pregnancy there are physiologic changes in both breasts and genitalia. An increase in breast size, because of changes in the vascular and glandular bed, is one of the earliest signs of pregnancy, particularly in the primipara. Sexual tension in the nulliparous woman also results in vasocongestion, which can increase breast size by 20 to 25 per cent. When these changes in relation to sexual stimulation are superimposed on the changes of pregnancy, it is not surprising that many women, particularly primiparas, complain of tenderness and pain in their breasts during intercourse. The area of the areola and nipple is especially sensitive. It is helpful for the mother to know that this discomfort is greatest during the first trimester and that it will be reduced considerably during the remainder of her pregnancy.

Pregnancy affects the normal female genital response to sex in three major ways. First, as with the breasts, the vascular bed of the genitalia is increased. During the first and second trimesters, there is additional engorgement caused by sexual tension. In the third trimester the genitalia are so chronically engorged that sexual tension appears to bring little change.

Second, the increased production of vaginal lubrication and a light mucoid discharge, beginning toward the end of the first trimester, appears to be greater in multiparas than in primiparas.

Third, using both intrauterine and abdominal electrode placement, Masters and Johnson have demonstrated that uterine muscle contractions occur during the orgasmic phase of the female sexual cycle.[26] During the third trimester, tonic spasm, lasting as long as 1 minute, may occur during orgasm

rather than the regular contractions that normally occur. Fetal heart rate may slow at this time, but it quickly returns to normal levels. In some instances uterine contractions were observed to last as long as half an hour after orgasm during the last month of pregnancy.

Changes in Female Sexual Drive During Pregnancy

A second major consideration is the way in which pregnancy affects the emotional component of sexuality for women, recognizing that the emotional and physical components are very closely interrelated. Many factors certainly influence a woman's feelings about sexual intercourse when she is pregnant, including the beliefs of her cultural group, the attitudes of the significant people around her, and her own fears and misconceptions.

Table 7–1 summarizes the findings of three separate studies.

In the women interviewed by Masters and Johnson, decreased interest in sex was reported by three-quarters of the nulliparous women during the first trimester, but there was little change for most of the multiparas. Nausea and vomiting, sleepiness, and fatigue were present in many of those women who expressed a decreased interest. Others said they feared harming the baby.[26] In Falicov's group[12] 10 of 19 women expressed a fear of harming the fetus or of provoking miscarriage, a fear that is generally felt to be unrealistic for mothers who have no history of miscarriage. Couples may recognize this fear as groundless on an intellectual level but may still feel an emotional constraint. Some had pressing concerns about finances or other social problems that encroached on sexual interest.

Interest in sex markedly increased

Table 7–1   CHANGES IN SEXUAL PATTERNS DURING PREGNANCY

	Masters and Johnson[26]	Falicov[12]	Solberg, Butler, and Wagner[41]
Population studied	111 primiparas and multiparas; self-enrolled	19 primigravidas (16 college graduates)	260 women
When interviewed	4 interviews: 2nd, 6th, 8th month of pregnancy and 3 months postpartum	5 interviews: beginning in first trimester through 8 weeks postpartum	One interview 2nd or 3rd day postpartum
Sexual practices and feelings in first trimester	Decrease in sexual desire and coital frequency	Moderate to marked decrease in coital frequency	Decreased coital frequency
Sexual practices and feelings in second trimester	Marked increase in desire and coital frequency	Slightly increased coital frequency; below pregnancy levels	Continued decrease in coital frequency
Sexual practices and feelings in third trimester	Diminished interest	Fluctuation in desire in 7th and 8th months; 15 of 18 women* ceased intercourse by 8th month; 17 of 18 by 9th month (only 5 of 18 so advised by physician)	60 per cent abstained from intercourse during last month (only 29 per cent so advised by physician)

*One infant was delivered prior to 3rd trimester.

during the second trimester for virtually all of the women in the Masters and Johnson study. Sexual fantasies and dreams also increased. Falicov reported a slight increase in both coital frequency and sexual satisfaction although not to prepregnancy levels, while Solberg found a continuous decrease in interest. Falicov suggests that the difference in the results of Masters and Johnson may be related to the fact that women who enroll themselves in a study of sexuality may have a high level of sexual interest. There is an apparent association between the level of sexual interest prior to pregnancy and the level of sexual interest during pregnancy; high prenatal interest correlates with a higher level of interest during pregnancy. Women with low prenatal interest have a correspondingly lower interest during pregnancy, although the removal of the fear of pregnancy sometimes makes intercourse more appealing. During the second trimester, the increasing size of a woman's abdomen means that changes in coital position and movements will become necessary.

By the end of the third trimester, the frequency of coital activity is markedly diminished and often has ceased. Even women who are not advised by nurses or physicians to limit intercourse often do so because they have heard from others that sexual abstinence is advisable to prevent infection and/or premature labor (Chapter 9).

Pregnancy and the Male Partner's Sexual Activities

It is inevitable that pregnancy will have some effect on the male partner's sexual activities. Fear of harming the fetus causes some men to lessen the frequency of coitus. A variety of personal reasons influences others. But by far the most frequent reason for limiting intercourse was the constraint of their mate's physician. Of 71 men studied by Masters and Johnson whose partners' physicians limited intercourse for varying periods during and after pregnancy:

1. Twenty-one understood the reason and agreed with and honored the prohibition.

2. Twenty-three did not understand the reason, were not sure the doctor had really said it, or wished the doctor had explained the reason to them as well as to their wives.

3. Eighteen found other sexual partners; twelve during the prenatal and postnatal periods and six during the postnatal period only. Three of these men stated that this was the first time they had sought extramarital sex.[26]

Nursing roles in helping couples meet their sexual needs during pregnancy are discussed in Chapter 9.

ADOLESCENCE AND PREGNANCY

Although birth rates for the United States have decreased markedly in recent years, the numbers of births to teenaged mothers has increased. To effectively help teenagers cope with pregnancy, we need to consider the developmental aspects of adolescence, together with the ways in which pregnancy interfaces with those developmental needs. In doing so, we discover that for the teenager herself, her needs and concerns are principally directed toward her adolescence rather than toward her pregnancy.

Like the members of every group, adolescents who are pregnant are not a homogeneous group. Nor is every adolescent pregnancy necessarily a problem pregnancy, although many do present one or more special needs.

Mary Anne is 18 and a high school senior. Although she is not married to the man who is the father of her expected baby the relationship is close. He hopes to be with her during labor and delivery. Both his mother and her own plan to help care for the baby next year so that Mary Anne can attend the LPN program at the community college.

Janice is 16. She lives at home with her mother and sisters; two of her sisters, 17 and 18 years old, are also pregnant. She says she feels no long-term commitment to the father of this infant and would rather have her girlfriend with her during labor.

Cara is 17 and very much alone. Her parents live in a rural community approximately 50 miles from the city where she is now living. The baby's father is from that same community; she has not seen him since she discovered that she was pregnant and does not plan to tell him. Cara has not completed high school; she worked as a waitress when she first came to the city and is now a cashier in a movie theater from 2:00 P.M. until 10:00 P.M. each evening.

Needs of Adolescents Who Are Pregnant

Need for Acceptance by Peers. Observe any group of adolescents for an hour or so, and the importance of the peer group, i.e., their fellow adolescents, becomes apparent. Teens tend to dress alike, eat the same foods, participate in the same activities, use the same vocabulary, listen to the same music, and on and on. Few teens want to be different.

An understanding of this fact has a number of ramifications for our care of the pregnant teenager. If she is a part of a group in which pregnancy is frequent and accepted, *not* being pregnant or having never been pregnant may make her different. If she is part of a group that is looking toward college or a group in which out-of-wedlock pregnancy means "bad girl," being pregnant may be highly stressful. She may choose to terminate the pregnancy early and return to "normal" as quickly as possible.

If she chooses to continue the pregnancy, she may still attempt to remain like her peers in as many ways as possible. For example, she often continues to wear the same clothes that she wore before and to eat foods that are a part of the teenaged lifestyle (soft drinks and French fries, for example) even though we suggest to her that these foods are not ideal during pregnancy.

Need for Emancipation from Parents. One of the largest of all of the tasks of the teenager is achieving independence. For many girls, pregnancy can interrupt the process of becoming independent in a very disturbing way. Our nursing behavior can facilitate her developing independence or can be one more barrier to that independence.

Consider the following very familiar situation:

Mrs. Anderson has brought her 16 year old unmarried, pregnant daughter Sally to the obstetric clinic. Sally is quiet, occasionally biting her lip. She does what you ask, never smiling and saying little. Her mother has a great deal to say, most of which is not very complimentary to Sally.

Both Sally and her mother have needs, and Mrs. Anderson is pressing hers upon you very hard. It's very easy to get so drawn into dialogue with an adolescent's parents that we forget our first priority must be Sally herself—*Sally is our patient.* If we appear to be merely her mother's ally, we will not be very effective in helping Sally. The first rule is: *Remember who the patient is.*

This is not to say that her parents are not very important. A chance to express their feelings is very necessary, both for them and for their pregnant daughter. Ideally, this will come at a separate time and/or place—not during the daughter's prenatal visit. If a separate time is impossible, then a separate place to talk is needed.

Need to Express Feelings to a Nonjudgmental, Truly Interested Adult. Many pregnant adolescents have a need to express their feelings about their pregnancy. Few teenagers can share such feelings with their own parents; such discussions too often become punitive and judgmental.

For some, sharing in a group session may be easier than a face-to-face session with one individual. Here again, the support of the all-important peer group can be significant. Others may find it more difficult to express themselves in groups.

Cultural values will affect the degree to which individuals will share deeply felt emotions. When control of feelings is considered a value, sharing feelings may expose the individual to ridicule from her peers, as Lenocker and Daugherty demonstrated in their study of adolescent mothers.[22] Verbalization of feelings is largely a middle class value and a value of our profession. We need to be sensitive, however, to those groups that do not share this value and should not press our own values upon them.

One of the problems many nurses and other health professionals have in helping a teenager who is pregnant—especially the 14, 15, or 16 year old—is that we also often have very ambivalent feelings about her pregnancy. Thus it is difficult to be nonjudgmental. We may feel that her pregnancy is not a good idea, so that although a part of us truly wants to help her cope with pregnancy, another part of us may want her to understand that she shouldn't be pregnant in the first place. We may fear that being too accepting of her means that we condone her behavior.

We need to recognize our own feelings and to seek guidance in coping with them if we are to be the nonjudgmental professionals that patients have a right to expect us to be.

Need for Mutual Self-disclosures. Should a nurse or other professional person share her own experiences and values about pregnancy with her teenaged patients? Traditionally, we have been told that this is inappropriate and nonprofessional. However, Lenocker and Daugherty described their work with adolescents in which they consciously chose to be open with the teenaged mothers.[22] They found that the girls responded by questioning them about their attitudes toward many aspects of their (the authors) life—marriage, childrearing, men, birth control, and similar areas. The teenagers used this information not as a norm for their own life, but as a part of a process of forming perceptions about middle class white women. (The group of teens in the study were black and from low income homes.) The authors felt their openness, which included picnics at their homes, may also have demonstrated that self-revelation is an acceptable form of behavior.

Need to Be Understood Despite Language Barrier. An important characteristic of adolescent culture is a language by which teens communicate with one another. This language includes phrases that may mean something very different to the teenaged mother than they do to us. Moreover, many terms in general use are unfamiliar, especially if the teenager is from a different socioeconomic level and/or a different cultural background than the nurse.

By asking for frequent feedback and by checking out what we think we hear, we can overcome these language barriers and keep communication pathways open.

Need to Accept Changing Body. Accepting the changes in her own body is one of the developmental tasks that each teenager must achieve. The amount of time spent in front of the mirror is evidence of the importance of this task. The tremendously greater body changes that occur during pregnancy are superimposed upon this already major job.

How does she respond? Denial, exhibited by wearing a tightly buttoned coat or by refusing to wear maternity clothes, is one response. The 16 year old in her seventh month of pregnancy, sitting in the obstetrics clinic in a sweater and jeans, is not necessarily lacking funds to buy more appropriate clothing.

Need to Continue Education. Caring for the teenager who is pregnant will hopefully lead nurses to investigate what their community offers to meet the educational needs of adolescent gravidas. What happens to pregnant teenagers—married and unmarried—in your local school system? Do they have to drop out of school? Do they have an opportunity to learn about how to care for themselves and their babies? Is there a readily accessible person with whom they can talk?

In the past, and to this day in many parts of the United States, pregnancy has automatically meant exclusion from school, often not only during the prenatal period but for varying lengths of time after the baby is born. As a result, for most of the girls involved, pregnancy means an effective termination of their education. A survey by Gordon in 197 documents that local practices rather than statutes or regulations are the determinants of such customs.[14] Although arguments such as concern for the health of the teenaged gravida may be advanced as the basis of such policies, one suspects that the fact that these girls have violated community norms and the fear that they might, by their presence, encourage others to do so, seems closer to the real reason.

Recent court decisions suggest that this kind of exclusion may be a violation of legal rights. Whether or not this will ultimately be shown to be true, it is certain that the beginning of pregnancy is a poor time to interrupt a girl's education. To her increasingly important need for a basic education is now added a need for knowledge of pregnancy and child care. She needs more, not less, education and counseling.

A number of communities across the United States have dealt with the needs of the pregnant teenager in varying ways. Two of these programs are described below.

THE WINSTON-SALEM, NORTH CAROLINA PROGRAM. When a teenager attending public school in Winston-Salem thinks she is pregnant, she goes to her school guidance counselor. If it is her choice to continue her pregnancy, she may transfer to the Continuing Education Center or remain in her base school.

Prior to 1964, when the continuing education concept was originated, most girls terminated their schooling when they became pregnant. Few returned, since policies dictated that they must remain at home until after their baby's first birthday, a policy that was applied uniformly to married and unmarried students alike. Beginning with eight girls and one teacher, the program now serves more than 200 girls each year with a staff that includes a full-time director, a social worker, two nurses, seven teachers, the services of a vocational rehabilitation worker, a child development specialist, and college students who volunteer to tutor students in subjects not offered by the center. In addition to basic junior and senior high school subjects, students study the proc-

esses of pregnancy, newborn care and home economics and participate in group discussions, termed Laboratory for Effective Living, conducted by nurses, a social worker, and a child development specialist.

The nurses follow the students physically after their initial examination by a physician until the last month of pregnancy, when they return to the physician's care. The services of physicians are also available if any sign of complication arises.

After delivery, students usually return to classes within 2 weeks. They may return to regular school classes when a new semester begins or may remain at the Continuing Education Center until the end of the school year.

THE ATLANTA ADOLESCENT PREGNANCY PROGRAM. In Atlanta approximately 80 per cent of the pregnant students remain in their neighborhood schools throughout their pregnancy. They find this a feasible, workable, and inexpensive option. Special education classes are available, however, for the very young student in grammar school, who requires a greater degree of privacy and protection than regular school offers; for the student who does not plan to keep her baby; and for any student who feels a strong need for concealment.

Since this is a relatively new concept and one that may grow in the future, both opposing points of view and Atlanta's arguments for this type of program seem worth considering.

Reasons for Excluding Pregnant Students from Regular School Classes.

1. Pregnant students are unable, for medical reasons, to carry out the usual school program. The Atlanta program argues that this is not true for the majority of students, just as it is untrue for most women who are employed and/or care for their homes.

2. Allowing the student to remain in school makes it appear that the school board favors or approves of teenaged pregnancy.

3. The teenager who is pregnant needs teachers who are sympathetic and understanding. Experience in Atlanta showed that some teachers of regular classes were quite hostile, some quite sympathetic, but that the majority did not have strong feelings either way. It was not difficult to avoid the openly hostile teachers. It is also likely that the too sympathetic instructor might not be the most helpful, since the student must get along with the varied attitudes of people in the real world.

Reasons for Including Pregnant Students in Regular School Classes.

1. Relationships with teachers and friends are already built. At an age when peer relationships are very important, these ties are not broken by transfer to a special school.

2. Requiring a student to leave her regular school can be interpreted by the student as evidence that she is "undesirable" or "bad," creating or reinforcing a feeling of alienation. It is felt that it may be difficult for her to return to a school in which she feels she is not wanted.

3. The regular school can offer a wider range of educational and extracurricular activities. Although the small and specialized classes of a special school may seem ideal, what is the long-range gain once the student has returned to her regular classrooms?

4. Transportation problems are less likely when the student remains in her regular school.

5. The cost to the school system is less. Special facilities and teachers for small groups of students are not required.

6. School-aged pregnancy is visible, an important factor in helping

communities deal realistically with the needs of teenaged gravidas.

The Law and Patients Under 18 Years of Age

The basic legal theory that governs relationships between nurses and other givers of health care and patients under 18 years of age is that treatment of a minor without parental consent is assault.

However, exceptions to this theory are multiple. These exceptions are based on the laws of *states* (rather than federal law, which applies to all states) so that the illustrations given in this text may not apply to every nurse. It is very important that nurses know and understand the laws of their own state as they apply to the health care of minors. In some instances, local ordinances may apply as well.

Laws frequently use the term *emancipated minor,* which generally includes those under 18 who are married, serving in the Armed Forces, or living away from home, although the definition of an emancipated minor also varies somewhat from state to state. The law regarding emancipated minors often differs from the law that governs minors who live at home with their parents.

Perhaps the most widespread of the laws governing treatment of minors without parental consent is that dealing with the treatment of venereal disease. Because of the realistic recognition of the epidemic of venereal disease among adolescents (as well as among individuals over 18), most states allow a minor to seek treatment without parental consent.

On the other hand, giving family planning information to a minor without parental consent is not possible under many state laws. In some states, a teenager must have one pregnancy before she qualifies for family planning care.

Some states require parental consent for the care of a minor who is pregnant. Since many teenagers postpone "telling" their parents about pregnancy as long as possible, this means a delay in health care, often well past the important first trimester of embryologic development.

The inability of a minor to have an abortion without parental consent may delay the abortion until a time when a more complex procedure is necessary or when the abortion itself is not possible.

Not everyone is in favor of allowing adolescents to assume responsibility for their own health care. The major opposition has come from parents who see such efforts as one more assault on the family, by taking from the parents still another of their responsibilities.

We would encourage nurses to consider their experience with pregnant adolescents and the laws of their own states and then to actively lobby in their state legislature for any changes that they feel will facilitate improved health care for adolescents.

SUMMARY

Psychologic and social change is as much a part of pregnancy as physiologic change. Understanding psychosocial changes is therefore essential to the care of all childbearing families.

REFERENCES

1. Bell, R. R.: *Marriage and Family Interaction.* Homewood, Ill., The Dorsey Press, 1971.
2. Benedek, T.: Psychological Aspects of Pregnancy and Parent-Child Relationships. *In* Leibman, S. (ed.): *Emotional Problems of Childhood.* Philadelphia, J. B. Lippincott Co., 1958.
3. Benedek, T.: The Psychology of Pregnancy. *In* Anthony, E., and Benedek, T. (eds.): *Parenthood: Its Psychology and Psychopathology.* Boston, Little, Brown and Co., 1970.
4. Bibring, G.: Some Considerations of the Psychological Processes in Pregnancy. *In* Eissler, R. (ed.): *The Psychoanalytic Study of the Child.* Vol. XIV. New York, International University Press, 1959.
5. Brown, L. B.: Social and Attitudinal Concomitants of Illness in Pregnancy. *British Journal of Medical Psychology, 35*:311, 1962.
5a. Caplan, G.: Patterns of Parental Response to the Crisis of Premature Birth. *Psychiatry, 23*:365, 1960.
6. Caplan, G.: Psychological Aspects of Maternity Care. *American Journal of Public Health, 47*:25, 1957.
7. Cohen, M., and Friedman, S.: Nonsexual Motivation of Adolescent Sexual Behavior. *Medical Aspects of Human Sexuality,* September, 1975, p. 9.
8. Curtis, J. L.: A Psychiatric Study of 55 Expectant Fathers. *United States Armed Forces Medical Journal, 6*:937, 1955.
9. Deutsch, H.: *The Psychology of Women.* New York, Grune and Stratton, 1945.
10. Duvall, E.: *Family Development.* 2nd Edition. Philadelphia, J. B. Lippincott Co., 1962.
11. Dyer, E. D.: Parenthood as Crisis: A Re-Study. *Marriage and Family Living,* May, 1963, p. 196.
12. Falicov, C. T.: Sexual Adjustment During First Pregnancy and Post Partum. *American Journal of Obstetrics and Gynecology, 117*:991, 1973.
13. Foltz, A., Klerman, L., and Jekel, J.: Pregnancy and Special Education: Who Stays in School. *American Journal of Public Health, 62*:1612, 1972.
14. Gordon, L.: National Survey of Legislation Relative to Schoolage Parents. National Alliance Concerned with Schoolage Parents. Unpublished, 1971.
15. Grinder, R. G.: *Adolescence.* New York, John Wiley and Sons, Inc., 1973.
16. Havighurst, R.: *Human Development and Education.* New York, Longmans, Green and Co., 1953.
17. Hendricks, C.: Delivery Patterns and Reproductive Efficiency among Groups of Differing Socioeconomic Status and Ethnic Origins. *American Journal of Obstetrics and Gynecology, 97*:608, 1967.
18. Hill, R.: *Families Under Stress.* New York, Harper Books, 1949.
19. Katchadourian, A., and Lunde, D. T.: *Fundamentals of Human Sexuality.* New York, Holt, Rinehart and Winston, Inc., 1972.
20. Klaus, M., and Kennell, J.: *Maternal Infant Bonding.* St. Louis, C. V. Mosby Co., 1976.
20a. Koos, E. L.: *Families in Trouble.* New York, Kings Crown Press, 1946.

21. LeMasters, E. E.: Parenthood as Crisis. *Marriage and Family Living*. November, 1957, p. 352.

22. Lenocker, J., and Daugherty, M.: Adolescent Mothers' Social and Health-Related Interests: Report of a Project for Rural, Black Mothers. *JOGV Nursing, 5*:9, 1976.

23. Liebenberg, B.: Expectant Fathers. *Child and Family, 8*:3, Summer, 1969.

24. Loesch, J., and Greenberg, V.: Some Specific Areas of Conflicts Observed during Pregnancy: A Comparative Study of Married and Unmarried Pregnant Women. *American Journal of Orthopsychiatry, 32*:624, 1962.

25. Marquart, R.: Expectant Fathers: What Are Their Needs? *Men, 1*:32, 1976.

26. Masters, W., and Johnson, V.: *Human Sexual Response*. Boston, Little, Brown and Co., 1966.

27. Mercer, R.: Becoming a Mother at Sixteen. *MCN 1*:44, 1976.

28. Newton, H.: *Maternal Emotions*. New York, Harper Books, 1955.

29. Obeyesekere, G.: Pregnancy Cravings (Dola Duka) in Relation to Social Structure and Personality in a Sinhalese Village. *American Anthropologist, 65*:323, 1963.

30. Parsons, T.: *The Social System*. Glencoe, Ill., The Free Press, 1951.

31. Quirk, B., and Hassanein, R.: The Nurse's Role in Advising Patients on Coitus During Pregnancy. *Nursing Clinics of North America, 8*:501, 1973.

32. Rice, E. P.: Social Aspects of Maternity Care. *Obstetrics and Gynecology, 23*:307, 1964.

33. Richardson, L.: Unwed Mother. *American Journal of Nursing, 68*:2617, 1968.

34. Rosengren, W.: Social Sources of Pregnancy as Illness or Normality. *Social Forces, 39*:260, 1961.

35. Rosengren, W.: Social Status, Attitudes to-ward Pregnancy, and Child Rearing Attitude. *Social Forces, 41*:127, 1962.

36. Rubin, R.: Cognitive Style in Pregnancy. *American Journal of Nursing, 70*:502, 1970.

37. Rubin, R.: Maternal Tasks in Pregnancy. *Maternal-Child Nursing Journal, 4*(3): 143, 1975.

38. Sears, R. R., Maccoby, E., and Levine, H.: *Patterns of Child Rearing*. New York, Harper and Row, 1957.

39. Silberg, D., Butler, J., and Wagner, N.: Sexual Behavior in Pregnancy. *New England Journal of Medicine, 288*:1098, 1973.

40. Siler, M.: The Ministry of a Southern Baptist Church to Families at the Event of the Birth of a Child. Unpublished doctoral dissertation. Louisville, Ky., Southern Baptist Theological Seminary, 1967.

41. Solberg, D., Butler, J., and Wagner, N.: Sexual Behavior in Pregnancy. *New England Journal of Medicine, 288*:1098, 1973.

42. Trethowan, W., and Conlon, M.: The Couvade Syndrome. *British Journal of Psychiatry, 111*:57, 1965.

43. Turner, E. K.: The Syndrome in the Infant Resulting from Maternal Emotional Tension During Pregnancy. *The Medical Journal of Australia*, 1956 (1), p. 221.

44. Vincent, C.: *Sexual and Marital Health*. New York, McGraw-Hill Book Co., 1973.

45. Wapner, J.: The Attitudes, Feelings, and Behaviors of Expectant Fathers Attending Lamaze Classes. *Birth and the Family Journal, 3*(1):5, 1976.

46. Waters, J.: *The Atlanta Adolescent Pregnancy Program: Program Director's Report*. Atlanta, Emory University School of Medicine, 1971.

47. Ziegel, E., and Van Blarcom, C.: *Obstetric Nursing*. 6th Edition. New York, The Macmillan Co., 1972.

Chapter 8

THE PRENATAL FAMILY: NURSING ASSESSMENT

The nursing process—assessment, planning, intervention, and evaluation —is the framework for care of child-bearing families. *Assessment,* beginning at our first contact with the mother and other members of her family, and continuing throughout prgenancy, is the theme of this chapter.

THE FIRST CONTACT

Mother and Nurse

Consider the woman coming for her initial maternity examination. She may have only recently missed a menstrual period for the first time, or she may have considered herself pregnant for many months. She may suspect that she is pregnant and that is why she has come, but her pregnancy has probably not been confirmed. Her feelings about the possibility of pregnancy may easily be ambivalent, as noted in Chapter 7. If she has never had an obstetric evalua-tion, or perhaps even a pelvic examina-tion, she will almost always be anxious and fearful; many mothers show some anxiety at the time of initial examina-tion during second and subsequent pregnancies as well. For many young

women this visit may be their first con-tact with health care since they were children. Childhood fears of nurses and physicians may influence them uncon-sciously, if not consciously.

We will probably not be able to al-leviate all of a woman's anxiety, but we can do a great deal to lessen it by the way in which we interact with her dur-ing this first visit. Although there is a great deal that we will be trying to ac-complish at this visit, a first essential is allowing adequate time to make each woman feel comfortable in the clinical environment and to give us the oppor-tunity to establish a relationship with her.

The physical environment must be planned so that we can talk with her in some place that assures privacy. An ar-rangement of furniture that allows nurse and patient to sit facing one another directly is far better than the barrier of a desk between them. At-tempting to establish a relationship with a patient in a crowded waiting-room or while she is lying on her back on an uncomfortable examining table is poor nursing care.

How can we make a mother more relaxed and comfortable during her first

217

visit? Our approach, our manner, and our "therapeutic use of self" are difficult to codify into a set of rules. We can begin by introducing ourselves by name and by encouraging the woman to tell us something about herself before we begin to deal with specific questions. We want to convey the feeling that she is the focus of our concern at the moment and that we will take the time to answer any questions she may have.

The *goals* of the initial contact are seven:

1. To make the mother feel more comfortable by demonstrating our interest in her as a person and in her concerns, and by explaining to her what will happen during the rest of the initial visit (anticipatory guidance), along with the reason for each phase of the examination (these explanations will be reinforced as each step occurs).

2. To confirm the pregnancy by laboratory testing, if indicated.

3. To assess factors in the social, medical, and reproductive history that are pertinent to the course and outcome of this pregnancy.

4. To assess general and reproductive health by physical and laboratory examination.

5. To assess nutritional needs.

6. To assess pertinent social needs.

7. To assess the mother's feelings about the pregnancy, and also those of other significant people, usually the baby's father and/or other family members.

Father and Nurse

Note that we are discussing this first visit in relation to the mother, because most women come to clinics and offices without their husbands. We believe that the ideal situation is one in which both parents come together. Not only will both receive the same information, but we will have the opportunity to assess the needs and feelings of both man and woman. Often our only information about the father comes from the mother; what we hear, of course, is her perception of his feelings and attitudes. Her perception is important because it is a reality for her, but it should not be confused with the father's own perception of his feelings and concerns. In addition, observation of interaction between the couple, only possible if both are present, is important in understanding the couple's response to the pregnancy.

There is no reason why a father should automatically be banished to a waiting-room even during the physical examination. Just as many fathers sit at the head of the delivery table, talking with and supporting their wives, fathers can sit at the head of the table during the physical examination and support their wives during this initial assessment. Single mothers who desire to maintain a close relationship with their baby's father should have this same privilege.

Other Family Members

What about the mother of the unmarried daughter who comes with her for her initial visit? Vincent[16] suggests that we remember *who* the patient is, that it is the young woman who is pregnant and not her parents. If one or both of the young woman's parents are present during the initial interview, if indeed they are the major participants, their daughter may see us as an extension of her parents and her parents' attitudes. This may make it difficult for us to establish a relationship with her (see Chapter 7).

CONFIRMATION OF PREGNANCY

Jokes about pregnancy detection, particularly in old movies, often center on the rabbit test, in which urine from the woman is injected into a rabbit. Human chorionic gonadotropin (HCG), a hormone produced by the syncytiotrophoblast, is found only in the presence of trophoblastic tissue. If a woman is pregnant, the HCG in her urine causes formation of corpora lutea in the ovaries of the test animal.

Biologic tests for pregnancy include the Aschheim-Zondek test, first developed in 1928, which uses mature mice, the Friedman rabbit test, and others using young mice, frogs, and toads.

More common today than the biologic tests are the *immunologic tests,* which involve an antigen-antiserum reaction. This type of test requires: (1) antiserum against HCG, prepared by producing an antibody response in animals; (2) antigen, which consists of latex particles coated with HCG; and (3) urine from the mother.

If the mother's urine contains HCG, it will neutralize the antiserum and prevent the agglutination (clumping) of the latex particles. The test is considered positive, and the woman is felt to be pregnant. If the woman's urine does not contain HCG, the antiserum and the antigen will agglutinate. The test is negative, and it is assumed that she is not pregnant. The entire test takes only a few minutes.

False positive results are relatively rare. False negative results are more common, usually because the HCG level is insufficient or the urine is very dilute. The test may be positive 8 to 15 days after a missed period, but the likelihood of accurate results increases as levels of HCG rise.

A somewhat similar test, which takes about 2 hours to complete, is the *hemagglutination inhibition test,* which also utilizes maternal urine. If HCG is present, agglutination occurs between erythrocytes coated with antigen and gonadotropin antiserum. In both tests using urine, it is important that the urine container is a regular collection bottle and not a jar from home that may contain some substance that would interfere with accurate results.

A more recently developed test, *radioreceptor assay* (also called the Saxena test after developer Brij Saxena), has proved accurate as soon as the menstrual period is missed. A few drops of blood, taken from the woman's finger, are examined. In addition to early reliability, the Saxena test identifies which women may spontaneously abort and also determines the presence of ectopic pregnancy, information not available in earlier types of tests. Saxena has suggested that this test be done whenever any woman is admitted to the hospital prior to the use of X-ray, medication, anesthesia, or any other treatment potentially harmful to a fetus.

PSYCHOSOCIAL ASSESSMENT

Psychosocial assessment, like physical assessment, begins by gathering a data base at the first prenatal visit. Table 8–1 lists some basic questions that may be included in the initial data, along with some of the risk factors that may be associated with those questions.

Once the basic assessment is completed, potential problems can be identified and recorded, along with physical data, so that intervention can occur or referral can be made.

Horsley[7] has developed a system by which points are assigned to various risk factors. Two points are given for the

Table 8–1   PSYCHOSOCIAL ASSESSMENT

Data	Potential Risk Factors
MARITAL STATUS	
1. Married, single, separated, divorced, widowed	1. Single parent, bereavement, potential lack of emotional support
2. Date of marriage	2. Shotgun wedding
3. Husband's age, health, occupation, employed or unemployed	3. Disparity in age, stress of illness in family, economic problems
4. Husband's attitude about pregnancy	4. Source of conflict
5. Separation due to:	5. Potential lack of emotional support
a. Frequent need to travel (husband)	
b. Absent in military service	
c. Desertion	
FAMILY HISTORY	
1. Parents' ages, health; siblings' ages, health	1. Familial illness, stress of current family illness, fear of hereditary problem
2. Death, divorce, remarriage of parents	2. Broken home, bereavement
3. Relationship with mother, father	3. Effect on perceptions of parent role
4. Obstetric problems of female relatives	4. Fear of complications
5. Communication with parents	5. Isolation
CURRENT PREGNANCY	
1. Planned/unplanned	1. Either may be associated with psychosocial risks but of different type (see text)
2. How long attempting to conceive	2. Relative infertility
STATUS OF MOTHER	
1. Employed: plans for continuation of employment	1. Economic problems, baby as interference in career plans
2. Feelings about bodily changes*	2. Denial of bodily changes
3. Physical symptoms*	3. Possible relationship between marked physical symptoms and attitudes and feelings
4. Relationship to fetus*	4. Potential problems in mother-baby relationship
a. Marked preference for one sex	
b. Signs of attachment	

*Depending on the stage of pregnancy during which initial assessment takes place, may not be evident until later.

following: unmarried mother, attempted abortion or miscarriage, bereavement during this pregnancy, no emotional support, no financial support, and isolation. One point is accorded for: old for childbearing, shotgun wedding, relative infertility, serious illness or abnormality, maternal or sibling obstetric complications, broken home in childhood, economic insecurity, or concealed fears.

Horsley considers mothers with 0 or 1 point as being at low risk of severe emotional stress in pregnancy; two points indicate a high risk mother and three or more points a very high risk mother. Such an evaluation does not indicate that attention to the emotional needs of the *low* risk or *no* risk mothers is not important but that special attention is necessary for mothers recognized as being at high risk.

A potential risk factor must be evaluated within the total context of each woman's life. For example, a woman who has no communication with her parents, or whose parents are dead, may lack other support systems or may have many other sources of support. The potential problem is a red flag that says, "Explore this further!"

HEALTH HISTORY ASSESSMENT

A mother with a lifelong history of good physical and mental health is far more likely to have a healthy pregnancy with a successful outcome than is the mother with a chronic disease or frequent acute illnesses. Just as healthy mothers produce healthy babies, healthy babies, with proper care, are likely to grow to become healthy parents. Unfortunately, the opposite is also true. Mothers who are not healthy produce babies who are less likely to be healthy and who will grow to be parents who are not healthy. Generation after generation of poor or marginal health is hard to correct during the months of pregnancy. Good health (and good health care) prior to conception and in the period between pregnancies could probably improve pregnancy outcome for many mothers. Those of us who are concerned about the outcome of pregnancy need to focus attention on both research and designs for care during these periods, as well as during pregnancy itself.

General Medical History

Some disease states are known to have specific effects on pregnancy; they include diabetes mellitus, chronic hypertension, severe anemias and other blood dyscrasias, obesity, heart disease (including a past history of rheumatic fever), and venereal disease. A family history of certain of these conditions, diabetes mellitus for example, will alert us to the possibility that the disease itself may appear during pregnancy, even though it has not been previously detected. Pregnancy may have a deleterious effect on some of the mother's health problems. The mother with valvular damage from rheumatic fever may have difficulty because of the increased cardiac workload of pregnancy.

Other factors in the general medical history that should be noted include urinary tract disease; chronic lung problems such as asthma, emphysema, and tuberculosis; ulcers; phlebitis; varicosities; thyroid disease; hepatitis; gallbladder problems; seizure disorders; allergies and drug sensitivities; and major surgery or accidents.

Note should be made of what immunizations the woman has had, particularly for rubella (Chapter 6). Women who are not sure whether they have had either rubella or rubella immunization should have their rubella titer evaluated. Rubella vaccine is not given to women who are pregnant. Any medications taken by the mother, either self-prescribed or prescribed by a physician, must be noted and evaluated (Chapter 6).

Reproductive History

In addition to general health, reproductive health is assessed during the initial visit. Menstrual history includes the date of menarche (i.e., the onset of menstruation), a description of usual periods (interval, duration, amount of flow), and the date of the last menstrual period. Any gynecologic problems or surgery should be noted.

Certain specific terms are used to describe reproductive history. *Gravida* refers to the number of times a woman has been pregnant, regardless of the outcome of the pregnancy.

Para refers to the number of pregnancies that last beyond 20 weeks; it does not refer to the number of infants born. A woman who is para III has had three pregnancies that lasted at least 20 weeks. She may have more than three children; multiple births, such as twins, are counted as a single pregnancy. She may have no living children, if she delivered three stillborn infants after 20 weeks of pregnancy.

The following terms are used:

Abortion: a pregnancy that terminated prior to the twentieth week (miscarriage).

Nulligravida: a woman who has never been pregnant.

Nullipara: a woman who has never delivered a viable infant (legally an infant of 20 weeks' gestation or more).

Primigravida: a woman during her first pregnancy (gravida I, para 0).

Primipara: a woman who has delivered one viable infant (gravida I, para I).

Multigravida: a woman pregnant for the second or subsequent time (gravida II, para I).

Multipara: a woman who has delivered two or more viable infants (gravida II, para II, etc.).

In practice, one may hear the terms primigravida and primipara interchanged, as well as the terms multigravida and multipara. For example, a woman pregnant for the second time (gravida II, para I) is often referred to as a multipara.

Each pregnant woman, thus, is described briefly as gr____, p____, a____. A woman pregnant for the fifth time who has had two miscarriages and two pregnancies that lasted beyond 20 weeks, one of which resulted in a stillborn infant and one of which re-

sulted in a live infant, would be described as gr V, p II, a II.

An alternate system has been suggested, using four digits—first digit: full term deliveries; second digit: premature deliveries; third digit: abortions; and fourth digit: living children. Thus 2102 would mean two full-term deliveries, one premature birth, no abortions, and two living children. This system gives more information than the system in common use.

It is equally important to know if the mother had complications during a previous pregnancy and if she had any pregnancy terminated by induced abortion.

Factors in a mother's reproductive history that suggest the possibility of a problem during pregnancy or the birth of a high-risk infant include:

1. Two or more consecutive spontaneous abortions.
2. A previous perinatal death.
3. Previous premature labor.
4. Five or more pregnancies.
5. Previous cesarean section.
6. Multiple pregnancy (twins, triplets, and so on).
7. A previous baby with a major congenital anomaly.
8. Rh_D incompatibility in a previous pregnancy.
9. A previous baby weighing 4000 grams or more.
10. A previous baby with intrauterine growth retardation.
11. Two or more years of infertility.

In addition to the mother's own reproductive health, some aspects of reproductive health in other members of her family—mother, aunts, sisters—may also be significant. For example, if there have been frequent miscarriages in her family, there may be some geetic basis. If several women relatives have had cesarean delivery because of a small pelvis, she may share this characteristic. She may not know why they have had a cesarean section, but may report that all the women in her family have had a cesarean birth.

PHYSICAL ASSESSMENT

General Health

Key factors in the general physical examination include assessment of height and weight, temperature, pulse, blood pressure, heart, lungs, and abdomen. Although this examination is ideally performed early in pregnancy, in reality it may occur at almost any time, so it is important to try to establish the prepregnancy weight as well as the weight at the time of the examination. In general, mothers who weigh less than 100 pounds or more than 250 pounds prior to pregnancy are at higher risk for problems (Chapter 9). Each

woman's weight must be evaluated in relation to her height.

Blood pressure evaluation will be important throughout pregnancy. Early identification and correction of hypertension are essential if serious problems are to be averted. Recent studies have shown that *mean arterial pressure* has value in predicting which mothers are likely to have hypertension. The mean arterial pressure is determined by adding one-third of the pulse pressure to the diastolic pressure. For example, if a woman's blood pressure is 120/60, her pulse pressure (the difference between the systolic and diastolic pressures) is 60. One-third of 60 is 20. The mean arterial pressure is thus 80. Normally, mean arterial pressure reaches its lowest point about 22 weeks after the last menstrual period (Fig. 8-1) and then rises slowly until term. Mean arterial pressures of 90 or more in the second trimester or 105 or more in the third trimester indicate hypertension.

MEAN ARTERIAL PRESSURE BY GESTATIONAL AGE
FOR SINGLE WHITE TERM LIVE BIRTHS
(nulliparae, age 25-34)

Figure 8-1 Mean arterial pressure in pregnancy. (From Page, Villee, and Villee: *Human Reproduction: The Core Content of Obstetrics, Gynecology and Perinatal Medicine.* 2nd Edition. Philadelphia, W. B. Saunders Co., 1976.)

Evidence of heart disease or thyroid disease may be noted on physical examination, even though no previous history has been reported.

An examination of the teeth and gums should be included in the general physical examination, not as a substitute for an evaluation by a dentist but to emphasize the importance of dental care during pregnancy. Because many women believe that dental care is contraindicated during pregnancy, this brief check-up gives us the opportunity to assure them that this is not true. For patients unable to afford private dental care, appropriate referral should be made.

Breast Examination

Careful examination of the breasts provides an opportunity for evaluation and for some beginning instruction in self-examination. Because breast changes begin early in pregnancy, we can assure the mother that the increased size and tenderness, the darkening of the areola, and so forth, are normal. We will want to observe the protrusion of the nipples (are they protruding, flat, or inverted?), the general contour of the breasts, and the presence of any lumps or painful areas.

Laboratory Studies

Significant laboratory studies include urinalysis, a complete blood count, blood typing and Rh determination, a serologic test for syphilis, and both a smear for gonorrhea and a Papanicolaou smear.

Urinalysis. A complete urinalysis at the time of the first visit is followed by checks for glucose and protein in the urine at each subsequent visit throughout pregnancy. The presence of glucose may indicate gestational diabetes; protein in the urine is a symptom of pre-eclampsia. Both conditions are discussed in Chapter 10.

Blood Tests. Iron deficiency anemia is the most common nutritional complication of pregnancy. All mothers should have a complete blood count, including hemoglobin and hematocrit, during their initial prenatal visit. Norms for these indices are summarized in Table 8–2. The slight decrease in the norms for hemoglobin and hematocrit during pregnancy reflects expanded blood volume; the number of red cells is actually increased. When values fall below these levels, further studies are important to discover the reason for anemia. In addition to iron deficiency anemia, the mother may have megaloblastic anemia due to folate deficiency (fairly common in combination with iron deficiency anemia—see Chapter 9), or she may have anemia due to blood loss or infection, hemolytic anemia, or anemia due to other causes.

Black women should be tested for sickle cell disease or sickle cell trait.

The mother's blood type and Rh status are determined to identify those mothers who are potentially at risk for problems of Rh and ABO incompatibility. Should the mother be Rh negative and the father Rh positive, antibody

Table 8–2   NORMAL RED BLOOD CELL VALUES

	Nonpregnant	Pregnant
Hemoglobin	>12 grams/100 ml.	>11 grams/100 ml.
Hematocrit	>36%	>33%

titers will be followed throughout pregnancy (Chapter 10).

A laboratory test for tuberculosis is frequently performed and cases may be discovered in this way, probably because pregnancy is the first contact the mother has with the health care system in a number of years.

Venereal Disease Testing. Since both syphilis and gonorrhea affect the fetus and the newborn infant, a serologic test for syphilis (VDRL or RPR) and a vaginal smear for gonorrhea should be part of the initial examination of all pregnant women. The laws of many states require testing for syphilis, both during pregnancy and prior to marriage. A second test for syphilis during the third trimester is recommended for women who might become infected during pregnancy.

If a woman acquires syphilis shortly before, during, or soon after conception and is not treated, fetal infection is nearly certain. The result may be fetal death, premature labor and birth, and/or congenital syphilis. The spirochetes cross the placenta between the eighteenth week of pregnancy and the time of delivery.

The baby is most likely to be affected by gonorrhea during his passage through the birth canal at the time of delivery. Ophthalmia neonatorum, a gonococcal infection of the infant's eyes, was formerly a major cause of neonatal blindness. Prophylactic treatment for ophthalmia neonatorum is mandatory in most states at the time of birth (Chapter 15).

Penicillin is the treatment for both syphilis and gonorrhea. If the mother is allergic to penicillin, erythromycin is used. Although tetracycline is given in place of penicillin for treatment of syphilis in nonpregnant women, it is not recommended during pregnancy because it is widely deposited in the fetal skeleton and teeth and may cause inhibition of bone growth and discoloration of fetal teeth. Since the efficacy of drugs other than penicillin in the treatment of syphilis has not been established, careful documentation of penicillin allergy is important.

After the pregnant woman has been treated for syphilis, she should have monthly serologic tests for the remainder of pregnancy. Many months may elapse before a negative serology is obtained (245 days is the average), but some drop in titer should be evident. (This is why a mother may come to delivery with a positive test for syphilis, yet her baby will not be syphilitic.) Treatment early in pregnancy will prevent fetal infection; penicillin given late in pregnancy will cross the placenta and treat the fetus as well as the mother. A fourfold rise in titer for syphilis indicates reinfection and the need for re-treatment.

Smears and cultures for gonorrheal organisms are also repeated monthly when gonorrhea has been detected, and the woman is re-treated if gonococci reappear. When a woman with known, untreated, or resistant gonorrhea is in labor, vaginal exploration is kept as minimal as possible. Silver nitrate is instilled in the baby's eyes once each day for 3 days following delivery; the baby is also treated with penicillin.

Papanicolaou Test. The Papanicolaou test (Pap smear) for cervical cancer, introduced by Papanicolaou and Traut in 1943, is an important part of the prenatal examination because for many women pregnancy may be their only contact with health care during this period of their lives. Ideally, Pap smears should be performed each year for women over 18 years old and for younger women who are sexually active. After 35 years of age a semiannual test is often recommended. Thus it is not enough to perform the test; we need to explain its purpose and the importance of annual tests to each woman. Because of the strong emotions of most women during this initial examination, which may interfere with learning, our teaching needs to be reinforced at a later date.

The test consists of "scraping" the ectocervix, the endocervix, and the vaginal pool in the posterior fornix with a wooden spatula and spreading the material obtained on slides that are then sprayed with a fixative. Analysis of the cervical scrapings is about 98 per cent accurate in detecting cervical dysplasia, carcinoma in situ, and invasive cancer. Analysis of the vaginal pool scrapings is about 75 per cent accurate in detecting adenocarcinoma of the endometrium and will detect cancer of the ovary 25 per cent of the time. Certain vaginal infections can also be recognized.

Pap specimens were originally grouped into five classes; today they may be described rather than classified, but many institutions still report in terms of these classifications:

Class I: Absence of atypical or abnormal cells.
Class II: Atypical cytology but no evidence of malignancy.
Class III: Cytology suggestive of, but not conclusive for, malignancy.
Class IV: Cytology strongly suggestive of malignancy.
Class V: Cytology conclusive for malignancy.

Evaluation of the External and Internal Genitalia

Many women dread examination of their genitalia, in part because of life-long conditioning that tells them (and us) that genitalia should not be exposed, and in part because of the fear of discomfort or the experience of discomfort during a previous examination. In some parts of the world pelvic examinations are not performed during pregnancy or are performed only by women. Because of these feelings, many women fear and even postpone an initial pregnancy examination.

How can we support and reassure women in preparation for a vaginal examination? As already noted, we can explain what will happen and why. We can give them an opportunity to express their fears and bring them into the open by a statement such as, "Many women have told me they do not look forward to a vaginal exam. How are you feeling about it right now?" We can assure them of our presence during the examination. We can drape them to provide minimum exposure. Examining-room furniture can be placed so that the woman's head, and not her genitalia, is placed in the direction of a door that could possibly be opened during the examination. The number of people in the room can be minimized, a somewhat difficult task in a teaching clinic of a large medical center but not impossible with good planning.

An empty bladder is essential before the examination begins. Examination of the external genitalia includes inspection for the presence of a cystocele or rectocele (Chapter 3) and palpation of Bartholin's glands and the urethra. The character of any vaginal discharge is noted. A thin, greenish-gray, foul-smelling discharge that is very irritating is probably caused by *Trichomonas vaginalis* (trichomoniasis vaginitis); microscopic examination of the discharge will show motile trichomonads. Metronidazole (Flagyl), used for trichomonas infection in nonpregnant women, is contraindicated in pregnancy. Topical agents will relieve symptoms, but the condition may recur and require re-treatment. The woman's sexual partner should also be treated since the infection is transmitted during coitus; he can, of course, take metronidazole.

Because of the high glycogen content of the vaginal mucosa during pregnancy, Candida vaginitis is not uncommon. There is intense burning and itching with candidiasis but not necessarily a discharge. When discharge is present, it tends to be thick and tenacious, resembling cottage cheese. White patches are seen on the vaginal walls about 50 per cent of the time. Treatment is topical, and may include the use of gentian violet, nystatin, or candicidin. The preparation is applied twice a day during the first week and then at bedtime during the next 2 to 3 weeks. When gentian violet is used, the mother should be alerted to protect clothing and linens. Candidiasis is also difficult to relieve during pregnancy. Should the mother have candidiasis at the time of a vaginal delivery, her baby may have *thrush* (Chapter 16). Further discussion of vaginal discharge in pregnancy is found in Chapter 9.

The vaginal speculum, used for the internal examination, is always warmed before insertion. The cervix is examined through the speculum (Chapter 3). After the speculum is removed, two gloved, lubricated fingers are inserted in the vagina for palpation of size, shape, and consistency of the uterus. With the middle finger in the rectum and the index finger in the vagina, the examiner palpates the lateral pelvic walls and the parametrial areas.

Evaluation of the Bony Pelvis

In order for vaginal delivery to be possible, the bony pelvis must be large enough to accommodate the passage of the baby. The pelvis is often evaluated early in pregnancy as an aid for planning delivery. Sometimes measurement of the diagonal conjugate is deferred until the vagina and perineum become more elastic at midpregnancy. Evaluation of pelvic capacity can be repeated near term when fetal size can also be estimated.

Three areas, the inlet, the midpelvis, and the outlet, must be adequate for the descent of the fetal head. The two largest diameters of the head in the flexed position, in which it usually passes through the pelvis, are the biparietal and the suboccipitobregmatic (Fig. 8–2). Both of these diameters measure approximately 9.5 cm. in a fetus weighing approximately 3400 grams (7.5 pounds).

The major measure of the pelvic inlet is the *diagonal conjugate*. From this measure the true conjugate is estimated (Table 8–3). The average measure of the true conjugate, 11 cm., is adequate for the 9.5 cm. fetal head.

Direct measurement of the midpelvis is possible only by X-ray; because of the danger of radiation to the fetus, X-ray is usually deferred until the time of labor. Such X-ray is necessary only when there is a question about the adequacy of the pelvis for delivery. During vaginal examination, however, the examiner can feel the prominence of the ischial spines, the way in which the walls of the pelvis slope, the curve of the sacrum, and the width of the sacrosciatic notch.

The outlet is measured by the distance between the ischial tuberosities, which averages 11 cm. If the distance is 8 cm. or less, the posterior sagittal measurement is particularly important. The sum of the intertuberous and the posterior sagittal measurements should be at least 15 cm. in order for the pelvis to be adequate for vaginal delivery. The mobility of the coccyx, which is pressed back during delivery, and the

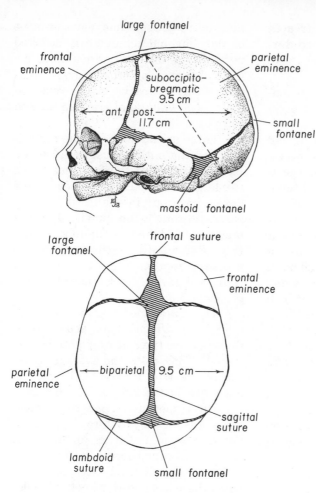

Figure 8–2 Average measurements of the full-term fetal head. (From Page, Villee, and Villee: *Human Reproduction: The Core Content of Obstetrics, Gynecology and Perinatal Medicine.* 2nd Edition. Philadelphia, W. B. Saunders Co., 1976.)

shape of the suprapubic arch are also noted in the evaluation of the outlet.

ASSESSING FEELINGS

Chapter 7 has described many feelings of pregnant women and their partners. The myths of our culture suggest that women should be happy that they are pregnant, although studies indicate that both women and men may be at least initially ambivalent and that some may continue to have mixed feelings or be unhappy through much of their pregnancy. Certainly many other women and couples accept the idea of pregnancy and the birth of their child with joy.

Since few of us are going to share deep feelings with strangers, the verbal expression of feelings about pregnancy during an initial visit may be infrequent. Nonverbal cues, such as facial expression and posture, may be helpful but are not as easy to interpret as they will be when we know the woman better.

It is customary to ask if the pregnancy was planned, the answer to which may give us some clue about the wom-

Table 8–3   MAJOR PELVIC MEASUREMENTS

Measure	Area Measured	Method	Normal Measure	Comment
True conjugate (conjugata vera)	Upper margin of symphysis pubis to sacral promontory (Fig. 8–3)	Subtract 1.5 to 2.0 cm. from diagonal conjugate measurement (below). Cannot be measured directly.	11 cm.	—
Diagonal conjugate	Inferior margin of symphysis pubis to sacral promontory	First two fingers in vagina until tip of 2nd finger touches sacral promontory (Fig. 8–4). Point at which lower margin of symphysis pubis rests on finger is marked with fingernail and measured.	12.5 cm.	Examiner must know own reach. Not all examiners will be able to reach sacral promontory; record "diagonal conjugate reached at 12.0 cm." or "diagonal conjugate not reached at 11.5 cm." May be uncomfortable for patient; reassure.
Intertuberous diameter	Plane of the outlet. Distance between ischial tuberosities	Measured with pelvimeter (Fig. 8–5) or with four knuckles of hand.	Should be 9 cm. or greater; average is 11 cm.	Measurement of outlet is best indication of midplane diameters, through which passage may be most difficult.
Posterior sagittal	Distance between midpoint of intertuberous diameter and tip of sacrum	Measured with pelvimeter	7.5 cm.	—
Shape of the suprapubic arch	—	Palpation	Arch should be wide (Fig. 8–6)	A narrow arch, as found in male pelvis, may indicate other characteristics of narrow male pelvis.

an's feelings. However, unplanned pregnancies are not always unwelcome, nor is a planned pregnancy necessarily a happy one (as, for example, a pregnancy planned by a woman to hold a shaky marriage together). One way to elicit this information in a manner nonthreatening to the patient is to ask if she was using contraceptives at the time that she conceived. Questions about desired family size may also lead to some indication from the mother about her feelings regarding the pregnancy.

CONTINUING MATERNAL ASSESSMENT

At the conclusion of her first visit, the course of a mother's pregnancy may be considered "normal" or "high risk." The plan of care during pregnancy will vary according to each mother's special needs. Continuing evaluation will designate some mothers as high risk later in pregnancy or may remove other mothers from the high risk category. Continuing assessment for the high risk mother is discussed in Chapter 11.

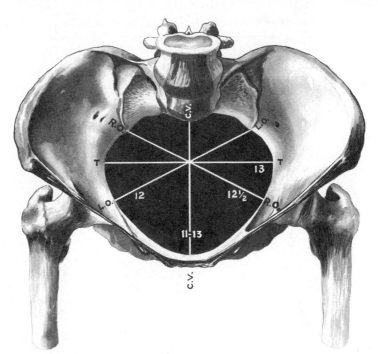

Figure 8–3   The pelvic inlet. *C.V.*, conjugata vera; *T.*, widest transverse; *L.O.*, left oblique; and *R.O.*, right oblique. (From Greenhill and Friedman: *Biological Principles and Modern Practice of Obstetrics.* Philadelphia, W. B. Saunders Co., 1974.)

Figure 8–4   Measuring the diagonal conjugate. (From Eastman and Hellman: *Williams Textbook of Obstetrics.* 13th Edition. New York, Appleton-Century-Crofts, 1966.)

Figure 8–5 Measuring the pelvic outlet with the Thoms pelvimeter. (From Eastman and Hellman: *Williams Textbook of Obstetrics.* 13th Edition. New York, Appleton-Century-Crofts, 1966.)

Figure 8–6 The pelvic outlet viewed from below. It passes through the arch of the pubic rami, the ischial tuberosities, and the tip of the coccyx, forming two triangles bent at their mutually shared base, the intertuberous diameter. (From Greenhill and Friedman: *Biological Principles and Modern Practice of Obstetrics.* Philadelphia, W. B. Saunders Co., 1974.)

For mothers with no apparent major problems during pregnancy, a common pattern of return visits is: monthly until the twenty-eighth week, biweekly from 28 to 36 weeks, and weekly from 36 weeks until delivery.

A return visit within a week of the initial visit is ideal to begin implementation of a nursing care plan early in pregnancy. This visit need not include physician examination, but gives nurses a chance to begin a teaching program after the mother (and father) have had a few days to become accustomed to the idea of pregnancy.

Assessment during these visits follows a plan similar to the initial assessment, in that we will be concerned with general health, course of pregnancy, nutritional status, and social and emotional status.

The Mother's Assessment of Her Pregnancy

As important as the physical examination or laboratory testing is what the mother tells us about her reactions to the pregnancy since the time of her last visit.

Has she been "feeling well" since her last visit, or has she been tired and listless? Has nausea limited her diet?

Table 8–4 SUMMARY OF SIGNS INDICATING NEED FOR IMMEDIATE INTERVENTION

Genital bleeding
Puffiness in face, hands, and in feet and legs in morning
Sudden increase in abdominal size
Sudden weight gain
Decrease in urinary output
Persistent or severe headache
Blurred vision, spots or flashes of light, abdominal pain, back pain, epigastric pain
Chills and fever
Muscle twitching or torpor

Has she been constipated? Has she been having marital problems or problems with her children? Or is she finding this pregnancy to be one of the most satisfying times of her life?

We want particularly to note any danger signs that she may report (summarized in Table 8–4) and to refer these to her physician for immediate care. The significance of these symptoms is discussed in Chapter 10.

Other aspects of the mother's evaluation are mentioned in the sections below.

Certain specific assessment procedures will be a part of each return visit.

Continuing Physical and Laboratory Assessment

A great deal of attention has been focused on *weight gain* during pregnancy in the last three decades. It is believed now that the limitations placed on weight gain in the 1950's and 1960's, and still to a large extent in the 1970's, are harmful to the developing fetus. Because there is a close relationship between the total weight gain of the mother and the birth weight of the baby, a weight gain of 22 to 27 pounds is considered advisable for *all* patients, even those who are obese. The highest incidence of low birth weight babies occurs in mothers who gain less than 11 pounds.

The distribution of the weight gain in pregnancy is summarized in Table 8–5.

Weight gain should follow a pattern; a graph as illustrated in Figure 8–7 should be on each patient's chart to aid in evaluating weight gain. Approximate rates of gain at various stages of pregnancy have also been noted in Chapter 6.

When weight gain varies from the standard pattern, the cause should be

Table 8–5   DISTRIBUTION OF WEIGHT GAINED IN PREGNANCY

	Pounds (Approximate)	Grams (Approximate)
Fetus	7–8	3200–3600
Placenta	1.5	700
Amniotic fluid	2.0	900
Uterine mass	2.0	900
Blood volume	3–4	1400–1800
Breasts	1–3	450–1400
Maternal stores	7.5–8.5	3400–3800
	24	11,000

assessed and an attempt made to correct it. It is particularly important to differentiate between acute weight gain, which is caused by fluid retention and may be related to pre-eclampsia (Chapter 10), and long-term weight gain, which is normal. A gradual, long-term weight gain of as much as 30 pounds may be perfectly healthy, while a total gain of 22 pounds, if 10 of those pounds are gained in a 2 to 3 week period, is potentially dangerous. Weight gain is discussed further in the nutrition section of Chapter 9.

Urine is checked at each visit for sugar and acetone, which may indicate gestational diabetes, and for protein, an indication of pre-eclampsia. These high risk conditions are discussed in Chapter 10.

Blood pressure elevation, as noted above, is also a warning sign of pre-eclampsia; therefore blood pressure is carefully monitored at each visit.

Continuing Nutritional Assessment

In addition to the monitoring of weight gain, nutrition is assessed by interview with the mother-to-be throughout pregnancy. The amount of time spent in re-evaluating nutritional intake will be determined largely by the mother's needs. Adolescents, for example, will probably need more intensive counseling than a 25 year old school-teacher. *Hemoglobin* is often re-evaluated in the eighth month to assure an adequate level at the time of delivery (see also Chapter 10).

Continuing Social Assessment

The primary nurse caring for each mother needs to keep herself informed about social problems that may have been referred to other professionals. For example, has a plan been made for a teenager's continuing education, and is it being followed? Is the eligible mother receiving food stamps? Have financial arrangements been made for hospital delivery? It is not unusual for the best of ideas to get lost in bureaucratic red tape if someone—the primary nurse—does not continue to monitor them.

New social problems, unanticipated at the initial interview, also arise during the months of pregnancy. The illness of another family member, the unexpected loss of a job, or a sudden need to move one's residence are examples. Anxiety related to such changes may affect feelings about pregnancy and may make the period of pregnancy a most difficult time.

Continuing Emotional Assessment

As noted in Chapter 7, a woman's feelings about pregnancy, and those of her husband, may change appreciably

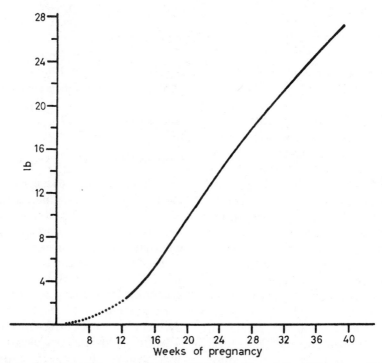

Figure 8–7 Graph charting prenatal weight gain. (From Greenhill and Friedman: *Biological Principles of Obstetrics.* Philadelphia, W. B. Saunders Co., 1974.)

during the course of 9 months. Finding time at each visit to talk at least briefly about feelings not only is essential to evaluation but indicates to the woman (or couple) that changes in feelings are normal. When a woman's comments, or her husband's, indicate particular stress, more time from us, or perhaps referral to another professional may be indicated. We might say, "You seem particularly concerned about _____. Would you like to make an appointment to discuss this on Wednesday afternoon?" or " _____ has talked with many women (couples) with similar concerns. Would you like an appointment to talk with her?"

FETAL ASSESSMENT

After the thirteenth week of pregnancy, abdominal palpation will ascertain the *height of the fundus*. An approximation of the correlation of fundal height with the duration of pregnancy is known as Bartholomew's "rule of fourths," which describes the uterus as being at the pubis at the end of the first month, one-quarter of the way to the umbilicus each successive month, at the level of the umbilicus at the end of the fifth month (20 weeks), and then one-quarter of the distance of the ensiform process at the end of each of the following months (Fig. 8–8). There may be a slight drop in the height of the fundus in the ninth month as the time of delivery approaches. When the height of the fundus does not correlate with the mother's menstrual dates, the duration of pregnancy may need to be re-evaluated. Ultrasound measurements (Chapter 10) may give additional information.

A more rapid increase in fundal height than would ordinarily be expected may indicate multiple pregnancy (twins, and so on); excess amniotic fluid (hydramnios), which in turn may be caused by one of several factors (Chapter 10); the presence of tumors or a hydatidiform mole (Chapter 10); or internal hemorrhage, as in abruptio placentae (Chapter 10).

When the fundal height is lower than expected, possibilities such as intrauterine growth retardation, death of the fetus, fetal abnormality, or decreased amniotic fluid (oligohydramnios) must be considered.

Fetal Outline

By 30 weeks the fetal outline is also palpable. Note in Figures 8–9 through 8–12 that palpation is done with the fingers and palms and not with the fingertips.

In palpating for fetal position, first palpate the fundus (Fig. 8–9). If you feel

Figure 8–8 The relative level of the fundus of the gravid uterus during each successive month of pregnancy according to Bartholomew's "rule of fourths." Beginning with the uterus at the level of the pubis at the end of the first month of pregnancy, it is expected to grow one quarter of the way to the umbilicus each month until the fifth month (with slight positive variation from the dotted line at the end of the fourth month) and one quarter of the remaining distance to the ensiform process (with slight negative variation in the last month) with each succeeding month. (From Greenhill and Friedman: *Biological Principles and Modern Practice of Obstetrics.* Philadelphia, W. B. Saunders Co., 1974.)

Figure 8–9   What is the fundus? Palpation of the uterine fundus will disclose the presence of the breech or the head. (From Greenhill and Friedman: *Biological Principles and Modern Practice of Obstetrics.* Philadelphia, W. B. Saunders Co., 1974.)

a hard, smooth, round body, this is likely to be the fetal head. If you feel an irregularly shaped structure, this is very likely the breech, i.e., the fetal buttocks and legs. Verify your assessment by ascertaining what is over the inlet (Fig. 8–10). In either instance the fetus is said to have a *longitudinal lie* (Chapter 11). If neither the head nor the breech can be palpated, the lie is said to be *transverse;* one must palpate the head and breech at the sides of the uterus (Fig. 8–11).

After 32 weeks, most commonly the breech will be felt in the fundus, and the lie will be longitudinal.

When the lie is ascertained, the position of the fetal spine and "small parts" (hands and feet) may be felt (Fig. 8–12).

Next check for *engagement* of the *presenting part.* Engagement means that the largest section of the presenting part of the fetus has passed the pelvic inlet and entered the true pelvis (Chapter 11). The extent of engagement can be determined by placing both hands on the presenting part (Fig. 8–13) and trying to move the part from side to side. If it is movable, or if the fingers can meet below the presenting part, the part is not engaged.

Fetal Heart Rate

Between 20 and 24 weeks, fetal heart rate (FHR) or fetal heart tones

Figure 8–10 What is over the inlet? By pressing deeply into the pelvis on either side, one learns whether the hard fetal head or soft breech is presenting. (From Greenhill and Friedman: *Biological Principles and Modern Practice of Obstetrics.* Philadelphia, W. B. Saunders Co., 1974.)

(FHT) can be heard by stethoscope. (As noted in Chapter 6, FHR may be heard as early as 10 weeks by Doppler effect.) After the fetal outline is determined, FHR is best heard at the position of the anterior shoulder. FHR is approximately 140 beats per minute with a normal range of 120 to 160 beats per minute. As noted in Chapter 6, the FHR can be differentiated from the maternal heart rate by checking the mother's pulse simultaneously. The quadrant on the mother's abdomen where FHR is heard, as well as the rate, may be recorded as shown here.

This indicates that a FHR of 145 is heard in the left lower quadrant.

Further Assessment of the Fetus

In many pregnancies, the assessment techniques described above will be adequate to assure both caretakers and parents that the fetus is growing normally and is healthy.

Under certain circumstances, however, further assessment of the fetus is desirable. These circumstances include:

1. A mother with a condition that may affect the fetus, such as diabetes or pre-eclampsia.

2. Multiple pregnancy.

3. A mother with complications in a former pregnancy (a stillbirth, for example, or a congenital defect that was detectable in utero).

4. A mother who is to have a cesarean section.

Figure 8–11   Is the ovoid longitudinal or transverse? Facing the patient's head, the nurse applies her hands to the sides of the uterus to determine the fetal lie. (From Greenhill and Friedman: *Biological Principles and Modern Practice of Obstetrics.* Philadelphia, W. B. Saunders Co., 1974.)

Figure 8–12   Method of determining the greater cephalic prominence, here shown on the mother's right side. As both hands are passed along the abdomen toward the pelvis, one is impeded by the fetal forehead and the other one descends until the occiput is reached. The forehead is the greater cephalic prominence in well-flexed vertex presentations, but in face and brow presentations, the occiput is the greater cephalic prominence because the head is deflexed. (From Greenhill and Friedman: *Biological Principles and Modern Practice of Obstetrics.* Philadelphia, W. B. Saunders Co., 1974.)

Figure 8–13   A method of determining overriding of the head. The head is grasped with one hand and pushed down toward the pelvic cavity, while with the other hand over the symphysis pubis, it is determined whether the head sinks into the pelvic cavity or overrides the symphysis. (From Greenhill and Friedman: *Biological Principles and Modern Practice of Obstetrics.* Philadelphia, W. B. Saunders Co., 1974.)

More extensive fetal assessment is done for one of three reasons:

1. To determine the possibility that the fetus may have a particular congenital defect.

2. To assess fetal well-being.

3. To assess fetal maturity.

The techniques for further assessment of the fetus are described in Chapter 10.

SUMMARY

Nursing assessment is the basis of care of the prenatal family. This assessment is multifaceted, involving physical, reproductive, nutritional, social, and emotional aspects on an initial and a continuing basis.

REFERENCES

1. Benson, R. C., Berendes, H., and Weiss, W.: Fetal Compromise During Elective Cesarean Section. *American Journal of Obstetrics and Gynecology, 105*:579, 1969.
2. Brock, D. J. H., and Sutcliffe, R. G.: Alpha-fetoprotein in the Antenatal Diagnosis of Anencephaly and Spina Bifida. Lancet, *II*:197, 1972.
3. Chard, T.: Monitoring of High-Risk Pregnancies by Alpha-Fetoprotein. *In* Spellacy, W. N. (ed.): *Management of the High-Risk Pregnancy.* Baltimore, University Park Press, 1976.

4. Gant, N. F., Chand, S., Warley, R. J., et al: Clinical Test Useful for Predicting the Development of Acute Hypertension in Pregnancy. *American Journal of Obstetrics and Gynecology, 120*:1, 1974.
5. Gluck, L.: Fetal Maturity and Amniotic Fluid Surfactant Determinations. *In* Spellacy, W. N. (ed.): *Management of the High-Risk Pregnancy.* Baltimore, University Park Press, 1976.
6. Greenhill, J., and Freedman, E.: *Biological Principles and Modern Practice of Obstetrics.* Philadelphia, W. B. Saunders Co., 1974.
7. Horsley, S.: Psychological Management of the Pre-Natal Period. *In* Howells, J. (ed.): *Modern Perspectives in Psycho-Obstetrics.* New York, Brunner/Mazel, 1972.
8. Mandelbaum, B., LaCroix, G., and Robinson, A. R.: Determination of Fetal Maturity by Spectrophotometric Analysis of Amniotic Fluid. *Obstetrics and Gynecology, 29*:471, 1967.
9. Page, G., Villee, C., and Villee, D.: *Human Reproduction: The Core Content of Obstetrics, Gynecology and Perinatal Medicine.* 2nd Edition. Philadelphia, W. B. Saunders Co., 1976.
10. Pitkin, R. M.: Fetal Maturity: Nonlipid Amniotic Fluid Assessment. *In* Spellacy, W. N. (ed.): *Management of the High-Risk Pregnancy.* Baltimore, University Park Press, 1976.
11. Pitkin, R. M., and Zwirek, S. J.: Amniotic Fluid Creatinine. *American Journal of Obstetrics and Gynecology, 98*:1135, 1967.
12. Sabbagha, R. E.: Ultrasound in Managing the High-Risk Pregnancy. *In* Spellacy, W. N. (ed.): *Management of the High-Risk Pregnancy.* Baltimore, University Park Press, 1976.
13. Seller, M.: Alpha-fetoprotein and the Prenatal Diagnosis of Neural Tube Defects. *Developmental Medicine Child Neurology, 16*:369, 1974.
14. Spellacy, W. N.: *Management of the High-Risk Pregnancy.* Baltimore, University Park Press, 1976.
15. Tulchinsky, D.: The Value of Estrogens in High Risk Pregnancy. *In* Spellacy, W. N. (ed.): *Management of the High-Risk Pregnancy.* Baltimore, University Park Press, 1976.
16. Vincent, C.: *Sexual and Marital Health.* New York, McGraw-Hill Book Co., 1973.

Chapter 9

THE PRENATAL FAMILY: TEACHING AND COUNSELING

When the mother is physically and emotionally healthy throughout pregnancy, nursing care is focused on teaching and counseling. Antenatal teaching and counseling involve three basic areas:

1. Coping with the physical, social, and emotional changes and needs related to the pregnancy itself.

2. Preparing for the process of labor and delivery.

3. Preparing for parenting.

HOW NURSES CAN HELP PARENTS LEARN TO BE PARENTS

Classes taught in high school and colleges, and many of the textbooks that accompany these courses, seem to stress preparation for and adjustment to marriage much more thoroughly then they explore pregnancy and parenthood. Popular media often romanticize the lives of young mothers and fathers. And with relatively few large and/or extended families in our society, most of us come to pregnancy with neither a realistic idea of what will be demanded of us nor the knowledge that will help us cope.

Mothers (and fathers, as well) are seeking different kinds of information at various stages of pregnancy. During the first weeks and months, principal concerns are for the woman herself—the changes that are occurring within her body, the changes in her feelings, and the fluctuations in the couple's relationship. Later, particularly after quickening, interest in the baby will heighten, and she will be more interested in learning about infant needs and care. Some mothers, especially adolescents, may not show any interest in baby care until after the time of delivery; their own needs seem to outweigh those of an infant who hardly seems real. At this later stage of pregnancy, a mother will also be concerned about the process of labor and delivery—about what is going to happen to her. In the days following delivery, interest in baby care and in her own recovery is intensified. Table 9–1 summarizes learning interests by trimester.

We teach best when we take these general interests into account, always individualizing them for each mother or

242

Table 9–1   LEARNING INTERESTS DURING PREGNANCY

First Trimester	Second Trimester	Third Trimester
LEARNING NEEDS CENTERED ON MOTHER	INTEREST IN FETUS GROWS	PREPARATION FOR LABOR AND PARENTING
The expected date of delivery	Fetal growth	Fetal growth
Fetal growth	Physiologic changes of second trimester	Physiologic changes of third trimester
Physiologic changes of first trimester	Alleviation of maternal discomfort related to growing fetus	Alleviation of maternal discomfort
Emotional changes of men and women during first trimester	Emotional changes of second trimester	Emotional changes as time of labor approaches
Changes in family relationships	Maternal nutrition	Labor: signs, progress, the experience of labor
Nutritional needs	Infant feeding plans and other preparation for baby	Preparation for labor: relaxation and breathing techniques
Exercises for comfort and conditioning	Danger signs	Analgesia and anesthesia
Danger signs		Hospital tour; hospital policies
Available resources		Provision for others in family (e.g., other children) during hospitalization
		Preparation for homecoming
		Care of new baby

couple. Although that would seem to be only common sense, how often we hear of a mother with whom contraception is discussed during the initial visit at which the pregnancy is confirmed, as if to say, "Why didn't you know better?"

How do parents learn best? Obviously there is no single answer. At times a one-to-one relationship is very important. Groups, either of mothers alone or of couples, are ideal at other times; the sharing of feelings as well as of information makes the classes themselves assets to learning. Nurses leading groups need to watch for the shy mother who never asks a question or volunteers a comment; she may need some individual attention at another time.

The length of a group session will vary with the setting and the needs and interests of the group. Classes for couples that are held in the evening are frequently 2 hours long. On the other hand, classes for a group of mothers waiting their turn for examination will often be as short as 15 minutes and rarely longer than 30 minutes.

Many childbirth education classes have focused on the middle class couple. Attendance is dependent on knowledge that the classes exist, the value to be gained, transportation, and often a fee, which is small ($20 to $30, for example) but nevertheless prohibitive for many poorer people. One of the challenges of the next years in maternity nursing will be to extend classes to a broader group—mothers from lower income groups, teenaged mothers, unwed mothers, and mothers in rural areas, for example.

Nurses may not always be the best persons to teach classes when socioeconomic background of the parents is vastly different from their own. For example, if a mother in a Mexican-American community can be trained to teach parents in ways that are both in harmony with their cultural beliefs and consistent with our best knowledge, she may be far more effective than the nurse who is an "outsider."

Another type of prenatal learning experience described by Flapan and Schoenfeld,[13] is a "maternal role practicum" in which pregnant women visit homes of women with infants "to observe, ask questions, practice child care tasks, and experience the realities of ministering to an infant." Each woman visits a number of different homes in order to observe many different styles of mothering and thus to feel more free to develop a pattern that suits her best. Regular group meetings with other mothers give them a chance to discuss their reactions.

By visiting and volunteering to babysit for friends with small children, prospective parents accomplish much the same objective. We can encourage this trying on of the role of mother and father and can use it as a basis for both individual and group teaching.

Basic Principles for Prenatal Classes

1. Because women in prenatal classes are usually pregnant, and often in their third trimester, sitting for long periods of time is uncomfortable. There should be a break after 45 or 50 minutes of class. Moreover, mothers should be encouraged to get up and walk around or go to the bathroom whenever they need to do so.

2. One of the greatest values of prenatal classes is the chance to share feelings with other mothers and couples. A mother-to-be said, "None of my friends have been pregnant yet, and it's hard to talk with them about the way I feel sometimes. It's been great to be with other couples who are pregnant." Ten to 12 couples, or 15 mothers, is an ideal group size for discussion. The physical arrangement of the room, with

group members facing one another rather than sitting in rows facing an instructor, is also important (Fig. 9–1).

Most childbirth instructors have couples wear name tags; first names are used in class to promote an atmosphere of informality and cohesiveness.

3. Most childbirth education series last six to eight sessions, sometimes meeting once a week, sometimes twice a week. Couples' classes meet in the evening; classes for women only in the daytime as a rule. This type of scheduling tends to overlook the woman who will be coming to classes alone for any of a variety of reasons (single, husband travels in his work, husband chooses not to come) but who works during the daytime.

It has been our practice to include both couples and mothers whose husbands cannot be present in our classes. A woman will often ask, "Is it all right to come even if my husband can't (won't)?" Once they are assured that every class has both couples and individual women, they seem quite comfortable in being present.

4. Young teenagers who are not married rarely choose to attend traditional classes. Although we would certainly not exclude them if they wanted to come, we find that classes that deal with their special needs (e.g., nutritional, emotional, and so on) are probably more appropriate.

The Nurse's Role in Prenatal Classes

The most effective role for nurses in parent education classes in not that of an authoritative teacher but of a group facilitator. This does not mean that the nurse has no plan for the series of classes, but rather that her plan is flexible and can be adapted to the needs and interests of the class. For example, she

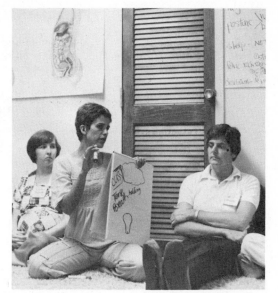

Figure 9–1 A group of mothers and fathers in a prenatal class. Notice that both the teacher, Brenda McBride, R.N., and the couples are seated on the floor. The drawing on the pad illustrates the brain and the uterus.

will plan at some point to talk about signs of labor, but she would not interrupt a very active discussion about how relationships in marriage change when the couple become parents because her preplanned schedule says she must discuss signs of labor that particular evening.

Nurse leaders need to be accepting of opinions and lifestyles different from their own and at times may need to help the group accept the right of an individual to express a point of view that is different from the majority.

Nurse leaders need to be comfortable in discussing sexuality (see below). If the nurse is obviously uncomfortable, the entire class will have difficulty in discussing their feelings.

HELPING THE MOTHER COPE WITH PHYSIOLOGIC CHANGES

In Chapter 6 physiologic changes that pregnancy produces in the mother's body were discussed. As a re-

sult of these changes, many mothers have symptoms that are often described as "minor" discomforts of pregnancy. Although these symptoms are minor in that they are not life-threatening to either mother or fetus, they can be a *major source of discomfort* to an individual woman.

GASTROINTESTINAL PROBLEMS

Gastrointestinal problems are often major sources of discomfort to women during pregnancy. In addition, they can interfere with a woman's ability to meet her nutritional needs. Table 9–2 summarizes the relationship between the gastrointestinal problems discussed below, nutrition, and the relief of symptoms.

Nausea and Vomiting

Nausea, with or without vomiting, is closely associated with pregnancy in the minds of most people in our society,

Table 9–2   GASTROINTESTINAL PROBLEMS DURING PREGNANCY

Gastrointestinal Problem	Interference with Nutrition	Relief of Symptoms
Nausea and vomiting	Nausea may interfere with appetite and consumption of essential foods. Vomiting may lead to loss of nutrients.	Fatty foods may enhance nausea; avoid at time of day nausea occurs. Dry carbohydrate foods (e.g., crackers) before rising help many women with morning nausea. Limiting fluids at mealtime may be helpful (take adequate fluids between meals to meet body's needs).
Heartburn and indigestion	May interfere with appetite and consumption of essential foods.	Smaller, more frequent meals; defer dinner dessert. Decrease fats. Eliminate highly sweetened foods and drinks. Avoid recumbent and "bending over" positions after eating.
Constipation	May interfere with appetite and consumption of essential foods.	Daily exercise. Include foods with fiber (whole grains, raw fruits and vegetables) at each meal. Adequate water intake. Include foods that are laxative, such as prunes.
Flatulence	May interfere with appetite and consumption of essential foods.	Daily bowel movements. Avoid gas-producing foods (cabbage and bean families, fried foods, highly sweetened foods).

so much so that "morning sickness" constitutes a confirmation of pregnancy for many women. It is important, however, to recognize that nausea of pregnancy seems totally absent in some societies. Burrows[4] reports that he was unable to find any evidence of nausea among Ifaluk women of the South Pacific, either by listening to their conversation or by direct questioning. Holmberg,[15] who lived among the Siriono of eastern Bolivia for many months, was unable to observe any cases of "morning sickness" or to find any recognition of it among pregnant women he interviewed. In our society, some women never experience nausea, while others may have nausea and vomiting during one pregnancy but none at all in another.

No one knows why nausea occurs in pregnancy. Two persistent theories suggest that nausea:

1. Is caused by hormonal imbalance, involving human chorionic gonadotropin and/or estrogens and/or progesterone.

2. Is related to emotional factors and perhaps to a rejection of pregnancy. (Remember that a high percentage of women are initially ambivalent about being pregnant.)

Although nausea and/or vomiting may begin as early as the second week of pregnancy, they are most common during the fifth to twelfth weeks.

Nausea may occur in the morning ("morning sickness"), at which time it may be aggravated by an empty stomach, or at any time during the day. Frequently, it is associated with excess salivation.

A dry carbohydrate snack before getting out of bed may help the mother with early morning nausea. Fatty foods and fluids exacerbate nausea and vomiting for many women; fluids can be taken between meals rather than with meals. Cooking odors are often enough to stimulate feelings of nausea.

When nausea is prolonged and so severe that no food is retained, the condition is known as *hyperemesis gravidarum*. Complete anorexia may also be present. Women with hyperemesis will lose weight, become dehydrated, and eventually become severely ill if their vomiting is not stopped. Years ago hyperemesis could lead to death, but this would be highly unusual today. As with nausea and vomiting, the basis is unknown, although many feel that there is a major emotional component to hyperemesis.

Initial treatment is similar to that of nausea and vomiting—small, frequent meals and fluids taken between meals. Rest after meals may be helpful. Tranquilizers are sometimes prescribed. If these measures are inadequate, the mother may be hospitalized, with oral intake stopped and intravenous fluids given. Feeding by mouth is gradually resumed 48 hours after vomiting has ceased.

Nausea and vomiting that *begin* after the first trimester probably have some basis other than the pregnancy; pyelonephritis is one possibility. This should never be ignored as "just nausea of pregnancy."

Heartburn

The combination of decreased gastric motility, increased intra-abdominal pressure caused by the enlarging uterus, and relaxation of the cardiac sphincter may allow gastric contents to reflux into the esophagus (gastroesophageal reflux). The mother experiences "heartburn" and indigestion, which may be relieved, at least partially, by eating smaller meals containing fewer fatty or highly sweetened foods.

Remaining upright for 3 to 4 hours following a meal or resting propped with pillows may alleviate some discomfort. Bending over shortly after mealtime should be avoided. Some women will find sleeping with additional pillows (a semi-Fowler's position) helpful.

If antacids are taken, those that contain sodium, including baking soda, should be avoided. Aluminum antacids are considered safe (Maalox, Amphojel, milk of magnesia, or Gelusil, for example). Often the other methods described can eliminate the need for antacids.

Constipation

Decreased muscle motility together with the pressure of the enlarging uterus on the descending colon and rectum are factors in constipation. The oral iron preparation commonly (and appropriately) taken by pregnant women also contributes to this common problem.

Mineral oil (which depletes the body of fat-soluble vitamins) and enemas and harsh laxatives (which may stimulate premature labor) are contraindicated in pregnant women.

Effective remedies for constipation during pregnancy include daily exercise, such as walking; an adequate fluid intake (6 to 8 glasses each day); and menus that include foods with fiber and laxative properties (Table 9–2). A bulk-producing agent or "wetting agent," for example, dioctyl sodium sulfosuccinate (Colace), is safe to use if proper diet and exercise do not resolve the problem.

Flatulence, also common, is again related to decreased motility, which retards peristalsis and allows gas to accumulate (just as it may after surgery). Avoiding gas-producing foods (fried foods, members of the cabbage and bean families, and highly sweetened foods are the major offenders) and having daily bowel movements should be helpful.

MUSCULOSKELETAL PROBLEMS

Backache

The center of gravity progressively shifts during pregnancy. In addition, an increased level of hormones leads to a softening of ligaments and pelvic joints, which is important in preparation for labor and delivery. These changes lead to a characteristic walk during the later months of pregnancy (the waddle) and often to backache, as pelvic ligaments are stretched.

Women who have maintained good posture since they were girls are likely to have fewer problems with backache. Good posture during pregnancy will also be helpful. Because high-heeled shoes increase the pressure on the already strained pelvic ligaments, wearing shoes with moderate heels will also help to prevent backache.

Tailor sitting and pelvic rocking are two exercises that we can teach mothers that can be helpful in minimizing backache. Tailor sitting (Fig. 9–2) involves sitting on the floor with the feet crossed at the ankles. A woman can sit "tailor style" during some of her everyday activities, such as sewing, preparing fruits or vegetables for a meal, or watching television. In the tailor position, knees can be pushed toward the floor to stretch the thigh muscles in preparation for delivery (Fig. 9–3).

Figure 9–2 Susan finds tailor-sitting comfortable a week before delivery.

Stretching three times, twice a day, is adequate.

Pelvic rock may be performed in several positions. In the most common, the woman lies on her back with her legs bent and her feet flat on the floor (Fig. 9–4). The buttocks are contracted, the back is pushed against the floor, and the abdominal muscles are contracted to tip the pelvis forward (Fig. 9–5). The woman then relaxes. Practicing pelvic rock three times, twice a day, can relieve a good proportion of back strain.

Rocking is also possible in a standing position; again it can be combined with other tasks.

Leg Cramps

Painful spasm of the gastrocnemius muscle in the back of the calf may occur during the late months of pregnancy. Such spasms are likely to occur when the woman has been lying down and pointing with her toes. As a preventive, each woman should be taught to always stretch her leg by pointing with her heel rather than with her toe.

The level of ionizable calcium in the woman's plasma has been implicated in

Figure 9–3 Mother practicing stretching thigh muscles in prenatal class.

leg cramps. If calcium intake is too low, levels will obviously be low. However, an excessive intake of milk, with its high levels of phosphorus as well as of calcium, may also lead to low levels of ionizable calcium. If leg cramps become a major problem, calcium lactate may be given at bedtime.

When a cramp occurs, straightening the muscle will alleviate it. Standing on the affected leg is the easiest way to relieve the cramp. Any way in which the toe can be forced upward while the knee is kept straight will be helpful.

RESPIRATORY SYMPTOMS

Dyspnea

As the fetus grows larger and the uterus begins to encroach on the thoracic cavity, a certain amount of shortness of breath occurs. For some mothers dyspnea becomes sufficiently marked to make lying flat in bed difficult and to limit certain activities. The mother may need to sleep in a semi-Fowler's position with her head elevated.

Lying on her back with her arms stretched out above her head will maximize the area of the mother's thorax and allow the fullest possible lung expansion. This position will frequently relieve dyspnea.

GENITOURINARY SYMPTOMS

Urinary Frequency

It was noted in Chapter 6 that urinary frequency occurs early in pregnancy as the growing uterus presses on the bladder, is relieved during the third month as the uterus rises into the ab-

Figure 9–4 Pelvic rocking with the small of the back against the mat. (From Davis and Rubin: *De Lee's Obstetrics for Nurses.* 18th Edition. Philadelphia, W. B. Saunders Co., 1966.)

domen, and reappears late in pregnancy as the greatly enlarged uterus again compresses the bladder.

Frequency cannot be avoided; limiting fluids is not healthy. We can, however, explain the reason for frequency to the mother and, during the early period of pregnancy, assure her that the condition will improve.

Vaginal Discharge

A normal increase of white or yellowish vaginal discharge is to be expected during the last months of pregnancy, caused by an increase in mucus produced by the cervical glands, increased cervical vascularity, and in-

creased cervical desquamation. These secretions are less acid than the vaginal secretions of nonpregnant women.

Douching is not recommended for removing these normal secretions. Daily bathing and wearing cotton underpants, rather than nylon, will help keep the mother-to-be comfortable.

Vaginal secretions caused by infection are summarized in Table 9–3. Gonorrhea, candidiasis and trichomoniasis have already been discussed in Chapter 8. Herpes, one of the TORCH organisms that can lead to fetal damage, was discussed in Chapter 6.

Because of the tremendous discomfort caused by trichomoniasis, a douche prepared with 3 tablespoons of vinegar

Figure 9–5 Pelvic rocking with the small of the back arched. (From Davis and Rubin: *De Lee's Obstetrics for Nurses.* 18th Edition. Philadelphia, W. B. Saunders Co., 1966.)

to 2 quarts of warm water may be recommended. A douche bag should be used to hold the solution; bulb syringes may cause an air embolus and death. The bag should not be more than 2 feet above hip level, nor should the nozzle be inserted more than 3 inches into the vagina. These instructions should be given to the mother in a clearly understood form. It is never adequate to tell her "to take a vinegar douche" and send her home.

GENERAL SYMPTOMS

Edema of the Feet and Legs

Edema of the feet and legs toward the end of the day can be frightening to the mother who has been told that "swelling" is a danger sign during pregnancy. This dependent edema is not unusual during late pregnancy and is often prevented or relieved by resting, with the feet elevated, several times during the day.

Edema that causes concern is present in the early morning as well as the late afternoon, is found in the face, hands, and pretibial area, and may be accompanied by sudden weight gain (Chapter 10).

Pruritus (Itching) of the Skin

Pruritus is not uncommon; it may be due to overactive sebaceous glands. Daily bathing, adequate fluid intake, and the use of bland soaps usually will relieve pruritus. A starch bath or some baking soda in the bath water may also be helpful.

Varicosities of the Legs and of the Anus (Hemorrhoids)

Increased pressure from the enlarging uterus that may obstruct venous re-

Table 9–3   VAGINAL SECRETIONS DURING PREGNANCY

Cause	Description of Secretions	Accompanying Symptoms
Normal	Yellowish or white; often profuse	
Candidiasis (moniliasis)	Resembles cottage cheese; thick and tenacious	Itching Dysuria Discomfort during intercourse (dyspareunia) Vulva edematous and irritated
Trichomoniasis	Thin Frothy, "bubbly" Greenish or variously colored	Itching Burning Highly irritating Hemorrhagic areas on cervix and vagina
Gonorrhea	Purulent	Infection may be noted in cervix and urethral glands
Herpes, Type II	Nonremarkable	Painful vesicular rash Dysuria

turn from the legs and perineal area, combined with decreased tone in the smooth muscles of vein walls, predisposes about 20 per cent of all pregnant women to varicosities in the legs or around the anus (hemorrhoids). The vulva and perineum may also be affected.

Varicosities may be prevented or their severity decreased by some simple measures that should be suggested to all mothers:

1. Garters or stockings with elastic bands around the calf should not be worn during pregnancy (or at all). Maternity garter belts are available. Support hose should be worn if previous varicosities have occurred or if much standing is done. Support hose should be put on before arising and worn throughout the day.

2. Do not wear clothes that are too constricting.

3. Standing for long periods of time causes blood to pool in the lower veins. Sit when possible, with feet elevated.

4. Avoid crossing legs in such a way as to restrict blood flow. Crossing legs at the ankles with the barest of touching is all right.

5. Try to find some time each day to lie on the floor or on a bed next to a wall with your legs at right angles to your body resting against the wall. Elevating hips on a pillow may help avoid hemorrhoids and varicosities of the vulva.

Surgery for either hemorrhoids or leg varicosities is not performed during pregnancy. Occasionally, a clot in an external hemorrhoid may be evacuated as an office procedure. Hemorrhoids usually improve so markedly following delivery that no further treatment is necessary. Varicose veins should be evaluated and, if necessary, treated after the baby is delivered, or they may continue to be a source of problems for the mother, particularly during subsequent pregnancies.

Variations in Sleep Patterns: Excessive Sleep and Insomnia

During the early weeks of pregnancy, some mothers find themselves constantly tired and sleepy. The desire is strong to spend most of the day and night sleeping. A mother may report feeling very disgusted with herself. Our assurance that many other mothers experience the same fatigue and that this excess fatigue will usually disappear near the end of the first trimester is important.

By contrast, other mothers, and even the same mother at a different stage of pregnancy, may have periods of insomnia. The cause may be a combination of physical discomfort, especially during the last trimester, and a measure of anxiety, which may be present at any stage. Dreams are not unusual. Many babies become very active just as the mother lies down and begins to be comfortable.

The most comfortable position for sleeping for many mothers is a side-lying position (Fig. 9–6). Old remedies such as warm milk or cocoa at bedtime and limited tea, coffee, or "cola" after dinner may help. If anxiety is the problem, an alert nurse may be able to note this and help the mother express her concerns.

Short rest periods and naps during the day can help, because extreme exhaustion can make sleep difficult. Sleeping medications should be avoided.

ACTIVITIES OF DAILY LIVING DURING PREGNANCY

Many of the changes in a mother's activities of daily living during preg-

Figure 9–6 This position is comfortable for rest and sleep during pregnancy and is often a comfortable position for much of labor.

nancy have been noted in the section immediately preceding. These needs are summarized in Table 9–4.

usual is not uncommon. Extra rest may also be required during the third trimester.

Rest

Many women who consider themselves to be in excellent health during pregnancy nevertheless find that they tire more easily. During the first trimester, a desire to sleep more than

Exercise

As noted in Table 9–4, daily exercise in some form is desirable during pregnancy, just as it is during all of life. The amount and kind of exercise will vary with a woman's lifestyle. Women

Table 9–4 CHANGES IN ACTIVITIES OF DAILY LIVING

Need	Meeting the Need
Proper clothing	Nonrestrictive clothing Moderately low-heeled shoes Maternity garter belt Support hose, if varicosities present
Adequate rest	Frequent rest periods, with feet elevated, during day A minimum of 8 hours sleep at night
Daily exercise	Exercise should not be carried to the point of fatigue* Formal exercises, such as pelvic rock, may alleviate backache
Bathing	Tub bathing allowed throughout pregnancy; care must be taken to avoid slipping Daily bathing aids comfort

*See section on exercise.

who have been active in sports such as swimming and golf, for example, may continue to enjoy these activities throughout most of their pregnancy. It would be a mistake, however, for a woman who has led an extremely sedentary life to begin strenuous exercise. Walking is one example of an exercise more appropriate for her. For some women, the exercise involved in caring for a home may be adequate.

How much exercise? Exercise that leads to fatigue exhaustion is *too much*. Moderate exercise, on the other hand, often results in a feeling of both physical and mental well-being.

As the woman's center of gravity shifts during the last months of pregnancy, she should avoid exercise in which she might lose her balance; active tennis is an example. A woman with a previous history of spontaneous abortion or premature labor is usually advised to limit her activity for part or all of her pregnancy.

Employment

Employment during pregnancy is common today; many women work away from their home until very close to their expected delivery date with no apparent adverse effects. For some women the income from the job is vital; for others the satisfaction of the job itself is equally important. We do, however, want to discuss certain precautions for each mother.

1. Becoming overly tired should not be allowed.

2. Heavy lifting and straining must be avoided.

3. Good body mechanics are as important on the job as at home. If the mother is asked to describe the activities involved in her job, we may be able to suggest ways in which she can utilize good body mechanics.

4. Both prolonged sitting and prolonged standing in one spot should be avoided.

5. Pregnant women should not work around radiation or chemicals. Women with jobs that expose them to these potential teratogens should discuss the possibility of hazard with their employers.

6. Some arrangement for rest periods during the working day should be planned. Is it possible for her to lie down or sit with her feet elevated during coffee break?

Nurses might begin to become aware of employers' attitudes toward and provisions for pregnant employees by examining practices in hospitals and health agencies. An awareness of policies of other community employers, particularly those that employ large numbers of women, is also important for nurses who care for childbearing couples.

Travel

The basic principle governing travel is the same as for exercise and employment: fatigue should be avoided.

For women with a history of spontaneous abortion, travel is usually contraindicated in the early months of pregnancy. As the date of delivery approaches, travel may mean delivery in another community if labor begins earlier than expected.

NUTRITION DURING PREGNANCY

Nutrition is a keystone of health at any period in life, but particularly so during pregnancy. Both maternal health and fetal development, including brain development, may be affected by malnutrition.

Currently, nutritional guidance during pregnancy is delegated mainly to nurses. Few physicians take the time or have the practical knowledge of foods and their preparation that can be helpful to a mother. Nutritionists are not currently available in adequate numbers to see each pregnant woman even once during 9 months, much less on a continuing basis. Patients of private physicians may have no access at all to a nutritionist.

Nutritional guidance for pregnant women begins with general and nutritional assessments (Chapter 8). A number of factors in general and reproductive health that may be related to nutritional status are summarized in Table 9–5.

Nutrition guidance during preg-

Table 9–5 FACTORS IN GENERAL AND REPRODUCTIVE HEALTH THAT MAY BE RELATED TO NUTRITIONAL STATUS

Factors	Relation to Nutritional Status
Age	Young adolescents have increased nutrient needs for growth; often have poor food habits.
Age at menarche	Average age at menarche: 12.5 years. Delayed onset may be associated with poor childhood nutrition.
Prepregnancy weight	Weight less than 100 pounds or greater than 200 pounds correlates with poor pregnancy outcome. Recent substantial weight loss from dieting may deplete nutritional reserves.
Addiction to drugs, alcohol, cigarette smoking	Women addicted to drugs and alcohol often have nutritional deficiencies; cigarette smoking correlates with low birth weight.
Chronic disease	Effects of metabolic diseases are intensified during pregnancy; nutrient requirements of some disease states may affect pregnancy.
Weight gain in previous pregnancies	Previous patterns of low or excessive weight gain may indicate special nutrition learning needs.
Outcome in previous pregnancies	Low birth weight may suggest previous nutritional problem that is still present; large for gestational age infant (Chapter 15), stillbirths, congenital malformations may suggest pre- or gestational diabetes.
Length of interconceptual period	Interval between end of lactation and subsequent pregnancy of less than a year may deplete nutritional stores in undernourished mothers.
Steroid contraception	May inhibit folic acid absorption.
EDC (Estimated Date of Confinement)	Nutritional planning is keyed to stage of pregnancy.
Anemia: iron deficiency or megaloblastic	Inadequate nutrition.

nancy serves not only to help both mother and fetus during the months of pregnancy but hopefully will help to establish patterns that will carry over into the period of lactation, if the mother is breast-feeding, and into the care of her children as they grow.

The problems of helping mothers with nutritional needs are complex for several reasons:

1. Her diet during her entire life, as well as during the 38 weeks of gestation, has a bearing on the outcome of pregnancy.

2. There is no clear indication of just what the nutritional needs of pregnancy are for a number of important food constituents.

3. Eating patterns are cultural practices that are often deeply ingrained and difficult to change.

4. Economic factors, physiologic status, cooking facilities, and other related factors limit the diets of many women.

In order to help mothers meet their nutritional needs during pregnancy, nurses need to know:

1. The relationship between nutrition and the outcome of pregnancy.

2. The specific nutritional needs of mothers and what foods will meet these needs within the framework of the mothers' cultural, physiologic, and economic environment.

3. How to assess the nutritional needs of women during pregnancy (Chapter 8).

NUTRITION AND THE OUTCOME OF PREGNANCY

Several specific concepts describe the relationship between nutrition and the outcome of pregnancy.

1. There is a strong positive association between the total weight gain of the mother and the birth weight of the baby. This concept has been discussed in Chapter 8 in relation to assessment of maternal weight gain.

2. There is a strong positive association between the prepregnancy weight of the mother and the birth weight of the baby. The highest incidence of low birth weight babies occurs when infants are born to mothers with a prepregnancy weight of less than 100 pounds or more than 10 per cent below the standard weight for height.

Low prepregnancy weight may indicate long-term malnutrition and depleted stores. The mother who has severely restricted her diet during her teenaged and early adult years in order to be fashionably slim may have inadequate nutritional stores, just the same as the mother who is underweight from chronic malnourishment.

It has been postulated that men with severe nutritional depletion require 16 weeks of good diet to return to their level of function prior to nutritional deprivation. This emphasizes the importance of adequate nutrition not only from the beginning of pregnancy but at every stage of life, a point we can emphasize in all of our nutritional teaching.

Mothers with a prepregnancy weight of greater than 200 pounds or more than 20 per cent above the standard weight for their height are also at higher risk of developing complications. However, no attempt at reduction should be undertaken during pregnancy; these mothers should gain between 22 and 27 pounds during their pregnancy. While obese women consume large quantities of food, the quality of their diet is often poor. If good nutritional practices can be developed during pregnancy, they may form the basis of a sound postpregnancy reduction diet. Breast-feeding can also contribute to postpartum weight reduction.

No other postpartum weight reduction should be undertaken until the baby is off the breast.

In addition to compromising essential intake, attempts at weight reduction during pregnancy can lead to acidosis, which may place the fetus at risk.

3. The concept that the fetus will be able to supply its needs from maternal stores, regardless of the nutritional status of the mother, is invalid. As noted above, the mother may not have adequate stores.

4. Pregnancies involving more than one fetus (twins, for example) increase nutritional needs, particularly for iron and folic acid.

5. When pregnancies are closely spaced, particularly if there is reason to believe that nutritional needs have been unmet or marginally met in prior pregnancies, the mother is nutritionally at risk.

MEETING NUTRITIONAL NEEDS

During pregnancy, women have specific needs for calories, protein, fats, iron, calcium and phosphorus, sodium, iodine, trace elements, vitamins, and folic acid. The need for many of these essentials is increased during adolescence, when growth needs for mother as well as for the fetus must be considered, as indicated in the tables that follow.

For convenience, the needs of the lactating mother are also included.

The Need for Calories

The need for adequate calories to provide optimal weight gain has already been discussed. Calories are needed for the growth of the fetus, placenta, and associated maternal tissues. An increased maternal basal metabolism also requires additional calories. If the mother's daily activities become more limited, this will partially offset her caloric needs. Calories are also important to protect protein. When calorie intake is not adequate, the body will utilize protein for energy; protein then becomes unavailable for necessary growth. In addition, the breakdown of protein leads to acidosis. Caloric needs are summarized in Table 9–6.

The Need for Protein

It should not be surprising that the need for protein, so essential for all growth, is increased during pregnancy (Table 9–7). Proteins are the only food substances that contain nitrogen, phosphorus, and sulfur; fats and carbohydrates do not. Protein is essential for the synthesis of hemoglobin; iron alone will not alleviate anemia.

Proteins consist of 22 known amino acids, the amount of a single amino acid

Table 9–6   DAILY CALORIC NEEDS*

Age	Normal	Pregnancy	Lactation
11–14	2400	2700	2900
15–22	2100	2400	2600
23–50	2000	2300	2500

*From *Recommended Dietary Allowances*. 8th Edition. Dietary Allowance Committee and Food and Nutrition Board. Washington, D.C., National Academy of Sciences, 1974.

Table 9–7   PROTEIN*

Recommended Daily Dietary Allowance (Grams)

	11–14 Years	15–18 Years	19–50 Years
Nonpregnant	44	48	46
Pregnant	74	78	76
Lactating	64	68	66

Foods	Size of Serving	Approximate Grams of Protein
Turkey (combination dark and light)	3 ounces (3 pieces)	26.8
Chicken	Thigh or half breast	25.7
Tuna fish†	3¹/₂ ounces (small can)	27.7
Great northern dried beans (raw)	¹/₂ cup dried (raw)	20
Canned salmon (various kinds)	1 cup	47
Cottage cheese (large or small curd)	¹/₂ cup	16.6
Beef (chuck roast, e.g.)	3 ounces (1 slice)	19–26
Fish (perch, haddock, e.g.; not seafood)	3¹/₂ ounces (1 piece)	17–19
Hamburger (cooked)	3 ounces	19–23
Milk†	8 ounces (1 cup)	8.5
Eggs	1 medium	5.7
	1 large	6.5
	1 X-large	7.4
Peanut butter	1 tablespoon	4.0
Bread	1 slice	2.2–2.4

*From Adams: *Nutritive Value of American Foods in Common Units.* Agriculture Handbook #456, Washington, D.C., United States Dept. of Agriculture, November 1975.

†Most economical in terms of amount and quality of protein in relation to cost.

and the combinations of amino acids varying from one protein to another. Nine of these amino acids are called "essential" because they cannot be synthesized within the adult human body. Of the nine essential amino acids, the need for histidine for adults has not yet been established. It is necessary for infants. Not only must the essential amino acids be ingested, they must be ingested *simultaneously* and in *proper balance*.

Proteins that contain all eight essential adult amino acids in a balance usable by the body are called *complete* proteins. In general, animal proteins are complete proteins. When one or more amino acids are limited in amount, the usefulness of all the other amino acids is limited in the same proportion. Proteins lacking or having a limited amount of an essential amino acid are called *incomplete*; most plant protein is incomplete. However, all eight essential adult amino acids are contained in one plant or another, so that it is possible to eat meals containing the necessary amino acids using plant sources rather than animal sources by a proper combination of foods. When the amino acids in one protein complete the amino acids in another, these are called *complementary* protein combinations. Basic complementary combinations are grains and legumes, grains and milk, and seeds and legumes. Table 9–8 illustrates some complementary combi-

Table 9–8 COMPLEMENTARY VEGETABLE PROTEIN

Serve	At the Same Meal with One of These Foods
Rice	Beans Soy products Sesame seeds Milk Wheat and soy combinations
Whole wheat	Milk Beans Soy products Peanuts and milk Peanuts and soy products Soy and sesame products
Cornmeal	Beans Soy products and milk
Peanuts	Milk Sunflower seeds Soy and sesame products
Beans	Rice Cornmeal Milk Whole wheat bread
Potatoes	Milk

nations using commonly available foods. It is interesting that the traditional dishes of many cultures combine plant foods that complement one another to make a complete protein. For example, Latin American black beans and rice, Creole red beans and rice, the Hopping John of the Carolina low country (cow peas and rice), New England baked beans and brown bread, and the corn bread and pinto beans of the South.

Although knowledge of complementary proteins is essential in counseling women who choose to be vegetarians (see below), it is also useful in helping any mother supplement the protein in her diet. Many plant proteins are less expensive than animal proteins and can be used to stretch animal proteins for maximum effectiveness. Just adding milk, for example, to a meal that contains rice, whole wheat, peanuts (peanut butter), beans, or potatoes complements the incomplete protein in these foods and boosts the mother's intake of usable protein.

The Need for Fats

Large amounts of fats are not tolerated well by many women during pregnancy (see gastrointestinal disturbances above), nor are large amounts necessary. Some fat is necessary to supply essential fatty acids and fat-soluble vitamins; margarine on a piece of toast will supply this need. Many popular foods, such as peanut butter, contain fat as well as protein.

The Need for Iron

Iron is essential during pregnancy for both mother and fetus. Few mothers have iron stores sufficient to meet their own needs and those of the fetus. Beginning in the fifth month, the fetus begins to store iron that will serve him during the first 4 to 6 months of his life. If the mother's iron intake is inadequate or if the baby is born prior to term, the newborn's iron stores will be inadequate, and he will be at risk of developing iron deficiency anemia during his first year of life. Inadequate iron intake during pregnancy will also leave the mother with iron deficiency anemia in the weeks following delivery; she may find herself weak and chronically tired and find mothering a difficult task.

The increased need for iron during pregnancy is caused by:

1. Increased maternal red cell volume—300 mg.
2. Fetal iron stores—300 mg.
3. Iron stored in the placenta—70 mg.
4. Iron in blood lost at the time of delivery—50 mg.

A small amount of iron (about 150 mg.) is conserved by the body during pregnancy because of the cessation of menstruation.

Iron is available in small quantities in a large variety of foods (Table 9–9). When the diet habits of many Americans are considered, these foods are not eaten in quantities sufficient to meet iron needs. Since these needs are greater during pregnancy, mothers should be encouraged to eat those foods high in iron. An iron supplement (30 to 60 mg. per day) is also recommended during pregnancy to help the mother in meeting these increased needs. However, supplements should not be relied upon to correct improper food habits. Good eating patterns formed during pregnancy can be the basis for good eating patterns that will last after pregnancy and that can influence the food habits of other family members.

The Need for Calcium and Phosphorus

Calcium needs during pregnancy are increased by 50 per cent because of the needs of the fetus for calcium in skeletal development and because of the role of calcium in muscle function and blood coagulation.

Four glasses of milk will meet the need for calcium; a piece of cheddar cheese weighing 1¼ ounces substitutes for 8 ounces of milk. Green leafy vegetables are also good sources of calcium (Table 9–10). Outside of these foods, calcium amounts in single servings are more limited. For the woman who does not drink milk or utilize sufficient quantities of milk in her cooking, calcium supplementation, usually calcium gluconate (1000 mg. in the first and second trimesters; 1500 mg. in the third trimester) is necessary. The mother with lactose intolerance has a dual problem because of low calcium intake and a decreased calcium absorption.

Maternal stores of calcium are more difficult to monitor than iron stores unless deficiency is severe because the body maintains equilibrium of calcium and other minerals in the plasma.

Needs for phosphorus are met when calcium needs are adequately served.

The Need for Sodium

Sodium needs are adequately met through normal eating patterns. The problem with sodium intake is *iatrogenic* (i.e., caused by faulty health care), in this instance the result of faulty health teaching. For several decades we have urged women to restrict

Table 9–9   IRON

Recommended Dietary Allowance		

ADOLESCENT AND ADULT (AGES 11–50)		
Nonpregnant	18 mg. per day	
Pregnant	18 plus mg. per day*	
Lactating	18 mg. per day	

Foods	Size of Serving	Mg.
Liver, pork	3 ounces	24.7
Liver, beef	3 ounces	7.5
Variety meats:		
Kidney	4 ounces	14.8
Heart	4 ounces	6.8
Turkey (combination light and dark)	3 ounces	1.5
Beef (chuck)	3 ounces	2–3
Soybean flour (low fat)	½ cup	4
Grits†	½ cup	0.4
		(based on minimum level of enrichment)
Dark green vegetables		
Mustard greens	½ cup cooked	1.2
Turnip greens	½ cup cooked	0.8
Spinach	½ cup cooked	2.0
Bread (enriched)	1 slice	0.3–0.7
Eggs·	1 X-large	1.3
	1 large	1.2
	1 medium	1.0
Cereals—may be fortified (see individual packages)		

*The Committee on Maternal Nutrition, National Research Council, recommends supplementation with 30 to 60 mg. of elemental iron per day.
†Can be blended with other flours in making breads and used as ground meat extender.

their salt intake as a precaution against edema and pre-eclampsia. It is now recognized that:

1. Some edema of the ankles and feet is normal during pregnancy and is not a sign of impending pre-eclampsia.

2. Sodium is essential to maintain normal sodium levels in plasma, bone, brain, and muscle, as both tissue and fluid expand during the prenatal period.

Sodium restriction is now considered potentially hazardous. Therefore, sodium *should not be restricted*. Diuretics, which can lead to sodium loss, should not be used.

The Need for Iodine

The need for iodine, an essential nutrient, can be met by encouraging the use of iodized salt. Women who buy most of their foods at "natural food" stores should know that sea salt is not iodized. However, seafoods such as shrimp, scallops, and clams are good sources of iodine.

The Need for Trace Elements

There is a great deal yet to be learned about trace elements, those

Table 9–10   CALCIUM

Recommended Daily Dietary Allowance		
Adolescent and Adult	11–18 Years	19–50 Years
Nonpregnant	1200 mg.	800 mg.
Pregnant	1200 mg.	1200 mg.
Lactating	1200 mg.	1200 mg.

Foods	Size of Serving	Mg.
Milk	1 cup	288
Cheese, cheddar	1 ounce	213
Dark green vegetables		
Mustard greens	½ cup cooked	97
Turnip greens	½ cup cooked	134
Broccoli	½ cup cooked	68
Spinach	½ cup cooked	84
Soybean flour	½ cup	116
Grits (cooked) enriched*	½ cup	1

*Can be blended with other flours in making breads and used as ground meat extender.

nutrients that appear in foods in small "traces" but that are nevertheless essential. One of the fallacies of relying on vitamin preparations rather than foods to supply essential nutrients is that we may not even be aware of all of our needs. For example, when breads and cereals are enriched, intake of B vitamins and iron may be sufficiently increased, but the content of magnesium and zinc will be less than that in whole grain products.

The Need for Vitamin A

Vitamin A is abundant in a number of foods (Table 9–11). Many of these foods are not included in American diets, which tend to skimp on liver and dark green and yellow vegetables. Whole milk contains limited amounts of vitamin A, but nonfat dry milk to which vitamin A has been added can be a good source.

The fetus stores about 7000 I.U. of vitamin A in his liver during the last half of pregnancy, a need met adequately if the required intake is achieved. The increased need for vitamin A during lactation provides for the vitamin A excreted in breast milk.

The Need for B Vitamins

Thiamine, riboflavin, niacin, B_6 and B_{12} are components of the B complex vitamins. During pregnancy, the need for these vitamins is increased slightly as caloric intake is increased because of their essential role in metabolism. When foods are cooked properly and eaten in the recommended amounts for pregnancy, the B complex vitamin needs will be met (Table 9–12)

Good food sources of thiamine are pork, dried beans and peas, liver, and nuts. Up to 50 per cent of thiamine may be destroyed by heat. From 12 to 24 per cent of the thiamine in meat may be in the gravy by the time the meat is served.

Riboflavin, like thiamine, is affected by heat, with 10 to 30 per cent being lost in the cooking liquid of

Table 9–11   VITAMIN A

Recommended Daily Allowance

ADOLESCENT AND ADULT (AGES 11–50)
Nonpregnant   4000 I.U.
Pregnant   5000 I.U.
Lactating   6000 I.U.

Foods	Size of Serving	Vitamin A Content (I.U.)
Spinach (cooked)	½ cup	11,000–23,000*
Other leafy green vegetables	½ cup	Up to 12,000
Broccoli	½ cup	1900–2400
Liver (beef)	3 ounces	5000–10,000
Sweet potatoes	1 medium	9000–11,000
Squash, yellow	½ cup	790–1060
Carrots	½ cup	7600–12,000
Apricots (dried or fresh)	2	1570–2200
Peaches, fresh yellow	1 medium	1000–2000
Nonfat dry milk:		
Vitamin A added	1 cup reconstituted	2000
No added vitamin A	1 cup reconstituted	30
Whole milk (not fortified with vitamin A)	1 cup	350

*Content varies; in general, the deeper the color, the more vitamin A.

vegetables. The old custom of dunking cornbread in the liquid in which greens were cooked ("pot-licker") saved vitamins for our grandfathers' generation, but is rare today. Riboflavin is also lost when foods are left in the light. Foods that are high in riboflavin are liver, milk, meat, and cottage cheese.

Although niacin is not affected by heat, it is still lost in the water in which vegetables are cooked. Liver, fish, poultry, meat, and peanut butter are all good sources of niacin. The body is also able to convert a small amount of the amino acid tryptophan into niacin.

Vitamin B_6 (pyridoxine) plays an essential role in metabolism; it is required by all animals. The need is increased as protein needs are increased, because it is a coenzyme in many phases of amino acid metabolism. Meat, cereals, nuts, lentils, and some fruits and vegetables are good sources of vitamin B_6.

Vitamin B_{12} plays an important role in normal growth and in the main-

Table 9–12   B VITAMINS

	Thiamine (mg.)			Riboflavin (mg.)			Niacin (mg.)		
AGES	11–14	15–22	23–50	11–14	15–22	23–50	11–14	15–22	23–50
Nonpregnant	1.2	1.1	1.0	1.3	1.4	1.2	16.0	14.0	13.0
Pregnant	1.5	1.4	1.3	1.6	1.7	1.5	18.0	16.0	15.0
Lactating	1.5	1.4	1.3	1.8	1.9	1.7	20.0	18.0	17.0

tenance of epithelial cells and the myelin sheath of the nervous system. It helps to maintain erythropoiesis (in combination with folic acid) and leukopoiesis. Like several other vitamins, it is heat labile and some is lost in cooking. Vitamin B_{12} is found primarily in animal products. Therefore, a strict vegetarian must receive supplementary B_{12}. A serum B_{12} determination is advisable for women who are vegetarians.

The Need for Vitamin C

Because water-soluble vitamin C is not stored in the body, daily intake is essential (Table 9–13). Meeting the requirement for vitamin C is not as difficult as for some other vitamins, at least for middle class mothers, who choose daily citrus fruits and juices. Fortunately, in the summer when citrus fruit is more expensive, tomatoes, cabbage, and green peppers are fairly abundant. Heat affects vitamin C.

The Need for Vitamin D

Vitamin D is necessary to ensure calcium absorption and utilization. The normal need for vitamin D, 400 I.U., is apparently not increased during pregnancy or lactation. Ever since margarine, butter, and milk have been fortified with vitamin D, and because even a few minutes of sunshine each day will lead to the manufacture of vitamin D in the body, deficiencies of this vitamin are not a major problem in the United States unless the diet is very severely limited.

The Need for Vitamin E

Vitamin E plays roles in both growth and metabolism. Vitamin E is found chiefly in vegetable and seed oils. When food needs have been properly met, vitamin E needs will be met as well.

The Need for Folic Acid (Folacin)

Folic acid is involved in a number of metabolic processes. A deficiency of folic acid leads to several types of anemia, including megaloblastic anemia, which is relatively common in pregnancy. Folic acid deficiency also affects the normal response of female reproductive

Table 9–13   VITAMIN C

Recommended Daily Allowance		
ADOLESCENT AND ADULT (AGES 11–50)		
Nonpregnant	45 mg.	
Pregnant	60 mg.	
Lactating	80 mg.	
Foods	**Size of Serving**	**Mg.**
Orange juice	4 ounces (½ cup)	50–60
Grapefruit	½	30–67
Green vegetables:		
Broccoli	½ cup	50–70
Green, leafy vegetables	½ cup	20–50
Green peppers	½ cup	20–50
Tomatoes	1	20–40
Cabbage, raw	½ cup	15–35

organs to estrogens. Folic acid is provided by intestinal synthesis in man. Of the folic acid ingested, 75 per cent is excreted in the urine.

Serum folacin levels are measured in some pregnant patients. The desired level is 6 nanograms per ml. Folic acid is available in a wide variety of foods, especially liver, leafy vegetables, fruit, and yeast. Folic acid requirements during pregnancy are greatly increased (Table 9–14). Many nutritionists and the American College of Obstetrics and Gynecology (ACOG) advise supplementation of the diet with folic acid (200–400 mg. per day).

A DIET PLAN

Nurses must understand basic food needs before they can counsel patients. But basic needs must be translated into the kind of meals that patients eat. The following pattern (Table 9–15) is suggested because it can be adapted by women from every cultural background (Table 9–16).

Applying Principles to an Individual Patient

Doris C. is 20 years old, a black woman pregnant for the first time. She finished eleventh grade before dropping out of school. Ms. C. is 5′3″ tall and weighs 133 pounds in her fifth month of pregnancy. She says that her prepregnancy weight was "about" 125 pounds, which is slightly overweight for her

Table 9–14   FOLIC ACID (AGES 11–50)

Nonpregnant	400 mg.
Pregnant	800 mg.
Lactating	600 mg.

Table 9–15   BASIC MEAL PLAN

Vitamin C fruit or vegetable	1 serving
Vitamin A fruit or vegetable	1 serving
Other fruits or vegetables	2 servings
Meat	3 servings
Milk	3–4 cups
Grain	3–4 servings

height. A weight gain of 8 pounds at 20 weeks is "right on target."

Breakfast:	1 slice toast
	1 soda (soft drink)
Lunch:	2 beef sandwiches
Dinner:	2 pork chops
	½ cup snap beans
	2 slices light bread
Snacks:	2 sodas
	3 donuts
	4 cups cracked ice
	¼ cup starch
	(laundry starch)

She reports that she has approximately $16 to spend each week on groceries for herself and her husband. She is eligible for and uses food stamps.

An analysis of Doris C.'s diet indicates an adequate intake of protein and an excessive intake of grains. She had one nonleafy green vegetable. Milk; a vitamin C fruit or vegetable; and leafy, green vegetables are lacking.

This mother indicated, however, that she likes milk and often drinks as much as 6 glasses a day; that she eats oranges and apples two to three times a week, and that she likes both broccoli and spinach. Using foods she likes, it should not be too difficult to modify her diet to meet her basic needs. The amount of money she has to spend for food would be a real constraint without food stamps; however, with stamps and careful spending, she can manage adequately.

One of the biggest problems for Doris C. is the large number of "empty"

Table 9–16   ADAPTATION OF BASIC NEEDS IN SELECTED CULTURES

	Basic	Southern	Mexican-American	Oriental
BREAKFAST				
Fruit or vegetable containing vitamin C*	Orange	Orange	Orange	Orange
	Cereal or toast	Grits or biscuits	Tortilla	Rice
Grain product (bread, cereal)	Milk		Milk in coffee	(Limited milk taken as beverage)
	Egg	Buttermilk	Egg	
Milk product		Egg		Egg
Protein food				
LUNCH				
Grain product (2 servings, e.g., 2 slices bread)	Grilled cheese sandwich	Cornbread	Tortillas†	Rice
	Apple	Pinto beans	Pinto beans	Fish
Protein food	Milk	Greens	Apple or tomatoes	Bean sprouts
Fruit or vegetable		Milk		Tofu‡
Milk product			Custard	
DINNER				
Protein food (2 servings)	Hamburger	Chicken	Chicken	Chicken
	Spinach (2)	Collards	(Few green and yellow vegetables eaten; suggest carrots)	Chinese broccoli
Leafy green vegetables (2 servings)*	Roll	Broccoli		Mustard greens
	Milk	Biscuits		Rice
Grain product		Milk		Cheese
Milk product			Rice pudding	
BETWEEN MEALS AND AT BEDTIME				
Milk product	Cottage cheese or milk	Cottage cheese or milk	Cheese	Tofu

*Could be eaten at another meal.
†Suggest nonfat dry milk in preparing tortillas.
‡Tofu is soybean curd; it contains protein and also calcium, the latter often deficient in Oriental diets because of low milk intake.

calories she consumes from laundry starch (see pica, below), sodas (soft drinks), and donuts. These habits will be difficult to change, but if they are not changed, her baby will probably also be eating these foods before his first birthday.

A follow-up interview 2 weeks later showed the addition of orange juice, milk, and "greens" to the day's menus, but continued to show intake of both starch and "junk food."

MOTHERS WITH SPECIAL NEEDS

Many mothers will need special help in planning meals during pregnancy. The reason may be cultural, economic, or physiologic (lactose intolerance, gastrointestinal problems during pregnancy, or a medical complication such as diabetes or toxemia). Nutritional problems related to high risk conditions such as diabetes and toxemia are discussed in Chapter 10.

Cultural Variations in Food Preferences

There is no standard diet in the United States. Many groups of peoples have special foods and special ways of preparing food that add welcome variety to our dining.

During pregnancy, some ethnic variations in diet may present problems in achieving optimum nutrition. Several large ethnic groups are discussed here by way of example. In our practice, we must become familiar with both customs in our own communities and also with the ways in which each individual woman conforms to or varies from cultural practice of her group.

The Spanish-American Mother. The Spanish-speaking mother may be a Mexican-American in California or Texas, a Cuban-American in Miami, or an American of Puerto Rican descent in New York City (Chapter 4). Although food preferences vary, there are some similar areas. Special considerations concerning Spanish-American diets are:

1. Milk is not commonly used as a beverage, and only fairly small amounts are used in cooking. Cheese, however, is popular, but the amount is often not adequate for calcium needs. Some milk is used in puddings.

2. Consumption of carbonated beverages and other foods with high calories but low nutritive value is common.

3. Tomatoes and chili peppers are popular vegetables. Few yellow and green, leafy vegetables are used. Vegetables may be cooked for long periods of time.

The Mother of Asian Heritage. Mothers of Asian heritage—Japanese, Chinese, Filipino, and Indian, for example—like Spanish-speaking mothers represent a diverse heritage, but may share some characteristics.

Oriental cuisine varies from one nationality to another; the longer a family has been in the United States, the less strict is adherence to traditional diet patterns. There are some common practices that are important to note when planning a diet during pregnancy and lactation.

1. Milk is used in limited quantities; it is rarely used as a beverage. Thus calcium and vitamin D intake may need to be supplemented. Six ounces of tofu (soybean curd), a popular dish, contains the same amount of calcium as a cup of milk.

2. Since rice is such a basic staple, it is important that enriched rice be used and that it not be washed before cooking.

3. A large assortment of fruits and vegetables are used.

4. Stir frying, a popular method of preparing vegetables, meats, and fish, results in minimal vitamin loss.

5. Meats and fish may be eaten in such small quantities that protein and calorie intake is often inadequate.

American Indian Mothers. Every American Indian tribe has had its own traditional diet modifications in years gone by. Today Indian diets tend to be "Americanized" and vary with location. Coastal Indians will eat more seafood, for example, but so do non-Indian peoples living in coastal areas.

Because of poverty (Chapter 4), rather than of Indian traditions, the diets of many American Indian mothers may be limited. Protein, fruits, vegetables, and milk may be limited and carbohydrate intake high.

Traditional Southern Cooking. All of the necessities of excellent basic nutrition are present in the traditional Southern diet. Proteins are available not only in meats but in popular pinto beans, black-eyed peas, and the like. Probably few people eat as many leafy, green vegetables (collards, mustard greens and turnip greens, for example) as do Southerners. Unfortunately, these vegetables are cooked for a long period of time, and if the cooking water (pot-licker) is discarded, much food value is lost. The old custom of dipping bread in the pot-licker was commendable from a vitamin standpoint. Both buttermilk and "sweet milk" are popular. Peaches, strawberries, and apples are grown and eaten.

Disadvantages include a high consumption of carbonated beverages and a somewhat limited intake of citrus fruits. The popularity of pica among many Southern black women is discussed below.

The Mother Who Is a Vegetarian. Vegetarianism is popular with many young couples. Unknowledgeable vegetarianism, with limited intake of complete proteins, can present hazards to the growing fetus and to the mother herself. Ideally, women who are vegetarians should be counseled by nutritionists during pregnancy and lactation. The aim of counseling is not to convince the mother to give up vegetarianism but to be sure that she is eating combinations of plant products that will assure adequate nutrition.

There are three basic types of vegetarian diets:

1. The strict or pure vegetarian diet, which excludes all foods of animal origin.

2. The lactovegetarian diet, which includes milk, cheese, and other dairy products, but not eggs, meat, poultry, and fish.

3. The lacto-ovo-vegetarian diet, which includes eggs and sometimes fish, as well as dairy products, but excludes meat and poultry.

Obviously the more limited the diet, the greater the potential hazard. The macrobiotic diet eaten by some families, which contains no fresh fruits

or vegetables as well as no animal protein, is extremely limited and dangerous. Vegetarian diets lack vitamin B_{12} unless four glasses of cow's milk are consumed daily; otherwise vitamin B_{12} (4 micrograms) must be given as a supplement. An iron supplement is recommended, as it is for all pregnant women. Vegetarians who do not drink milk must have supplemental calcium (see calcium, above) and vitamin D (400 I.U. per day). Iodized salt should be used during pregnancy.

Special Physiologic Needs

The Mother Who Is Lactose Intolerant. In talking with patients about diet, it is not unusual for a woman to tell us, "I can't drink milk; it makes me sick." For many years this was translated as either (1) the individual just didn't like milk or (2) she was allergic to milk. A third possibility is the presence of lactose intolerance.

Lactose is the sugar in milk; lactase is the enzyme that breaks down lactose into simple sugars (glucose and galactose) that are then utilized by the body. Adult mammals other than man lack lactase; kittens and puppies drink milk for example, but cats and dogs do not. Many humans after the age of two to four years are also lactase deficient and therefore lactose intolerant. The reason that this has not been recognized widely until very recently is that approximately 90 per cent of individuals of northern European ancestry are exceptions, and much of scientific research has dealt with northern Europeans. Another exception are the members of certain pastoral tribes in Africa, tribes that use fresh milk as a major contribution to their diet; about 8 per cent of the people in these tribes are lactose intolerant.

Why this difference in lactose tol

erance? There are two theories, each of which may be a partial explanation. In terms of evolution, those individuals who were able to digest milk in societies in which milk was available had a survival advantage over those individuals who were not able to do so. It may also be that the drinking of milk by men and women in those societies stimulated lactase activity. Experiments in rats suggest that this may be so.

In the United States one might expect to find more lactose intolerance among blacks than among whites. Most of the black people brought to the United States were West Africans, people originally intolerant to lactose. Kretchmer[17] suggests that in the 10 to 15 generations that black men and women have been in this country a certain amount of northern European genes have entered the black population; he estimates that approximately 70 per cent of American blacks may be lactose intolerant. So, too, may white persons from many areas of the world, and Indian and Asian peoples as well.

Symptoms of lactose intolerance include a bloated feeling, flatulence, cramps, and watery diarrhea after the ingestion of milk. (These symptoms are also seen in some newborns who are lactose intolerant either because of a congenital deficiency or as a secondary reaction to a variety of conditions, including surgery, drugs, or even nonspecific diarrhea.)

Some lactose intolerant people can drink small amounts of milk or eat milk products, which can be helpful in planning their diets. In Nigeria, for example, pastoral Fulani drink fresh milk and prepare a partially fermented yogurt-like milk drink, with reduced lactose content, for sale in the marketplace to villagers who cannot digest milk. Mothers who tell us they cannot drink milk may be able to include cheeses in their diet in order to receive the nutrients contained in milk.

An awareness and appreciation of lactose intolerance is important not only in helping people in the United States but in nutrition assistance to peoples in other parts of the world. Large scale dissemination of standard powdered milk to a lactose intolerant people is of no value; lactose-free powder would be far more useful.

Mothers who are lactose intolerant should receive supplemental calcium (1200 mg.) and vitamin D (400 I.U.) each day during pregnancy. They will also need to increase their intake of other protein foods, since milk is such a major source of dietary protein.

The Mother with Food Allergies. Mothers who have specific food allergies must have meals planned or supplements provided to supply the nutrients in the foods they must avoid. Orange juice is a fairly common allergen, as are yeast, wheat, eggs, and milk. Although it is important to help women recognize the difference between their dislikes and true allergies, the practical results of both are the same—the food will not be eaten, and the nutrient will therefore be missed.

The Mother Who Ingests Pica. Nonfood substances that are eaten are called *pica*. Varieties of pica common in the United States include laundry starch, white flour (considered a nonfood in the raw form), and clay. The excessive consumption of cracked ice is a similar practice.

The ingestion of pica is increased during pregnancy but occurs at other times as well. It is also practiced by men, although apparently less frequently in the United States than in other countries. The ingestion of pica is high among poor black women in both the South and in northern cities. Li and White[20a] found that 45 of 49 pregnant teenagers, all black, admitted having eaten starch at one time or another. Twelve had also eaten clay or expressed a preference for clay over starch.

In a smaller sample of thirteen women in another community, Hochstein[14a] found that one-fourth ate clay, half favored starch, and the remaining women preferred raw flour.

Various reasons have been offered to explain the phenomenon of pica. They include the relief of spasms due to hunger, the relief of menstrual cramps or uterine sensations that occur during pregnancy, and the belief that the clay may contain substances essential to the well-being of mother or child. Hochstein points out that just as the physician may recommend soda crackers to the middle class mother who is nauseated during early pregnancy, neighbors and relatives of the poorer mother may guide her to clay or starch for the same purpose.

Regardless of the historically reported reasons for pica, Li[20a] found that the girls in her study ate clay because it was "good," "gummy," "crunchy," or "bitter." Their descriptions of starch included "good," "smooth," "sweet," "bitter," and "thick." In short, they enjoyed eating the clay or the starch, just as the woman who smokes or chews gum enjoys that particular habit. In no way did the girls in the study attribute any special food value to either starch or clay. The habit seemed so natural to them that there was no reluctance to discuss it; it was no different than expressing a preference for a candy bar. The findings of other researchers support this matter-of-fact attitude.

Is the ingestion of pica harmful? One potential harm is the substitution of "empty calories" for food that contains essential nutrients. Anemia is not unusual among mothers who ingest pica, probably due in part to socioeconomic status as well as to the pica itself. Eating clay is thought to interfere with the absorption of iron in the gastrointestinal tract; anemia in a mother who continues to eat clay is treated with parenteral rather than oral iron. Fecal impaction is a potential hazard to clay eaters; the attempt to relieve the impaction with enemas may lead to premature labor.

It is not easy to persuade a woman to give up the ingestion of pica, just as it is not easy to persuade many people to give up cigarettes.

The Mother with a Limited Income

The foods that pregnant women need most—foods high in animal protein and rich in vitamins and minerals—often appear to be the most expensive in the grocery store. Certainly though, when one looks at food value in relation to cost, they are not; a quarter spent for a soft drink is wasted in terms of nutrition. However, many people on limited incomes, with little knowledge of nutritional needs, eat foods that fill their stomachs and keep them from feeling hungry—usually foods high in carbohydrate and often little else.

It is more difficult for the mother with limited income to buy the foods she needs, not only because of the number of dollars she has to spend but because of several other related factors. She may be forced to shop in a neighborhood "Mom and Pop" store, in which prices are higher as a result of small volume, because she has no transportation to a less expensive supermarket. In addition, she may be charging food at the small neighborhood grocery and, as a result, spending part of her food dollars paying interest on the bills she owes for last month's food. She may not have proper storage facilities for what she buys, which not only limits her purchase of "specials" at reduced prices but may also mean spoilage and waste. The low income mother may also not have cooking facilities to prepare a variety of foods.

Changing any of these factors involves a change in lifestyle that may not be possible for many women. The time required to bring about such change may not be available to the nurse working with a large number of women, all of whom need help. Resource people are essential. In addition to a nutritionist who may be attached to the same facility where the nurse is working, homeworkers from extension services or the county agricultural services are available in many urban as well as rural communities. These home economists welcome referrals from obstetric clinics and have more time than we usually do to help families improve their practices of buying, storing, and preparing food.

Concurrently, as we assess nutritional needs (see below), we may be able to begin to make one or two changes within the framework of the mother's budget. Information, of the kind described below, which is related to the specific community, can be incorporated into information given to patients during pregnancy.

Milk. In reviewing the nutritional components of food, it is obvious that milk plays a major role in meeting the nutritional needs of pregnancy. Some low income mothers receive milk free through federally-sponsored programs such as WIC (Women, Infants and Children Supplemental Food Program). Nonfat dry milk, now fortified with fat-soluble vitamins A and D, is very useful for the mother who does not like to drink milk, because it can be so easily incorporated into cooking. For example, if a recipe for pudding or macaroni and cheese calls for a cup of milk, 1/2 cup of powder can be used instead of the 1/3 cup of powder that is ordinarily used to reconstitute a cup of milk. Hence, milk intake is increased by using the most inexpensive variety of milk. For those women who will drink milk but who do not enjoy the taste of reconstituted powdered milk, the powder can be combined with fresh whole milk (1:1 ratio) for good taste at a reduced price.

Cheeses. Many processed cheese foods have the nutritional value of more expensive varieties. Cheese is a good value because there is no waste; even the smallest scrap can be used in salads or sauces, for example.

Meats. Comparing meat prices should be on a cost per *serving* basis, not cost per pound. There are approximately four servings per pound in boneless meat and fish (hamburger, canned tuna, or canned chicken), two servings per pound in meat and fish with moderate bones (chicken, turkey, pot roast of beef) and one serving per pound in meats with a large amount of bone (spare ribs, short ribs).

Eggs. Eggs can be the protein food at lunch or dinner, as well as at breakfast.

Fish. Fish often gives more protein per ounce and per unit cost than meat and can be a big help in stretching budgets. (See *Meats* above for serving information.)

Fruits and Vegetables. Farmer's markets, seasonal specials, and home gardens can help provide these foods, sometimes more difficult to include in the diet than the high protein foods in some parts of the country. Fruits and vegetables may be particularly difficult for the inner city mother to find at a good price at certain times of the year.

Cereals. Cooked cereals, many of which require only the briefest of cooking or merely the addition of hot water, are not only less expensive but are usually better sources of nutrition than cold cereals. They are excellent and economical foods for a growing baby, another important reason for making the mother more aware of them during pregnancy.

PREPARATION FOR INFANT FEEDING

As parents prepare for birth, one significant decision that they must make is the manner in which they will feed their infant—a decision that should be made in advance of the day of delivery.

What influences the choice of breast- or bottle-feeding? The choice is almost always a cultural decision, rather than a medical one. In societies that are just beginning to develop technologically, there is no real choice but breast-feeding, either by the infant's own mother or by another lactating female. But even in traditional societies, breast-feeding is on the decline as mothers become aware of Western practices. This is hardly surprising; cultural change in some aspects of life does not take place in isolation from the rest of life. But it is unfortunate that the switch from breast- to bottle-feeding has taken place in many instances before water has become safe and before adequate sanitary conditions and practices are established. Thus gastrointestinal disease remains the major cause of infant mortality in many developing nations.

There was also little choice in the manner of feeding infants in our own country until late in the nineteenth century when technology made bottle-feeding a reasonably safe alternative to breast-feeding. As recently as 1946 ap-

proximately 65 per cent of American infants were breast-fed during the newborn period. By 1965 the figure had dropped to 26 per cent. However, in the seventies, the incidence of breast-feeding appears to be increasing.

In the early twentieth century breast-feeding was more common among women from the lower socioeconomic classes. Today, however, the reverse is true; the incidence is higher among upper and middle class women. In the process of cultural change, innovations are usually accepted by the best educated people of the community and later by the economically poorer peoples who have limited access to new ideas. The trend toward bottle-feeding followed this pattern; it may be that the current increased incidence of breast-feeding among better educated women will, in time, affect the practices of the rest of the community.

Schmitt[26] emphasizes that the cultural values of nurses, as articulated by the nursing literature, are strongly in favor of breast-feeding. In her review of the literature on breast-feeding, from the social as well as the biologic sciences, she sees this bias as resting on no firm scientific evidence, a premise that many would contest. She also feels that such strong predispositions can interfere with good nursing care, and in this we feel she is correct. If a mother who prefers to bottle-feed feels that nurses expect her to breast-feed, she may do so while she is in the hospital, but will switch very quickly to bottle-feeding when she returns to her own home.

There are several disadvantages to this. Having changed her baby to the bottle, the mother may subsequently feel uncomfortable in the presence of nurses who favor breast-feeding. She may equate the attitudes of hospital nurses with those nurses in the clinic or doctor's office or with the public health nurse who comes to her home. It is not too difficult to imagine the mother's fearing the nurse's disapproval in other aspects of child care. Thus a barrier arises between mother and nurse, and the infant receives less than the best of medical care.

Moreover, too strong an insistence on breast-feeding may create some nagging measure of guilt or feeling of inadequacy in mothers who really prefer bottle-feeding, particularly in the mother whose feelings are ambivalent to begin with. Since the mother who has really decided to bottle-feed will probably do so shortly after she returns home, regardless of what she has done in hospital, it would be much wiser to spend the time that is available in the hospital instructing her about bottle-feeding rather than teaching her a technique that she plans to discard.

Recognizing the validity of these arguments, it is also important to face some other realities. It is easy to say that breast-feeding from the standpoint of infant health is important today only in developing nations in which environmental standards in terms of water and sanitation are low. This argument fails to recognize that for a significant proportion of our own population, both sanitary and economic resources are limited. There are homes, both rural and urban (and I have visited them), in which mothers feed their babies from "coke" and whiskey bottles topped with nipples because these are these are the only kinds of bottles available; in which a hungry, runny-nosed toddler drinks from the baby's bottle that has dropped from the crib to the floor and then puts the bottle back in the baby's mouth; and in which refrigeration is inadequate and a pan for sterilization of equipment just doesn't exist, even if the mother had the time, energy,

and knowledge to carry out daily formula preparation. That some middle and upper class mothers can purchase presterilized, individually packaged formula is virtually as remote for these mothers as it is for a Southeast Asia tribeswoman or an Australian aborigine mother. The babies of these mothers suffer a high rate of neonatal and postneonatal mortality and could certainly benefit from breast-feeding during their early months, but as we have already pointed out, they are the least likely to be breast-fed.

It would be tremendously worthwhile if we could find some effective way to encourage poor mothers to breast-feed their babies, not only because poor techniques of bottle-feeding increase the likelihood of introducing infection into milk but also because the lactobacillus flora in the gastrointestinal tract of breast-fed babies produces an environment unfavorable to *Escherichia coli,* the organism most commonly associated with infection in infants. Low pH produced by the lactobacillus is thought to be the primary inhibiting factor. Cow milk, on the other hand, produces an environment favorable to the growth of enteric bacteria.

Perhaps the kind of techniques used by cultural-change agents (public health nurses, agriculturalists, sanitary engineers, anthropologists, and others), who work in developing nations, can offer some ideas. One or two key members of a neighborhood group are won to the new idea, and it is they, rather than the change agent, who bring about change on a larger scale. Nurses who work with programs that aim to bring about significant change need to know the neighborhoods in which they work; they need to be able to recognize who the leaders in the neighborhood are, and they need to have a large measure of rapport with the people for whom they care.

PRENATAL EDUCATION ABOUT INFANT FEEDING

All parents deserve information about the relative advantages and disadvantages of different methods of infant feeding during the prenatal period.

Advantages of Breast-feeding

No formula can duplicate exactly the composition of human milk. Not only do the nutritional components vary, but there are nonnutritional components, such as macrophages and immunoglobulins that can never be incorporated in formulas. (See Chapter 17 for comparison of human milk and cow milk.)

For the baby with a family history of allergy, there is the possibility of allergy to formula, but not to breast milk. Occasionally a baby may develop an allergic reaction to some food his nursing mother has eaten that is transmitted in the milk, but the symptoms subside when the mother discontinues the food.

Breast-feeding is less expensive. The small additions to the mother's diet are not as expensive as are infant formula and equipment. In some areas, supplemental feeding programs for mothers and infants will provide food to nursing mothers for a longer time than to mothers who are bottle-feeding.

Not only is it virtually impossible for breast milk to become contaminated, there is a marked difference in the intestinal flora of the breast-fed baby. The *Lactobacillus bifidus* nonpathogenic organism is the major bacteria in the gastrointestinal tract of the breast-fed baby; a variety of bacteria may be found in the stools of bottle-fed infants.

The different growth rate of the breast-fed infant, once considered a possible disadvantage, seems now to be still another advantage, as we examine the relationship between infant feeding and adult obesity (Chapter 17).

Sucking at the breast varies from sucking at the bottle in a manner that appears to be significant for tooth and jaw development. The energy required to suck at the breast is as much as 60 times greater than that required to suck from a bottle. This muscle exercise encourages the development of the jaws and teeth. Not only does sucking a nipple fail to require as strong exercise as nursing at the breast, but the easy flow of milk from the bottle's nipple may cause the baby to use his tongue to protect himself from a too rapid flow of milk. Dentists have suggested that this forward thrust of the tongue may lead to a variety of problems, including mouth breathing, disease of the gums, and problems in tooth alignment. An "orthodontic nipple" has been designed to help correct the problem of "tongue thrust."

The physiologic benefits of breast-feeding to the mother are described in Chapter 19.

For both mother and baby, the experience of breast-feeding is often immensely satisfying. The emotional benefits are difficult to quantify, but are reflected in the statements of many mothers and in the apparent contentment of their infants.

The Environmental Contamination of Milk

In recent years concern for potential environmental contamination of everything that humans eat and drink has grown. Included in that concern has been the level of contaminants present in human milk. From time to time articles in newspapers and magazines and programs on television have suggested that human milk may be a potential cause of cancer, genetic defects, liver damage, and central nervous system disorders in breast-fed infants. There have been hearings by a subcommittee of the United States Senate about the possible dangers of human milk. Many parents are puzzled and confused by conflicting information.

Some pollutants do appear to exist in greater concentration in human milk than in cow milk. This is because animals, including poultry and fish, store certain chemicals in their tissues and pass them on to humans. Some chemicals are also secreted in higher concentration in human milk. Even after a specific pollutant has been banned, it may continue in the food chain for many years.

However, no one at this time is suggesting that women abandon breast-feeding. Other foods contain many of the same pollutants that have been found in human milk. Some of these pollutants (DDT, for example) also cross the placenta, so that even prior to birth they may be stored in the baby's tissues.

Moreover, the content of milk varies from one woman to another, and even from the beginning of a particular feeding until the end, the last part of the feeding having the highest fat content and therefore the highest level of contaminants.

Infant formulas are also subject to most of the pollutants suspect in human milk.

As nurses, we need to be aware of the continuing research in this field and of efforts to reduce environmental pollution for all individuals. Without more concrete data than are presently available, we believe we can continue to recommend breast-feeding to mothers who are interested.

Breast-feeding and the Working Mother

In our society in which many mothers return to work, often within 4 to 6 weeks after the birth of their infants, a very frequent question is, "Can a mother who works away from home breast-feed her baby?"

Certainly she can for a few weeks, and this is worthwhile for both mother and baby. Breast-feeding is usually well established by the time the mother returns to work at 4 to 6 weeks. She may then nurse while she is at home and express her milk during the hours that she is at work (see Expression, Chapter 18). If refrigeration is available, the expressed milk can be given to the baby in her absence the next day. If necessary, the expressed milk can be discarded and formula given when the mother is at work. She should continue to express her milk about midway through her work period, however, to maintain her supply.

A mother who prefers to wean her baby as she returns to work should do so gradually, one feeding at a time. For example, she may first switch the baby to formula at feedings when she will be away, then an early morning feeding, and then evening and night feedings. Not only will the gradual change be easier for baby but it will be much more comfortable for her.

Breast Care During Pregnancy

Whether or not a mother plans to breast-feed her baby, her breasts will enlarge during pregnancy. By the fifth month, and sometimes earlier, she will need a larger bra. If she is planning to breast-feed, it is more economical to buy nursing bras and wear them for the rest of pregnancy, rather than purchase a larger size of a regular bra now and nursing bras later. The cup of the bra should support the entire breast in a comfortable natural position. If there are pressure marks on the shoulders or under the arms or breasts, the bra is too tight. Wide straps are more comfortable and offer better support than narrow straps.

Nursing bras have plastic liners that trap moisture and will often cause sore nipples even before the baby is born, as well as afterward. It is a good idea to remove these liners.

Striae appear on the breasts, just as they do on the abdomen; there is no way to prevent them.

Prenatal Preparation for Breast-feeding

Throughout most of the world, women do nothing to prepare their nipples for breast-feeding and have no problems after the baby is born. But because of our lifestyle, some special preparation may be helpful.

During the last trimester (and as long as the baby is nursing) washing the breasts with plain water, rather than with soap, is preferable. Soap is drying; if the mother insists on using soap, it must be thoroughly rinsed away.

After washing, the nipples can be rubbed with a rough washcloth or towel. In contrast to many societies our custom of wearing brassieres prevents nipples from receiving any friction. Rubbing with a towel and allowing clothing to rub against the nipple by not wearing a bra during part of the day or cutting a nipple hole in a bra will help "toughen" the nipple in preparation.

If nipples are inverted, a Woolwich breast shield (not a nipple shield) can be placed inside the bra; the nipple will eventually be drawn into the shield. The Woolwich shield should be worn for 1 or 2 hours at first; later they can be left in place all day. If not available locally Woolwich shields may be ordered from La Leche League (address in appendix).

Nipple rolling is also helpful in preparing breasts for nursing. The nipple is held between the thumb and forefinger and gently pulled out and rolled for 1 to 2 minutes.

Opinions differ on the value of breast massage in prenatal preparation. Massage is done for the purpose of bringing colostrum from alveoli into the lactiferous sinuses (see Figure 3–14 in Chapter 3). The mother encircles the breast with the fingers and thumbs of both hands and closes them together gently.

Massage may be followed by hand expression of colostrum with the hands held at the edge of the areola. Again, the value of regular manual expression prenatally is debated, but the prenatal period is an excellent time to learn the technique that will be useful to many mothers at some time after the baby is born.

SEXUAL RELATIONSHIPS DURING PREGNANCY

Basic physiologic and psychologic factors influencing sexual relationships during pregnancy were discussed in Chapter 7.

The Nurse's Feelings About Discussing Sexuality

"I'm not sure I can discuss sex with a group of expectant mothers and fathers," a very excellent nurse told me as we were planning a series of prenatal classes. Many nurses, as well as others

A.

B.

Figure 9–7 Hoffman's exercise to make the nipple more protractile. *A,* The nipple is stimulated by opposing thumbs in a horizontal plane. *B,* The procedure is repeated with thumbs in a vertical plane. (From Applebaum: *Pediatric Clinics of N. America, 17*:207, 1970.)

in and out of the health field, share these feelings, although not everyone is as open about confessing their discomfort.

The ability to discuss sexual concerns with patients is related to: (1) comfort about our own sexuality and (2) experience in talking about sexual feelings and practices.

Providing an opportunity for students and registered nurses to discuss their own feelings about sex is an important facet of basic and continuing education, not only for nurses who care for couples during childbearing but for all nurses. Fortunately, this need is becoming more widely recognized in both the nursing literature and in conferences, workshops, and other continuing education programs.

Role playing, on a one-to-one or a group basis, can help nurses gain experience and feel more comfortable. The following example of the beginning of a discussion with a group of expectant parents could be used as a role play.

Nurse: "Many couples find their sex life changes during pregnancy. I wonder if any of you have noticed changes?" (No one responds verbally, but couples exchange glances with one another, which indicate that your comments are appropriate to their concerns.)

Nurse (continuing): "While every couple's experience is unique in some ways, many couples find they have intercourse less frequently during pregnancy. This does not mean that they care less about each other, although they may be afraid that it does."

The nurse can go on to talk about specific fears, such as fear of harming the baby or fear of beginning premature labor (see below). Her manner can convey, or she may verbally indicate, that anyone in the group may interrupt at any time. In our own experience, we find many glances and even whispered comments shared by couples, but some reluctance to share comments with the group as a whole. How often the group has met together, how much they feel they have in common, and other variables will influence their participation.

Similar comments can be used to introduce sexual counseling with individual mothers or, ideally, with couples.

Specific Concerns

Some specific concerns are so common that they are worthy of close scrutiny to separate fear from fact.

The Fear of Harming the Baby. There is no indication that intercourse is harmful to the fetus. However, when the presenting part has become engaged, intercourse is not recommended.

The Fear of Infection. As noted in Chapter 6, the baby can be affected by maternal infection, but the route is transplacental, via the maternal bloodstream, rather than vaginal. Any vaginal infection should, of course, be treated, but as long as the maternal membranes are intact, fear of infection need not be a contraindication to intercourse. Once membranes have ruptured, women should not have intercourse.

The Fear of Premature Labor. As already mentioned, sexual intercourse does indeed cause uterine contractions. Some women who are *near term* have reported that labor began following intercourse. In Solberg's study[26a] of 260 women, not one woman reported the onset of labor following intercourse.

However, there is currently no good data concerning sexual practices and the onset of premature labor, a very significant question that needs to be investigated. When intercourse is limited, many women substitute masturbation and/or other sexual manipulation. However, these activities produce more intense contractions than does intercourse. In oral sex there is a danger of air embolism.

Currently, it is suggested that women who have a history of miscarriage or premature labor should limit intercourse during pregnancy. Intercourse may be permissible for these women at certain stages of pregnancy; the decision is based on individual physician evaluation.

A woman who is bleeding should refrain from intercourse.

PREPARATION FOR LABOR AND DELIVERY

Preparation for labor and delivery has many components. Mothers and fathers need to know:

1. The signs of labor and delivery.
2. What happens during each stage of labor and delivery.
3. Preparation for coping with labor and delivery.
4. Practices in local hospitals.

Some parents have questions about alternatives to labor and delivery in the hospital which should be discussed.

The Signs of Labor and Delivery

Signs that indicate that the time of labor is approaching, but is not necessarily immediately imminent, include lightening, intensifying of Braxton Hicks contractions, cervical changes, and the presence of *show*. Occasionally rupture of the membranes may occur several days before true labor begins, although spontaneous rupture may not occur until well after labor has begun.

Bloody show and rupture of the membranes, together with regularly spaced contractions that increase in frequency and duration, are usually signs of true labor.

Lightening. Lightening, the process that indicates that the presenting part has descended into the pelvis, has been described in Chapter 7. Since lightening may not occur in multiparas, and does not always occur in primiparas, the absence of lightening has little significance. The presence of lightening indicates that the time of labor is approaching, but it may yet be a week or more in the future. Urinary frequency, due to the pressure of the uterus on the bladder, usually occurs after lightening.

Intensifying of Braxton Hicks Contractions. Contractions of the uterine muscles occur throughout pregnancy, but in the early months they are so slight that they are usually not noticed by the mother. During the last trimester, and chiefly during the last 6 weeks of a first pregnancy, Braxton Hicks contractions become more frequent and more intense. As the time of labor approaches, mothers may find it difficult to distinguish Braxton Hicks contrac-

tions, termed false labor, from the contractions of true labor. These differences are summarized herewith.

Many mothers enter the hospital with false labor. Prenatally, we can reassure mothers that no one will be angry with them if they come to the hospital in false labor and that it is, in fact, quite a common occurrence. Labor room nurses must be supportive of the often highly embarrassed mother with false labor.

Cervical Changes. As the time of labor approaches, the cervix becomes shorter and softer; it may begin to dilate 1 to 2 cm. prior to the actual beginning of labor.

Show. Vaginal secretions increase as the time of labor approaches. As the cervix softens and shortens, the mucous plug that has occupied the cervical canal is discharged; this discharge is called *show*. Show may be blood-streaked or blood-tinged. The appearance of show usually indicates that labor will begin within 1 to 2 days; however, show may not appear until after labor has begun.

The bloody tinge of show, which is from the rupture of superficial blood vessels, must be differentiated from true bleeding, which may be due to a placenta previa or abruptio placentae,

DIFFERENTIATION OF TRUE AND FALSE LABOR		
	True Labor	**False Labor**
Contractions	Regular	Irregular
	Increase in intensity	Fail to increase in intensity
	Increase in frequency	Fail to increase in frequency
	May intensify with activity	Often lessen with activity
Discomfort	Most of discomfort in back	Most of discomfort in abdomen
Cervix	Cervix becomes thinner and dilates	Cervix does not change in thickness or dilate

very serious complications (Chapter 10).

Rupture of the Membranes. In about 15 per cent of patients, membranes rupture an hour or more before th onset of the first stage of labor. In another 15 per cent, rupture occurs about the time that painful contractions begin. For the remaining 70 per cent, spontaneous or artificial rupture will occur late in the first stage of labor or early in the second stage. (Stages of labor are discussed in Chapter 11.)

The rupture of the membranes may be accompanied by a sudden gush of amniotic fluid, or, occasionally, fluid may only "dribble" out slowly. Since amniotic fluid continues to be produced until delivery, the myth of a "dry labor" if the amniotic sac ruptures early is unfounded.

Once membranes have ruptured, the mother should come to the hospital. If labor has not started, it is frequently initiated, because the incidence of infection in the newborn infant increases when membranes have been ruptured more than 24 hours.

Coming to the Hospital

Mothers are told to be prepared to come to hospital (1) when membranes rupture and/or (2) when they believe they are having contractions of true labor.

Hospitals differ in determining what the mother brings with her. Some prefer that her personal suitcase be brought after the time of delivery because they have no place to keep it while she is in the labor room. In other hospitals her mother brings her own clothes with her, but is advised to wait until the time of discharge to bring her baby's clothes. In either event, she does need to have everything ready prior to the time she herself goes to the hospital.

Basic needs for mother and baby are listed below.

BASIC NEEDS FOR MOTHER AND BABY IN HOSPITAL

Mother

Gowns
Robe
Firm slippers or shoes
Toilet articles

Baby

Two diapers
Safety pins
Shirt
Gown
Blankets
(Fancy dresses, shoes are not necessary)

Useful articles to bring include: hard candy, such as sour balls; Chapstick, because lips get dry during long hours of labor; talcum powder, for effleurage; and warm socks, because feet often feel cold during labor. Depending on hospital facilities and policies, food for the father may be brought along. Many hospitals will not permit food to be brought into the labor area. Couples should know about this and similar policies in advance (see hospital tour, below).

The Stages of Labor

The stages of labor are discussed in detail in Chapter 11, along with suggestions about the information that is helpful to prenatal families.

Films of Labor and Birth

Because couples pregnant for the first time will rarely have witnessed the process of labor and delivery, many nurses who teach prenatal classes use films to help parents anticipate what their experience may be like. Individuals and couples have varying reactions to films of birth. Some parents find birth films very helpful; others seem to feel more anxious about labor and delivery than they did before seeing the film. Sometimes it is hard for a nurse who has seen both films and births many times to appreciate the impact of these films on some prospective parents. Student nurses who may be witnessing birth and/or birth films for the first time can evaluate their own feelings and, in sharing them with their classmates and with faculty, gain an appreciation of how a first-time parent may feel.

In general, it has been found that films (whatever their subject) that reinforce previous knowledge and attitudes are influential in attitude change, while films antagonistic to attitudes held by the viewer are less influential.[20] This would indicate several important considerations:

1. Films of labor and delivery must be preceded by a discussion of labor and delivery and by a very clear explanation of what will be seen in the film. (All films should be presented in this way.)

2. The film itself should be chosen carefully. Films helpful to medical personnel (student nurses, for example) are not necessarily the best for parents. Films emphasizing husband participation would not be a good choice for a group of single mothers. In general, we have found films with a minimal number of views of the perineum most acceptable to parents.

3. The instructor should know her class and have a "feeling" for their attitudes about labor and birth.

4. Class participants should feel comfortable in choosing not to see a particular film. Usually we have to give them "permission" to refrain from witnessing a showing. For example, labor and delivery may be discussed during one class meeting. During this period the film can be dicussed and announced (a) for a special time other than class time or (b) for a specific hour of the next class. Mothers and fathers can be told that sometimes couples choose not to see birth films and that this is quite all right or that some couples prefer to wait until closer to the time of delivery. By scheduling the film at a particular time, couples are free to come or not to come without feeling the need for explaining their reasons to other class members or to the instructor.

5. Films should be followed by a discussion that involves both questions about the material portrayed and a sharing of feelings about what was seen. Sometimes scenes viewed are misconstrued and need to be clarified. After seeing a film couples may have questions that they had not previously considered. Both women and men need a chance to say what the film meant to them in terms of their own experience.

Following these guidelines, our own experience in using birth films in prenatal classes has been very good. But we are aware of other situations in which the showing of similar films has been distressing, so we continue to urge thoughtfulness in planning this teaching.

SPECIFIC PREPARATION FOR LABOR

In the decade of the seventies, more and more women have sought to be awake, aware, and in control of themselves during labor and at the time of delivery. In response to these desires, several methods and systems of preparation for childbirth, although not new, have become far more popular and widespread.

The basis of each of these methods is a combination of physical and psychologic techniques that help each pregnant woman, with the help of her mate or another person, cope with labor and delivery in a manner acceptable to her. The normality of childbirth is emphasized as the mother is helped to prepare herself to consciously and effectively participate in birth. The term *psychoprophylaxis,* which literally means prevention (prophylaxis) by the mind (psyche) is used to describe Lamaze training, probably the most popular method in the United States. The Bradley method and the Read method are other examples of psychophysical preparation for birth.

Historical Background

Methods practiced today are an outgrowth of a search that began over 50 years ago (or many centuries ago, if the varied proscriptions of tribal and folk medicine are considered). Although contemporary psychoprophylaxis as practiced in the United States neither guarantees painless childbirth nor rules out the use of medication, the techniques did evolve from a search for a method of painless childbirth that began in the Soviet Union in the 1920's.

Hypnosis was first investigated as a possible answer. The researchers were strongly influenced by Pavlov's principles of conditioned response, and when hypnosis as a general method proved disappointing, the basic principles of psychoprophylaxis were developed in 1930, although the applications were not introduced into practice until 1947 to 1949. The sociocultural climate of the Soviet Union in these years following World War II was ideal for the acceptance of these new ideas. Both money and physicians were limited, emphasizing the necessity of making childbirth easier for the mother. Initially the Russians taught the mother during labor itself, but this made demands upon hospital staff time that were difficult to meet. The current method of training before labor was then developed.

The Work of Grantly Dick-Read

It was in the 1930's that an English physican Grantly Dick-Read suggested that childbirth was a beautiful emotional experience, divinely intended, and as such was never meant to be painful. Read observed childbirth in both traditional and contemporary societies. He suggested that at some point in history, anxiety and fear became a part of childbirth. Because of this, muscle tension resulted, which made dilatation more difficult and caused pain by tension-stimulation of nerve endings in the uterus—a syndrome of fear leading to tension leading to pain.

Read believed that by replacing fear and tension with a calm attitude and the ability to relax, childbirth would become the wonderful experience it was meant to be. This childbirth would be "natural," i.e., as nature intended.

To eliminate fear, Read began to educate mothers about birth and brought them to the hospital to visit before the time of labor. To eliminate tension, he developed a series of exercises in mental and physical relaxation and breathing.

The Read method has been helpful to many women since its introduction. The concepts of education, relaxation, and breathing were a tremendous advance.

One difficulty with the Read method is the tendency to deny the possibility of pain altogether, rather than assisting women to cope with discomfort. Both women and labors vary widely; the woman who has a difficult labor or the woman who does not find labor to be the joyous, spiritual experience described in a Read class, may feel disappointed and cheated.

The Bradley method, similar to the Read method, emphasizes husband-coached childbirth. Here again the possibility of pain is usually denied.

Psychoprophylaxis: The Lamaze Method

The goal of contemporary Lamaze training is the preparation of parents to participate actively and knowledgeably in their baby's birth. Based on the principle of the conditioned response, preparation substitutes controlled breathing and relaxation for tension as an automatic response to uterine contractions. By concentrating on the technique, rather than on the contraction, mothers are better able to control their bodies during labor.

Lamaze training does not guarantee childbirth without pain; many factors influence the amount of discomfort an individual mother may experience (Chapter 13). However, the trained mother is better able to cope with pain.

Some Lamaze mothers may need no medication for pain or no anesthesia; other mothers may choose to have medication. A mother does not "fail" Lamaze by asking for medication; this concept needs to be emphasized in prenatal training and affirmed during labor.

Exercises in Psychoprophylactic Preparation

Exercises are an important part of psychoprophylactic preparation for childbirth. There are different types of exercises that serve different purposes; they are summarized in Table 9–17. The role of posture, pelvic rock, and tailor position have been described previously. Because understanding the role of breathing during labor is so closely related to understanding labor itself, breathing exercises are described in Chapter 13 and are shown in Figure 9–8.

Kegal Exercise. The Kegal exercise for strengthening of the vaginal muscles is not just for pregnancy and the postpartum period, but for all women during their lifetime. Fortunately, it can be practiced while washing dishes, watching television, talking on the phone, riding in a car—almost any time and any place. One only has to remember to do it. The result should be improved muscle tone that may add to sexual enjoyment and prevent gynecologic difficulties later in life.

The Kegal exercise is valuable as a preparation for vaginal examinations and for labor because a woman learns to consciously relax her vaginal opening.

One of the easiest ways to learn the Kegal exercise is to practice stopping the flow of urine during voiding. The actual exercise involves simply relaxing, as if voiding, and then contracting, as if to stop the flow. Hold the muscle for a moment while it is contracted; then relax and repeat.

Exercising the Muscles of the Pelvic Floor. This exercise is done lying on the back with arms at the side and legs crossed at the ankles. Contract the buttocks and hold. Squeeze the legs together, contracting the thigh muscles, and hold. Contract the muscles of the urethra, vagina, and rectum. Hold all muscle groups contracted and then relax.

Exercising the Abdominal Muscles. An exercise called "blowing out the candle" is helpful in strengthening the abdominal muscles. The mother lies on the floor with her legs bent, her feet flat against the floor, and a pillow beneath

Table 9-17   EXERCISES IN PSYCHOPROPHYLACTIC PREPARATION

Type of Exercise	Specific Exercise	Purpose	Frequency
Body building	Good posture		At all times
	Kegal	Firms muscles in front of and behind vagina	
	Pelvic floor muscles	Firms muscles of pelvic floor	3 times, twice a day
	Pelvic rock	Relieves backache	3 times, twice a day
	Blowing out the candle	Strengthens abdominal muscles	3 times, twice a day
Stretching	Tailor position		
Controlled relaxation	Contraction of specific muscle groups along with relaxation of other groups	Learning to consciously relax specific muscle groups	Twice a day
Controlled breathing	Effacement breathing (slow, deep)	Learning to respond to contractions with controlled breathing	Daily
	Dilation breathing (shallow accelerated-decelerated)		
	Transition breathing (shallow with forced blowing out)		
	Expulsion breathing		
Massage	Effleurage (light massage)	Aid in relaxation	Daily
	Deep massage		

her head. She holds her finger, as if it were a lighted candle, about 12 inches from her lips; takes a deep breath; and exhales. Then, without taking another breath, she continues to "blow out the candle," blowing and blowing as she feels her abdominal muscles contract.

Exercising to Achieve Relaxation Through Neuromuscular Control

Relaxation may be passive or active. Most of us, when we relax, relax passively; we flop down in a chair or stretch out on a bed. We are not consciously thinking about what we are doing.

Active relaxation, however, does require conscious thought. If you stretch out your leg; tighten your leg muscles; and then consciously relax first your toes, then your foot, your ankle, your calf, and your thigh—concentrating all the while and feeling the muscles relax—this is active relaxation.

Mothers practice actively relaxing one part of their body while contracting other parts (Fig. 9-9). As Braxton Hicks contractions become more noticeable, mothers can use them as a stimulus to practice relaxing other areas of the body. By the time labor has started, the mother will be able consciously to relax the other muscles of her body instead of tensing them (the "natural" response to a painful stimulus). The smooth, involuntary muscles of the uterus cannot

Figure 9–8 Couples practice breathing during a prenatal class. Notice the father's intense concentration.

be controlled by relaxation techniques. But concentrating on relaxation, along with concentrating on breathing, effectively helps women to control their bodies during contractions.

Massage

Both light massage (effleurage) and deep massage are helpful to many women in coping with labor. Husbands and others who stay with the mother during labor often help by using both massage techniques.

Effleurage is a light massage that can be felt by the mother but is not so heavy as to irritate the uterus. The movement of the hands is from the pubic area upward and outward toward the hip bones (Fig. 9–10). During a contrac-

Figure 9–9 Fathers and mothers have switched roles for a few minutes. The men are trying to relax and the women are checking to see how relaxed they are. Each should be better able to appreciate the task of the other during labor.

Figure 9–10 Brenda McBride, R.N., demonstrates effleurage to a class of mothers and fathers.

tion that lasts about a minute, from 10 to 20 effleurage movements are average. The massage should begin as the contraction begins and should continue until it is completed.

Deep massage of the back from the coccyx to the lower back is very comforting during labor. Both of these techniques will be more effective if practiced antenatally.

A Hospital Tour in Preparation for Labor and Delivery

Rarely have first-time parents ever seen a labor and delivery suite. Many have never seen a newborn nursery. In our mobile society many parents may have a second baby delivered in a city far removed from the area of their first delivery. Thus a valuable part of preparation for childbirth can be a visit to the maternity unit of the hospital at which the couple will deliver. This tour can be particularly helpful if many of the following points are observed:

1. Give mothers or couples an overview of what they will see before they go. If the hospital is a large medical center with many parking areas and entrances, arrange for them to enter at the same entrance they will use when they come for delivery. Very specific directions and/or a map may be necessary. Be sure to note if entrances used at night are different from those used during the day.

2. Point out the place and procedure for registration and admission.

3. Show them the labor and delivery rooms. Explain how various pieces of equipment may make them more comfortable and protect mother and baby. Receiving a warm greeting from nurses in various areas, and especially in the labor and delivery suites, helps to lessen the anxiety some parents feel about approaching delivery.

4. Seeing babies in the nursery helps to prepare parents for the appearance of newborn infants—an appearance that surprises many of them. (Even in hospitals with rooming-in, there are still usually some babies in the nursery at most times.) Many questions about newborns and newborn care arise from even a brief view of the nursery.

5. On the postpartal unit, policies about visiting, rooming-in, and learning opportunities can be reviewed.

Following the tour, there are often many questions. The ideal time to answer them is immediately, but this is not always possible. The nurse who is teaching childbirth preparation classes may not be able to participate in the tour if the mothers in her classes are to be delivered at many different hospitals. The nursing staff in the hospital may be having a busy day and may be unable to spend as much time with touring couples as they would like. Couples can be encouraged to have a note pad and pencil with them so that they can write down questions that occur to them at the time or after they return home. These questions can then be a basis for discussion at a subsequent class.

Because all parents will forget some of the information they have heard discussed on a hospital tour, written information about the policies of the hospital is also essential. A booklet, which reviews policies from admission to discharge, is helpful. The more specific this information is, the more helpful it will be. Here is an example of introductory paragraphs from one such booklet.

It is our pleasure to welcome you to our maternity unit. Our aim is to provide physical and emotional support during your hospitalization. We value your cooperation and suggestions as we work together.

Before your expectant admission date, you will receive pre-admission forms that should be completed and returned to the hospital. This preparation will hasten and simplify the admission process.

When labor starts you do not have to call the hospital. Come to the hospital using the emergency entrance. There a nurse will direct you or have someone take you to the labor and delivery suite.

All jewelry, valuables and other personal items should be left at home. Neither is it necessary for you to bring your luggage with you when you are admitted since you will not need any personal items until after your baby is born. The hospital cannot assume the responsibility for valuables brought with you to the hospital.

Upon arrival at the labor and delivery suite on the second floor, notify the nursing staff that you are ready to be admitted by using the buzzer at the door. A nurse will talk with you through the intercom system and will ask you if she can help you. Please respond by telling her your name and that your need to be admitted.[22]

This 18 page booklet, developed by nurses working in the maternity unit, describes all phases of the hospital experience. Photographs complement the text.

PREPARATION FOR HOME DELIVERY

The current and controversial area of home delivery is discussed in Chapter 23. In areas where planned home deliveries occur, there may be classes that prepare parents. A series of classes in the Washington, D.C. area, sponsored by H.O.M.E. (Home Oriented Maternity Experience) include five meetings:

1. Positive aspects of home birth.
2. Practical aspects of home birth.
3. Psychologic aspects of home birth.
4. Medical aspects of home birth, including contraindications and emergencies.
5. Postpartal care and breastfeeding.

Home Oriented Maternity Experiences: A Comprehensive Guide to Home Birth[12] is recommended to nurses who would like additional information about preparation for home delivery.

REFERENCES

1. Adams, C.: *Nutritive Value of American Foods in Common Units.* Agricultural Handbook #456. United States Depart. of Agriculture, 1975.
2. Bing, E.: *Six Practical Lessons for an Easier Childbirth.* New York, Bantam Books, 1969.
3. Bradley, R.: *Husband-Coached Childbirth.* New York, Harper and Row, Publishers, 1965.
4. Burrows, E., and Spiro, M.: *An Atoll Culture. Ethnography of the Ifaluk in the Central Carolines.* New Haven, Human Relations Area Files, 1957.
5. Chabon, I.: *Awake and Aware.* New York, Dell Publishing Co., 1966.
6. Dick-Read, G.: *Childbirth Without Fear.* Second Revised Edition. New York, Harper and Row, Publishers, 1959.

7. Doering, S. C., and Entwisle, D. R.: Preparation During Pregnancy and Ability to Cope with Labor and Delivery. *American Journal of Orthopsychiatry, 45*:825, 1975.

8. Eiger, M., and Olds, S.: *The Complete Book of Breastfeeding*. New York, Bantam Books, 1973.

9. Emerson, K., Saxena, B., and Poindexter, E.: Caloric Cost of Normal Pregnancy. *Obstetrics and Gynecology, 40*:768, 1972.

10. Enkin, M.: An Adequately Controlled Study of the Effectiveness of P.P.M. Training. *In* Morris, N. (ed.): *Psychosomatic Medicine in Obstetrics and Gynecology*. Basel, S. Karger, 1972.

11. Ewy, D., and Ewy, R.: *Preparation for Childbirth*. New York, New American Library, 1972.

12. Fitzgerald, D., Herman, E., Ventre, F., et al.: *Home Oriented Maternity Experience. A Comprehensive Guide to Home Birth*. Washington, D.C., H.O.M.E., Inc. 511 New York Ave., Takoma Park, Washington, D.C., 20012, 1976.

13. Flapan, M., and Schoenfeld, H.: Procedures for Exploring Women's Childbearing Motivations, Alleviating Childbearing Conflicts and Enhancing Maternal Role Development. *American Journal of Orthopsychiatry,* 42:389, 1972.

14. Hawkins, M.: Fitting a Prenatal Education Program into the Crowded Inner City Clinic. *MCN, 1*:226, 1976.

14a. Hochstein, G.: Pica: A Study in Medical and Anthropological Explanation. *In* Weaver, T. (ed.): *Essays in Medical Anthropology*. Athens, University of Georgia Press, 1968.

15. Homberg, A.: *Nomads of the Long Bow*. New York, The Natural History Press, 1969.

16. Karmel, M.: *Thank You, Dr. Lamaze*. Philadelphia, J. B. Lippincott, Co., 1959.

17. Kretchmer, N.: Lactose and Lactase. *Scientific American, 227*:71, October, 1972.

18. Laird, M., and Hogan, M.: An Elective Program on Preparation for Childbirth at the Sloane Hospital for Women. *American Journal of Obstetrics and Gynecology, 72*:641, 1956.

19. Lamaze, F.: *Painless Childbirth: The Lamaze Method*. New York, Pocket Books, 1972.

19a. Lappe, F.: *Diet for a Small Planet*. New York, Ballantine Books, 1971.

20. Leppert, P., and Williams, B.: Birth Films May Miscarry. *American Journal of Nursing, 68*:2181, 1968.

20a. Li, S., and White, R.: The Presence of Geophagy in North Carolina. Unpublished manuscript.

21. Luke, B.: Lactose Intolerance During Pregnancy: Significance and Solutions. *MCN, 2*:92, 1977.

22. *Maternity Care Book*. Winston-Salem, N. C., Forsyth Memorial Hospital OB-GYN Ongoing Education Committee, Ollie S. Taylor, R.N., Chairperson, 1976.

23. *Nutrition During Pregnancy and Lactation*. Sacramento, California Department of Health, 1975.

24. Recommended Treatment Schedules for Syphilis. *Resident and Staff Physician,* September, 1976, p. 60.

25. Roberts, J.: Priorities in Prenatal Education. *JOGN, 5*(3):17, 1975.

26. Schmitt, M. H.: Superiority of Breast-Feeding: Fact or Fancy. *American Journal of Nursing, 70*:1488, 1970.

26a. Solberg, D., Butler, J., and Wagner, N.: Sexual behavior in pregnancy. *New England Journal of Medicine, 288*:1098, 1973.

27. Sumner, G.: Giving Expectant Parents the Help They Need: The ABC's of Prenatal Education. *MCN 1*:220, 1976.

28. Thomas, H., and Wyatt, R.: One Thousand Consecutive Deliveries Under a Training for Childbirth Program. *American Journal of Obstetrics and Gynecology, 61*:205, 1951.

Chapter 10

THE HIGH RISK MOTHER AND HER FETUS

Who is the high risk mother? In the broadest sense, any mother who has a problem or condition—physiologic, emotional, or social—that may adversely affect the delivery of a healthy, full term infant may be considered high risk.

Physiologic conditions that designate a mother/newborn as high risk may exist before the mother becomes pregnant (diabetes mellitus, heart disease, and hypertension are three examples) or may be directly related to the pregnancy (eclampsia, for example). Certain conditions, such as ectopic pregnancy or a spontaneous abortion, prevent the completion of pregnancy. Others, such as the TORCH diseases described in Chapter 6, go unnoticed by the mother until a baby is born with characteristic problems. Mothers who have a multiple gestation (twins, for example), mothers who have previously delivered a child with a congenital abnormality, and mothers who have been trying to conceive for a number of years prior to becoming pregnant are examples of women who are classified as high risk because *statistics* indicate that their chances of having difficulty in their current pregnancy are greater

than the chances of the mother who has had no previous reproductive problems.

Psychosocial factors are equally as important as physiologic factors as criteria for identifying the potentially high risk mothers. Psychosocial factors are usually interrelated with physiologic factors as, for example, in the adolescent mother who may have poor nutritional stores, poor dietary habits, and at the same time a psychologic denial of the fact of her pregnancy.

The purpose of this chapter is to examine:

1. The major factors that designate a pregnancy as high risk.
2. The ways in which the special needs of high risk mothers can be met.
3. The concept of regionalization as a strategy for improving the care of high risk mothers.

IDENTIFYING HIGH RISK MOTHERS

A variety of studies, each approaching the issue with a somewhat different perspective, have attempted to identify the percentage of all mothers who can be considered high risk. Table 10–1 summarizes findings of several studies. Note that in the Harbor Hospital study,[10] a total of 55 per cent of mothers were considered at risk at some time during the prenatal or intrapartum period. Moreover, these studies indicate only risk associated with physiologic morbidity or mortality. They do not include emotional and social risks that are far more difficult to measure but are highly important in caring for whole families during childbearing.

The number of women at risk will vary from one population to another. Socioeconomic factors, for example, appear to be an important influence. There are likely to be more high risk mothers, even in a strictly physiologic sense, in an inner city clinic than in a suburban private office.

MORTALITY AND MORBIDITY

Mortality indicates death; morbidity indicates illness. Measurements of mortality and morbidity are one parameter of care given to mothers and infants.

In order to communicate with others who care for childbearing families, we must understand certain commonly used terms and use these terms in the same way.

Maternal mortality is expressed as the number of maternal deaths per 100,000 live births. (Prior to 1960, maternal mortality was expressed in deaths per 10,000 live births. The rates are now so low that the higher base is used. In comparing maternal mortality rates, it is important to note the way in which the rate is expressed.)

Several terms are used to describe fetal and neonatal death. Unfortunately, these terms are not defined identically by all professionals, which makes comparisons very difficult.

Fetal death (stillbirth) refers to the death of a fetus or an infant weighing at least 500 grams or of at least 20 weeks gestation. Weight is felt to be a preferable criterion because estimates of ges-

Table 10–1   IDENTIFYING HIGH RISK MOTHERS AND INFANTS

Study	Date Published	No. of Pregnancies	Time Included	Criteria	Per Cent at Risk	
					MOTHER	INFANT
Prechtl[22]	1967	1378	Prenatal, intrapartum, neonatal	7 or more non-optimum conditions	12	
Nesbitt and Aubry[15]	1969	1001	Prenatal	Weighed 29 adverse prenatal factors	29	
Stembera, Zezvlakova, and Dittrichova[27]	1975	3500	Prenatal, intrapartum, neonatal		23	20
Harbor Hospital[10]	1976	1417	Prenatal, intrapartum, neonatal		Prenatal risk only—16 Intrapartum risk only—23 Prenatal and intrapartum risk—16	12.5 to prenatal only 23.2 to intrapartum only 39.9 to both

tional age vary. A fetus weighing less than 500 grams is considered an abortus. The *fetal death rate* is the number of fetal deaths per 1000 births.*

Neonatal death is death of a newborn who has shown any sign of life (such as heartbeat or respiratory effort) within 28 days following birth. The *neonatal death rate* is the number of neonatal deaths per 1000 births.*

The term *perinatal death* is frequently used today, reflecting the concept that both fetal and neonatal deaths are often related to similar problems. The *perinatal death rate* is the sum of the fetal death rate plus the neonatal death rate.

On a worldwide basis, perinatal and neonatal statistics are not always available for comparison. *Infant mortality* rates are more readily available. The infant mortality rate is the number of deaths in the first year of life per 1000 live births. A comparison of infant mortality in the United States as compared with other nations is discussed in Chapter 23.

WHAT DOES BEING A HIGH RISK MOTHER MEAN?

Having considered the emotional and social tasks of pregnancy when the pregnancy is viewed as "normal" (Chapter 7), one might easily suspect that the mother designated as "high risk" must face even more complex feelings.

As these feelings are explored, remember that our designation of a mother as being at risk does not necessarily mean that she feels herself at risk. The teenager who is pregnant and considered at risk from a health point of

view may feel herself quite normal, particularly if she has friends who are also pregnant. Moreover, if *her* mother was also a teenaged mother, the mother may not feel that her daughter's pregnancy is particularly unusual or hazardous.

Some mothers enter pregnancy knowing they are at risk—the mother with diabetes who has had a previous pregnancy, for example. (The diabetic mother who has not previously been pregnant may not be aware of all the implications that her diabetic condition may have for her pregnancy.) For other mothers, events during the course of pregnancy may classify her as high risk, sometimes quite suddenly.

Thus, pregnancy for the high risk mother, just as pregnancy for all mothers, will have varied meanings. Nevertheless, it is possible to identify feelings that many of these mothers and fathers may share.

Grief Reactions

Just as the person who learns that he has a serious or terminal illness or just as the parents who deliver a malformed or sick infant, high risk parents exhibit many of the same manifestations of grief: anger, guilt, questions of "why me," and, in time, acceptance.

"Why me," for the mother with a chronic condition, may revive old feelings present when the diagnosis of the condition (diabetes, for example) was originally discovered. Self-esteem, threatened then, is now again attacked. "Other women are able to have normal pregnancies; it is unfair for me to have these problems," will not often be spoken but will underlie behavior.

The mother and/or father may express guilt feelings through questions ("What did I do to cause this?") or statements ("I suppose this is my punishment—for not wanting a

---

*These rates are sometimes expressed per 100 *live* births, rather than births. Before rates can be compared, it is essential to ascertain that one is comparing identical rates.

baby—for having sex when I wasn't married," and so on). "I am going to eat properly during *this* pregnancy" or "we are not going to have intercourse *this time*" are statements indicating guilt for an unhappy outcome in a prior pregnancy.

Anger may be directed at nurses or physicians, or at one another. It may be expressed directly in relation to the care during pregnancy ("If my care had been better, *this* might not have happened,") or less directly ("The nurses don't care about me" or "I have to wait too long"). Anger may lead to blaming the partner ("I didn't want another baby but *he* insisted" or "If *she* would rest when she should, she wouldn't be sick").

Before there can be any degree of acceptance of high risk pregnancy, these feelings must be recognized—a major nursing goal. Because they may not be verbalized directly, a primary nurse who can come to know a couple is very important. She may be the nurse in the high risk clinic; the public health nurse; or the school nurse, who may be the one most likely to see adolescents on a continuing basis.

Good records that describe feelings as well as physiology are also essential to helping families recognize and cope with these feelings.

Communication between the mother and father and the nurse is important; communication between the mother and the father themselves is even more significant and is behavior that we can encourage. It would be ideal, perhaps, to have the father present at each prenatal visit, but this is rarely possible. But we can encourage the mother to share her feelings with her partner, a suggestion that may seem obvious but that, in actuality, may be unusual for some couples. Galloway suggests role playing between the mother and the nurse as preparation for a discussion with her husband, if the mother feels this will be difficult for her.[7]

Developmental Tasks in High Risk Pregnancy

In Chapter 7 maternal development tasks were identified as accepting the pregnancy, assuring safe passage, acceptance of the child by significant others, attachment, and giving of oneself. Each of these tasks has special meaning for the high risk mother, although every mother and couple will not necessarily achieve each task with the same degree of difficulty (Table 10–2).

Accepting the Pregnancy. Accepting a pregnancy with risks involved means accepting the idea of being a less than perfect bearer of children; this can be a blow to feelings about oneself as a woman. For a woman who defines her femininity in terms of childbearing, the possibility that she will not be successful is difficult to accept. For some mothers there will have been previous unsuccessful pregnancies—pregnancies that ended in spontaneous abortion or stillbirth or a malformed infant. The anxiety that this pregnancy may also come to a less than perfect conclusion is ever present.

Denial is one way that a mother or father may fail to accept the fact of high risk pregnancy. In denying the reality of the pregnancy with risk, the mother and/or father may behave as if there were no problem. Specific needs in terms of rest or diet or keeping appointments may be ignored.

Once the pregnancy has been accepted, the mother is ready to deal with additional tasks.

Assuring Safe Passage. For the high risk mother, assuring safe passage for her baby is a major task. It may

Table 10-2 COMPARISON OF DEVELOPMENTAL TASKS FOR ALL MOTHERS AND FOR HIGH RISK MOTHERS

Tasks for All Mothers	Special Tasks for High Risk Mothers
Accepting the pregnancy	Pregnancy may not be successfully completed
Assuring safe passage	Long term hospitalization
	More frequent outpatient visits
	Special proscriptions
	Added expense
	Fear of potential problems
Acceptance of the child by significant others	Fear that the baby may die or may be abnormal and thus unacceptable
Attachment	Fear of attachment because child may die or be abnormal.
	Postponement of nesting behavior
Giving of oneself	Extensive sacrifice to protect fetus
	Need for recognition of her sacrifice

involve inconvenience and a considerable expenditure of time and money. The mother living in a small community may need to travel to a medical center for specialized care. Hospitalization may be required for 1 or more weeks, or even months, during the course of the pregnancy. The mother, and the father as well, may have to make major adjustments in their lives.

The willingness of mothers to do this—to sometimes spend days in the hospital awaiting the appropriate time for delivery, to submit to multiple amniocenteses and other tests, and to comply with all the other proscriptions we place upon them—testifies to the strong drive of most mothers to assure safe passage for their baby.

We can reinforce this need by recognizing the mother's efforts and praising her for them. This can also be helpful later, if the pregnancy does not result in the birth of a healthy infant, by assuring the mother that she did everything she possibly could.

Acceptance of the Child by Significant Others. It is important to all mothers to feel that the father of their child, the grandparents, or whoever is important to them accepts their unborn child. People important to the high risk mother may be reluctant to talk with the mother about her coming child or to become too attached to the idea of the child's birth, lest something happen to the baby.

Added to the mother's anxiety about rejection of her baby is the concern that she too may be rejected if she is unable to produce a healthy child.

Although these thoughts may be almost continually on the mother's mind, the father may not even suspect her concern. Our opportunity to talk with both parents together may help her share her concern; lacking this, we can encourage her communication.

Attachment. Just as the mother fears that others may not accept her baby if he is less than perfect, she may also be afraid to become attached to him during the prenatal period. The assessment of prenatal attachment behavior (described in Chapter 7) is an important tool in recognizing this fear. Once recognized, it is appropriate to help the mother cope with her feelings. We believe that attachment to the baby after birth, even if the baby is going to die, is necessary to healthy grieving (Chapter 22); we wonder if prenatal attachment may also be important to a healthy grief process—grief for the perfect baby who was not born, should the baby have some type of abnormality, as well as grief for the baby who dies, either in utero or following delivery.

Not every baby born to a high risk mother will die or will even be ill following delivery. What effect might failure to form a prenatal attachment have on the mother's relationship with her subsequently healthy infant?

Giving of Oneself. Pregnancy makes certain demands on all women, but the demands placed upon the high risk mother to give may be overwhelming. She may have to give up time for favorite or necessary activities for hospitalization or for periods in bed at home. She may have excessive costs for care. The experience of the fetus as her gift to others may be tempered by concerns about the status of the fetus.

Her need for evidence of concern from those around her—husband, friends, relatives—is frequently heightened. Yet at the same time, she may reject some of the traditional signs of concern and affection (a baby shower, for example) because of her fear of attachment.

Thus, just as the high risk mother has specific and special physiologic needs, she also has particular social and emotional needs. Helping her to cope with these needs is as important as the care we give to support the physiologic demands of her pregnancy.

AGE AS A RISK FACTOR

From a biologic perspective, and in many ways from social and psychologic perspectives, the ideal age range for reproduction is the twenties to early thir-

ties. Although many women, both younger and older, may successfully bear and care for children, there is good evidence that at either end of the reproductive years both mortality and morbidity are increased. For this reason, the particular needs of adolescents and women over 35 require special attention.

ADOLESCENCE AND PREGNANCY

The psychosocial needs of adolescents who are pregnant have been discussed in Chapter 7. Adolescents, especially those under 16, are statistically at risk for physiologic complications during pregnancy.

Physical Development during Adolescence

The physical changes of adolescence have their beginning in the increased output of the gonadotropic hormones of the anterior pituitary gland, which in turn stimulates increased production of testosterone in males and estrogens in females (Chapter 3).

As a result, body growth and development accelerates rapidly, being most marked in girls between the ages of 11 and 13 years and in boys between the ages of 13 and 15½ years. Between the ages of 11 and 16 a girl achieves 8 per cent of her total physical development. At no other period in life after the first birthday does growth occur so rapidly.

To keep pace with this rapid development, nutritional demands both in the 11 to 14 and 15 to 18 age groups are increased in terms of extra calories, protein, minerals, and vitamins. Only during pregnancy and lactation will nutritional needs be as high (Chapter 9). Because of cultural influences, however, girls between 11 and 18 may have the poorest diets of any group in our society.

Physical Complications of Pregnancy during Adolescence

From a physiologic perspective, adolescents have higher rates of several complications of pregnancy that are discussed in more detail later in this chapter. These complications include: pre-eclampsia and eclampsia, anemia, prolonged labor, preterm delivery, and delivery of a low birth weight infant. The higher incidence of preterm and low birth weight infants, in turn, leads to higher rates of infant mortality and morbidity.

One factor that many of these complications would appear to have in common is poor nutrition. The role of nutritional inadequacy in causing iron deficiency anemia is direct. While the causes of pre-eclampsia, eclampsia, and prematurity are not known, the incidence is higher in low income groups of people who may also eat nutritionally inadequate diets.

When the nutritional demands of pregnancy are imposed upon the nutritional demands of adolescence, it is not surprising that these demands go unmet unless they are a specific focus of attention in a program designed for adolescent or high risk mothers.

THE MOTHER OVER 35

Although it is certainly possible for a mother older than 35, and even older than 40, to deliver a healthy infant, the mathematical possibility that there may be a problem is increased.

As the hormonal regulation of the menstrual cycle becomes less regular, the internal environment becomes less optimal for the development of both egg and endometrium. The incidence of multiple pregnancy increases because more than one egg is released. The egg itself may be defective, with chromosomal abnormalities.

Down's syndrome, described in Chapter 2 is due to a chromosomal abnormality. The risk increases dramatically with age (Table 10–3). Because of this, some physicians suggest that all mothers over 35 have an amniocentesis to screen for Down's syndrome.

Many "older" mothers are aware of the increased risks and this is a source of concern during their pregnancy. Although most mothers worry about "will my baby be normal?" they feel they have added reason for concern. Even though amniocentesis assures them that their baby is not likely to have Down's syndrome, they are concerned about other possible problems.

Some older mothers are very self-conscious about their pregnancy. They

Table 10–3   RISK OF DOWN'S SYNDROME

Age of Mother	In Any Pregnancy	After Birth of Baby with Down's Syndrome
–29	1 in 3000	1 in 1000
30–34	1 in 600	1 in 200
35–39	1 in 280	1 in 100
40–44	1 in 70	1 in 25
45–49	1 in 40	1 in 15
All mothers	1 in 665	1 in 200

sit in the office or clinic waiting-room with women much, much younger. They joke half-heartedly about being the grandmother at the Parent-Teachers' Association or about reaching retirement age when the child is still in college. Careful listening to small comments will help us to assess this mother's needs realistically and thereby to help her cope with her pregnancy.

HIGH RISK PREGNANCY DUE TO PRE-EXISTING MATERNAL CONDITIONS

DIABETES MELLITUS

The number of mothers with diabetes mellitus is increasing steadily. Prior to the discovery of insulin in 1923, most women with diabetes were sterile. Young girls who acquired diabetes early in childhood often did not live to their reproductive years. For those who did become pregnant, there was a 25 per cent maternal mortality and a 50 per cent fetal mortality.

Now mothers with diabetes rarely die when they are pregnant; maternal mortality is less than 1 per cent. But mortality for the fetus and infant remains far higher than for the general population (see below). Moreover, as the number of mothers with diabetes increases, the number of potential diabetic mothers in succeeding generations increases. For these reasons, an understanding of the relationship between diabetes and pregnancy is extremely important.

Table 10–4 describes the classifications that are commonly used to group mothers with diabetes. The term *gestational* diabetes is used for mothers who have diabetes during pregnancy but who have no apparent symptoms after their baby's birth. Mothers who have babies that resemble infants of diabetic mothers (IDM) or who have a history of stillborn infants and who subsequently develop diabetes at some later time in their life are, in retrospect, considered *prediabetic,* although the diagnosis is not made at the time. Recognizing the possibility of future diabetes in these mothers is important in health counseling.

The goal in the care of a mother with diabetes is good health for both mother and baby. The mother may have problems because of the effect of her diabetes on the pregnancy or because of the effect of the pregnancy on her diabetes. The fetus faces multiple risks, including an increased possibility of intrauterine death, of congenital abnor-

Table 10–4   WHITE'S CLASSIFICATION OF DIABETES IN PREGNANCY*

Group A:	Abnormal glucose tolerance test only.
Group B:	Onset of clinical diabetes after age 20, duration less than 10 years, no demonstrable vascular disease.
Group C:	Onset between ages 10 and 20, duration 10 to 19 years, no X-ray evidence of vascular disease.
Group D:	Onset before age 10 or duration over 20 years, X-ray diagnosis of vascular disease in legs, retinal changes.
Group E:	Same as Group D with addition of calcifications of pelvic arteries by X-ray examination.
Group F:	Diabetic nephropathy.
Group R:	Active retinitis proliferans.

*Adapted from White: *Medical Clinics of North America, 49*:1015, 1965.

mality, and of a difficult delivery if he is oversized and if vaginal delivery is attempted. In the hours following birth, the newly born infant is also at risk (Chapter 18).

The frequency of complications for both mother and baby is reduced when excellent care is given by nurse-physician-nutritionist teams. The large, fat baby still considered typical of Group A, B, and C diabetic mothers is less frequent with proper prenatal care and is now considered an unnecessary outcome by many.

The Effect of Pregnancy on Diabetes

We have noted in earlier chapters that pregnancy affects the hormonal system of the body. One of the effects of the mother's accelerated endocrine activity is increased insulin production by the islet cells of the pancreas. If this increased insulin output were to go unchecked, progressively increased hypoglycemia would result. The mother's body, however, is also producing estrogen, progesterone, cortisol, and human chorionic somatomammotropin (HCS, or placental lactogen), all of which are antagonistic to insulin. Moreover, glucocorticoids from the adrenal cortex and human growth hormone from the anterior pituitary are produced in increased amounts; these hormones increase the mother's tendency to hyperglycemia.

The net result of all of these changes is an increased insulin requirement in over two-thirds of mothers who have diabetes; some diabetic mothers have a decreased requirement, however, so that all mothers must be individually evaluated throughout pregnancy (see below).

The increase in glomerular filtration rate, which occurs in all pregnant women, along with a decrease in glucose reabsorption (i.e., a decreased renal threshold), makes glycosuria rather common in all pregnant women and makes the evaluation of the meaning of urine sugar more difficult.

The Effect of Diabetes on Pregnancy

Diabetes mellitus may affect pregnancy in several specific ways. Even with good care, perinatal mortality for the fetus-infant is as much as eight to ten times higher than in normal pregnancy. More than 10 per cent of fetuses may die in utero, and neonatal mortality is greater than 8 per cent. In addition, the likelihood of the infant's having one or more congenital anomalies is three times greater than in the general population, and brain damage from hypoglycemia following birth does occur, although this is largely preventable with proper care (Chapter 18). Respiratory distress syndrome is far more common in infants of diabetic mothers (Chapter 18). Vaginal delivery is complicated when the infant is oversized.

The likelihood of *toxemia* (below) is five times greater in mothers with diabetes than in the general population; approximately one diabetic mother in every four will have pre-eclampsia, eclampsia, or hypertensive disease.

Maternal hydramnios (amniotic fluid in excess of 2000 ml.) occurs about 20 per cent of the time. Hydramnios may cause maternal distress because of the pressure of an enlarged uterus on the diaphragm, the gastrointestinal tract, or the venous system returning blood from the lower extremities.

Recognizing the Mother at Risk

The woman who has previously diagnosed diabetes is clearly recognizable. Over half of the women with diabetes in pregnancy, however, will be in Group A, i.e., they will not have been diabetic prior to pregnancy. A number of factors in these women's history make them suspect:

1. A family history of diabetes.
2. The birth of a previous infant weighing more than 9 pounds or 4000 grams.
3. The birth of a previous infant who was stillborn or who had a congenital anomaly.
4. Hydramnios during a previous pregnancy.
5. Maternal weight of more than 200 pounds.
6. A positive test for glycosuria during pregnancy, particularly on more than one occasion.

None of these characteristics in themselves is absolutely predictive of gestational diabetes, although when two or more exist the likelihood is increased. Women with any of these characteristics should have a glucose tolerance test. If the test is normal, it may be repeated during the third trimester. If it is abnormal (values for an abnormal test will vary slightly with the procedures used in different institutions), the mother will be followed as a high risk patient with more frequent visits and care appropriate to her individual requirements (below). As high risk patients, these women should be under the supervision of an obstetrician trained in high risk obstetrics rather than a general practitioner or a nurse-midwife.

The Basic Plan of Care

The prevention of hyperglycemia is the basic principle underlying the plan of care for pregnant women with diabetes. Women with Group A through Group C diabetes who maintain blood sugars below 120 mg. per 100 ml. usu-ally will have babies with normal weight and low morbidity.

Diet. Diet is important for anyone who has diabetes and for any woman who is pregnant; it should therefore not be surprising that good diet control is essential for the pregnant diabetic woman. Many obstetricians will choose to hospitalize a woman for a few days early in pregnancy for diet instruction and stabilization of the woman's carbohydrate metabolism. The mother, especially if this is her first pregnancy and she is feeling well, may have difficulty understanding the reason for and the importance of this hospitalization. Both before her admission and while she is in the hospital, we can help her by encouraging her to express her feelings about this hospitalization and by using her time and ours to teach her as much as possible about the special requirements of her pregnancy. She should not remain in bed during the time she is in the hospital but should be as normally active as possible during the time that diet and insulin requirements are being regulated. Diabetic mothers who have experienced difficulties during a previous pregnancy may better recognize the reason for early hospitalization.

For the diabetic mother with normal weight and activity, a diet of approximately 2000 to 2400 calories is usually recommended; about 400 additional calories per day are needed for mothers under 18 years of age. Protein is calculated at 1.5 grams per kg. of body weight per day (roughly 90 grams for a 130 pound woman, carbohydrate at 3.0 grams per kg. per day, and fat in quantities sufficient to make up the total caloric needs. (Note that the protein intake is considerably higher than that of the average pregnant woman for whom approximately 65 grams of protein are recommended.)

Mothers receiving insulin usually

receive four meals with the total food intake divided as follows: 2/7 at breakfast, 2/7 at lunch, 2/7 at dinner, and 1/7 at bedtime. For mothers who do not require insulin, nutritional requirements are divided into relatively equal thirds. Even distribution of the calories is important, so that blood glucose will remain as constant as possible and fetal equilibrium will be maintained with no marked episodes of either hypoglycemia or hyperglycemia.

The diabetic mother who is overweight should not attempt to reduce during pregnancy; inadequate calories will result in fatty acid breakdown, which, in turn, will lead to acidosis.

A "diet diary" will help the mother become aware of what and when she is eating; it will help us in assessing her diet and in counseling her about subsequent planning. Again, this may seem like a lot of extra "trouble" to the mother unless she understands the reason and the importance. She is not likely to keep records accurately just because we ask her to do so.

Insulin. Insulin is regulated so that the fasting blood sugar level is maintained between 80 and 110 mg. per 100 ml. or the 2 hour postprandial blood sugar level between 110 and 145 mg. per 100 ml. Values considered acceptable will vary somewhat from one institution to another. Testing is usually done once every 2 weeks, although a specific plan will be made for each patient.

A common insulin regimen combines intermediate or long-acting insulin plus regular insulin taken in the morning, with only regular insulin taken again in the evening. Insulin requirements may be lower for some women in the first trimester; by the third trimester insulin will usually be increased by as much as 50 to 75 per cent, although again there are individual variations.

Oral hypoglycemic agents are not used during pregnancy, even if the mother has taken them previously. These agents stimulate the beta cells, not only in the maternal pancreas but in the fetal pancreas as well.

Because insulin is inactivated by the placenta, failure to require an increased amount of insulin after the first trimester or a sudden drop in insulin requirement may mean some problem in placental function.

Urine Checks. Diabetic mothers are asked to check urine sugar levels four times a day and to keep a record of urine tests, insulin taken, and unusual activities. These records can be used to help the mother recognize variations that affect her, such as the interaction between a favorite activity and her urine sugar level, and thus can help her to become better able to plan for herself. Sugar levels of 4+ should be reported to her nurse or physician immediately. Urine sugar levels are not the basis on which insulin is adjusted; variations in urine sugar levels may, however, indicate the need for a check of blood glucose levels.

Monitoring the Fetus

In the third trimester, beginning at 32 to 34 weeks, urinary estriol levels and oxytocin challenge testing to determine fetal well-being and evaluation of the lecithin/sphingomyelin (L/S) ratio and creatinine levels to assess fetal maturity become a part of care. These procedures, important to high risk mothers with many kinds of problems, are discussed below.

Note in the discussion of the L/S ratio on page 330 that a ratio of 2.0 or greater is usually considered an indication of lung maturity. Experience indicates that in certain laboratories, at least, the infant of a diabetic mother may need a higher ratio (at least 2.5 to 3.0) to indicate lung maturity.

HEART DISEASE

The cardiac-related changes that occur in all pregnant women have been discussed in Chapter 6. To review these briefly, there is an increase in both blood volume and heart rate, with a resultant increase in cardiac output of from 40 to 50 per cent. For the mother who has a diseased heart, this increased workload may compromise her health.

About 1.5 to 3 per cent of all pregnant women have some form of heart disease. As a cause of maternal mortality, heart disease ranks fourth or fifth, depending on the study. The most common cardiac problem of women who become pregnant is rheumatic heart disease, with mitral stenosis the most common lesion. Over 80 per cent of pregnant women with heart disease will have rheumatic heart disease. Ten to 15 per cent (figures vary from study to study) will have some form of congenital heart defect. All other forms of heart disease account for only 2 per cent of cardiac maternity patients.

For some mothers with heart disease, there may have been no prior symptoms; the diagnosis of cardiac disease is made during the pregnancy. This is not always an easy diagnosis because:

1. The apex of the heart rotates laterally during pregnancy, and, therefore, it is normal for the heart to *appear* larger in an X-ray film.

2. A systolic murmur is common in pregnant women (as frequent as 96 per cent of the time in some studies) and a diastolic murmur may be present as often as 18 per cent of the time.

3. Tachycardia is not unusual.

It is not difficult to imagine the anxiety of a woman who must adjust not only to pregnancy but also to the possibility of heart disease as well. Difficulty in diagnosis will add to her anxiety; it is essential that we understand and explain why the diagnosis is not always easy. Symptoms that clearly indicate heart disease include:

1. A continuous diastolic or presystolic murmur.

2. A loud, harsh systolic murmur especially with a thrill.

3. Definite heart enlargement.

4. Severe arrhythmia, such as bigeminy.

The Effect of Heart Disease on Pregnant Women

In assessing the status and needs of the mother with heart disease, the classification of the New York Heart Association is commonly used (Table 10–5). This classification is one indication of the extent to which pregnancy will affect the mother.

Also important is the mother's age. The incidence of congestive heart failure increases with age; mothers over 30 often do not tolerate pregnancy as well as younger mothers. Therapeutic abortion may be suggested for some older mothers.

The longer the mother has had heart disease, the greater her likelihood of problems. Previous atrial fibrillation, previous heart failure, and cardiomegaly are also serious signs.

Although we cannot change the mother's age or cardiac status, there are a number of other factors that can be controlled in helping her to experience a safe pregnancy. If the mother is obese, weight reduction prior to pregnancy will improve her chances for a good outcome. Anemia must be prevented; anemia alone can lead to congestive heart failure.

Toxemia (below) can also cause congestive failure, even if the mother has mild heart disease (and can, in fact, cause congestive failure in the mother with no heart disease). Many physicians

Table 10–5   CLASSIFICATION OF HEART DISEASE IN PREGNANCY*

Class	Criteria	Possible Course of Pregnancy
I	No discomfort during normal activity.	Generally few problems during pregnancy.
II	May have transient angina during normal activity.	Generally few problems during pregnancy.
III	Activity brings discomfort (fatigue, angina, dyspnea). Comfortable only at rest.	Often advised against pregnancy, but may choose to become pregnant. Should be hospitalized if signs of cardiac decompensation develop.
IV	Barely comfortable even at rest; may have symptoms of angina or congestive heart failure at rest. Unable to perform any activity without discomfort.	High maternal mortality. Postpartum period particularly hazardous. Usually advised against pregnancy.

*Adapted from New York Heart Association: *Nomenclature and Criteria for Diagnosis of Diseases of the Heart and Blood Vessels.* 5th Edition. New York, Peter F. Mallon, Inc., 1953.

will digitalize a woman with heart disease who shows signs of toxemia. Infection may also contribute to heart failure. Congestive heart failure is a cause of death in pregnant women with heart disease.

Cardiac Workload in Pregnancy

Cardiac output increases slightly during the first 8 weeks of pregnancy and then increases more sharply until the period of maximum output, about 28 to 32 weeks. It then levels off from 32 weeks until the time of delivery.

During labor, cardiac output increases slightly with each uterine contraction. Following delivery, cardiac output increases markedly within the first day or two, as fluid in the mother's tissues returns to the circulatory system (Chapter 19). The first days postpartum are critical, and the mother must be watched closely for the signs of congestive heart failure described below. By the third to fourth postpartal day, marked diuresis has occurred, and the risk of heart failure decreases.

The Plan of Care during the Prenatal Period

The goal of care for the pregnant woman with heart disease is reduction of the workload on the heart.

Activity is limited in relation to the extent of the heart disease. If the mother is short of breath and dyspneic or tachypneic, she is doing too much. For mothers in Classes I and II, limitation may mean a rest period midmorning and midafternoon. Ten hours of sleep are recommended at night, as well as a rest period after each meal. Mothers in Class IV may require complete bed rest throughout pregnancy.

Reduced physical activity is so important, particularly for Class III and IV mothers, that time spent in helping the mother plan her daily schedule is a significant part of her care. If appropriate, perhaps some type of household help can be arranged; many communities have "homemaker" services as part of the Department of Social Services or of another community agency. Another resource is a home economist (a county extension agent, for example) who will visit the home and help the mother plan her work with a minimum amount of effort.

The frustration of inactivity, particularly for the mother who must have complete bed rest, must also be faced. She will need frequent opportunities to share her feelings about this pregnancy and the changes it is making in her family life. For many mothers hospitalization for rest may be required at some time during pregnancy.

Sodium intake is usually limited to 2 grams. If a mother is restricting her sodium intake and still gaining excessive weight, a diuretic such as hydrochlorothiazide may be prescribed.

Any *infection* is promptly treated with antibiotics. Upper respiratory infections, if complicated by bronchitis and pneumonia, are important as contributory causes of heart failure. Infection may also lead to bacterial endocarditis in a patient with diseased heart valves. Because of this, prophylactic antibiotics may be given during labor and following delivery.

The avoidance of *anxiety* is important. A certain amount of anxiety is present during every pregnancy. That anxiety is easily compounded when the mother knows she has "complications." Frequent visits to the clinic or office, careful explanations of what is happening and the reasons for care, and, again, the opportunity to talk with a concerned and interested listener are essentials. Frequent visits are particularly important as the period of maximum cardiac output is reached. Output increases rapidly beginning about 20 weeks and peaks from 28 to 32 weeks.

Assessment of the Gravida with Heart Disease

Weight gain—A gain in weight in excess of the normally expected gain may indicate accumulating fluid and the potential for congestive heart failure.

Heart rate—A heart rate of 110 or more when the woman is resting may be a sign of early heart failure or of infection.

Respiratory rate—Respirations greater than 20 to 24 per minute may be a preliminary to heart failure. Ask about dyspnea, orthopnea, and coughing.

Unexplained cough—An unexplained cough may be a first sign of congestive failure.

Hemoptysis, distention of neck veins, rales and *wheezes,* and *pulmonary edema*—These are signs of congestive heart failure.

The treatment for congestive heart failure is medical; it is almost never the termination of the pregnancy. As in the nonpregnant patient, treatment includes rest, digitalis, diuretics, oxygen, sedatives, and restricted sodium and fluids.

The Woman with a Cardiac Valve Prosthesis

Since a cardiac valve prosthesis is only inserted in patients with significant cardiac impairment, these patients are not particularly good candidates for successful pregnancy. In addition, such a woman has special problems during pregnancy. She normally uses an anticoagulant because thrombosis and thromboembolism are problems with all prostheses currently available. The coumarin derivatives, often prescribed for these patients, cross the placenta and (1) may be teratogenic

(Chapter 6) and (2) may cause bleeding in the newborn infant (especially cerebral bleeding) if given to the mother late in pregnancy. Heparin is the anticoagulant of choice during pregnancy because it does not cross the placenta. (Oral anticoagulants are sometimes used after the first trimester until the thirty-seventh week.)

Mothers with a cardiac prosthesis are at increased risk of endocarditis; they may be given prophylactic antibiotics during labor for this reason.

Prostheses may limit the blood flow and make it difficult to meet the higher tissue needs for oxygen during pregnancy.

Valve prostheses also cause some trauma to red blood cells, which may be sufficiently extensive to cause anemia.

URINARY TRACT AND/OR RENAL DISEASE

Urinary tract infections are a fairly common complication of pregnancy. Asymptomatic bacteriuria occurs in approximately 5 per cent of pregnancies, chiefly because ureteral dilatation and urinary stasis are frequent. The diagnosis is based on examination of a clean, midstream urine specimen. The mother should wash her vulva with soap and water prior to obtaining the specimen. If the specimen cannot be cultured immediately, it should be refrigerated. A count of 10,000 bacterial colonies per ml. is considered significant.

Even though they are asymptomatic, bacterial infections are treated (commonly with sulfonamides or ampicillin) because (1) they may lead to acute pyelonephritis, and (2) they may represent chronic pyelonephritis.

Acute pyelonephritis, which occurs in 1 to 2 per cent of all pregnant or puerperal women, is a serious and sometimes fatal complication, but one that responds dramatically to ampicillin. Signs include chills, fever, flank pain, pyuria, and tenderness over one or both kidneys.

Renal disease, in which there is impairment of kidney function, is associated with both eclampsia and premature labor. Some studies indicate that asymptomatic bacterial infections also may be associated with premature labor, while others find no similar relationship.

The effect of chronic renal disease on pregnancy is related to the presence of hypertension. When there is no hypertension, a successful pregnancy and good fetal outcome are possible even if there is impaired renal function. However, if the mother is hypertensive, intrauterine growth retardation is common, and the incidence of pre-eclampsia and perinatal mortality is very high.

ESSENTIAL HYPERTENSION

Essential hypertension is defined as a resting blood pressure of 140/90 on several occasions. The cause is complex; heredity appears to be one important factor.

What happens when the woman with essential hypertension becomes pregnant? Approximately 15 to 30 per cent of gravidas with essential hypertension will develop pre-eclampsia. The higher the blood pressure, the greater the risk of both pre-eclampsia and a poor fetal outcome.

For some women, pregnancy is a stimulus to the development of latent essential hypertension, just as pregnancy may stimulate latent diabetes (gestational diabetes). The hypertension may disappear following delivery only to reappear during subsequent pregnancies and eventually become chronic hypertension.

Antihypertensive medications are given when hypertension is severe. Although they help to protect the mother, they are less successful in protecting the fetus.

SICKLE CELL DISEASE

No condition complicating pregnancy carries as great a risk as sickle cell disease. Maternal mortality is as high as 10 to 20 per cent, and perinatal mortality is in the range of 50 per cent in the severe forms of the disease. (There are several forms of sickle cell disease, such as sickle cell disease (SS), hemoglobin SC disease, homozygous hemoglobin C disease, and so on, the description of which is beyond the scope of this book.)

Approximately 8 per cent of black gravidas have sickle cell trait (SA) (Chapter 2). Although they do not have the severe problems of the mother with sickle cell disease, their fetuses may be at risk of hypoxic stress.

The mother with sickle cell trait or sickle cell disease should ideally be identified prior to pregnancy by community screening programs. (The mother with sickle cell disease may have been identified because of recurrent illness throughout her life.) If a woman has never been tested, this should be a part of her prenatal assessment, along with testing of the baby's father for purposes of genetic counseling.

Care of the mother with sickle cell disease who wishes to complete a pregnancy includes careful observation of hemoglobin levels. A hemoglobin level in the range of 6 to 8 grams per 100 ml. is normal for these mothers; no attempt is made to raise the hemoglobin level

beyond the mother's normal range during the course of pregnancy. A rapidly falling hemoglobin value is a sign of sickle cell crisis. At term or during labor, transfusions of whole blood or packed red blood cells are usually given as a measure of protection for mother and infant.

Iron is not given to mothers with sickle cell disease. Folic acid needs are increased during and following crises.

Sterilization is frequently recommended for a mother with severe sickle cell disease because of the risk pregnancy carries to her own life.

RH ISOIMMUNIZATION

When a mother lacks the D factor in her blood, she is said to be Rh negative. If her fetus has the D factor and is thus Rh positive, Rh isoimmunization is possible.

The genetic basis of Rh disease has been discussed in Chapter 2.

In about 10 per cent of all pregnancies, an Rh negative mother is carrying an Rh positive fetus. Theoretically, each Rh positive fetus of an Rh negative mother is a candidate for *erythroblastosis fetalis,* in which the red blood cells of the fetus and newborn are destroyed by a process described below. However, in only 5 per cent of pregnancies in which there is a potential problem does the mother develop antibodies to the fetal red blood cells.

Erythroblastosis occurs in from 4 to 10 pregnancies per every 1000. The problem could be eliminated in the vast majority of these babies by applying our current knowledge.

The physiologic basis of erythroblastosis is an antigen-antibody reaction. The Rh_D negative mother (genotype dd) has no Rh_D antigen in her body. When her fetus is Rh_D positive, any fetal blood (containing D antigen) that enters her system is treated as a "foreign substance," i.e., she develops antibodies to protect her system against the "intruder." Her antibodies attach themselves to the fetal red blood cells and destroy them.

Since fetal blood and maternal blood do not mix, normally fetal red blood cells do not enter the maternal system during the prenatal period. Thus the first D-positive infant of a D-negative mother does not usually have problems, *unless* at some prior time the mother was transfused with D-positive blood (rare) or has had a spontaneous or an induced abortion of a D-positive fetus without the use of passive-antibody (RhoGAM), as described below.

At the time of delivery (or abortion), fetal red blood cells do enter the maternal circulation. The mother's immune system develops anti-Rh_D antibodies. Once the immune response begins, antibody production may continue for many years without additional stimulus.

When the Rh_D negative mother next becomes pregnant with an Rh_D positive fetus, those antibodies cross the placenta, coat the red blood cells of the fetus, and cause their destruction.

In the most severe form, red blood cell destruction in the fetus results first in marked anemia and subsequently in an attempt to raise red cell production and in heart failure, as the heart tries harder and harder to oxygenate the body with a limited number of red blood cells. The fetus develops edema with pleural effusion and ascites. Intrauterine hypoxia, hypoproteinemia, and lowered oncotic pressure probably are factors in causing edema, in addition to the anemia. This condition is termed *hydrops fetalis*. The fetus may die in utero or, if born alive, frequently dies in the first days after birth. Once a mother has delivered a stillborn infant whose death was caused by Rh sensitization, the chances are less than 30 per cent that she will ever be able to deliver a living child.

Fortunately, not every infant of a sensitized mother is so seriously affected. With a more moderate course, the infant may be delivered and then develop erythroblastosis fetalis postnatally, with characteristic jaundice and anemia caused by the breakdown of red blood cells. The needs and care of the infant with erythroblastosis are discussed in Chapter 18.

Caring for the Sensitized Mother

Determination of the level of anti-D antibody in the serum of an Rh_D negative mother (when the father is Rh_D positive) is basic to her continued assessment. This test, known as the antibody-titer or anti-Rh titer, is repeated every 4 weeks, even if there is no indication of antibody. As long as there is no antibody present, the mother's prenatal care and delivery will be the same as that of any woman with no special problems.

If antibodies are detected but titers remain below or at low levels throughout pregnancy (the critical levels will vary according to the laboratory technique used), again pregnancy care is essentially "normal." The mother will, however, need information and reassurance about the meaning of antibody testing. She needs to understand why testing is important and why she should return for testing at prescribed intervals, without being unduly alarmed.

If titers rise above a level determined as critical in a particular laboratory (commonly 1:32 or 1:64), amniocentesis is performed to determine the level of bilirubin in amniotic fluid by a technique called spectrophotometric analysis. The amount of bilirubin in amniotic fluid more accurately reflects fetal involvement than does mother's antibody titer. The optical density (expressed as ΔOD_{450} and read delta OD_{450}) of the amniotic fluid indicates the amount of bilirubin and thus the severity of fetal disease.

If the ΔOD_{450} is low, the fetus will probably be only mildly affected. If the ΔOD_{450} is moderate at the time of the first amniocentesis, amniotic fluid analysis will be repeated every 2 to 3 weeks thereafter. It may subsequently:

1. Fall to a low zone, with a mildly affected infant delivered at or near term.

2. Fall slowly, but remain in a middle zone, with a moderately affected infant delivered at approximately 37 weeks.

3. Increase to a high level.

When the ΔOD_{450} is at a level deemed critical on initial or subsequent examination, one of two courses is chosen. If the parameters of gestational age indicate that the baby could survive, he is delivered, with preparations made for a very sick infant. When it is at all possible, the mother should be transferred to a major medical center for delivery, rather than attempting to transfer a very sick newborn after delivery.

If the baby is too immature for extrauterine survival, he may receive an intrauterine transfusion. Intrauterine transfusion does not always save the baby's life. If the fetus already has hydrops fetalis, the infused blood is not absorbed. Fetal organs such as the liver or bladder may be perforated. However, since it is used only for a fetus already severely sick and in danger of death, any success is welcomed.

Radiopaque material is injected into the amniotic fluid approximately five hours prior to the transfusion. Because the fetus is continually swallowing amniotic fluid, the radiopaque material will concentrate sufficiently in the fetal bowel to outline the bowel. A needle is then inserted into the fetal peritoneal cavity, further dye is injected, and the position of the needle is verified by X-ray. From 80 to 150 ml. of fresh O-negative packed red blood cells that have been cross-matched with the mother's serum is injected, the amount being approximately 15 per cent of the estimated fetal weight.

It is believed that the injected red blood cells enter the fetal circulation by way of the lymphatics below the diaphragm. Fetal hemoglobin levels rise. The procedure can be repeated every 1 to 2 weeks, if necessary, until the fetus has reached a gestational age at which extrauterine existence is possible.

Nursing Support for the Sensitized Mother

The sensitized Rh_D negative mother has realistic fears that her unborn or newborn infant may die or may be neurologically damaged (see Chapter 8). She may have lost one or more infants in previous pregnancies.

She may feel guilty and/or angry about her baby's condition. For example, if she became sensitized as a result of an induced abortion after which she was not given RhoGAM, she may feel that sensitization was her fault for having had the abortion or may be angry at the caretakers who failed to give her RhoGAM.

Like the mother of any sick fetus or newborn, she needs the opportunity to talk out her feelings and feel our concern. She needs to be informed about what is happening to the fetus, with hope for survival offered as long as it is appropriate.

The Prevention of Sensitization

Techniques for treating the affected fetus and newborn of sensitized mothers have certainly improved during the past decade. Far more significant in terms of eliminating the problem is the successful prevention of antibody formation.

The product RhoGAM, already mentioned, is gamma globulin containing anti-D antibody. Remember that when the fetal Rh_D-positive cells enter the mother's circulation, she produces antibodies to destroy the positive cells. If she is given antibodies to destroy these cells, her system will not produce antibodies. The antibodies given in this way are not permanent; the positive red blood cells are destroyed and the antibodies, as in all passive immunization, are short-lived. With certain exceptions described below, sensitization can be prevented and each pregnancy for an RH_D negative mother can be as safe as a first pregnancy.

Treatment with RhoGAM is required within 72 hours of delivery. We do not know the exact time at which the mother's body begins to produce anti-D antibodies; it is apparently longer than 72 hours. Some researchers believe that if the mother has not been given RhoGAM in the first days following delivery, it may be given up to 3 to 4 weeks postpartum. Mothers should be tested for the presence of antibodies 4 to 6 months postpartum (or postabortion). Once a mother has been sensitized, RhoGAM is of no value. RhoGAM can only prevent sensitization; it cannot eliminate actively acquired anti-D antibodies.

Two types of problems prevent the elimination of Rh sensitization as a cause of infant mortality and morbidity. The first is physiologic; the second a problem of utilization of RhoGAM.

Physiologic Problems. About 10 per cent of women given RhoGAM are sensitized nevertheless. This may be caused by bleeding from the mother to the fetus prior to delivery, during a threatened abortion, for example, or during amniocentesis in which the placenta is entered by mistake. A massive hemorrhage at the time of delivery, so large that the amount of RhoGAM given is inadequate to destroy the large numbers of cells that have entered the circulation, may also result in sensitization.

The Rh_D negative daughter of an Rh_D positive mother may become sensitized at the time of her own birth if some maternal cells enter her bloodstream; there may be no indication that she has been sensitized until Rh titers are performed, perhaps 20 years later when she herself becomes pregnant.

Some women may become sensitized without even knowing they have been pregnant. For example, a woman may have a spontaneous abortion during the early weeks of pregnancy and believe she has had a delayed, heavy menstrual period.

Problems in Utilization of RhoGAM. It is estimated that 15 to 20 per cent of the women who should receive RhoGAM each year do not. The rate of utilization is poorer in women following abortion than in women following delivery. Nurses play a vital role in making certain that every woman who should get RhoGAM is treated.

ABO INCOMPATIBILITY

If the husband is blood type A or B and the wife is type O, ABO incompatibility is possible. Severe anemia, hydrops, and stillbirth are rare in ABO incompatibility. No special antenatal care is necessary. Care of the baby is discussed in Chapter 18.

If both Rh$_D$ and ABO incompatibility exists in a mother-infant pair, the ABO incompatibility may act as a protection for Rh sensitization. The mechanism may be the destruction of the fetal red cells in the mother before they can stimulate Rh antibody formation.

OTHER PRE-EXISTING CONDITIONS

In addition to the pre-existing conditions described above, any mother with a health problem, physical or emotional, needs special attention. Medications for thyroid disease, tuberculosis, carcinoma, and a variety of other conditions may affect the course of pregnancy more than the illness per se. Then the effect of the disease must be considered, as well as the effect of the medication.

COMPLICATIONS OF PREGNANCY THAT CONTRIBUTE TO RISK

HYPERTENSIVE STATES OF PREGNANCY

One of the terms most commonly used by nurses, physicians, and others who care for childbearing families is *toxemia*. The use of this term is discouraged today because it has long been used, and misused, to mean so many different things to different people. Old habits are hard to change, however, and student nurses may hear the word frequently.

More appropriate is the phrase *hypertensive states of pregnancy;* this term is recommended by the American College of Obstetricians and Gynecologists to describe a group of conditions that are a significant cause of maternal and perinatal death. The principal symptoms of these conditions are edema, proteinuria, and hypertension.

Table 10–6 summarizes basic information about the hypertensive states of pregnancy.

PRE-ECLAMPSIA AND ECLAMPSIA

Approximately 90 per cent of hypertension in pregnancy is related to pre-eclampsia.

Etiology

The etiology of pre-eclampsia and eclampsia is unknown, although many theories exist. Pre-eclampsia:

1. Requires the presence of trophoblastic tissue, but not necessarily of a fetus (preeclampsia often occurs when there is a hydatidiform mole).

2. Occurs after the twentieth week of pregnancy, characteristically in the third trimester.

3. Is most common in young nulliparas.

4. Most frequently occurs in the southern states.

5. More frequently occurs in multiple gestation pregnancies.

6. Disappears after delivery or fetal death.

7. Seldom recurs in subsequent pregnancies.

Theories of the cause of preeclampsia include speculations that the condition may be related to such factors as inadequate nutrition, metabolic disease, or an immunologic process. None of these theories adequately explains the characteristics of the condition. For example, if poor diet is the basis, why is pre-eclampsia primarily a disease of a first pregnancy?

Table 10–6 CLASSIFICATION OF HYPERTENSIVE STATES OF PREGNANCY

Condition	Definition	Time of Occurrence	Incidence	Comments
Pre-eclampsia	Hypertension with protein-uria, edema, or both	After the 20th week	6 to 7% of pregnant women in U.S., primarily in primigravidas	May occur earlier than 20 weeks in presence of trophoblastic disease
Eclampsia	Occurrence of one or more convulsions, not attributable to other cerebral conditions (e.g., epilepsy) in woman with pre-eclampsia	After 20 weeks	1:2000	
Chronic hypertensive vascular disease	Persistent hypertension from whatever cause	Before pregnancy; before the 20th week of gestation; beyond the 42nd postpartum day		Incidence is 3 times higher among black gravidas than white gravidas
Superimposed pre-eclampsia or eclampsia	Proteinuria and/or edema; a rise in blood pressure of 30 mm. Hg systolic or 15 mm. Hg diastolic in a woman with chronic hypertensive vascular disease	After 20 weeks		

Some societies are apparently free of pre-eclampsia. Soichet[25] reports little or no evidence of toxemia in certain African societies, Eskimo tribes in Greenland, and some tribes in the South Pacific. He suggests that in these societies:

1. Fertility is cherished by everyone in the society.

2. No stigma is attached to children born out of wedlock.

3. Babies of both sexes are welcomed.

4. Pregnant women are treated with tenderness and love.

We believe that the role of psychosocial factors is worthy of further exploration. In the interrelationship of psychosocial and physiologic antece-

dents, clues to cause and thus to prevention may be discovered.

Pathophysiology

An understanding of the pathophysiology of pre-eclampsia and eclampsia is essential to understanding both the medical plan of care and the nursing intervention.

Blood vessel spasm is postulated as the underlying mechanism. When vessels are in spasm, less blood perfuses all body tissues. This basic problem leads to a number of other physiologic changes that account for the classic symptoms of edema, hypertension, and proteinuria.

1. The delivery of oxygen and glucose is decreased to all tissues.

2. Fluid shifts from the vascular compartment (i.e., from within the blood vessels) to the intracellular space. Protein and electrolytes also shift into the intracellular space. Particularly significant is the leakage of sodium.

3. Because of the fluid shift, the blood becomes "thicker," with a tendency to sludge and coagulate. Intravascular coagulation leads to diminished blood flow to all organs, including, of course, the uterus, placenta, and fetus. In addition, peripheral resistance is increased when blood is thicker; the heart must work harder and the blood pressure becomes high. The increased workload of the heart in the presence of a decreased blood supply leads to heart failure.

4. Decreased blood supply to the kidneys leads to a loss of integrity in the glomeruli and a consequent spillage of protein into the urine.

5. In the brain, loss of fluid from the blood vessels leads to cerebral edema.

Table 10–7 summarizes the relationship between the pathophysiology and the three major symptoms of pre-eclampsia and eclampsia.

Major Signs: Assessment and Intervention

The principal signs of pre-eclampsia, already noted, are edema, proteinuria, and hypertension.

Edema. In Chapter 9 the normal dependent edema of pregnancy was described. This normal edema usually disappears with elevation of the feet or after a night in bed. Edema that does not disappear after 12 hours of rest in bed; or pitting edema of the face, hands, sacral area, abdominal wall; or a weekly gain of more than 5 pounds suggests a need for careful evaluation of a woman's condition. However, it is possible to have even extensive edema without pre-eclampsia, just as it is possible to have pre-eclampsia without edema. About 10 per cent of women who have eclampsia (i.e., convulsions) do not have pitting edema.

The classic treatment of edema, i.e., diuretics, is *not* currently felt to be of

Table 10–7   RELATIONSHIP BETWEEN SYMPTOMS AND PATHOPHYSIOLOGY
OF PRE-ECLAMPSIA AND ECLAMPSIA

Symptom	Pathophysiologic Basis	Criteria for Assessment*
Edema	Fluid moves from intravascular to intracellular space.	Pitting edema after 12 hours rest in bed; weight gain of 5 pounds or more in 1 week.
Hypertension	Increased peripheral vascular resistance, increased blood viscosity leads to increased cardiac load.	Elevation of blood pressure of 30 mm. Hg systolic and 15 mm. Hg diastolic or levels above 140/90. Levels of 125/85 at 32 weeks or at term. Blood pressure must be abnormal on at least two occasions 6 hours apart.
Proteinuria	Loss of integrity in the glomeruli from decreased blood supply allows spillage of protein.	Urine protein 1+ or greater (Ketostix) on two occasions 6 hours apart; protein in excess of 300 mg. in 24 hour urine specimen.

*See also text.

value in pre-eclampsia or eclampsia, and may even be harmful.

Because excess body fluids and electrolytes are in the tissues rather than within the blood vessels (intravascular compartment), giving diuretics without expanding blood volume and supplying electrolytes will further complicate electrolyte imbalance, and lead to possible neonatal hyponatremia and other complications. Diuretics may also mask the appearance of early warning signs of pre-eclampsia by preventing fluid retention and edema, thus postponing detection until the condition is further advanced.

Salt, like fluid, is in the tissues, not the vascular tree. Low serum sodium levels lead to increased sodium reabsorption in the kidney tubules. Several studies report that increasing salt intake may relieve manifestations of pre-eclampsia. Nevertheless, restriction of salt is still practiced for patients with pre-eclampsia.

Albumin may be given to increase oncotic pressure and thus bring fluid back into the intravascular system from the tissues. Women receiving albumin must be observed very closely. If too much albumin is given or if the solution is given too quickly, the oncotic pressure may become too high, and pulmonary edema may result. Blood pressure and urine specific gravity are checked frequently. If the woman has had central nervous system changes, such as mental confusion and hyperactive reflexes caused by cerebral edema, these symptoms will improve. As fluid is drawn back into the bloodstream and perfuses the kidneys, urinary output should improve. Careful intake-output records are important.

In addition to those measures already mentioned, the progress of edema is also checked by daily recording of weight and by determinations of hematocrit, which will indicate decreased intravascular fluid.

Proteinuria. Small quantities of protein (less than 1+ by Ketostix) are found in the urine of many pregnant women. Strenuous exercise or work, exposure to cold, and other factors tend to increase proteinuria. Two specimens at 6 hour intervals that are 1+ or greater or more than 300 mg. of protein in a 24 hour specimen is considered beyond the range of normal (Table 10–7).

Urine that is to be tested for protein must be either a clean, midstream voided specimen or obtained by catheterization, because contamination with either blood or vaginal discharge will give falsely high protein determinations.

Hypertension. Several criteria are helpful in identifying hypertension during pregnancy:

---

1. An elevation of 30 mm. Hg or more systolic or 15 mm. Hg diastolic blood pressure.
2. A blood pressure level above 140 mm. Hg systolic or 90 mm. Hg diastolic.
3. A blood pressure level above 125 mm. Hg systolic or 75 mm. Hg diastolic prior to 32 weeks, or at term.
4. A mean arterial pressure greater than 90 (Chapter 8).
5. A positive response to the rollover test.

A positive roll-over test, performed between 28 and 32 weeks of pregnancy, is 90 per cent accurate in predicting pre-eclampsia. With the woman resting on her side, blood pressure is recorded until it is stable. The woman then lies on her back; blood pressure is again recorded until stable. A rise of more than 20 mm. Hg indicates a positive test.

Progression of Pre-eclampsia

Pre-eclampsia may progress from mild to severe symptoms over a period of weeks or within a period of hours. Signs of a more severe pre-eclampsia include:

---

1. Increasing edema, proteinuria, and hypertension.
2. Oliguria, anuria, and hemoconcentration.
3. Headache.
4. Blurring of vision.
5. Clouding of consciousness.
6. Epigastric pain.
7. Nausea and vomiting.
8. Hyperactive reflexes.
9. Jaundice.
10. Evidence of cardiac impairment.

Once seizures have occurred, the condition is eclampsia. With optimum care, many instances of eclampsia are probably preventable by early recognition of symptoms of pre-eclampsia, when pre-eclampsia is mild and more easily treatable.

Caring for the Mother with Pre-eclampsia

When pre-eclampsia is recognized in a woman, she is usually hospitalized. Bed rest is the principal treatment for mild pre-eclampsia. Since a reversal of the pathophysiology is the goal, the woman rests on her side to increase both renal and uterine blood flow. Diuresis should follow improved perfusion of the kidneys, with a subsequent drop in blood pressure.

Careful assessment of blood pressure, urinary output, weight, and hematocrit is essential. Deep tendon reflexes and ocular fundi are evaluated.

Sedation may be prescribed to ensure quiet rest. Whether medication for sedation is prescribed or not, nursing care must be carefully planned so that vitally important assessment does not conflict with the need for rest. Examinations, for example, should be performed shortly before the time that medication is given for sedation, not afterward. Not only must nurses plan their own care to provide maximum periods of rest, but they must coordinate the actions of physicians, laboratory technicians seeking blood specimens, and others who might enter the woman's room.

As diuresis occurs and symptoms return to more normal levels, the woman is allowed out of bed. If the fetus is assessed to be mature by the parameters described below, the mother will be delivered (vaginally unless there are obstetric indications for cesarean section). If the fetus is not sufficiently mature, the mother may be discharged but must continue to be followed closely. Labor may be induced when the fetus has matured, on the premise that pre-eclampsia has not been "cured."

If more severe symptoms of pre-eclampsia appear, magnesium sulfate is given intramuscularly or, more frequently, intravenously. Magnesium sulfate decreases neuromuscular irritability by depressing action at the myoneural junction (i.e., the junction of muscle and nerve). Magnesium sulfate does *not* lower blood pressure. Excess magnesium sulfate will depress respirations and can lead to cardiac arrest.

While magnesium sulfate is slowly administered, respirations are carefully observed, and the knee jerk reflex is tested. Once the knee jerk reflex is hypoactive, no further magnesium sulfate is given. *Calcium gluconate* is the metabolic antagonist for magnesium sulfate; the two drugs bind to the same receptor sites. Therefore, calcium gluconate is kept instantly available whenever magnesium sulfate is given, in the event of overdosage.

Traditionally, once women with severe pre-eclampsia were stabilized for a period of 24 hours, the fetus was delivered by cesarean section; this practice is still common.

However, in institutions with staff and facilities for perinatal intensive care, more vigorous treatment of the mother, along with the assessment of fetal maturity and well-being, is possible if the baby is less than 34 to 35 weeks gestational age.

The mother may be treated with hydralazine hydrochloride (Apresoline), which relaxes the smooth muscle of the blood vessels. The vascular bed then dilates, and, as a result, blood pressure falls, and there is better perfusion of the body's organs, including the kidneys. Hypotension is the danger of too much hydralazine. The antidote for hydralazine hypotension is *metaraminol bitartrate*.

Constant attention is paid to the woman herself and to:

1. Central venous pressure.
2. Arterial blood pressure.
3. Temperature, pulse, and respiration.
4. Urinary output and fluid intake.
5. Weight (each day).
6. Urine creatinine and estriol.
7. Urine protein (every 1 or 2 hours).
8. The presence of jaundice or cyanosis.

Should one or more convulsions occur, the condition is eclampsia. The treatment of a woman with eclampsia requires constant and excellent nursing care closely correlated with medical management. The goals are:

1. No further convulsions.
2. Insurance of adequate ventilation.
3. Control of blood pressure.
4. Prevention of cardiac failure.
5. Continuing assessment of the fetus.

Once the woman is stable for 6 to 12 hours, pregnancy is terminated by cesarean section. It is felt that not only is the mother at risk of further disease but that the severity of the mother's condition probably indicates that the well-being of the fetus is compromised by placental insufficiency.

Convulsions: Prevention and Care. A woman with eclampsia is cared for in a dark, quiet room. She lies on her side to prevent possible aspiration of vomitus and other secretions. Standard precautions for patients with convulsions are essential: a padded tongue blade and padded side rails are required.

The foot of the bed is elevated to permit drainage of mucus. Suction equipment must be immediately available, as an additional precaution against aspiration.

Should a convulsion occur, the tongue blade is placed between her teeth. It is often necessary to give oxygen for cyanosis.

Drugs used for the control of seizures include thiopental sodium (Pentothal Sodium), amobarbital sodium (Amytal Sodium), and diazepam (Valium).

PRENATAL BLEEDING

One of the most feared symptoms during pregnancy is bleeding. Bleeding has meant "something is wrong" to most of us throughout our lives. Vaginal bleeding during pregnancy, other than the slightest spotting, is a serious or potentially serious complication that deserves immediate attention.

From a physiologic standpoint, hemorrhage may be sufficiently serious to be life-threatening to the mother, requiring rapid intervention. From an emotional standpoint, bleeding often indicates the potential or actual loss of the fetus and demands skilled care to deal with the associated anxiety and grief.

In this segment we will examine some major causes of bleeding during pregnancy and the appropriate interventions to meet physiologic and psychosocial needs.

Ectopic Pregnancy

First trimester bleeding is usually related to *ectopic* pregnancy or to the potential or actual loss of the fetus by spontaneous abortion. Ectopic or extrauterine pregnancy refers to gestation outside of the uterine cavity, most commonly in the uterine tube and in the distal portion of the tube.

Initially, the ovum burrows into the muscular wall of the tube. As the ovum grows, the wall at the placental site becomes weakened and eventually bursts from overdistention. This occurs in the second or third month after conception if the ovum is in the isthmus of the tube, and somewhat later if the ovum is in the ampulla or in the interstitial portion of the tube, because those areas are more easily distended.

Signs of Ectopic Pregnancy. The woman may complain of cramping pains on *one side* of her lower abdomen. Pregnancy may have been diagnosed, or she may only have noticed menstrual irregularity. If the ectopic pregnancy ruptures, more definite symptoms are sudden, exruciating pelvic pain, dizziness, and/or shock. The woman often appears pale and slightly cyanotic; her pulse is rapid and thready. Bleeding occurs at the placental site; when blood reaches the level of the diaphragm, shoulder pain may occur.

Rupture may be more gradual, with symptoms including abdominal pain and tenderness, nausea, vomiting, and diarrhea.

Intervention. Surgical intervention is the treatment for an ectopic pregnancy. Ideally, the condition is recognized before rupture, and the affected tube is removed. If the woman has only one functioning tube, occasionally the surgeon may try to remove the ovum and leave the tube, but this is uncommon because the risk of a subsequent ectopic pregnancy is high.

If the tube has ruptured, a salpingectomy is performed immediately. When the abdomen is opened, the intestines may be found floating in blood. Blood loss is replaced during and following surgery.

Spontaneous Abortion

The term *abortion* refers to the process by which a nonviable fetus is expelled from the uterus. By convention, a fetus of less than 20 weeks' gestation or less than 500 grams in weight is considered an *abortus*.

Probably one in every five to seven conceptions ends in abortion. In many instances the abortion occurs in the first weeks at a time when the mother may not even know she is pregnant. The bleeding may appear to be a somewhat delayed and perhaps heavier than normal menstrual period.

A variety of terms are used by laymen and professionals to describe events related to abortion.

Miscarriage is the word most commonly used by laymen to describe a spontaneous abortion. The word abortion, for many, implies an event that is sinful or criminal. A mother or couple may be terribly upset to hear their problem referred to as an abortion. If we ask a mother if she has ever had an abortion, she will assure us that she has not.

Spontaneous abortion occurs with no apparent interference.

Threatened abortion refers to

transcervical bleeding. Uterine contractions may or may not be present, but the cervix is not dilated, and the conceptus has not been expelled.

In *inevitable abortion*, bleeding, uterine contractions, and progressive cervical dilatation are present.

Abortion is *incomplete* when only part of the products of the conception are expelled. For example, the fetus may be expelled, but portions of the fetal membrane may remain.

In *complete abortion*, all of the uterine contents are expelled.

Missed abortion refers to the situation in which the fetus dies but is retained in the uterus for 8 weeks or longer following death.

When a woman has three or more consecutive spontaneous abortions, she is said to have *habitual abortions.*

Deliberate interruption of pregnancy is termed *induced abortion*.

Why Spontaneous Abortion? A major concern of mothers who have had a spontaneous abortion is "Why did this happen to me?" In most spontaneous abortions the cause is unknown. Trauma is rarely a cause. Abnormalities of the fetus and of the umbilical cord, fetal chromosomal abnormalities, inadequate levels of progesterone to support implantation and development, acute maternal infection, diseases of the decidua, and an incompetent cervix (see below) are some factors that have been shown to cause abortion.

An incompetent cervix begins to dilate for no apparent reason, often during the second trimester. Once an incompetent cervix has been diagnosed as the cause of abortion, a cerclage surgical procedure is performed, either between pregnancies or when the cervix begins to dilate.

Intervention. The traditional advice to a woman in whom abortion is suspected is to go to bed and to avoid coitus. Although these prohibitions may be harmless, there is no evidence that they are effective. Nor is there good evidence that bleeding or abortion is more likely at the time that menstruation would normally occur, which is another popular belief.

If bleeding continues in spite of bed rest, the woman may be allowed to be out of bed on the premise that the gestation may best be terminated. If and when the abortion occurs, it is important that the uterus be completely emptied; remaining fragments of fetal or placental tissue can cause infection and/or continued bleeding. The method used varies with such factors as the length of gestation.

Aftercare. Following spontaneous abortion, observation for bleeding and signs of sepsis is important. Equally critical is emotional support, described at the conclusion of this section on bleeding problems.

Hydatidiform Mole

In one of 2000 pregnancies, hydatidiform mole will be the cause of bleeding. Hydatidiform mole is a developmental anomaly of the placenta. Some or all of the chorionic villi degenerate into transparent vesicles (Fig. 10-1) that may fill the uterus. This anomaly is classified as a trophoblastic disease.

Signs that a possible mole may be present include:

---

1. Bloody discharge beginning at the tenth to twelfth week of pregnancy.
2. Enlargement of the uterus out of proportion to the estimated gestational age of the fetus.
3. Absence of fetal heart tone.
4. A high level of serum human chorionic gonadotropin (HCG) 100

days or more after the last menstrual period.

5. An ultrasound evaluation unique and characteristic of a mole (Fig. 10–2).

6. The edema, proteinuria, and hypertension of pre-eclampsia.

The bleeding of a molar pregnancy may be bright red, but is frequently brownish and often not profuse. It may be continuous or intermittent.

Human chorionic gonadotropin is produced in the second week of pregnancy (Chapter 6). In normal pregnancy, HCG declines after 100 days. However, when trophoblastic tissue proliferates, levels of HCG continue to be high or to rise further.

The treatment for hydatidiform mole is evacuation of the uterus. If the woman is already undergoing spon-

taneous abortion, it will be completed. Otherwise a procedure appropriate to the size of the uterus, such as dilatation and curettage, suction curettage, or intra-amniotic saline (Chapter 23), is used.

Evacuation does not end the mother's need for care, however. Trophoblastic tissue may remain and may metastasize to other areas of the body. The continued presence of trophoblastic tissue is indicated by the presence of HCG in the urine. Metastases are most frequent to the lung and may be apparent on chest X-ray; the vagina, liver, kidneys, and brain are other possible sites. Treatment of metastasis is most commonly by chemotherapy today.

The finding of a negative HCG level is recommended strongly for 1 year before another pregnancy is planned.

Figure 10–1 Drawing of a uterus containing a hydatidiform mole. (From Page, Villee, and Villee: *Human Reproduction: The Core Content of Obstetrics, Gynecology and Perinatal Medicine.* 2nd Edition. Philadelphia, W. B. Saunders Co., 1976.)

Figure 10–2   Ultrasonograms reveal the snowflake pattern typical of hydatidiform mole (top) in a 16 week size uterus, showing trophoblastic hyperplasia, and a normal 14 week pregnant uterus (bottom), showing fetal bone and tissue. (From Perdue: *American J. of Nursing*, 77:836, 1977.)

Placenta Previa

Placenta previa is the development of the placenta in part of, or entirely in, the lower uterine segment. A placenta previa occurs in approximately 8 of 1000 pregnancies; about 75 per cent occur in multiparas, although the age of the mother, rather than parity, appears to be more significant.

Figure 10–3 illustrates the difference between (A) low implantation of the placenta, in which the edge of the placenta can be palpated through the cervix, but the placenta itself barely extends to the margin of the internal os;

(B) partial placenta previa, in which the placenta partially covers the internal os; and (C) total placenta previa, in which the placenta entirely covers the internal os.

Why does placenta previa occur? It is probable that the ovum is implanted low in the uterus. Because the nutritional support of the lower uterine segment is not as great as that of the body of the uterus, the placenta will spread further in its search for nourishment. A placenta previa is usually both larger and thinner than the usual placenta.

Symptoms of Placenta Previa. The first and only symptom of a pla-

Low implantation
of placenta

A

C

Total and central
placenta previa

Total placenta
previa

B

D

Partial placenta previa
with placental separation
and bleeding following
beginning cervical
effacement

Figure 10–3 Some variations of placenta previa.

centa previa may occur when the woman awakens one morning and finds herself lying in a pool of blood. Or she may first notice blood in the toilet bowl. The bleeding is painless. Although bleeding caused by placenta previa is most common in the third trimester, particularly in the eighth month, bleeding may begin before this time. The earlier bleeding occurs, the more likely it is that the placenta previa is total. Partial placenta previa may not cause bleeding until the cervix dilates during labor.

Dangers of Placenta Previa.   Placenta previa presents major dangers both to the mother before and after delivery and to the fetus. For the mother, the loss of large amounts of blood can lead to hemorrhagic shock, fibrinogenopenia (see below), thrombocytopenia, and marked anemia.

Other complications that may be related to placenta previa are:

1. Premature rupture of the membranes.

2. Premature labor.

3. Malposition and/or malpresentation of the fetus.

4. Air embolism (because the uterine sinuses are exposed to external air).

5. Rupture of the uterus (because the uterine musculature is weakened by placental ingrowth).

6. Postpartum hemorrhage (because the thin, weakened uterine wall does not contract firmly and quickly to prevent hemorrhage from the large venous sinuses at the placental site).

7. Postpartum infection (because pieces of placenta may adhere to the uterine wall and become infected as a result of the close proximity of the placental site to the cervix and vagina).

The fetus is also at risk. Anoxia resulting from the premature separation of the placenta is the most common cause of fetal death. There may also be fetal blood loss, largely preventable if proper care is given (see below). Because a bleeding placenta previa may force early delivery, prematurity is an additional problem.

The Recognition and Immediate Care of a Mother with Suspected Placenta Previa. As noted in Chapter 9, mothers should be told early during their pregnancy to call the physician or nurse if bleeding occurs. The mother should be hospitalized immediately. She should not be examined in a clinic or office first. Rectal or vaginal examination can lead to uncontrollable hemorrhage. An ambulance is preferred for transportation to the hospital.

When the mother arrives at hospital, blood is immediately typed, and a minimum of 1000 cc. of blood is matched. If the mother is anemic, she is immediately transfused. Even though the mother may not be bleeding profusely at the time she is admitted, she should be treated as if she might begin to hemorrhage.

A rapid physical assessment is necessary, both to establish the woman's status at admission and to evaluate any future changes. This assessment includes:

---

1. Vital signs, with particular attention to the character as well as the rate of the pulse. A central venous pressure line may be inserted for continuous assessment.
2. The condition of the abdomen. Is pain present? Is the abdomen tender?
3. The condition of the uterus: size, contour, irritability, relaxation, fetal presentation.
4. Engagement of the presenting part.
5. Presence of a placental souffle just above the symphysis pubis.
6. Urinary output, a measure of both fluid and kidney perfusion.

The placenta is localized by an ultrasound technique. Placental localization is necessary before the course of action can be determined.

No vaginal examination is done until:

1. Blood for transfusion is available.
2. The delivery room is totally prepared for both abdominal and pelvic delivery (called a "double set-up"). Not only must all equipment and personnel be available, including a physician or nurse competent to manage anesthesia, but equipment must be ready for use (i.e., trays and tables "opened" so that their contents are instantly available).

At this point a speculum may be inserted into the vagina; sometimes a reason for bleeding other than placenta previa (a cervical polyp or a laceration, for example) is detected.

Intervention Following the Definite Diagnosis of Placenta Previa. Medical intervention will vary with the severity of the bleeding. If bleeding is profuse and the mother has signs of shock (decreasing blood pressure and increasing pulse rate), emergency measures are undertaken. Blood must be replaced, and blood pressure, cardiac output, and tissue perfusion must be maintained. Oxygen is administered. Simultaneously, cesarean section is performed. Obviously, these mothers must be carefully observed following delivery for signs of shock, hemorrhage, and infection for reasons already noted.

Fortunately, the majority of mothers with placenta previa do not arrive with such life-threatening symptoms. For these other mothers, *expectant management* has improved fetal survival, mainly by allowing the fetus to become more mature. Expectant management involves putting the mother to bed, close observation for signs of bleeding, and both physiologic (e.g., blood replacement) and emotional support.

Should the mother begin to hemorrhage at any time, surgical intervention will be necessary.

The Newborn Infant of a Mother with Placenta Previa. Anemia is possible in the infant of a mother who has had placenta previa. Hemoglobin and hematocrit levels should be checked during the first days and weeks of life.

Abruptio Placentae

Abruptio placentae is defined as premature separation of a normally implanted placenta. Studies indicate that major abruption occurs in from 1 in 85 deliveries to 1 in 139 deliveries.

What Causes Abruptio Placentae? The mechanism of abruptio placentae is apparently degeneration of the spiral arterioles that nourish the endometrium and supply blood to the placenta (Chapter 3). This degeneration leads to necrosis of the decidua beneath the placenta; hemorrhage follows, and the placenta becomes detached.

The area of detachment may be a small one at first; the resulting hemorrhage may then further separate the placenta from the decidua.

The more basic question of why changes occur in the spiral arterioles has not been answered definitely. Similar changes have been experimentally produced by elevating venous pressure; this would explain why mothers with pre-eclampsia and eclampsia have a higher rate of abruption.

Abruption may occur during labor because of a sudden loss of a large amount of amniotic fluid, a shearing effect that may follow the birth of a first twin, or traction on the placenta.

Types of Abruptio Placentae. Table 10–8 summarizes types of abruptio placentae. Note that in the first three instances, vaginal bleeding is unlikely, at least initially (Fig. 10–4). The flow of blood may be blocked by the fetal head or by a clot. In most patients, external hemorrhage eventually follows internal bleeding. (Fig. 10–5).

Assessing the Symptoms of Abruptio Placentae. Abruption of the placenta may be so mild that there are no recognizable symptoms in the antepartum period; the sole evidence may be a scar on the maternal surface of the placenta, indicating a separation that may have occurred weeks or months before. The woman may or may not have reported symptoms such as uterine tenderness or pain and vaginal bleeding at the time. The fetus apparently had not been jeopardized.

In more serious instances of abruption, sudden and severe abdominal pain is usually the first sign. The pain is often at the site of the placenta and is often described by mothers as "knifelike" at first and later as varying between "dull" and "colicky." The mother may be nauseated or may vomit.

Table 10–8   TYPES OF ABRUPTIO PLACENTAE

Type	Description	Hemorrhage
I	Placenta edges attached to uterus (most rare)	Concealed (internal)
II	All membranes around placenta severed from uterine wall	Concealed (internal)
III	Hemorrhage into the amniotic sac	Concealed (internal)
IV	Hemorrhage outward under the edge of the placenta	Apparent (external)

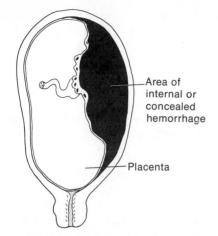

Figure 10–4 Abruptio placentae with internal or concealed hemorrhage.

Blood pressure readings may indicate shock, but if the mother has preeclampsia or eclampsia, blood pressure may remain high.

Abdominal examination will usually reveal an enlarged uterus; repeated examinations will indicate that the uterus is enlarging each hour as blood collects behind the placenta. The uterus is often boardlike; fetal parts cannot be palpated. The mother reports uterine

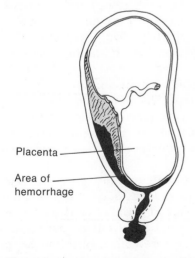

Figure 10–5 Abruptio placentae with external (revealed) hemorrhage.

tenderness when palpation is attempted.

In severe abruption, fetal movement may no longer be felt by the mother, nor can fetal heart tones be heard by the examiner.

Laboratory examination reveals increasing anemia.

Intervention. Unlike placenta previa, in which expectant management is often appropriate, moderate to severe abruptions of the placenta require rapid intervention. Time is important. Delay may result in severe hemorrhage with anemia and fibrinogenopenia, leading to shock and fetal and maternal death.

The mother who is admitted with potential abruptio placentae is often in pain and always anxious. She may not understand exactly what has happened, but she feels that it is "something terrible." In our haste to perform the many tasks that her physiologic condition requires, we must not forget her or her husband's emotional concerns.

Blood is drawn for examination (hemoglobin, hematocrit, clotting time, prothrombin time, type and cross match) and from four to six units of blood are prepared for transfusion.

A central venous pressure line is inserted to monitor blood pressure. A careful record of intake and output is essential; oliguria indicates poor kidney perfusion and depleted intravascular fluid.

Subsequent intervention varies with the condition of both mother and fetus.

If the fetus is alive but in apparent distress, if the bleeding appears to be increasing, if the mother has tachycardia and hypotension, and/or if fibrinogen levels are falling (see below), immediate cesarean section is almost always performed.

However, if the condition of the

mother and fetus appears good, if no coagulation problem is present, and if coagulation can be monitored closely, labor may be induced. No more than 6 to 8 hours should be allowed for the progress of labor, during which both mother and baby are intensively monitored. Any deterioration in the condition of either mother or fetus would indicate immediate cesarean intervention.

If the fetus is known to be dead, the decision is made on the basis of the mother's condition, often allowing labor if the mother's physiologic status appears stable, or intervening with cesarean section if the mother's life is in jeopardy.

FIBRINOGENOPENIA. As fibrin forms in the retroplacental clot following an abruption of the placenta, the level of fibrinogen in the blood decreases and thus interferes with normal clotting mechanisms. Disseminated intravascular coagulation (DIC) may result, with widespread bleeding. Any woman in whom abruptio placentae is suspected should have levels of fibrinogen checked.

Rapid information is obtained from observing carefully drawn blood placed in a clean test tube. The blood should clot quickly; the clot should be firm and retract well. In many hospitals plasma fibrinogen levels are obtained. If the level is below 100 mg. per 100 ml., clotting mechanisms are abnormal. (Normal levels during pregnancy exceed 300 mg. per 100 ml.).

Intervention includes: (1) prompt treatment of the cause, (2) replacement of lost blood, (3) use of heparin to block the consumption of fibrinogen, and/or (4) replacement of lost fibrinogen with 4 grams or more of fibrinogen.

It is obviously essential that fibrinogen be available in the delivery room.

Other obstetric conditions that may cause fibrinogenopenia include retention of a dead fetus, as in a missed abortion; amniotic fluid embolism; bacteremia; and any instance of massive hemorrhage.

Emotional Support of the Mother with Bleeding

The physiologic support of the pregnant woman with bleeding can be, in some instances, truly a matter of life and death. In every instance, considerable attention must be paid to blood loss and replacement, monitoring of vital signs, and the other care that has been described. In the necessary haste, it is easy to forget the monumental fear and sadness that the mother and her husband are experiencing. Mary Ross Osborn, a nurse and mother, describes her own feelings, "Frantic over my extreme discomfort and terrified of the bleeding, I called the nurse again."[12]

How can we help women and their families cope with this experience?

1. The mother should not be left alone if she is having contractions and/or active bleeding. Even if the father or another family member is with her, she needs close nursing attention. If no one else is present, a nurse should stay with her. Ideally, no mother should labor alone, but if staffing needs make it impossible for every mother to have constant attention, this mother has priority. She should be made as comfortable as possible; clean bedding, back rubs, and cool cloths can convey emotional support as well as physical comfort.

A woman may cry, quietly or loudly; she may moan softly or call out. This is appropriate behavior. She may talk about her feelings, but often she will be receiving medication for pain and will not be able to communicate effectively until the next day.

2. Should the mother see her dead baby? Only she should make that decision. Neither physicians nor nurses should make it, nor should the father decide for her. The decision need not be made immediately; it can be deferred until the next day. Consider the following conversation in the paper by Kowalski and Osborn:

"Would you like to see the baby?" I asked.

"I don't know, Karren," she replied hesitantly . . . "No, I don't think I want to."

"Think about it, Mary. I'll do whatever you want. But please remember how angry you were that you did not see John" (a previous child who had died almost immediately after birth).

There was a pause. Mary looked intently at me.

"Would you like me to find her?" I asked.

Mary nodded. I squeezed her hand and went in search of the baby.[12]

Are there advantages to a mother and father in seeing their dead fetus or baby? In Chapter 22 the importance of parents' becoming "attached" to their high risk newborns, even when it is highly likely that the baby is going to die, is discussed. Attachment under these circumstances is felt to lead to a more normal resolution of grief.

Can seeing and touching a formed but nonviable fetus, a fetus of 16 to 20 weeks' gestation, for example, serve a similar function? Kowalski and Osborn commented about "feelings of peace and calm after having seen the baby."[12]

The baby was wrapped in blankets to be taken to the mother. Before the nurse showed the baby to the mother, she prepared her for what she would see. The mother should be told that the baby will feel cold; he will probably be blue. If there is an abnormality or bruising, she should know this. But normality can be stressed. "Your baby is small but seems perfectly formed . . . or has perfect hands and feet . . . or a perfect face."

Many parents fantasize a deformed fetus. Particularly in relation to abortion, they may have been told that a spontaneous abortion is nature's way of "getting rid of an imperfect fetus" or, more bluntly, "getting rid of a mistake."

The mother and nurse then talked about similarities between the baby and other members of the family as the mother touched first the baby's hands and then her trunk and her back. They spent about 20 to 25 minutes examining the baby and then another 30 to 45 minutes talking about feelings after the baby was taken away.

The value of similar nursing intervention for other mothers who deliver a nonviable or dead fetus seems worth exploring.

3. A future pregnancy may or may not be possible for an individual mother. Even if a subsequent pregnancy is highly likely (as for example, a first spontaneous abortion), it is inappropriate at this point to say, "You can always have another baby." Parents need to resolve their grief for this baby before they can contemplate another.

Should the parents ask or appear to be anxious about the possibility of a similar occurrence in a future pregnancy, their questions should be answered. For many parents, follow-up counseling may be the best time to explore this issue.

For some parents, future pregnancy obviously may be impossible. A single functioning uterine tube may have been removed because of an ectopic pregnancy. Hysterectomy may have been performed following the rupture of the uterus. Self-image and lifetime goals may have been shattered in a few hours. Not only must these parents grieve for their lost baby, but perhaps also for their hopes and dreams of a future family.

4. The resolution of grief may begin in the hospital, as we take the time to encourage and allow both the mother and father to talk about their feelings, to cry, to be angry. But further opportunities for expressing feelings must be available following discharge, and a plan for utilizing resources in each family's community should be a part of discharge planning. So acutely do some families feel this need that they travel many miles to have the opportunity to talk about their feelings.

MULTIPLE PREGNANCY

Approximately one in 90 births in the United States is a twin birth. The frequency of triplets is roughly 1 in 90^2 births and of quadruplets 1 in 90^3 births. The use of "fertility drugs" (Chapter 5) has somewhat increased the frequency of multiple births in recent years.

Twins, the most common multiple birth, are more commonly born to black women (1 of 39 births) than to white women (1 of 54 births). Multiple births are more frequent as maternal age increases.

Monozygotic and Dizygotic Twins

Monozygotic twins, often called identical twins, occur when a single fertilized ovum divides to form two embryos at an early stage of development. Monozygotic twins will thus have the same genetic make-up, the same sex, and the same blood type and will be very similar in physical appearance. About one-third of twins born are monozygotic; the ratio of monozygotic twins to all births is similar throughout the world.

Dizygotic twins, often called fraternal twins, result when two eggs are fertilized. These twins have no more in common than siblings born at different times. They may or may not be of the same sex.

The frequency of dizygotic twins varies with ethnic group and maternal age. The tendency for multiple ovulation is governed by genotype, and thus dizygotic twins tend to recur in families.

It is not always possible to tell at the time of brith if twins are monozygotic or dizygotic. If there is a single placenta, amnion, and chorion, the twins are definitely monozygotic. But monozygotic twins may have two placentas and membranes. If the twins are of different sexes, they must be dizygotic, but dizygotic twins may also be of the same sex.

Prenatal Diagnosis of Multiple Birth

Not every multiple pregnancy is diagnosed prenatally. There are some indications during the prenatal period. The uterus may be larger than expected for the gestational age and/or the rate of growth more rapid. Palpation may be difficult, but feeling two heads or an excessive number of small parts may be possible. Two fetal heart rates may be heard.

When multiple pregnancy is suspected, ultrasound techniques may reveal two or more gestational sacs as early as the tenth week.

Intrauterine Development

The intrauterine environment is not necessarily identical for twin fetuses. Placental exchange may vary, with one twin receiving less than the other. Recently we saw a twin weighing approximately 700 grams while his brother weighed over 2500 grams. In all cases of disparate size the smaller twin is particularly at risk of hypoglycemia (Chapter 18) following birth.

In monozygotic twins with a circulatory connection between the two placentas, twin-to-twin transfusion occurs about 15 per cent of the time. The donor twin will be pale at birth and may be stillborn. Twin-to-twin transfusion is suspected in identical twins with a difference in hemoglobin levels of more than 5 grams per 100 ml.

Hydramnios is ten times as frequent in twin pregnancies as in single pregnancy, but often only one sac is involved.

When the combined weight of the fetuses reaches 7 to 8 pounds (about 32 weeks' gestation in twin pregnancies and even earlier when there are three or more fetuses), fetal growth is usually slowed because the placenta cannot nourish the babies adequately.

Antenatal Problems

Classically, the problems of multiple pregnancies have been described in terms of six *P*'s (Table 10–9). We have added a seventh *P*, psychosocial concerns, because in our experience we have found these to be significant factors.

Many of the psychosocial problems of the high risk mother described earlier in this chapter are applicable. She often recognizes that twins are premature and may be ill. One mother who knew she was to deliver twins wanted to see

Table 10–9 SPECIAL PROBLEMS IN MULTIPLE PREGNANCY

Problem	Description/Basis	Intervention
Prematurity	Mean duration of pregnancy: twins: 260 days triplets: 246 days quadruplets: 238 days	Activity is restricted
Pre-eclampsia	20% of all twin pregnancies (4 times greater than singleton)	More frequent, careful assessment
Pressure symptoms	Increased uterine size Hydramnios 10 times more frequent, usually involving one sac only	Position changes to decrease pressure Small, frequent feedings rather than large meals Placement of pillows to support uterus during rest
Primary anemia (and secondary anemia)	Increased fetal demands for iron and folic acid	Increased protein, supplementary iron, vitamins, folic acid
Placenta previa	Area of placental attachment twice as great as singleton pregnancy	Careful assessment of bleeding
Postpartum hemorrhage	Uterine overdistention predisposes to atony (Chapter 13)	Blood ready Intravenous fluids during second and third stage Birth interval no longer than 15 to 20 minutes
Psychosocial concerns	High risk pregnancy Ability to care for more than one newborn	Provision of opportunity to share fears Anticipatory guidance

the intensive care nursery rather than the newborn nursery when she toured the hospital, because she expected her babies to be there (they were). She also planned to attend Lamaze classes during the second trimester, in anticipation of restricted activity and early delivery during the third trimester.

Although each pregnant woman ponders her adequacy as a future mother, the mother expecting more than one infant often has appropriately heightened concerns about how she will be able to care for more than one baby.

The opportunity to talk with another mother who has twins (some communities have formed groups of mothers with twins) may be helpful. Increased costs, beginning with a potentially longer period of hospitalization and extending ad infinitum, will be a worry for many families and will make financial counseling desirable.

FETAL ASSESSMENT IN HIGH RISK PREGNANCY

ULTRASONOGRAPHY

Ultrasonography is a technique by which sound waves, too high in frequency to be audible, are beamed into the body. Different body tissues reflect the sound waves in different ways, and thus as the sound waves "bounce off" or echo from different tissues, they can be captured and displayed on an oscilloscope and, if desired, preserved permanently in Polaroid photographs. By using real-time ultrasound techniques, continuous activity can be observed; watching real-time ultrasonography is like watching a motion picture. One can observe the fetal heart beating and even fetal thumb-sucking.

Through ultrasonography, the fetus can be observed within the uterus approximately five weeks after the last menstrual period; at 6 to 7 weeks, with certain techniques, the beating of the fetal heart can be observed. After 14 weeks, measurement of the biparietal diameter of the fetal head is possible; this measurement is a major use of ultrasonography (see below). Ultrasound examination is also used to localize the placenta prior to amniocentesis; to diagnose placenta previa; to detect multiple pregnancy, polyhydramnios, and fetal anomalies; and to determine fetal death.

Ultrasonography has the advantage of being a noninvasive procedure. No harmful effects to either the mother or the fetus have been discovered.

Unlike many procedures that require that a woman empty her bladder before examination, ultrasonography requires a full bladder, which then functions as an amplifier to transmit sounds. Beginning approximately 1½ hours before the test, the woman is asked to drink an 8 ounce glass of water every 15 minutes.

AMNIOCENTESIS

The term *amniocentesis* is derived from the Greek words *amnion* (sac), the inner lining of the fetal membranes, and *kentesis,* which means puncture. Amniocentesis may be done in the clinic or office; hospitalization is not required.

The mother voids in preparation for amniocentesis and then lies supine on the examining table. If this is a first amniocentesis during a particular pregnancy, ultrasound examination may precede amniocentesis, so that the position of the placenta will be located and the placenta will not be penetrated by the needle. The position of the fetus can be determined by palpation; the fetal heart rate is recorded.

After the abdomen is prepped with antiseptic solution and draped and the skin is infiltrated with anesthetic solution, a spinal needle is inserted transabdominally into the amniotic cavity over the fetal small parts or in the area behind the fetal neck.

Amniotic fluid that is withdrawn can be used for a variety of tests that are described in the section below.

The risks of amniocentesis are slight but possible. Maternal complications include hemorrhage (minimized if the placenta and fetus are located by ultrasonography); infection; and Rh sensitization, if fetal blood enters the maternal circulation. In several studies one amniocentesis in 100 has resulted in spontaneous abortion. Fetal infection and trauma are rare complications.

Because of these attendant risks, amniocentesis is not used as a routine "screening" procedure. When there is a specific reason for the amniocentesis, the birth of a previous child with a neural tube defect or Down's syndrome, for example, or the need to accurately determine fetal maturity, the benefits would easily appear to outweigh the risks. But when there is no reason to suspect an abnormality, even small risks would be considered unjustified.

When amniocentesis is to be done to detect a potentially anomalous fetus, a fetus with Down's syndrome, for example, it is usually expected that if the anomaly is detected, the mother will choose to have a therapeutic abortion. Should the amniocentesis be performed if the parents do not plan to have an abortion? Opinions differ. Those who say "no" argue that such exposure serves no useful purpose. Others feel that parents cannot truly make an informed decision until they know the results of amniocentesis. In addition, should they continue the pregnancy, it has been suggested that they may be better prepared emotionally for an infant with a major defect.

STUDIES TO DETERMINE POSSIBLE CONGENITAL DEFECTS

Although not every congenital defect can be detected in utero, many can be, including several that are associated with major physical and mental abnormalities.

Amniotic Fluid Studies

Alpha-fetoprotein (AFP) Studies. Alpha-fetoprotein is the major circulating protein of the early human fetus. In 1972 Brock and Sutcliffe[2] first described the association between fetal neural tube defects and highly elevated AFP levels in the amniotic fluid. A number of other investigators have since confirmed their work. Approximately 95 per cent of all instances of anencephaly and 65 per cent of all instances of "open" spina bifida can be detected in this way. It is suspected that leakage of fetal cerebrospinal fluid or transudation from fetal capillaries directly exposed to amniotic fluid is the cause.

Researchers are attempting to develop practical and reliable methods of determining AFP in maternal blood, a test that could then be used for screening all pregnant women. For reasons already discussed, amniocentesis is not desirable for mass screening. Other investigators are studying the value of AFP determinations in detecting intrauterine death and severe fetoplacental dysfunction.

The Detection of Chromosomal Abnormalities. Amniotic fluid cells grown in culture can be karyotyped (Chapter 2) to detect chromosomal abnormalities (such as Down's syndrome) approximately 3 weeks after the amniocentesis is performed. In a competent laboratory, accurate prediction rates are very high. Because the risk of Down's syndrome increases significantly with maternal age, many physicians and clinics now routinely screen mothers over 37 to 40 years old in the fourteenth to fifteenth week of pregnancy.

Timing is important in relation to the successful growth of the amniotic fluid cells in culture. Because of the 3 week time period necessary for cell growth and because the mother may choose abortion should the test show the fetus to have Down's syndrome, the test is not usually performed much later in pregnancy than the fourteenth to fifteenth week.

Chromosomal Studies to Detect Sex. Although many parents may wonder about the sex of their coming child, for those mothers known to be carriers of X-linked recessive traits, the baby's sex is especially important. Daughters will not inherit the condition (certain types of muscular dystrophy or hemophilia, for example) but sons have a 50:50 chance of inheritance (Chapter 2). Amniotic fluid studies to identify the fetal sex may be important to these parents.

The Detection of Genetic Defects. Cultured cells from amniotic fluid are used to detect the presence or absence of certain enzymes and thereby to predict such inborn errors of metabolism as galactosemia. Early detection combined with early treatment can prevent deleterious side effects.

THE ASSESSMENT OF FETAL WELL-BEING

Assessment of fetal well-being and assessment of fetal maturity must be integrated for those mothers for whom an optimum time for delivery must be selected. The mother with diabetes mellitus or pre-eclampsia is an example. If the infant remains in utero for too long a period of time, his condition often deteriorates. However, if he is delivered too soon, he may be too immature either to survive or to survive as a mentally and physically intact human being. Fortunately, there are now tools to help us assess both fetal well-being and fetal maturity.

Amniotic Fluid Studies

Bilirubin in Amniotic Fluid. Mothers with Rh-isoimmunization will have a series of amniocenteses during the second half of pregnancy to follow the level of bilirubin pigment in the amniotic fluid. In this way the severity of their disease may be assessed and the fetus identified as having: (1) very mild disease or no problem, (2) moderate disease that may necessitate early delivery, or (3) severe disease.

Meconium Staining of Amniotic Fluid. Meconium is not normally present in amniotic fluid. If meconium is present, it is considered a sign of current and/or previous fetal anoxia that causes the anal sphincter to relax.

Blood and Urine Studies

Estriol Determination. The measurement of estrogens in the urine is one of the chief methods of determining fetal well-being. During the first 6 to 8 weeks of pregnancy, estrone (E_1) and estradiol (E_2) are produced by the corpus luteum. After the sixth week the corpus luteum begins to regress (Chapter 6), but the levels of estrogens continue to rise as the placenta becomes the producer. Estrogen precursors are produced in the mother's adrenal gland in the first trimester. These precursors are the basic substances from which estrogen is produced; the principal precursor is dehydroepiandrosterone (DHEA).

In the third trimester, the fetal adrenal glands become a significant source of estrogen precursors; at term the fetal adrenals provide more than 60 per cent of E_1 and E_2 precursors. The placenta secretes E_1 and E_2 into the maternal and fetal circulation. In the maternal bloodstream, E_2 is further metabolized to estriol (E_3) and other estrogens that are excreted in the urine. Estradiol may also undergo further change in the fetal liver to form estetrol (E_4), which is transported to maternal circulation and excreted in maternal urine as estetrol glucuronide.

Because of this physiologic sequence, measurement of estriol (E_3) is thought to be a measure of the activity of the fetal adrenals and thus of fetal well-being.

Estriol is most commonly measured in a 24 hour urine specimen. A single estriol level is of limited value, but serial estriol levels on consecutive days are helpful. Because E_3 levels normally continue to rise until delivery, a fall in these levels is one indication of fetal distress, especially if that fall is marked.

Estriol levels are not universally useful; they are evaluated along with other criteria described below. In Rh disease, levels may be high even if the fetus is sick, because the placenta is both hypertrophied and efficient in converting precursors to estriol. The test is unreliable in a mother with renal disease or a mother receiving ampicillin.

Researchers have recently developed feasible methods of determining estriol levels from blood rather than from a 24 hour urine specimen, which has the advantage of much more rapid results.

Human Placental Lactogen. Human placental lactogen (HPL), also called human chorionic somatomammotropin (HCS) and several other names, is a hormone produced by the placenta. HPL can be detected in serum as early as the twenty-eighth to thirty-fourth day of pregnancy. Levels rise gradually until the thirty-sixth week of pregnancy. During the remaining weeks, levels tend to remain stable.

In normal pregnancy, values of less than 4 micrograms per 100 ml. are rarely found in the last 10 weeks of pregnancy. When HPL values are low, fetal distress is possible. This possibility is even more likely when other tests, such as estriol levels, also suggest fetal distress. There is evidence that using HPL values to recognize a fetus in distress can lower perinatal mortality.

HPL values can also aid in detecting other problems of both mother and fetus. Values are low in threatened abortion, toxemia, intrauterine growth retardation, and postmaturity. They may be high in a multiple gestation, maternal diabetes mellitus, Rh sensitization, maternal liver disease, and maternal sickle cell disease.

Fetal Stress and Oxytocin Challenge Tests

In assessing fetal well-being, it is important to know how the fetus will respond to stress. We are particularly concerned with how he will respond to the stress of labor.

One way of measuring this reaction is to give the synthetic hormone oxytocin, which stimulates the uterus to contract (Chapter 14). Oxytocin is given until the mother has three contractions within a 10 minute period. Both the contractions and the fetal heart rate are monitored. If the heart rate remains essentially stable during the contractions, the test is negative, a reassuring sign. If late decelerations (Chapter 13) are noted, the baby may not be able to tolerate labor without becoming hypoxic. Positive tests are interpreted along with other measures of fetal well-being. They may be repeated, since it is possible for a test to be falsely positive.

Mothers may also be monitored without the use of oxytocin during late pregnancy, utilizing Braxton Hicks contractions (normally occurring uterine contractions) as the point of reference.

The monitor tracing is also observed for beat-to-beat variability in the fetal heart rate (Chapter 13). Disappearance of beat-to-beat variability is considered an ominous sign, indicating major fetal distress.

When the fetus moves about in the uterus, the fetal heart rate should increase. Absence of this increase in fetal heart rate is another sign of fetal danger.

THE ASSESSMENT OF FETAL MATURITY

We have already noted that obstetricians must sometimes balance fetal well-being against fetal maturity. Estimates of fetal maturity are also important in selecting the date for an elective cesarean section. In a study published in 1969,[1] before the studies of fetal maturity described below were in use, it was found that 8.4 per cent of all infants delivered by *elective* cesarean section weighed less than 2500 grams. Thus a large number of newborns each year were unnecessarily exposed to the hazards of prematurity, not only to problems in the immediate postnatal period but some, undoubtedly, to long-term problems such as learning disability, which may not even become evident until the child is of school age.

It is probable that tests of fetal maturity will ultimately be required before every elective cesarean section. This is already the practice in some centers.

Amniotic Fluid Studies

Amniotic Fluid Surfactant. When an infant is born before he is able to synthesize a substance called *surfactant*, a complex of phospholipids, he will develop respiratory distress syndrome (RDS). RDS is a major cause of death in immature babies and is discussed in detail in Chapter 18.

Lecithin is the predominant phospholipid in surfactant. Early in pregnancy the concentration of sphingomyelin in amniotic fluid is greater than the concentration of lecithin. From about 30 to 32 weeks, the two are approximately equal. After 32 weeks, the concentration of lecithin exceeds that of sphingomyelin; at 35 weeks the rise becomes abrupt.

In 1971 Gluck demonstrated that the relationship between lecithin and sphingomyelin could serve as an index of fetal lung maturity.[8] This discovery is the basis of a now widely used test of fetal maturity, the L/S ratio. When the ratio of lecithin to sphingomyelin is 2.0 or greater, the lung is considered mature. One exception, in some laboratories, has been testing the diabetic mother; her fetus may still have immature lungs until the ratio is higher than 2.0.

The *shake test* is a more rapid determination of phospholipids in amniotic fluid. In the shake test, amniotic fluid in several dilutions is shaken in a test tube containing alcohol. If bubbles are present 15 minutes later in a 1:4 dilution of amniotic fluid, the probability of respiratory distress is considered very low.

Creatinine Levels. Levels of creatinine in amniotic fluid rise gradually until the thirty-second to thirty-fourth week of pregnancy and then rise more rapidly until term, when levels are two to four times greater than at midpregnancy. This rise is generally believed to be related to the increasing muscle mass of the fetus; it may also be due to maturing renal function. Creatinine levels of 2 mg. per 100 ml. or greater are considered to indicate a fetal age of 37 weeks or more.

Cytologic Changes. Epithelial cells, probably from the skin of the fetus, are normally present in amniotic fluid during the second and third trimesters of pregnancy. As the fetus becomes more mature, the percentage of cells containing lipid increases. By staining amniotic fluid cells with Nile blue stain, lipid cells can be identified. At 34 weeks less than 1 per cent of the cells are lipid cells; by 38 to 40 weeks from 10 to 50 per cent are lipid cells. After 40 weeks' gestation, more than 50 per cent are lipid. One advantage of this test is that it can be done without sophisticated laboratory equipment.

Maturity is also assessed by identifying types of cells present. Basal cells are the major type of cell present until approximately 32 weeks; precornified cells predominate between 32 and 36 weeks. After 36 weeks cornified cells begin to appear; they predominate after 38 weeks.

Bilirubin Levels. In studying the amniotic fluid of mothers who were Rh-sensitized, it was recognized that in normal pregnancy bilirubin levels in amniotic fluid reach a peak between 20 and 24 weeks and then decline. When levels reach zero, the fetus is assumed to be mature.[13] This test is of no value if the mother is Rh-isoimmunized.

Measurement of Fetal Biparietal Diameter

The fetal biparietal diameter, determined by ultrasound scanning, serves as a measure both of fetal maturity and of fetal well-being.

Careful studies have established tables correlating biparietal diameter with the age of the fetus in weeks. On this basis an expected date of delivery can be established that will fall within 11 days of 40 weeks 95 per cent of the time. (An expected date of delivery based on menstrual history will fall within 14 days of 40 weeks in only 84 per cent of women.)

Fetal head growth well above or below established norms indicates abnormality. A series of measurements at 2 to 3 week intervals is far more useful in evaluating an abnormality such as hydrocephalus or intrauterine growth retardation than a single measurement.

PERINATAL REGIONALIZATION

In this chapter's discussion of the needs of high risk mothers and their infants, hopefully it is obvious that optimum care for these mothers involves intensive professional nursing coordinated with medical care; a laboratory that is immediately available 24 hours a day, 7 days a week; and other supportive services.

This level of care is not available at every hospital in the United States, nor should it be. Even if it were possible to provide highly sophisticated care at every community hospital and outpatient clinic in order to serve one or two high risk mothers each month, the cost would be prohibitive and unwarranted.

The concept of regionalization is a strategy to provide each family with the level of maternity care they need in the most effective way. The goal of regionalization is reduction in maternal and perinatal mortality and morbidity. Originally, regionalization developed as a neonatal program, transferring small and/or sick newborns from community hospitals to medical centers for specialized care. It is on this basis that regionalization exists in several states today.

It is increasingly apparent, however, that transfer of a high risk mother to a regional center in advance of delivery may prevent complications and reduce perinatal mortality and morbidity. Thus the concept of *perinatal regionalization*, rather than neonatal regionalization, is the goal of many states during the next decade.

Plans for regionalization vary somewhat from state to state, but the basic features are similar. A number of regions are designated within the state, taking population, geography, traditional patterns of care, and other factors into consideration. Within each region one center offers highly specialized inpatient and outpatient care for the most critically ill mothers and infants. This center (sometimes called a regional center or a Level III center) is also active in perinatal education for the entire region and in perinatal research. Level II or district centers offer an intermediate level of care for many complications of both the period of pregnancy and the neonatal period. Level I centers, usually located in smaller communities, care for mothers and infants without complications.

Implementing this concept is no easy task. Nurses, social workers, nutritionists, administrators, obstetricians, pediatricians, and consumers must work together to plan and coordinate regionalization on both state and regional levels.

Many issues must be faced:

Financial Support. Upgrading the quality of care costs money—money for equipment, money for additional professional personnel, money to help alleviate the very high cost of maternal and neonatal intensive care, and money

for transportation for high risk mothers and infants from the communities in which they live to the regional or district center best able to serve them.

The Committee on Perinatal Health* in 1976 estimated the cost of a Level III center caring for 1000 mothers and newborns each year as 2.6 million dollars annually and a Level II center dealing with 2000 births each year as 1.2 million dollars annually. Forty-nine per cent of the Level III Model Budget (1.3 million dollars) and 59 per cent of the Level II Model Budget (700,000 dollars) are for nursing salaries.[4] This Model Budget covers only in-hospital care, although outpatient care, with early recognition and more frequent and intensive care of mothers at risk, is crucial.

What are the sources for these large amounts of money?

(1) *Health and medical insurance:* Some types of health insurance do not provide coverage for newborn or high risk maternal care. State laws can be revised to require the inclusion of such benefits.

(2) *Public funds:* Federal, state, and local governments can have a direct influence on the availability and quality of care through the budgeting of tax dollars. Although this expense is costly if one looks only at immediate expenditure, over a period of years there may be a saving, not only in human terms but even in terms of actual dollars. The cost of prenatal and newborn care, even the cost of high risk neonatal care, which may be as high as $50,000 to $100,000 for a baby, is still far lower than the cost of lifelong institutionalization for a se-

---

*The Committee on Perinatal Health represented the American Academy of Family Physicians, the American Academy of Pediatrics, the American College of Obstetricians and Gynecologists, and the American Medical Association.

verely mentally retarded individual. Actual cost figures will vary from one state to another but can be compiled as a part of the effort to convince legislators at all levels of government of the value of perinatal care.

(3) *Private funds:* Both national and local foundations, philanthropic organizations, and service clubs have in the past been, and continue to be, valuable resources for equipment purchases, for the sponsorship of educational seminars, and for a variety of other types of support. Often a single specific purchase, such as an infant warmer for a delivery room or nursery or a modern transport incubator for use in transferring a sick infant to a medical center, can significantly improve the quality of care. Nurses can effectively explain such needs to community lay groups.

The members of community organizations who understand perinatal needs are also very helpful in supporting perinatal requests to governing bodies, such as state legislatures.

Availability of Nurses with Special Education in the Care of Mothers and Infants. Without an adequate number of nurses who have had, and continue to have, special education in the care of mothers and infants, quality of care cannot improve. The most sophisticated transport incubator is of little value if there is no nurse to accompany the baby or if the nurse is not adequately prepared to care for a very sick infant.

This is a nursing problem that can only be solved by nurses themselves. The basic problem of numbers of nurses is beyond the scope of this book. Continuing education needs can be met in a variety of ways. Because many community hospitals do not have staff adequate to provide continuing education, regional planning is essential. The opportunity for clinical experience as well as for lectures and discussions in the field of continuing education is valuable. In one type of plan, nurses from community hospitals may spend 1 day each week for a specific number of weeks at a regional center, the day being divided between clinical practice and classroom discussion.

A second type of program allows nurses from community hospitals to spend a specific number of weeks at a regional center, again with both clinical and classroom experience.

Nursing internship programs offer opportunities for beginning practitioners to acquire specialized knowledge and skills. More extensive programs to prepare nurse clinicians, clinical nurse specialists, and certified nurse midwives must be evaluated. Nurses with this type of advanced training play an essential role in quality care (see Chapter 23).

Both nurses in regional centers and nurses in community hospitals and health agencies must work together to plan and implement educational programs that meet their educational needs.

Continuing Education for Other Health Professionals. Although we have emphasized nursing education, continuing education for physicians, nutritionists, and all those who care for childbearing families is essential. Interdisciplinary programs meet a part of this need.

Establishment of Mechanisms for Coordinating Regionalization. Each state and region will coordinate regional activities in a somewhat different manner.

SUMMARY

A team approach is essential to the care of high risk mothers and their families. Nurses join with nutritionists, social workers, and physicians to meet the physical, social, and emotional needs of this group of parents.

REFERENCES

1. Benson, R., Berendes, H., and Weiss, W.: Fetal Compromise During Elective Cesarean Section. *American Journal of Obstetrics and Gynecology, 105:*579, 1969.
1a. Bonica, J. (ed.): *Principles and Practice of Obstetric Analgesia and Anesthesia.* Philadelphia, F. A. Davis Co., 1972.
2. Brock, D. J. H., and Sutcliffe, R. G.: Alphafetoprotein in the Antenatal Diagnosis of Anencephaly and Spina Bifida. *Lancet, II:*197, 1972.
3. Chard, T.: Monitoring of High-Risk Pregnancies by Alpha-Fetoprotein. *In* Spellacy, W.N. (ed.): *Management of the High Risk Pregnancy.* Baltimore, University Park Press, 1976.
4. Committee on Perinatal Health: *Toward Improving the Outcome of Pregnancy.* White Plains, N.Y., The National Foundation—March of Dimes, 1976.
5. Douglas, C.: Tubal Ectopic Pregnancy. *British Medical Journal, 2:*838, 1963.
6. Galloway, K.: Placental Evaluation Studies: Their Procedures, Their Purposes and the Nursing Care Involved. *MCN, 1:*300, 1976.
7. Galloway, K.: The Uncertainty and Stress of High Risk Pregnancy. *MCN, 1:*294, September/October, 1976.
8. Gluck, L.: Fetal Maturity and Amniotic Fluid Surfactant Determinations. *In* Spellacy, W. N. (ed.): *Management of the High Risk Pregnancy.* Baltimore, University Park Press, 1976.
9. Greenhill, J., and Friedman, E.: *Biological Principles and Modern Practice of Obstetrics.* Philadelphia, W. B. Saunders Co., 1974.
10. Hobel, C. J.: Recognition of the High Risk Pregnant Woman. *In* Spellacy, W. N. (ed.): *Management of the High Risk Pregnancy.* Baltimore, University Park Press, 1976.
11. Jasper, M.: Pregnancy Complicated by Diabetes—A Case Study. *MCN, 1:*307, 1976.
12. Kowalski, K., and Osborn, M.: Helping Mothers of Stillborn Infants to Grieve. *MCN, 2:*29, 1977.
13. Mandelbaum, D., LaCroix, G., and Robinson, A. R.: Determination of Fetal Maturity by Spectrophotometric Analysis of Amniotic Fluid. *Obstetrics and Gynecology, 29:*471, 1967.
14. Nelson, B., Gillespie, L., and White, P.: Pregnancy Complicated by Diabetes Mellitus. *Obstetrics and Gynecology, 1:*219, 1953.
15. Nesbitt, R., and Aubry, R.: High Risk Obstetrics. Value of a Semi-objective Grading System in Identifying the Vulnerable Group. *American Journal of Obstetrics and Gynecology, 103:*972, 1969.
16. *Nomenclature and Criteria for Diagnosis of Diseases of the Heart and Blood Vessels.* Fifth Edition. New York, The New York Heart Association, 1955.
17. Page, E., Villee, C., and Villee, D.: *Human Reproduction: The Core Content of Obstetrics, Gynecology and Perinatal Medicine.* 2nd Edition. Philadelphia, W. B. Saunders Co., 1976.
18. Pardue, S.: Hydatidiform Mole: A Pathological Pregnancy. *American Journal of Nursing, 77:*836, 1977.
19. Pilon, R.: Anesthesia for Uncomplicated Obstetric Delivery. *American Family Physician, 9:*113, 1974.
20. Pitkin, R. M.: Fetal Maturity: Nonlipid Amniotic Fluid Assessment. *In* Spellacy, W. N. (ed.): *Management of the High Risk Pregnancy.* Baltimore, University Park Press, 1976.
21. Pitkin, R. M., and Zwirek, S. J.: Amniotic Fluid Creatinine. *American Journal of Obstetrics and Gynecology, 98:*1135, 1967.
22. Prechtl, H. H.: Neurological Sequelae of Prenatal and Perinatal Complication. *British Medical Journal, 4:*763, 1967.
23. Sabbagha, R. W.: Ultrasound in Managing the High-Risk Pregnancy. *In* Spellacy, W. N. (ed.): *Management of the High Risk Pregnancy.* Baltimore, University Park Press, 1976.
24. Seller, M.: Alpha-fetoprotein and the Prenatal Diagnosis of Neural Tube Defects. *Developmental Medicine Child Neurology, 16:*369, 1974.
25. Soichet, S.: Emotional Factors in Toxemia of Pregnancy. *American Journal of Obstetrics and Gynecology, 77:*1065, 1959.
26. Spellacy, W. N.: (ed.) *Management of the High Risk Pregnancy.* Baltimore, University Park Press, 1976.
27. Stembera, Z., Zezvlakova, J., and Dittrichova, J.: Srovnani Vlivu Nekterych Faktorv Rizikoveho Tehotenstvi na Perinatalni Mortalitv a Morbiditv. *Cesk Gynekol, 40(6):*401, 1975.
28. Tulchensky, D.: The Value of Estrogens in High Risk Pregnancy. *In* Spellacy, W. N. (ed.): *Management of the High Risk Pregnancy.* Baltimore, University Park Press, 1976.
29. Webster, H. D., Barclay, C., and Fischer, C.: Ectopic Pregnancy: A 17-year Review. *American Journal of Obstetrics and Gynecology, 92:*23, 1965.
30. White, P.: Pregnancy and Diabetes, Medical Aspects. *Medical Clinics of North America, 49:*1015, 1965.

Chapter 11

THE PHYSIOLOGIC BASIS OF THE PROCESS OF LABOR

A number of concepts are used to explain that complex set of processes that result in the birth of each human infant. Understanding these concepts is basic to the understanding of our nursing role in supporting parents and their infants in the hours surrounding birth. In this chapter we will consider the:

1. Possible causes of the onset of labor.

2. Interrelationship between uterine contractions, the maternal pelvis, and the fetus.

3. Physiologic basis of pain during labor.

WHAT CAUSES LABOR TO BEGIN?

Roughly 40 weeks from the date of the last menstrual period (38 weeks after conception), human labor begins. The length of time varies for each mammalian species but is characteristic for that species. Why?

There is no satisfactory answer to this question, although there are a number of theories. The answer is important, however, not merely as a matter of academic curiosity but as a possi-

ble clue to better management for women who labor prematurely, women who do not labor spontaneously, and others. We will examine several theories briefly, keeping in mind that they are *theories*. It is probable that no one factor, but rather a combination of factors, is responsible for the onset of labor.

Uterine Distention. It is a fact that as the uterus expands, the muscles of the uterus become more irritable, and their contractility is enhanced. (This is also true of other muscle tissue.) When the uterus is more distended than usual at a given gestational age, as in the case of a twin pregnancy or *hydramnios* (excess amniotic fluid), early labor is frequent, but not universal. As the uterus becomes increasingly distended, intrauterine pressure and intramural tension increase, which *may*, in turn, contribute to a decreased oxygen supply and subsequent "aging" of the placenta. The possible changes in the placenta may influence the length of gestation (below).

Placental Aging. It has been suggested that progesterone, or an analog of progesterone, may inhibit uterine activity. As term approaches,

335

the placental production of progesterone falls, uterine inhibition is gradually decreased, and uterine contractions begin to increase. This parallels the menstrual cycle: when the corpus luteum begins to regress, blood levels of estrogen and progesterone fall, and menstruation occurs within a few days (Chapter 3). There is no evidence, however, that local tissue levels of progesterone fall prior to the onset of labor.

Oxytocin. As pregnancy approaches term, the uterus is increasingly sensitive to exogenous oxytocin, a fact confirmed in labor rooms daily when oxytocin is used to induce labor (Chapter 14). It may be that the enzyme *oxytocinase*, which inhibits oxytocin, is decreased as term approaches, allowing endogenous oxytocin to act upon the uterus, but this is unproved. The intermittent release of oxytocin may be more important in maintaining contractions than in initiating spontaneous labor.

Prostaglandins. Prostaglandins, present in the amniotic fluid during labor, are effective in inducing labor. Do they play a role in spontaneous labor? They have not been found in the plasma of pregnant women prior to the onset of labor.

Fetal Adrenal Production. Hippocrates thought that the fetus, when mature, initiated labor. The production of cortisone by the fetal adrenals may be a significant factor. Liggins[3] was able to manipulate the timing of the onset of labor in sheep by manipulating adrenal function. Anencephalic fetuses, who have retarded adrenal development secondary to hypofunction of their pituitary gland, have a delayed onset of labor about 40 per cent of the time.[5]

THE FOUR P's

Traditionally, descriptions of labor have described 3 *p*'s: powers, passage, and passenger. To these three we believe a fourth should be added: psyche. The first three are discussed below; the role of the psyche is discussed in Chapter 12.

POWERS

The power of labor comes from the force of contractions of the uterine muscles and the voluntary contractions of the abdominal muscles.

Uterine Contractions

The Physiology of a Uterine Contraction. A contraction begins as a result of "pacemaker" action in the myometrial cells near the right or left uterotubal junction. The contraction itself normally begins in one uterine cornu and spreads downward over a period of 15 seconds (Fig. 11–1). Although the contraction begins later in the lower uterus, it reaches its peak at the same time in all areas. The intensity of the contraction is directly proportional to the number of myometrial cells in that area of the uterus, being greatest at the fundus; less lower in the uterine body; and least at the cervix, where there are few muscle fibers. When contractions do not follow this normal pattern, various types of abnormalities are possible.

If the contraction begins in a lower segment and spreads upward, a *reverse gradient*, the cervix does not dilate and will contract during the contraction. This may be suspected if a woman complains of low back or low abdominal pain 5 to 10 seconds before the contraction is palpated at the fundus.

A *mild incoordination* occurs when there is more than one pacemaker and the pacemakers are asynchronous. Weak contractions may alternate with stronger ones. Mild incoordination is fairly common during early labor; often

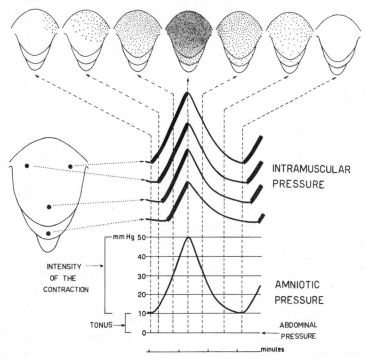

Figure 11–1 Schematic representation of the normal contractile wave of labor. Diagram of the uterus on the left shows the four points at which the intramyometrial pressure is recorded with microballoons. (From Caldeyro-Barcia: *Clinical Obstetrics and Gynecology*, 3:394, 1960.)

contractions become more coordinated as labor progesses.

If there are several pacemakers in various parts of the uterus, *severe incoordination* results. Labor does not progress; the mother is very uncomfortable and may become overly tired. Continued hypertonus can lead to fetal distress because of the interference with uteroplacental circulation. If sedation, analgesia, and regional anesthesia (Chapter 13) do not relieve the incoordination, cesarean section may be necessary.

Properties of Uterine Contractions. Uterine contractions have a number of specific properties.

PHASES. There are three phases in a contraction, the *increment,* during which intensity increases; the *acme,* or height of the contraction; and the *decrement,* or period of decreasing intensity (Fig. 11–2).

FREQUENCY, DURATION, INTENSITY. In describing contractions, the terms frequency, duration, and intensity are used.

Frequency is measured from the beginning of one contraction to the beginning of the next contraction (Fig. 11–2). The interval progessively decreases, and contractions become more frequent as labor progresses.

Duration is the length of the contraction. It is measured by abdominal palpation or by monitor from the time that the contraction is first perceived by the examiner (not the beginning of pain perceived by the laboring mother) until complete relaxation (Fig. 11–2).

Intensity, or strength, can be estimated by abdominal palpation or observed by monitor. When a contraction is strong, the uterus cannot be indented by examining fingers.

One measure of intensity is amni-

Figure 11-2   Terms used to describe uterine contractions.

otic fluid pressure. Table 11-1 summarizes the correlation between amniotic fluid pressure and certain clinical
signs.

Early in labor, contractions are
comparatively weak; the uterus is firm
but not hard, and the duration may be
about 30 seconds. As labor progresses,
the duration increases to about 45 seconds, and firmness also increases.
Strong contractions, of about 50 to 90
seconds' duration, occur as the time of
birth approaches. (See also Stages of
Labor, below.)

ABNORMAL VARIATION IN AMNIOTIC
FLUID PRESSURE. Certain abnormal
variations in labor patterns are defined
in relation to amniotic fluid pressure:

1. *Hypertonus:* resting pressure
from 12 to 30 or more mm. Hg (resting
pressures above 30 are dangerous to the
fetus; see below).

2. *Hyperactive labor:* contractions
that exceed 50 mm. Hg, or that occur
more frequently than every 2 minutes,
or both.

3. *Hypoactive labor:* contractior
with an intensity of less than 30 mm
Hg, or more than 5 minutes apart, c
both. When labor is hypoactive, there
little progress, and the length of labor
likely to be prolonged.

Abdominal Muscle
Contractions

During the second stage of labo
(see below), the voluntary contractior
of abdominal muscles, when coord
nated with uterine contractions, a
important in the expulsion of the bab
This coordination is facilitated b
skilled coaching from the nurse carir
for the woman, who tells her when
"bear down," i.e., when to contract h
abdominal muscles (Chapter 13). A
labor progresses and the fetus descen
to the floor of the perineum, the moth
feels such a great urge "to push" th
abdominal muscle contractions becom
difficult for the mother to control.

Table 11-1   CLINICAL CORRELATES OF AMNIOTIC FLUID PRESSURE

Amniotic Fluid Pressure (mm./Hg)	Clinical Correlates
10	Normal tonus
20	Contraction felt by abdominal palpation
25	Woman perceives "pain"; considerable individual variation
50	Height of contraction

THE PASSAGE: THE PELVIS

The four types of female pelves were briefly described and illustrated in Chapter 3. Here we will consider the effect of each type of pelvis on labor more specifically.

1. *Gynecoid pelvis:* Considered the most satisfactory for normal labor, the gynecoid pelvis allows effective uterine contractions and spontaneous delivery. Because the pubic arch is wide, the frequency of perineal tears is reduced.

2. *Anthropoid pelvis:* The head often engages in an occiput posterior position and may deliver in that position. Labor and delivery are usually without difficulty, and the fetus has a good prognosis.

3. *Android pelvis:* The head engages in a posterior or transverse diameter and may not rotate; forceps are often needed for both rotation and extraction. This is a difficult vaginal delivery, and the prognosis for the baby is often poor. Because the pubic arch is narrow, perineal tears are common.

4. *Platypelloid pelvis:* Because of the short anteroposterior, posterior sagittal, and anterior sagittal diameters, the baby may never be able to enter the pelvic inlet. The outlook for the fetus is poor unless the condition is recognized and cesarean section performed.

THE PASSENGER

The passenger is, of course, the fetus who must travel from the uterus through the vagina to the world outside his mother's body. The fetus is described in terms of lie, presentation, position, and station.

Lie

Consider first the fetus within the uterus in the days immediately prior to delivery. The relationship between the long axis of the fetus and the long axis of the mother is the lie. Lie may be longitudinal or transverse (Fig. 11–3). Labor cannot progress to vaginal delivery when the lie is transverse (see discussion under Shoulder Presentation, below).

Presentation

The part of the fetus that first enters the vagina is the *presenting part.*

Cephalic Presentation. At term, 95 per cent of presentations are *cephalic,* i.e., the head is the presenting part. It is necessary to understand the structure of the fetal head in order to appreciate the process of labor.

The landmarks of the cranium are illustrated in Figures 11–4 and 11–5. At the time of birth the bones of the cranium are joined only by a membrane; they are thin and easily compressed. These characteristics make it possible for them to overlap, changing the shape of the head to fit the pelvis, a process known as *molding.*

The *sutures,* the membranous spaces between the bones, serve a useful function in addition to permitting molding. The sutures can be identified on vaginal examination, and in this way an examiner can determine the position of the baby's head. At the intersection of the sutures are the fontanels, which also aid in identifying the position of the fetal head.

The anterior fontanel (bregma), at the junction of the frontal, sagittal, and coronal sutures, is diamond-shaped. Measuring about 2 by 3 cm., it is much larger than the posterior fontanel.

The sagittal and lambdoidal sutures meet to form the triangular posterior fontanel.

Several diameters of the fetal skull are important. These diameters were illustrated in Chapter 8 and are sum-

Figure 11–3 Schematic drawing of shoulder presentation, left acromion anterior position, in advanced labor with prolapsed right arm, head in the left iliac ala, and back down and anteriorly located. (From Greenhill and Friedman: *Biological Principles and Modern Practice of Obstetrics*. Philadelphia, W. B. Saunders Co., 1974.)

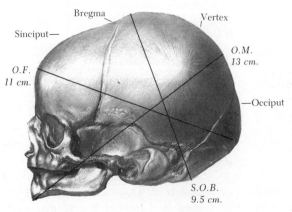

Figure 11–4 Lateral view of fetal skull showing cranial relationships, regional designations (reference points), and main diameters, including *O.F.*, occipitofrontal; *O.M.*, occipitomental; and *S.O.B.*, suboccipitobregmatic. (From Greenhill and Friedman: *Biological Principles and Modern Practice of Obstetrics*. Philadelphia, W. B. Saunders Co., 1974.)

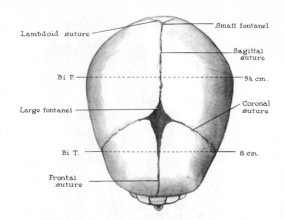

Figure 11–5 Top view of fetal skull, showing cranial bones, anterior (large lozenge shaped) and posterior (small triangular) fontanels and sutures. The important diameters, *Bi P.*, biparietal and *Bi T.*, bitemporal, are also designated. (From Greenhill and Friedman: *Biological Principles and Modern Practice of Obstetrics.* Philadelphia, W. B. Saunders Co., 1974.)

marized in Table 11–2. The diameter presenting to the pelvic inlet varies with the baby's position.

Breech Presentation. In 3 to 4 per cent of deliveries, the presenting part is the breech. Figures 11–6 and 11–7 illustrate the types of breech presentation.

In a breech presentation, lightening is rare; the presenting part is not engaged until after labor begins. Early rupture of the membranes is more common than in vertex presentations because the breech fits unevenly into the pelvis.

A number of circumstances make labor and delivery in the breech presentation more complex than in the vertex presentation.

1. Because the breech is not as effective as the head as a dilating wedge, labor is usually longer.

2. The breech, born first, is smaller than the head; the head must then pass through the pelvis quickly, with no time to mold.

3. Assisted delivery, a *breech extraction*, is often necessary.

4. *Prolapse* of the umbilical cord is more frequent than in vertex presentation (Chapter 14).

Because of the complexity of breech delivery, fetal and neonatal mortality and morbidity are higher than in vertex presentation. Potential complications include intracranial hemorrhage, injury to the brachial plexus, and fracture of the humerus and clavicle.

From 10 to 35 per cent of breech

Table 11–2 DIAMETERS OF THE FETAL SKULL

	Diameter	Location	Average Size at Term (in cm.)
Transverse diameters	Biparietal	Between parietal bosses	9.5
	Bitemporal	Between temporal bones	8.0
Anteroposterior diameters	Occipito-frontal	External occipital protuberance to glabella	11.0
	Suboccipito-bregmatic	Undersurface occipital bone to center of bregma	9.5
	Verticomental	Vertex to chin	13.5
	Submentobregmatic	Junction neck and lower jaw to bregma	9.5

Figure 11–6 Fetus in frank or single breech presentation, right sacrum posterior position, with lower extremities extended fully across the abdomen, chest, and face. (From Greenhill and Friedman: *Biological Principles and Modern Practice of Obstetrics*. Philadelphia, W. B. Saunders Co., 1974.)

Figure 11–7 Fetus shown in complete or double breech presentation with buttocks and both feet presenting in the pelvic inlet, right sacrum posterior position. Compare with Figure 11–6. (From Greenhill and Friedman: *Biological Principles and Modern Practice of Obstetrics*. Philadelphia, W. B. Saunders Co., 1974.)

presentations are delivered by cesarean section (Chapter 14). (See also Mechanisms of Labor in Breech Presentation, below.)

Shoulder Presentation. A shoulder presentation occurs when the lie is transverse, about once in every 300 to 400 deliveries. Predisposing causes include the pendulous abdomen of a grand multipara, placenta previa (Chapter 10), a very narrow pelvis, or a uterine anomaly.

Spontaneous version (change of direction) occurs only occasionally, with the *lie* changing to a longitudinal one (cephalic or breech presentation) shortly before or after labor begins. The obstetrician may try to "turn" the baby to a longitudinal lie by *external version* early in labor or by *internal podalic version* under general anesthesia if the longitudinal lie is not recognized until the second stage. Cesarean section is more common than version today.

If for some reason a transverse lie is not recognized, the following sequence is likely:

1. Uterine contractions are of poor quality, and the cervix dilates slowly.

2. Membranes rupture early.

3a. The fetal shoulder enters the pelvis, the uterus molds around the baby, and contractions cease. This leads to intrauterine sepsis and generalized sepsis,

or

3b. The upper segment of the uterus becomes shorter and thicker, the lower part becomes thinner and more and more stretched until it ruptures.

Either sequence leads to almost certain fetal death and possible maternal death. Thus, early recognition of a transverse lie and shoulder presentation is essential.

Describing the Presentation. In cephalic presentations the baby's head may be (1) flexed so that his chin is on his chest and the posterior occiput (O) presents (vertex presentation), (2) neither flexed nor extended (military attitude), so that the median portion of the occiput (O) presents (vertex presentation, (3) partially extended so that the forehead or frontum (F) presents (bregma or sincipital presentation), or (4) fully extended so that the face presents (face presentation) (Fig. 11–8). The chin, or mentum (M), is the point of reference. In the breech position the sacrum (S) is the point of reference in relation to the mother's pelvis; in a shoulder presentation it is the scapula (Sc).

Position

Position is the relationship between the presenting part and the mother's pelvis. The structure that is used as the point of reference (the occiput, the mentum, and so on) is described as being anterior (A), posterior (P), or transverse (T), and as facing the right (R) or the left (L) of the mother's pelvis.

All of the information about the position of the fetus in utero is then translated into a shorthand that in a brief form gives nurses and physicians very specific information about the position of the fetus. The components of the system of notation are summarized in Table 11–3. Figure 11–9 illustrates positions.

Consider the meaning of these examples.

1. LOA: the occiput, the presenting part, is facing the left anterior quadrant of the mother's pelvis (common position).

2. LOP: Here the occiput is facing the left posterior quadrant of the pelvis. This mother's labor will be longer and more difficult than that of the mother

Figure 11–8 Gamut of deflexion attitudes from *A*, sincipital and *B*, brow presentation to *C*, face presentation, showing altered presenting fetal diameters from occipitobregmatic to mentobregmatic to trachelobregmatic. (From Greenhill and Friedman: *Biological Principles and Modern Practice of Obstetrics.* Philadelphia, W. B. Saunders Co., 1974.)

with a baby in an anterior position because the baby must rotate to a greater extent prior to delivery.

3. SA: The presentation is breech; the sacrum is the presenting part, and it faces anteriorly, i.e., the mother's pubic bone. (The presenting part does not necessarily face the right or the left; hence, only two letters may be necessary.)

4. LMT: The face is the presenting part; the chin is toward the left and midway between the anterior and posterior quadrants of the pelvis, thus transverse.

Station

The progress of the fetus through the birth canal is also described in terms

Table 11–3   DESCRIBING FETAL POSITION

Right (R)	Occiput (O)	Anterior (A)
Left (L)	Sacrum (S)	Posterior (P)
	Mentum (M)	Transverse (T)
	Scapula (Sc)	

of *station*. Station refers to the level of the presenting part in relation to the maternal pelvis. When the presenting part is at the level of the ischial spines, the station is zero (0). Above the ischial spines the station is −1 if the lowest segment of the presenting part is 1 cm. above the spine, −2 if 2 cm. above, and so on. Below the ischial spines the station is +1 when the lowest portion of the presenting part is 1 cm. below the spine, and so on.

When the station is 0, the presenting part is *engaged*. At −1 and −2, the presenting part is *fixed*, but not engaged; a presenting part that is fixed is not movable. The station is +3 when the presenting part reaches the pelvic floor and +4 when the perineum is bulging (Figs. 11–10 and 11–11).

Normal Characteristics of the Fetus during Labor

Labor produces stress for the fetus. When the fetus is healthy and the labor is normal, the stress is not harmful and

A. Occiput.

B. Face.

C. Breech.

Figure 11–9   Position. (From Oxorn and Foote: *Human Labor and Birth*. 3rd Ed., 1975. Courtesy of Appleton-Century-Crofts, Publishing Division of Prentice-Hall, Inc., Englewood Cliffs, N.J.)

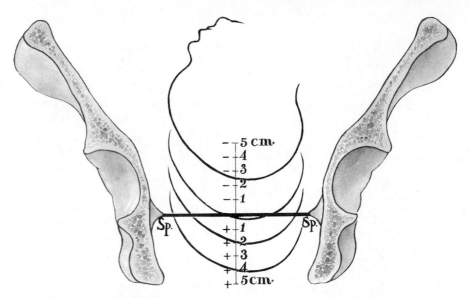

Figure 11–10 Diagrammatic presentation of the station or degree of engagement of the fetal head. The location of the forward leading edge or lowest part of the head is designated by centimeters above or below the plane of the interspinous line. (From Greenhill and Friedman: *Biological Principles and Modern Practice of Obstetrics.* Philadelphia, W. B. Saunders Co., 1974.)

Figure 11–11 Lateral planar representation of station designations comparable to those in Figure 11–10 along the pelvic axis. Each line shows the location of the leading edge of the fetal head above or below the interspinous plane (double line). Station lines are spaced 1 cm. apart at their midpoints. (From Greenhill and Friedman: *Biological Principles and Modern Practice of Obstetrics.* Philadelphia, W. B. Saunders Co., 1974.)

may even serve a useful purpose in the transition to extrauterine life.

How is the fetus affected during normal labor? Changes in amniotic fluid pressure have already been noted in this chapter. These changes bring pressure upon the flow of blood in the intervillous spaces and upon the fetal body. One manifestation of this stress noted in every labor is a brief fall in fetal heart rate that coincides with the contraction (see below). Research indicates that slight changes in fetal blood pressure also occur, although clinically fetal blood pressure is not monitored.

Physiologic Regulation of Fetal Heart Rate. Fetal heart rate is affected by several systems; recognizing this is fundamental to understanding fetal heart rate changes during labor. These systems are the parasympathetic, sympathetic, and central nervous systems; baroreceptors and chemoreceptors; and certain hormones. Figure 11–12 and Table 11–4 summarize these systems.

Baseline fetal heart rate is the rate between contractions or between transient changes that are unrelated to contractions. The baseline rate is usually between 120 and 160 beats per minute. As in older children and adults, the intrinsic pacemaker activity leads to rhythmic contractions.

Periodic fetal heart rate patterns are brief accelerations and decelera-

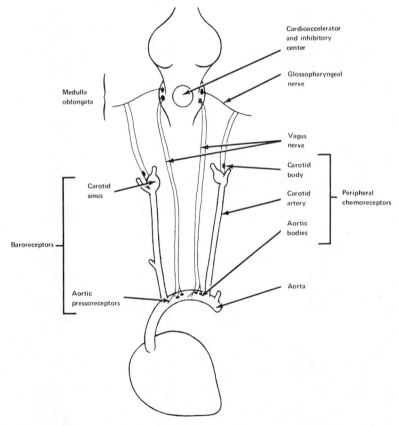

Figure 11–12   The baroreceptors and peripheral chemoreceptors and their input connections to the cardiac integrating center in the medulla oblongata. Fibers travel from this center to the heart. (From Perer: *JOGN Nursing (Supplement)*, 5:26s, 1976.)

Table 11–4 SYSTEMS INFLUENCING FETAL HEAT RATE (FHR) DURING LABOR

System	Location	Relevant Function	Effect of Stimulation	Effect of Blocking	Comments
Parasympathetic nervous system—vagus (10th cranial) nerve	Originates in medulla oblongata	Supplies sinoatrial (SA) node and atrioventricular (AV) node. Secretion of acetylcholine	↓ Firing SA node, therefore ↓ FHR, ↓ Atrioventricular transmission, therefore ↓ FHR. Causes beat-to-beat variability	↑ FHR. Eliminates beat-to-beat variability	Atropine blocks vagus by counteracting effects of acetylcholine. Even small amounts that do not increase FHR will eliminate beat-to-beat variability. Hypoxia depresses myocardial rhythm.
Sympathetic nervous system	Widely distributed in cardiac muscle	Secretion of norepinephrine	↑ FHR, ↑ Strength of contraction	↓ FHR	A reserve to improve cardiac output during stress. Propranolol blocks sympathetic nerves. Blocking does not influence FHR variability.
Baroreceptors (pressure receptors)	Arch of aorta; carotid sinus (Fig. 11–12)		↑ Blood pressure (BP) causes impulses from receptors via vagus or glossopharyngeal nerve → midbrain → vagus (Fig. 11–12) ↓ FHR		

Chemoreceptors Peripheral chemoreceptors: carotid and aortic bodies Central chemoreceptors: medulla	influence not well understood: Abrupt ↓ oxygen or ↑ carbon dioxide of peripheral receptors → ↓ FHR;* ↑ FHR variability. Mild ↓ oxygen or ↑ carbon dioxide → reflex tachycardia (↑ FHR). ↑ Carbon dioxide → ↑ arterial BP	
Central nervous system Nerve impulse to and from higher brain center believed to be mediated through hypothalamus	Emotional stimuli → ↑ FHR and ↑ BP	Experimental stimulation of hypothalamus in fetal lamb → ↑ FHR
Hormonal regulation Adrenal medulla: epinephrine, norepinephrine Adrenal cortex: aldosterone	↑ FHR ↑ Strength of contraction ↑ BP → ↓ FHR Role in fetus poorly understood	

*This response is opposite to that of the extrauterine infant or adult.

tions in rate, after which the rate returns to the baseline rate.

Uterine Contractions and the Fetus. When the uterus contracts, a vagal reflex, probably due to compression of the fetal head, may cause a brief deceleration in heart rate. The rate will not usually fall below 100, however, and will quickly return to a normal level of between 120 and 160. This pattern, and those described below, are discussed in more detail in the section on fetal monitoring in Chapter 13.

If uterine contractions interfere with the flow of blood to the fetus, hypoxia and acidosis may severely compromise the fetus. Careful monitoring of fetal heart rate in relation to uterine contractions, along with fetal scalp sampling, is important in recognizing the presence of these abnormal conditions (see Chapter 13).

THE STAGES OF LABOR

For convenience in communication, the process of labor is divided into four stages. These stages are briefly summarized in Table 11-5.

THE FIRST STAGE

Before a baby can be delivered through the vagina, the uterine cervix must become effaced and dilated. This is the purpose of the first stage of labor.

Effacement is the process by which the cervical canal becomes shorter and thinner until it no longer is present (Fig. 11-13). Physiologically, effacement occurs because the cervical muscle fibers closest to the internal os are pulled into the lower uterine segment.

The other major process of the first stage is *dilatation* of the cervix. At the beginning of labor, especially for the primigravida, the cervix is closed or just barely dilated (about 1 cm.). In multiparas the cervix may be dilated as much as 2 cm. (one fingertip passes through easily) at the beginning of labor (Fig. 11-14). During the first stage, the cervix dilates to an opening 10 cm. (4 inches) in diameter, in order to allow the baby to pass into the vagina.

This first stage is by far the most time-consuming of the labor process. Within the first stage are three distinct phases, the *latent* phase, the *active* phase, and the *transitional* phase, dia-

Table 11-5   THE STAGES OF LABOR

Stage	Beginning	Ending	Purpose
First	Onset of regular contractions of uterus	Cervix fully dilated (10 cm.)	Effacement and dilatation
Second	Cervix fully dilated (10 cm.)	Birth of infant	Delivery of infant
Third	Complete birth of baby	Delivery of placenta	Separation and expulsion of placenta
Fourth	Expulsion of placenta	Uterus contracted, vital signs stable, lochia moderate	Prevention of uterine atony

Figure 11–13   Effacement and dilatation in a primipara during labor. *A*, The cervical canal is closed; note the length of the canal. *B*, The cervix shortens, the internal os widens, and the cervical canal becomes funnel-shaped. *C*, Only a thin lip remains of the cervix—effacement is complete, and dilatation is beginning. *D*, Cervical dilatation completed.

grammed by means of Friedman's curve (Fig. 11–15).

The *latent* phase begins with the onset of regular contractions. These contractions are usually mild and are not perceived by the mother as being especially painful. They may last from 15 to 30 seconds and occur every 10 to 20 minutes. The latent phase may last more than 8 hours in primigravidas and a little more than 5 hours in multigravidas.

The *active* phase begins when the cervix is fully effaced. Contractions are now more frequent and of longer duration and greater intensity.

Almost all mothers find the period of *transition* the most difficult in labor. During transition, the cervix is retracting (being retracted) over the presenting part, which is pushing into the vagina. Contractions are strong, frequent (as often as every 2 minutes), and may last as long as 70 to 80 seconds. There is always a certain amount of individual variation.

Table 11–6 summarizes the first stage of labor.

THE SECOND STAGE

The second stage of labor begins when the cervix is fully dilated (10 cm.). It ends with the infant's birth. During the second stage, the baby descends through the vagina and is delivered. The second stage may be as brief as a few minutes or as long as an hour.

Physiologic Changes

Several physiologic changes facilitate the birth of the baby:

Soft Tissue Changes.   The soft tissues of the perineum hypertrophy; both blood supply and fluid content increase. These changes enable the tissues to stretch far more than they would be able to under ordinary circumstances. Changes are particularly marked in the *levator ani*, which will be markedly

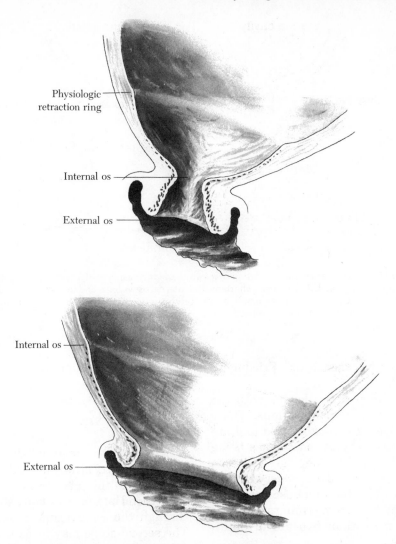

Physiologic retraction ring

Internal os

External os

Internal os

External os

Figure 11–14 Progressive effacement and dilatation of the cervix of a multipara, showing that dilatation may occur even if effacement is incomplete. (From Greenhill and Friedman: *Biological Principles and Modern Practice of Obstetrics.* Philadelphia, W. B. Saunders Co., 1974.)

stretched at delivery, and in the perineal body, which changes from a thick and wedge-shaped tissue to a thin tissue.

Uterine Changes. The uterus becomes longer as the lower uterine segment stretches and the transverse and anteroposterior diameters shorten. As the uterus changes, the position of the fetus becomes more nearly vertical. Contractions become longer (from 50 to 90 seconds), more frequent (at 1 to 3 minute intervals), and more intense.

Increased Show. As capillaries in the cervix rupture and the membranes separate from the decidua in the lower uterine segment, the amount of bloody show increases.

Bearing Down. As the presenting part of the fetus reaches the floor of the perineum, the mother has an uncontrollable desire to bear down, adding the

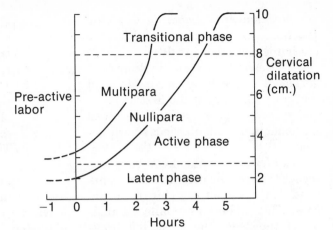

Figure 11–15 The Friedman curve diagrams the relationship between hours of active labor and cervical dilatation.

force of the abdominal muscles to the effect of uterine contractions.

The Mechanism of Labor

The way the fetus-passenger adapts himself to the maternal passage and passes through that passage is called the mechanism of labor. This mechanism consists of six movements, termed cardinal movements. Although these movements are described in sequence, many occur simultaneously, either entirely or in part. The fetus's position during each cardinal movement varies with his position at the onset of labor, but the mechanism itself is similar. Because LOA is a common position, the mechanism of labor described here is in that position. The mechanism of labor in a variety of positions is described in Oxorn and Foote's text.[6]

Table 11–6   THE FIRST STAGE OF LABOR

Phase	Begins	Ends	Time	Comments
Latent	Onset of regular contractions	Effacement complete Dilatation to 2–3 cm.	Primigravida— about 8½ hours	Woman usually comfortable
			Multigravida— about 5½ hours	
Active	Complete effacement Dilatation approximately 2–3 cm.	Approximately 8 cm. dilatation	Primigravida— 4 hours	Contractions more frequent, longer, and stronger
			Multigravida— 2 hours	Woman becomes increasingly restless
Transitional	Approximately 8 cm. dilatation	Cervix fully dilated	Primigravida— about 1 hour	Most difficult phase of labor for most women
			Multigravida— 10–15 minutes	

Mechanism of Labor in Cephalic Position. In the cephalic position the mechanism of labor involves:

1. *Descent.* Descent includes *engagement* of the head (page 344) and continues throughout the first and second stages of labor. All of the other movements are simultaneous with descent.

2. *Flexion.* As the LOA baby descends through the uterine passage, his head flexes so that his chin is on his chest. This enables the smallest diameter of the head (the suboccipitobregmatic, which is approximately 9.5 cm.) to present first. If flexion did not occur and the approximately 11.0 cm. occipitofrontal diameter presented, passage would be far more difficult (Fig. 11–16).

3. *Internal rotation.* Internal rotation usually occurs in the second stage of labor (i.e., after the cervix is fully dilated; see above and below) when the head reaches the pelvic floor or soon afterward. The reasons for internal rotation are three:

a. The pelvic *inlet* is usually a transverse oval; i.e., it is slightly longer from side to side (transverse diameter) than from front to back (anteroposterior diameter).

b. The pelvic outlet is an anteroposterior oval, being slightly longer from front to back.

c. The fetal head is an anteroposterior oval.

Thus, the head must enter the pelvic inlet in a transverse diameter and leave the pelvis in an anteroposterior diameter. Therefore, the head must rotate; the shoulders, however, do not (Fig. 11–17). Usually the head rotates so that the occiput is anterior.

4. *Extension.* As the baby reaches the pelvic floor, the combination of "push" from uterine contractions and abdominal muscles and resistance offered by the pelvic floor results in extension of the head. The perineum bulges, the head "crowns" (Fig. 11–18), and the baby is born—first the occiput, followed by the bregma, forehead, nose, mouth and chin.

The *Ritgen maneuver* is a method of

A   B

Figure 11–16 Reduction in the presenting fetal diameters as a result of flexion. The occipitofrontal diameter in a moderately deflexed sincipital presentation (*A*) is converted to the smaller suboccipitobregmatic in a well-flexed vertex presentation (*B*). (From Greenhill and Friedman: *Biological Principles and Modern Practice of Obstetrics.* Philadelphia, W. B. Saunders Co., 1974.)

A. Lateral view.

B. Vaginal view.

C. Anteroposterior view.

Figure 11–17 Internal rotation: LOA to OA. (From Oxorn and Foote: *Human Labor and Birth.* 3rd Ed., 1975. Courtesy of Appleton-Century-Crofts, Publishing Division of Prentice-Hall Inc., Englewood Cliffs, N.J.)

assisting the mechanism of extension and the birth of the head; its purpose is gradual delivery of the head between contractions, with minimal damage to the soft tissues (Fig. 11–19).

5. *Restitution.* Since the time of internal rotation, the neck has been twisted somewhat. After the head is born, it "restitutes" to a normal relationship with the shoulders. The baby

A. Vaginal view.

B. Lateral view.

Figure 11–18   Extension of the head: birth. (From Oxorn and Foote: *Human Labor and Birth*. 3rd Ed., 1975. Courtesy of Appleton-Century-Crofts, Publishing Division of Prentice-Hall Inc., Englewood Cliffs, N.J.)

Figure 11–19   The Ritgen maneuver *(A)* facilitates birth by encouraging extension of the fetal head. If the chin lodges against the perineum, it may be extracted as in *(B)*. (After Oxorn and Foote: *Human Labor and Birth*. 3rd Ed.)

thus returns to its original pelvic position (in this instance LOA). The head should be supported during restitution and external rotation (below).

6. *External rotation.* Just as the head rotated internally in order to pass through the pelvic outlet, so too must the shoulders. External rotation of the head is the visible evidence of internal rotation of the shoulders. The baby's position is now LOT. The anterior shoulder reaches the pelvic floor first, rotates anteriorly under the symphysis, and is born. The posterior shoulder is delivered as the mother "bears down," and the trunk and extremities follow.

Mechanism of Labor in Breech Presentation. In a breech presentation, there are mechanisms of labor for three segments of the fetus:

1. the buttocks and lower limbs.
2. the shoulders and arms.
3. the head.

If one imagines the fetus as a triangle (Fig. 11–20), with the head as the largest, most unyielding segment, the reason is easier to understand. In a cephalic presentation, the head is delivered first, and it is usually not difficult for the smaller shoulders and body to follow. In a breech presentation, each segment is larger and more difficult to deliver than the part of the fetal body that preceded it.

Consider this example of the mechanism of labor in the RSA position:

1. *Buttocks and lower limbs.* De-

scent may be delayed until the cervix is dilated and the membranes ruptured. Lateral *flexion* at the waist and *internal rotation* of the hips occur. Birth occurs by *lateral* flexion, the posterior hip first followed by the anterior hip.

2. *Shoulders and arms.* As the sacrum rotates (RST → RSA), the shoulders are engaged and rotate internally. The baby is lifted upward so that the posterior shoulder and arm are delivered over the perineum. The baby is then lowered, and the anterior shoulder and arm are delivered under the symphysis (Fig. 11–21).

3. *Head.* The head enters the pelvis as the posterior shoulder is born. The head *flexes* and *rotates internally* so that the occiput is under the symphysis and the back is anterior. The chin, mouth, nose, forehead, bregma, and occiput, in that order, are born over the perineum.

As in cephalic presentations, mechanisms for breech delivery in positions other than RSA vary (see Oxorn and Foote[6]).

THE THIRD STAGE

Uterine contractions begin again shortly after the baby's delivery, with a resultant retraction in the size of the uterus. This retraction decreases the area of placental attachment (Fig. 11–22), and the placenta separates from the uterine wall and is expelled through the vagina.

The lower edge of the placenta may appear first (Duncan method), or the placenta may resemble an inverted umbrella with the shiny fetal side appearing initially (Shultze method). Although the Shultze method may indicate the implantation of the placenta in the fundus and the Duncan method implantation in the uterine wall, this differentiation has no practical significance of which we are aware.

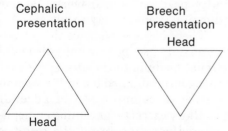

Cephalic presentation   Breech presentation

Head

Head

Figure 11–20 Breech presentation. Imagine the fetus as a triangle and the head as the largest segment. In a breech presentation, each segment is larger than the body part that precedes it.

Figure 11–21 Mechanisms of labor—breech presentation (RSA). *A,* Onset of labor; *B,* descent and internal rotation of buttocks; *C,* birth of posterior buttock; *D,* feet born, shoulder engaging; *E,* descent and internal rotation of shoulders; *F,* posterior shoulder born, head enters pelvis; *G,* anterior shoulder born, head descends; and *H,* flexion and birth of head. (After Oxorn and Foote: *Human Labor and Birth.* 3rd Ed.)

After placental separation the uterine muscles retract further, closing off the arterioles and venules that pass through the interlacing muscle fibers and controlling bleeding. If these muscles do not retract and remain retracted, hemorrhage will result.

DYSTOCIA

Difficult labor is termed *dystocia.* Dystocia may be due to a problem of the powers, the passage, or the passenger, or any combination of the three. Psychologic problems also may contribute to a difficult labor.

Hypoactive labor, with ineffective uterine contractions that are too weak and/or too infrequent, may lead to difficult labor. If there is disproportion between the size of the fetus and the size of the pelvic passage or if the fetus is in a faulty position (a transverse lie, for example), dystocia may result.

There is some evidence that excessive anxiety may be transmitted via the adrenal medulla to the uterus with resulting incoordinated labor. If a woman is given a combination of adrenal medullary extracts containing epinephrine and norepinephrine, the result is uterine incoordination.

Figure 11–22 Sequence of usual mechanism of expulsion of placenta. Early central separation with formation of retroplacental hematoma shown progressing to inversion of the placenta and expulsion with fetal surface leading, followed by membranes and blood that has accumulated. (From Greenhill and Friedman: *Biological Principles and Modern Practice of Obstetrics.* Philadelphia, W. B. Saunders Co., 1974.)

THE PHYSIOLOGIC BASIS OF PAIN DURING LABOR

From ancient times pain has been associated with labor. The expression "labor pains" is familiar to nearly every woman. Is labor always painful? If so, how painful?

Pain during labor has both a physiologic and psychosocial component, as has most pain. Both factors are interwoven so closely that it is difficult to say when the physiologic basis ends and the psychosocial component starts (or vice versa). The physiologic basis of pain during labor will be discussed here, whereas psychosocial factors will be discussed in Chapter 12. In Chapter 13 the adaptation of the physiologic and psychosocial concepts to nursing care during labor will be discussed.

Historically, a certain degree of pain during childbirth has been considered inevitable, at least in Western society, and apparently among most of the world's peoples. The idea of pain, including labor pain, as punishment has been expressed at various times in history and still may influence our perceptions. For example, we unfortunately find on occasion that some individuals are less sympathetic to discomfort during labor when the mother is unmarried. Comments such as "she should have thought about the pain 9 months ago" or "maybe next time she'll remember what it means to have a baby before she fools around" are still heard from time to time.

As "natural" childbirth and prepared childbirth concepts have become widely discussed, many women have come to wonder if pain during labor is largely psychosomatic. Sometimes women feel that they have "failed" if they require any medication at all during labor and/or delivery.

It is important to recognize that while fear, anxiety, and tension may play a significant role in the discomfort that is felt during labor, there is also a physiologic basis for that discomfort.

Basic Physiologic Stimuli

As noted in Chapter 3, ischemia with resultant anoxia and stretching are the two basic stimuli for pain in the uterus. Pressure is a third stimulus important for pain in areas adjacent to the uterus.

Anoxia occurs during prolonged muscle contraction because the blood supply to the muscle is compromised (ischemia). The longer the contraction, the greater the ischemia and anoxia and the more intense the pain. Moreover, when the period of relaxation between contractions is too short to allow adequate oxygenation, the intensity of the pain is increased.

Stretching occurs in the cervix during effacement and dilatation. The muscles of the pelvic floor and perineum are distended during the second stage of labor. There is also traction on and stretching of the ligaments supporting the pelvic organs.

Pressure is applied to nerve ganglia adjacent to the cervix and vagina, as well as to the urethra, bladder, and rectum.

Nerve Pathways Involved in Labor

The nerves supplying the pelvis have been illustrated in Chapter 3. Two major nerve pathways carry sensory information from the pelvis; one from the uterus and cervix and the other from the perineum, vulva, and vagina.

The sympathetic pathway carries sensations from the uterus and cervix via the structures indicated here.

Uterus-cervix
↓
via sensory sympathetic nerves
↓
uterine plexus
↓
pelvic plexus
↓
hypogastric plexus
↓
aortic plexus
↓
ventral rami (T_{10}, T_{11}, T_{12})

Sensations from the perineum travel via the pudendal nerve. The pudendal nerve arises from the anterior branches of the second, third, and fourth sacral nerves, which join into a single nerve approximately 0.5 to 1.0 cm. proximal to the ischial spine. The nerve then passes through the greater sciatic foramen; crosses the sacrospinous ligament to the lesser sciatic foramen; enters the pudendal canal medial and posterior to the inferior tip of the spine; and terminates at the second, third, and fourth sacral nerves. Relief of perineal pain may be achieved by blocking the pudendal nerve pathway near the time of delivery (Chapter 13).

Relationship between Type of Discomfort and Stage of Labor

The type of discomfort that a woman experiences will vary with the stage of labor. Table 11–7 summarizes the relationship between these two factors.

Other Physiologic Variables Influencing Discomfort

Several specific variables influence the discomfort that a mother experiences during labor.

The position of the baby makes a difference. Mothers with babies in a posterior position at the beginning of labor tend to have longer, more uncomfortable labors.

The duration of particular stages, as well as the overall duration of labor, is important. The transition stage, as noted above, is usually the most difficult. When transition is prolonged, the labor is felt to be difficult by the mother and by those working with her.

Table 11–7 RELATIONSHIP BETWEEN PAIN AND STAGE OF LABOR

Stage	Source of Discomfort	Pathway	Area of Pain
1	Effacement Dilatation of cervix Contraction of myometrium of uterus	Sensory sympathetic pathway → 10th, 11th, and 12th thoracic nerves and 1st lumbar nerve	Umbilical region Midsacral area Upper thighs
2	Stretching of vagina, vulva, perineum Contraction of myometrium	Sensory fibers of pudendal nerves → 2nd, 3rd, and 4th sacral nerves	Perineum and surrounding structures Urge to bear down
3	Passage of placenta through cervix Contraction of myometrium	Sensory sympathetic pathway→ 10th, 11th and 12th thoracic nerves and 1st lumbar nerve	Umbilical region Midsacral area Upper thighs

SUMMARY

This chapter has examined the physiologic accommodation of both mother and fetus during labor. This knowledge is the basis of nursing assessment of the mother-fetus, which is discussed in Chapter 13.

REFERENCES

1. Friedman, E.: *Labor: Clinical Evaluation and Management*. New York, Appleton-Century-Crofts, 1967.
2. Greenhill, J., and Friedman, E.: *Biological Principles and Modern Practice of Obstetrics*. Philadelphia, W. B. Saunders Co., 1974.
3. Liggins, G. C.: The Foetal Role in the Initiation of Parturition in the Ewe. *In* Wolstenholme, G. E. W., and O'Connor, M. (eds.): *Foetal Anatomy*. London, J. and A. Churchill, Ltd., 1969.
4. Martin, C., and Gingerich, B.: Factors Affecting the Fetal Heart Rate: Genesis of FHR Patterns, *JOGN Nursing*, 5(5): Suppl. 30s, 1976.
5. Milic, A. B., and Adamsons, K.: The Relationship between Anencephaly and Prolonged Pregnancy. *Journal of Obstetrics and Gynecology of the British Commonwealth*, 76:102, 1969.
6. Oxorn, H., and Foote, W.: *Human Labor and Birth*. New York, Appleton-Century-Crofts, 1975.
7. Page, E., Villee, C., and Villee, D.: *Human Reproduction: The Core Content of Obstetrics, Gynecology and Perinatal Medicine*. 2nd edition. Philadelphia, W. B. Saunders Co., 1976.
8. Pareri, J.: Physiological Regulation of Fetal Heart Rate. *JOGN Nursing* 5(5): Suppl. 26s, 1976.
9. Schifri, B. S.: Fetal Heart Rate Patterns Following Epidural Anesthesia and Oxytocin Infusion during Labour. *Journal of Obstetrics and Gynaecology of the British Commonwealth*, 79:332, 1972.

Chapter 12

SOCIAL AND EMOTIONAL CORRELATES OF LABOR

Labor and the birth of a child are universal, a part of every society. In terms of basic physiology, labor is similar for all women; the uterus contracts, the cervix is effaced and dilated, and the baby is expelled.

But the *experience* of labor differs from one society to another and also among women in an individual society. There is a physiologic basis for some differences; when the baby's position is posterior, for example, labor is usually more difficult. Physiologic differences were discussed in Chapter 11.

A significant difference lies in the *meaning of labor* for the society and for the individual mother and her family. A cross-cultural perspective is helpful in this regard. For example, one finds societies in which normal labor is largely nontraumatic, both physically and emotionally. Does this perhaps indicate that this potential may exist in other societies? Perhaps factors that contribute to a relatively easy labor can be identified.

LABOR IN OTHER SOCIETIES: SOME EXAMPLES

Tafel describes a birth in a Tibetan household.

During the night Mrs. Lobzang Dandudschumo gave birth to a son. She did it outside the tent in the goat stall which had no roof but a low protective wall of earth and frozen cow dung, which kept off the worst blasts of the wind. Inside the tent it would have been a few degrees warmer, but the nomad women avoid labor in the cook rooms, for religious reasons. All night long her husband prayed with a few lamas inside the tent, to the accompaniment of kettle drums and trumpets. The temperature during the night went down to −32. The next morning the mother was already busy at the stove in the tent.[18]

McDonald notes that Tibetan peasant mothers " . . . work in the fields up to the time of delivery, seldom resting for more than a couple of days after the child has been born." Moreover, "The Tibetan mother goes through her time of trial practically unassisted, but she seldom has any trouble in childbirth."[13]

Among the Australian aborigines "The actual physical experience in giving birth to a child is so minimized and the social implications of the result of the birth so magnified, that the former melts away into the obscure background before the all-embracing consequences of the latter."[1]

It must be noted in this connection that childbirth among the Australians, as among many aboriginal peoples who are relatively unmixed, is a comparatively light affair for

363

the woman, who is usually up and about her regular duties within a few hours after the delivery of the child. There is no period of confinement before the birth of the child, and there is no period of convalescence afterward, so that the actual experience of birth is by no means the traumatically impressive experience that it generally is for the white woman.[1]

Perhaps the reason that the physical experience of procreation is considered insignificant is that aboriginal beliefs about maternity regard the woman who gives birth as merely acting as a medium through whom the infant is conveyed into the proper moiety and section of the tribe. The conception, prenatal development, and birth of the child are matters completely independent of the mother in every physical sense. No association is recognized between intercourse and pregnancy. It is expected that "The physical act of intercourse between the sexes would have the effect of 'opening up' the womb of the mother, and thus, in the event of a spirit child electing to enter the particular woman it would find ingress easy and everything in order upon its arrival."[1]

The Ifaluk of the central Caroline Islands in the Pacific desire babies ". . . probably more than any other single thing. . . . A couple that does not have children is greatly pitied."[2] There are no midwives among the Ifaluk. The mother delivers her own infant, and although her own mother and her mother's sister are present at the delivery, they only assist if there is some difficulty. During delivery the mother kneels on a mat, catches the baby in her arms, and holds it until the placenta is delivered. She then severs the umbilical cord with a small ocean shell.[2]

Holmberg states that there are also no midwives among the Siriono of Eastern Bolivia, nor is any assistance by friends or relatives given to women in labor under ordinary conditions.[9] When labor pains begin, the mother ties a rope above the hammock in which she will lie to deliver the infant. She loosens the hard ground beneath the hammock with a digging stick and sometimes spreads it with ashes to make it still more soft, for as the baby is born, he will slide through the strings of the hammock to the earth below. Since the hammock is only a few inches above the ground, the fall is not so great as to harm the infant, yet is sufficient to induce breathing. In the births that Holmberg witnessed, all of the infants started to breathe immediately after the shock of birth. In no instance was one slapped to give it life.

It would be a mistake to believe, however, that difficulty in labor occurs only in industrialized societies and that in a more "natural environment" birth is always uncomplicated. Even in those societies in which birth is considered a casual and easy procedure, difficulties may occur. DuBois, commenting on the people of Alor, points out that the society had chosen not to emphasize the difficulties however.[8]

On the Pacific island of Bougainville, birth is considered a very painful experience; it is accompanied by anguished crying. Oliver describes this scene:

> When labor begins, the assisting women warn all boys and men to keep away from the place of birth. As labor pains increase the woman is made to sit in a low bed or log and hold onto a rope tied to an overhead beam or tree; then when birth begins she is encouraged to assist by pulling on the rope. Her mother or sister kneels behind her and massages her with heavy downward motions.[15]

CHANGE IN EMOTIONAL STATUS DURING LABOR

Just as there is variation in emotional response to labor among and within societies, there is also variation as labor progresses. To what extent the reactions described below are physiologically based and to what extent they are affected by social and emotional factors (including institutional and interactional factors) is an important question for future research.

The First Stage

Early in the first stage when the mother enters the hospital, she must cope with a new environment, unfamiliar procedures, and people who are to a large extent strangers to her. She surrenders her clothes and personal belongings. It is little wonder that she may feel that she has lost her identity and been separated from her normal existence—her family and familiar surroundings.

The desire to be in familiar surroundings is one major factor cited by women who opt for home birth (Chapter 23). All of us feel more in control when surroundings are familiar. When we are on someone else's "turf," we feel that they are in control, and when we feel we are losing control, we begin to lose self-esteem as well. As our self-esteem falls, we often become either aggressive because of our frustration or passive and dependent.

This sequence of feelings is not peculiar to labor; it affects all hospitalized patients as well as all persons at various stages of life. Much of our nursing intervention (Chapter 13) is directed toward helping the mother to cope and preventing this loss of control.

As the first stage progresses, mothers either cope or begin to lose control. For all mothers there is some loss of physiologic control that results in involuntary voiding or defecation.

Some mothers become increasingly passive as labor progresses. They feel they cannot help themselves and make statements such as "Please help me" or "Please give me something" or "Someone help me." Other mothers are able to retain control, or to regain control if it is briefly lost. Preparation appears to be a major factor in differentiating those mothers who move toward passive dependence from those who remain active participants in their own labor.

As nurses, we need to identify ways, both through personal observations and research, in which our intervention encourages maternal behavior to be either active or passive.

The Second Stage

During the second stage, emotions of individual mothers range from the mother who finds birth an exhilarating experience comparable to orgasm (see sexuality, below) to the mother who is unable to participate and sees herself as being "delivered" (recognizing that there are instances in which physiologic circumstances will not permit her active participation, discussed in Chapter 14).

The woman who is an active participant often expresses enjoyment of "pushing"; the work may be hard, but there are feelings of accomplishment, such as those that a runner or a swimmer feels after a good race.

The Third and Fourth Stages

The emotional components of the third and fourth stages are mediated by the events of the first and second stages, as well as by other factors discussed in this chapter.

Active participation usually leads to joy and heightened self-esteem for both mother and father—a "look what we did" kind of pride that is a sound basis for the completion of attachment. Lang[11] describes a feeling of elation following birth; Dick-Read[7] uses the term ecstasy; Klaus and Kennell[10] coin a term *ekstasis*.

Lang observed elation and attachment to the baby in others who observed the birth (friends and relatives present at home delivery). Klaus and Kennell suggest that in generations past, when maternal mortality was high, the attachment of observers (probably primarily women who were relatives or close friends) served the useful function of providing a substitute mother should the mother die.

Loss of self-esteem occurs if the mother and/or father feels that one of them behaved in an unacceptable manner. If their expectations of the labor or delivery were not fulfilled, this too will diminish self-esteem. These expectations may have been unrealistic (e.g., the mother who feels she has "failed" because she required medication) or may have been impossible because of unforeseen factors (e.g., the need for an unanticipated cesarean section because of difficult labor). Loss of self-esteem is particularly evident when the child is not full term or has a congenital abnormality (Chapter 22).

The psychologic work following delivery involves:

1. Recognizing the reality of the baby.

2. Integrating the birth experience into one's total life experience.

3. Furthering the attachment process.

Recognizing the Reality of the Baby. How frequently we hear immediately following the baby's birth "I can't believe he's really here" and even "Is he real?" As parents see and touch their baby, his reality, not just as a living baby but as a unique person, begins to emerge. Parents search for a characteristic that identifies him as a member of their family—a nose like his father's, dark hair like his mother's, or short little fingers like a sibling's.

Integrating the Birth Experience. During the fourth stage and again and again during the next days and weeks, the mother will talk about her labor to nearly anyone who will listen (just as patients often review a surgical experience with anyone who is available). This need to talk is an important concept, and a time must be provided for the mother to meet this need. Although friends and relatives are an important audience, a professional nurse as a listener is important as well, to reassure her that she did a good job during labor and to answer questions that she may have about her labor or delivery experience.

Furthering the Attachment Process. The first stages of the attachment process (planning, confirming, and accepting the pregnancy; perceiving fetal movement; and accepting the fetus as an individual) were described in Chapter 7.

Birth, followed by seeing and touching the baby, furthers attachment at the time of delivery. The concept of the fourth stage of labor as a sensitive period, during which parents and infants are bound together in complex ways, is discussed in Chapters 15 and 20.

SEXUALITY, LABOR, AND BIRTH

Niles Newton has suggested that labor and birth (and lactation as well) are all acts of female sexuality, closely interrelated both physiologically and psychologically.[14] At least three shared characteristics are the basis for this interrelationship.

First, labor, birth, and lactation are all influenced closely by related neurohormonal reflexes. Oxytocin is one of the substances involved, and probably one of the most significant. Second, environmental stimuli are highly important to each act. Interruption or fear of interruption, distracting sounds, and the like are inhibiting factors in the early stages of coitus, labor, and breast-feeding. Later on, as the woman becomes more involved, she becomes less aware of sensory stimuli. And third, each act is related to caretaking behavior.

Similarities between coitus and labor/delivery are summarized by Newton in Table 12–1.

DIFFICULTY DURING LABOR: PSYCHOSOCIAL CORRELATES

Some studies suggest a possible interrelationship between difficulties during labor and delivery and sociocultural and/or psychologic factors.

Davids and associates[6] predicted that women who show more signs of maladjustment during pregnancy would have more difficulties and complications in the delivery room and that women with difficult or complicated delivery would be more maladjusted than women with normal delivery.

In his study 48 women were given psychologic tests during their pregnancies. Twenty of the women were again tested postpartum. In addition, the degree of physical difficulty during each labor was classified on the basis of medical observations and records in the delivery room. Findings are tabulated in Table 12–2.

Crawford also studied relationships between anxiety and uterine dysfunction.[5] Her study included 504 clinic patients, over half of whom were nonwhite and one-third of whom chose a Spanish questionnaire to complete rather than one in English. Her instruments were a questionnaire on symptoms of muscle tension, completed by the patient at the time of admission to the labor room; an evaluation of emotional tension made by the admitting nurse in the labor room; and data from the patient's chart.

Crawford's major hypothesis ". . . that women who reported more than average symptoms of muscle tension during pregnancy and demonstrated at the beginning of labor more than average physiological and behavioral signs associated with anxiety would develop physiological disturbance related to uterine dysfunction" was confirmed. The infants of these same women also had a greater tendency to develop physiologic disturbances related to hypoxia.

Rosengren questioned the relationship between the tendency to take the sick role during pregnancy (Chapter 7) and subsequent difficulty during labor and delivery.[17] In a study of 94 expectant mothers (62 clinic patients and 32 private patients) Rosengren selected two major indices as criteria of delivery room difficulty:

1. Length of labor.
2. Evidence of gross complications (e.g., the use of forceps, complications involving the cord, abnormal fetal heart rate, and so on).

The women were also divided according to two bases:

1. Women with normal labor and delivery versus those with deliveries evidencing some kind of gross abnormality.
2. Women who had taken the sick role during pregnancy versus those who did not.

Rosengren's findings in this study suggest that the ". . . more a woman regarded herself as 'ill' during pregnancy the greater was the likelihood of a longer period of active labor."[17] He also found a trend toward longer labor in women of lower socioeconomic class, although not one he considered statistically significant. This might be expected in view of his previous findings

Table 12–1 SIMILARITIES BETWEEN CHILDBIRTH AND SEXUAL EXCITEMENT*

Undisturbed, Undrugged Childbirth	Sexual Excitement and Orgasm
Breathing: During early contractions, breathing becomes deeper. Second stage of labor brings deep breathing with breath holding.	During early stages of arousal, breathing becomes faster and deeper. As orgasm approaches, breathing may be interrupted.
Vocalization: Tendency to make noises, grunts, especially in second stage of labor.	Tendency to make gasping, sucking noises as orgasm nears.
Facial expression: As birth climax approaches, the face gets an intense, strained look: observers often assume the woman is suffering great pain.	As orgasm approaches, the face gets what Kinsey et al. call a "tortured expression": mouth open, eyes glassy, muscles tense.
The uterus: The upper segment of the uterus contracts rhythmically.	The upper segment of the uterus contracts rhythmically.
The cervix: Mucus plug from opening (os) of cervix loosens.	Cervical secretion may loosen mucus plug, thus opening cervix for sperm.
Abdominal muscles: Contract periodically in second stage of labor; a strong urge to bear down develops as delivery approaches.	Abdominal muscles contract periodically during sexual excitement.
Position: Woman flat on her back, legs bent and wide apart.	Typically, the "missionary position" (woman on her back, legs wide apart).

that the tendency to take the sick role during pregnancy varied inversely with socioeconomic class.

Rosengren also looked at the relationship between the mother and the physician. He concluded that:

Women who defined pregnancy as illness who were attended by a doctor who did not so define pregnancy tended to have significantly longer labor times than did women defining pregnancy in basically the same terms as did their doctors. The reverse also held; women who did not define pregnancy as illness who were attended by an obstetrician who did, tended to have longer periods of active labor than did women who had been involved in a doctor-patient relationship in which both individuals viewed pregnancy as an 'illness'. In fact, the mean

labor time of the doctor-patient role conflict subjects was over twice as long as that of the women whose doctor's perception of pregnancy was essentially the same as their own.[17]

Race as an independent variable in measuring the differential response to the pain experience of women in childbirth was investigated by Winsberg and Greenlick[19] in a study of 365 women (207 white; 158 black). Their findings were based on evaluations by obstetric interns and nurses in relation to cooperation, degree of pain, and response to pain. The findings indicated no difference between white and black patients of similar social

Table 12–1   SIMILARITIES BETWEEN CHILDBIRTH AND SEXUAL EXCITEMENT
(*Continued*)

Undisturbed, Undrugged Childbirth	Sexual Excitement and Orgasm
Central nervous system: Woman tends to become uninhibited, particularly as baby descends the birth canal. Veneers of conventional behavior disappear in later stages of labor.	Inhibitions and psychic blocks are relieved and often eliminated as orgasm nears.
Strength and flexibility: Delivery of the baby through the narrow passage requires unusual strength and body expansion.	Unusual muscular strength often develops. Many persons become capable of bending and distorting their bodies in ways they could not otherwise do.
Sensory perception: During labor the vulva becomes anesthetized with full dilation so that the woman often must be told of the emergence of the baby's head.	The whole body of the sexually aroused person becomes increasingly insensitive—even to sharp blows and severe injury.
There is a tendency to become oblivious to surroundings as delivery approaches. Amnesia develops. Suddenly, delivery complete, the woman becomes wide awake.	As orgasm approaches, there is a tendency to become oblivious to surroundings. There is loss of sensory perceptions, sometimes leading to moments of unconsciousness. After orgasm there is a sudden return of sensory acuity.
Emotional response: After birth, there is a flood of joyful emotion, which Dick-Read describes as "complete and careless ecstasy."	After coital orgasm there is a strong feeling of well-being in most persons.

*Newton: *Psychology Today,* July, 1971.

Table 12–2   SOME DIFFERENCES BETWEEN WOMEN WITH NORMAL AND
ABNORMAL DELIVERIES*

Criteria	Women with Normal Deliveries	Women with Abnormal Deliveries
Age	No significant difference in mean age	
Time in labor	Mean: 7.3 hours	Mean: 16.8 hours
I.Q.	During pregnancy: 102 Postpartum: 107	During pregnancy: 101 Postpartum: 91
Manifest anxiety score	During pregnancy: 16.5 (range: 8–26) Postpartum: 15	During pregnancy: 23.5 (range: 14–37) Postpartum: 18.5
Self-ratings		Less happy, more alienated; difference not statistically significant

*Davids, DeVault, and Talmadge: *Psychosomatic Medicine,* 23:93, 1961.

class on any of the three evaluations. Age and parity were found to be the significant factors influencing response to pain.

ANXIETY AND DIFFICULT LABOR

The relationship between anxiety and pain has been mentioned previously. If a woman customarily responds to anxiety with sympathomimetic symptoms, learned associations result. The symptoms themselves can then "elicit and reinforce further anxiety producing a self-generating, spiraling anxiety reaction."[5]

A variety of physiologic changes are initiated by the response of the sympathetic division of the autonomic nervous system—changes in heart rate; the constriction of blood vessels, other than coronary vessels, which dilate; decrease in gastrointestinal motility, and so on. The greater the anxiety, the more severe the sympathetic nervous system response is likely to be.

At the time of labor such response can inhibit uterine muscle contractions and/or constrict blood vessels, with resultant decreases in the oxygen supply to the fetus. In this latter relationship Crawford[5] has found that Apgar scores (Chapter 15) of infants whose mothers exhibited a high degree of anxiety were lower than those of infants whose mothers exhibited less anxiety (the higher the Apgar score, the healthier the infant).

PROBLEMS IN ASSESSMENT OF DISCOMFORT

One significant factor, both in cross-cultural comparisons and in comparing the experiences of women in our own society, is that it is difficult for an observer to evaluate objectively the level of discomfort experienced by another individual. This is particularly true when observer and observed do not share the same cultural heritage. As Zborowski[20] has demonstrated, people respond to discomfort in many different ways, some by "keeping a stiff upper lip," some by anguished cries, and some by silent tears. In caring for mothers during labor, as in caring for patients in many other situations, this is a basic concept of the assessment process.

VARIABLES AFFECTING ANXIETY DURING LABOR

Just as anxiety appears to be a part of pregnancy for all women, so too is anxiety a common denominator of labor. A number of factors influence the level of anxiety.

Customary Emotional Tone. Some individuals (men and women) are more anxious about every facet of their lives than are others. If one customarily feels positive about and in control of new situations, labor will not pose the threat that it does for the woman who feels "controlled by" and therefore helpless as she approaches an unknown experience.

Feelings about Femininity and Mothering. The birth of a baby is ultimately a feminine act. For the mother who has difficulty with her feminine identity, labor and birth may seem a difficult burden.

Attitude toward this Pregnancy. A resented pregnancy may mean that labor is resented as well. As one approaches the time for delivery of a baby, it is difficult to acknowledge that one still resents the fact of being pregnant. The need to express this resentment, and the counsel that resentment of a pregnancy does not necessarily mean rejection of the baby, is a significant part of nursing intervention.

Perception of Her Mother's Childbirth Experience. A woman's perception of her mother's childbirth experience influences her anxiety level in anticipation of labor and delivery, but not her evaluation of the actual delivery.[12] It would seem, therefore, worthwhile to assess the mother's perception of her own mother's labor experience prior to the time of labor and to include that information in her record.

Intensity of Communication about Childbirth Between Mother and Daughter. Levy and McGee report that the intensity of communication about childbirth between a mother and her daughter influences the daughter's feelings about childbirth (Table 12–3).

Levy and McGee postulated that those women who heard only highly favorable comments were unprepared for the discomfort that may accompany labor and thus were disappointed in their experience. This concept seems important for nurses who care for prenatal patients, i.e., stressing only the positive aspects of labor may lead to frustration and a negative experience.

The mother who receives no communication may also be unprepared for the labor experience.

An intensely negative communication may be difficult to overcome, although we believe that assessment early in pregnancy of whether such communication occurred and subsequent "appropriate" intervention might be possible. (Certainly this is an area for nursing research.)

Preparation for Labor. Few nurses who care for patients during labor fail to notice that preparation for labor does influence the level of anxiety for many women. The problem of raising unrealistic expectations, mentioned above and at other places in this text, along with the importance of assessment of individual needs and individualization of prenatal preparation, must guide preparation of parents for labor.

Physical Progress during Labor. Just as anxiety can influence the physical course of labor, physical factors (breech presentation, posterior position) can influence emotions. When labor is long and/or difficult or when there is concern for the well-being of the mother or fetus because of unusual circumstances, a heightened level of anxiety is inevitable.

COMPANIONSHIP DURING LABOR: MOTHER AND FATHER TOGETHER

During the past decade many couples have come to share the experience of labor and delivery. In the follow-

Table 12–3   EFFECT OF MATERNAL COMMUNICATION ON DAUGHTER'S EVALUATION OF HER OWN CHILDBIRTH

Communication from Mother to Daughter	Daughter's Evaluation of her Own Childbirth
Highly favorable	Negative
Highly unfavorable	Negative
No communication	Negative
Moderate communication	Positive

ing chapter specific ways in which couples can work together and along with the professional team are described. What has this experience meant to couples? Here are some responses in a study by Cook.[4]

The responses from mothers included:

"I didn't feel alone at all."

"My husband had not planned to be with me during labor and changed his mind at the last minute. Therefore his support during labor was even more meaningful."

"I could not have gone through labor without him there. He encouraged me, marked off time for me, and held my hand through it all. He was also able to help me when I forgot to breathe the correct way at particular times. He would remind me of things we learned in our course. But most of all, he was a companion; a comforter who assured me that *we* would make it" (italics mine).

"Our first child was the 'family' approach—the second child was born without father in attendance, due to hospital policy. I was frantic toward the end of labor—required more medication. With the first it was a beautiful experience; the second, a horrible one."

"We have always been a close twosome. This is our first child after nearly ten years of marriage. I wouldn't think of doing anything of such great moment without him."

The responses from fathers included:

"It was the most marvelous experience of my life. Susan and I have always done everything together. When we first became pregnant, I began to feel a little "left out" because this was something Susan would *have* to do on her own. But Lamaze changed that! We began the course—mainly for information—and we got very excited about doing this together. I visited Susan's doctor, the hospital, and all the classes. I feel closer to Susan than ever and love our son in a way that I don't think would have been possible without Lamaze."

"I was 'in the know' at all times—no wondering what was going on in some solarium. That would've driven me crazy."

"I was benefited in a way no one can understand except a father who has witnessed the birth of his child . . . beyond definition."

"I was somewhat afraid for some reason even though I thought we were prepared. Now after going through the experience I'm glad I did because I would still wonder about it if I hadn't."

One father, who was with his wife during labor but was not allowed to be present in the delivery room said, "The time they shoved me out for delivery was the worst time of all—it seemed forever."

A father who had no prior preparation but was allowed to be with his wife during labor said, "I didn't have any preparation, and so I felt really useless, except to be there and let Jenny squeeze my hand, but it left a real impact on me. I wouldn't have it any other way than to be with her."

Not every father or every mother chooses to share the experience of labor and birth, or is able to. Cultural values, as noted earlier, are one factor that will influence individual decisions. The demands of the father's job, noninvolvement between mother and father, and occasionally (although with increasing rarity) hospital policy may separate couples. Nevertheless, for many couples, being together offers many advantages and makes labor a truly special time.

SUMMARY

Throughout labor the physiologic process is influenced by cultural and individual emotional factors. These factors will be explored further as we examine nursing intervention for normal and high risk mothers and fathers.

REFERENCES

1. Ashley-Montagu, M.: *Coming Into Being Among the Australian Aborigines.* London, George Routledge and Sons, 1937.
2. Burrows, E., and Spiro, M.: *An Atoll Culture: Ethnography of the Ifaluk in the Central Carolines.* New Haven, Conn., Human Relations Area Files, 1957.

3. Cassidy, J.: A Nurse Looks at Childbirth Anxiety. *JOGN, 3*:52, 1974

4. Cook, M.: Father-Participation in Childbirth: A Study Presenting its Effectiveness. Unpublished paper. 1973.

5. Crawford, M.: Physiological and Behavioral Cues to Disturbances in Childbirth. *In: ANA Clinical Sessions.* New York, Appleton-Century-Crofts, 1968.

6. Davids, A., DeVault, S., and Talmadge, M.: Psychological Study of Emotional Factors in Pregnancy: A Preliminary Report. *Psychosomatic Medicine, 23*:93, 1961.

7. Dick-Read, G.: *Childbirth Without Fear.* 2nd edition. New York, Harper and Row Book Co., 1953.

8. DuBois, C.: *The People of Alor.* Minneapolis, The University of Minnesota Press, 1944.

9. Holmberg, A.: *Nomads of the Long Bow.* New York, The Natural History Press, 1969.

10. Klaus, M., and Kennell, J.: *Maternal-Infant Bonding.* St. Louis, The C. V. Mosby Co., 1976.

11. Lang, R.: Personal communication. *Cited in* Klaus, M., and Kennell, J.: *Maternal-Infant Bonding.* St. Louis, The C. V. Mosby Co., 1976.

12. Levy, J., and McGee, M.: Childbirth as Crisis: A Test of Janis's Theory of Communication and Stress Resolution. *Journal of Personality and Social Psychology, 31*:171, 1975.

13. McDonald, D.: *The Land of the Lama.* London, Seeley, Service and Company, Ltd., 1929 (Human Relations Area Files.)

14. Newton, N.: Trebly Sensuous Woman. *Psychology Today,* July, 1971, p. 68.

15. Oliver, D.: *A Solomon Island Society: Kinship and Leadership Among the Siuai of Bougainville.* Cambridge, Harvard University Press, 1955.

16. Rising, S.: The Fourth Stage of Labor: Family Integration. *American Journal of Nursing, 74*:870, 1974.

17. Rosengren, W.: Some Social Psychological Aspects of Delivery Room Difficulties. *Journal of Nervous and Mental Diseases, 132*:515, 1961.

18. Tafel, A.: *My Tibetan Trip.* Stuttgart, Germany, Union Deutsche Vertagegesellscheft, 1914.

19. Winsberg, B., and Greenlick, M.: Pain Response in Negro and White Obstetrical Patients. *Journal of Health and Social Behavior, 8*:220, 1967.

20. Zborowski, M.: Cultural Components in Response to Pain. *In* Apple, D. (ed.): *Sociological Studies of Health and Sickness.* New York, McGraw Hill Book Co., 1960.

Chapter 13

CARING FOR THE INTRAPARTUM FAMILY

A man and woman arrive at the door of the labor/delivery suite. The woman says she is in labor. The next hours will be among the most significant in their lives and in the life of the baby who is to be born. Our nursing care during these hours may provide the crucial difference between a physically and emotionally satisfying experience coupled with the delivery of a healthy infant or an experience long remembered with sadness and dissatisfaction. In the best of worlds, a nurse who has shared the prenatal period with the woman and her family will also be able to share labor with them.

The goals of nursing intervention during labor are to make the occasion as safe; as comfortable; and as satisfying, physically and emotionally, as possible. In order to do this, we must:

1. Assess the physiologic status of the mother and fetus throughout the four stages of labor.

2. Assess the emotional status of the mother and whoever accompanies her—father, friend, or other companion—throughout the four stages of labor.

3. Plan and intervene to:
   a. Facilitate the course of labor.
   b. Help the mother and her companion to cope with labor.
   c. Facilitate beginning parenting in the period immediately following delivery.

WHO ENTERS THE LABOR/DELIVERY SUITE?

Until the past decade, most labor/delivery suites were closed to all but the mother and the hospital personnel who attended her. The issue of fathers in the delivery room was hotly debated.

As more couples began preparing for childbirth, pressure was placed on hospitals to allow husbands to accompany their wives in order to support them and participate with them in labor and delivery. In many hospitals, although not in every one, husbands are today welcomed participants.

What about the woman who isn't married? What about the woman who does not wish to have her husband with her or whose husband is unable to be with her? Should every woman be able to have the companion of her choice

374

with her? Or should she, if she chooses, come alone?

We believe the choice should be hers, and an increasing number of hospitals share this belief. And so, in this text, even though we may use the word "husband," or "father," the same consideration should be given to anyone who accompanies the mother. Although some institutions require attendance at prenatal classes before the husband or other companion may enter the labor room, others place no prohibitions.

In a few labor settings, friends and siblings are now allowed to be present if the mother wishes (Chapter 23).

FIRST CONTACT

The mother entering the hospital for delivery is, understandably, excited and anxious about the coming hours. Her husband, or companion, may be supportive or, often, even more anxious than she. Although there will be wide individual variations in the levels of anxiety, these feelings will affect even basic physiologic assessment, such as assessment of blood pressure and pulse, for example. Our skill in enabling the mother, and her companion, to relax will benefit both her initial assessment and her entire course of labor.

Our actions, as much as our words, can convey interest in the individual couple. If we appear hurried and overwhelmed (and labor room nurses often *are* very rushed, with many demands made upon them), the anxiety of patients is intensified

Without compromising the tasks essential to initial assessment, we can make each woman/couple feel welcomed, make the woman feel that we will support her throughout her labor, and make this day a significant one for her/them.

INITIAL ASSESSMENT OF THE MOTHER

Initial assessment involves:

1. Reviewing the prenatal record.

2. Eliciting specific information from the mother about the course of this labor.

3. Assessing the physiologic status of the mother.

Reviewing the Prenatal Record

Prenatal records, whether from a physician's office or from a clinic, should be available in the labor suite. From the moment a woman is admitted, it is essential to know if there are any factors in her history that require special physical and/or emotional attention. High risk factors affecting labor and delivery and the care of mothers with these conditions are discussed in Chapter 14.

Even if the current pregnancy has apparently been normal in every way, a woman who has had complications during a previous labor will have memories that come rushing back to her, both throughout the pregnancy and particularly at the time of labor. We must know about these previous experiences in order to understand her behavior during this labor. For example, a mother whose fetus died during labor in a previous pregnancy is likely to appear very anxious about variations in fetal heart rate. If the present labor is progressing satisfactorily, her level of anxiety may seem inappropriate until one recognizes its true basis.

Additional essential information in the prenatal record includes the expected date of confinement (EDC) and the number of previous pregnancies and deliveries.

Eliciting Specific Information

The answers to specific questions about the course of this labor must be obtained and recorded in the woman's record.

1. When did contractions begin?

2. How often do contractions occur?

3. How long do contractions last?

4. Have the membranes (bag of waters) ruptured?

5. Has there been any bleeding?

6. When did you last eat?

If the prenatal record is not immediately available, questions about the EDC and the number of pregnancies must be asked.

Assessing the Physiologic Status

The mother usually changes into a hospital gown and is put to bed for initial assessment. Afterward, depending on her condition and on hospital policy, she may be allowed out of bed (see below).

Evaluation of general physical status includes checking the mother's:

1. Weight.

2. Vital signs (temperature, pulse, respiration, blood pressure).

3. General physical condition, including examination by a physician or a nurse-midwife, with special attention to cardiac and respiratory evaluation.

4. Blood and urine for laboratory examination.

The progress of labor is evaluated in relation to:

1. Frequency, duration, and intensity of uterine contractions (Chapter 11).

2. Vaginal examination to determine effacement and dilatation (below).

The status of the fetus is evaluated by:

1. Auscultation of fetal heart rate (below).

2. Abdominal palpation and vaginal examination to determine lie, presentation, and position (Chapter 11).

Vaginal Examination. Most assessment of effacement and dilatation is today done by vaginal examination, rather than by rectal examination, which was formerly used.

With a sterile glove on the examining hand, the labia are widely separated to avoid contamination, the lubricated index and second fingers are inserted into the vagina until they touch the cervix (Fig. 13-1). From the vaginal examination, one hopes to determine:

1. The degree of effacement.

2. The degree of dilatation.

3. Confirmation of the presenting part (as previously determined by Leopold's maneuvers).

4. Fetal position.

5. Fetal station.

Mothers are anxious for a report of the findings; the report should be in positive terms if there is anything positive to state.

The importance of sterile technique cannot be overemphasized. Vaginal examination should not be done if there is fresh bleeding because this may indicate a placenta previa (Chapter 10).

Rectal Examination. Rectal examination is not considered as accurate as vaginal examination, but it is still a matter of policy in some institutions. A clean but not sterile glove is worn for rectal examination. The lubricated index finger is gently inserted and the anterior wall of the rectum palpated until the cervix can be felt (Figs. 13-2 and 13-3).

Continuing Physiologic Assessment

Once baseline data are obtained, continuing physiologic assessment of the mother during the first stage of labor includes determination of:

1. Vital signs (temperature, pulse, respiration, blood pressure).

2. Frequency, duration, and intensity of contractions.

Figure 13–1	Vaginal examination. *A*, Method of making vaginal examination using sterile gloves. The labia are spread widely so that the examining fingers may be inserted without touching surrounding vulvar structures. Care must be exercised to avoid touching the anus. *B*, Vaginal examination with fingers inserted, wrist straight, and elbow sunk, to allow fingertips to point toward umbilicus. (From Greenhill and Friedman: *Biological Principles and Modern Practice of Obstetrics.* Philadelphia, W. B. Saunders Co., 1974.)

Figure 13–2   Ideal way of making a rectal examination. The introitus or the vulva must not be touched with the thumb. (From Greenhill and Friedman: *Biological Principles and Modern Practice of Obstetrics*. Philadelphia, W. B. Saunders Co., 1974.)

3. Progress of effacement and dilatation.

The progress of the fetus through the birth canal and the well-being of the fetus are also assessed on a continuing basis.

ASSESSMENT OF EMOTIONAL STATE

Mothers and fathers arrive, as noted above, excited and often anxious. Some become increasingly tense and nervous during admission activities, especially those women or couples who have had no preparation for labor other than the tales of their family and ac-

quaintances. In a totally different environment surrounded by strangers, they find themselves unable to cope.

It is not unusual for concerns other than the labor per se to be an additional source of anxiety. Perhaps the woman has not yet made plans to integrate the baby into her life. Perhaps there is difficulty with her marriage. For some women the reality of the coming baby is denied until the time of labor, when it can no longer be ignored.

If there are other children in the family, the parents may be concerned about their well-being at the moment, as well as their future reaction to the baby.

Couples well prepared for labor

Figure 13–3 Lateral view of rectal examination showing the technique for palpating the cervical dilatation and station through the rectovaginal wall. The thumb here is precariously close to the introitus. (From Greenhill and Friedman: *Biological Principles and Modern Practice of Obstetrics.* Philadelphia, W. B. Saunders Co., 1974.)

may seem confident as they begin previously practiced breathing patterns.

Emotional status should be noted in the record on admission and should be assessed and recorded on a continuing basis throughout labor.

In our observations we must not overlook the status (physical and emotional) of the father or other individual who accompanies the mother. It is often said that there are two patients to be cared for during labor, the mother and the fetus, but there are actually three. In addition, we need to be aware of the father. Is he tense? Is he fatigued? Do mother and father work together as a team, or do they appear to be at cross-purposes?

As labor progresses, most fathers need an occasional break—to go to the bathroom, to have something to eat. Yet a man may feel guilty about asking someone to stay with his wife while he "takes a break," since obviously there is no break for her. Our assessment of his needs, as well as hers, thus becomes part of the nursing care of this family.

ASSESSING FETAL WELL-BEING DURING LABOR

The most common assessment of fetal well-being is by observation of fetal heart rate. This assessment is for all mother-fetus pairs.

As labor progresses, or fails to progress, there may be a need for further assessment: fetal scalp sampling, X-ray studies, or ultrasound examination.

ASSESSING FETAL HEART RATE

The norms for and types of fetal heart rate have been discussed in Chapter 8. Heart rate is monitored intermittently by stethoscope and continuously by external or internal monitor. No one method is best under every circumstance.

Intermittent Auscultation by Stethoscope or Fetoscope

Auscultation by stethoscope or fetoscope is the traditional method of monitoring fetal heart rate, and is still the most widely used. It allows the mother to be up and about between contractions and to change her position easily. It is not frightening to mothers, as monitoring devices may be. Those couples and professionals who emphasize labor as a natural physiologic process feel that intermittent monitoring is satisfactory for the large numbers of mothers with normal labors. Some mothers resent continuous monitoring not merely because it is confining but on the philosophic basis that it focuses on abnormality rather than a normal, emotionally satisfying labor.

Intermittent monitoring does have the disadvantage of detecting only marked deviations from normal fetal heart rate. Moreover, the heart rate is often difficult to hear during a contraction, the most significant period.

The point at which fetal heart rate is best heard by fetoscope varies with the lie, presentation, and position of the fetus. Not surprisingly, tones are heard best in the area of the fetal chest or back. Figure 13–4 illustrates the approximate location of the fetal heart in several positions.

If the fetal heart rate appears to be 70 to 80 beats per minute, check to see if it is synchronous with the mother's pulse rate. The sound of the *uterine bruit,* the passage of blood through uterine blood vessels, is sometimes mistaken for the fetal heart rate.

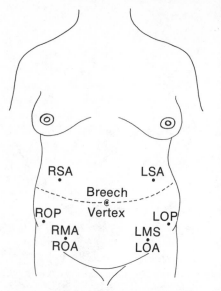

Figure 13–4 The position at which the fetal heart rate may be heard in relation to the fetal position.

Blood flowing through the umbilical arteries makes a sound called the *funic souffle*. The funic souffle is synchronous with the fetal heart rate.

When listening to the fetal heart, the rate and rhythm are assessed and recorded between contractions to ascertain the baseline rate, as well as during a contraction. The rate will usually fall during the contraction (Chapter 11; see also below) but should return to the baseline within 20 to 30 seconds following the contraction.

Fetal heart rate is checked at least every 30 minutes during early labor, at least every 15 minutes during the transition phase of the first stage, and every 5 minutes at the beginning of the second stage.

Continuous Monitoring of Fetal Heart Rate

Continuous monitoring of fetal heart rate (FHR) with simultaneous recording of uterine contractions is widely practiced today. Some professionals, both nurses and physicians, feel that it is desirable to monitor every mother during labor. Others feel that although monitoring offers obvious advantages for certain mothers—those who have recognized high risk conditions, those who show evidence of fetal distress, and perhaps all those who are primigravidas—there is no need to monitor all mothers.

For although the advantages of monitoring are obvious (the nurse or physician is continually aware of the pattern of fetal heart rate and uterine contractions, and thus variations from normal are readily recognized), there are potential disadvantages.

One disadvantage is in the way that the monitor is used. If we walk into the room and look at the monitor but not at the mother (and father), the monitor can be a barrier to good care rather than a way of enhancing care. This, of course, is a disadvantage over which nurses have control. Monitors *do not* reduce the number of nurses required to care for mothers in labor, although they may change the way in which nurses use their time (more time for coaching and support; less time for auscultation of fetal heart rate). Fathers, too, sometimes become so entranced with watching the monitor that they forget their coaching role.

Monitoring usually requires the mother to stay in bed, which may seem a disadvantage to some mothers and professionals. With external monitoring, position changes are more difficult, although this is not a problem with internal monitoring.

For some couples, and for some nurses, the *idea* of fetal monitoring conflicts with the idea of birth as a natural process.

Dulock and Herron[6] interviewed 71 women (36 primigravidas and 35 multiparas) concerning their knowledge of and attitudes toward fetal monitoring. In their group, only 21 per cent of the women came to labor without a prior knowledge of monitoring. Childbirth classes were the source of information for 38 per cent, the prenatal clinic for 14 per cent, and an antenatal tour of the maternity unit for 11 per cent. Previous labor experience, friends, or the media were the resource for 16 per cent. Thus for 63 per cent, health professionals were the source of information, underscoring the importance of our own attitude in the formation of mothers' attitudes.

The authors then asked the women about their initial feelings concerning monitoring, both before and after an explanation was given. Their results are summarized in Table 13–1.

Thirty-one of the 71 women initially interviewed by Dulock and Herron were monitored during delivery and were subsequently interviewed on the second or third postpartum day. Seventy-seven per cent (24 women) made some positive comments. Monitoring was helpful to these women in:

1. Anticipating a contraction and thus beginning controlled breathing and relaxation techniques early.

Table 13–1 PREDELIVERY REACTIONS TO FHR MONITORING AMONG 71 WOMEN BEFORE AND AFTER EXPLANATION OF MONITORING*

| | Before | | After | |
	No.	%	No.	%
Curious	28	39	15	21
Fearful	14	20	10	14
Secure	6	8	23	32
Intrusive	3	5	3	5
Impersonal	2	3	1	2
No response	18	25	19	26

*Dulock and Herron: *JOGN*, 5 (Suppl.) 69s, September–October, 1976.

2. Knowing when the peak of the contraction had passed.

3. Coordinating "pushing" with the peak of the contraction during the second stage.

4. Feeling secure that the baby's heart was beating.

5. Feeling that should something "go wrong" it would be noted immediately.

Seventy per cent (22) of the 31 women made some negative comments (obviously most women had some positive and some negative feelings). Negative comments centered on:

1. The discomfort and immobility of external belts.

2. The discomfort and feeling of "invasion" in the insertion of the internal monitor.

Total postdelivery response was reported as positive by 85 per cent; of these same 31 women, only 39 per cent had felt positively about monitoring before delivery. The common experience of the women who felt neutral about monitoring following delivery was a long, difficult labor or an unexpected cesarean section. No woman in this group reported feeling negative about monitoring following delivery (Table 13–2).

Table 13–2 COMPARISON OF BASIC ATTITUDES TOWARD MONITORING PRE- AND POSTDELIVERY AMONG 31 WOMEN WHOSE LABORS WERE MONITORED*

	Predelivery		Postdelivery	
	No.	%	No.	%
Positive	12	39	26	85
Neutral	9	29	5	15
Negative	3	10	0	0
No comment	7	22	0	0

*Dulock and Herron: *JOGN*, 5 (Suppl.) 70s, September–October, 1976.

Although we cannot generalize on the basis of such a small sample, this study both points the way for future studies and suggests that:

1. The nurse's own attitudes are important.

2. Explanations are important.

3. The mother's attitudes following delivery are more positive than their attitudes prior to delivery.

Four methods of continuous fetal heart rate monitoring are by phonocardiogram, abdominal wall electrocardiogram, Doppler ultrasound, and scalp electrode (Table 13–3). The first three methods are indirect, i.e., the fetus is monitored through the abdominal wall. In the fourth method, an electrode is attached directly to the fetal scalp; this is possible only after the membranes have ruptured.

Phonocardiogram. The *phonocardiogram* is a microphone that picks up the fetal heart sounds. However, it also picks up other sounds, including any sounds that the mother makes when she moves. These sounds make the noise level impractical for labor. The phonocardiogram is valuable in evaluating the fetus prior to labor, however.

If the fetal heart rate is very slow, it may be doubled by phonocardiogram; a very rapid rate may be halved. This is because no fetal monitor currently available can count rates slower than 30 to 60 beats per minute or more rapid than 240 to 250 beats per minute.

Abdominal Wall Electrocardiogram. An *abdominal wall electrocardiogram* is recorded with electrodes placed on the mother's abdomen. Both the maternal QRS complex and P waves and the fetal QRS complex are recorded. Usually the maternal QRS complex is larger and can be identified. Each brand of abdominal electrocardiogram monitor offers solutions for separating maternal and fetal patterns; more solu-

Table 13–3   METHODS FOR CONTINUOUS MONITORING OF FETAL HEART RATE

Indirect/Direct	Method	Description	When Used	Advantages	Disadvantages
Indirect	Phonocardiogram	Microphone	Antepartum	Noninvasive	Picks up many sounds; too noisy for labor Very slow rate may be doubled* Very fast rate may be halved*
Indirect	Abdominal wall electrocardiogram	Electrocardiogram	Antepartum Labor	Noninvasive	Picks up fetal and maternal QRS complex* Limited success early third trimester May count maternal rate
Indirect	Doppler ultrasound	Ultrahigh frequency sound waves "bounced" off moving heart or valves	Antepartum Labor	Noninvasive Satisfactory in 90–95% of laboring patients	1–3 beats/minute variability in rate Very slow rates may be doubled* Very high rates may be halved* Transducer may be uncomfortable Mother's position changes limited Constant repositioning necessary May count maternal rate
Direct	Fetal electrode	Electrode on fetal scalp detects fetal QRS	Labor	Most reliable Many noise signals filtered out Usually better tolerated by the mother Mother may change positions more easily	Invasive; membranes must be ruptured Cervix must be 1–2 cm. dilated Presenting part must be accessible

*Monitors currently available cannot count rates less than 30–60 beats/minute or greater than 210–250 beats/minute.

tions will undoubtedly become available in the years to come, because no totally satisfactory answer has yet been found.

Doppler Ultrasound. The principle of ultrasound was described in Chapter 8. When used to monitor the fetal heart, ultrasound waves are "bounced off" the walls of the moving heart or heart valves. Because two sets of heart valves are moving at different times (the bicuspid and the tricuspid valves), the system is designed so that once the movement of one valve is detected, the system will not respond for a specific period of time. Understanding this is important because:

1. If the fetal heart rate is very rapid, every beat may not be detected.

2. If the fetal heart rate is very slow, the movement of both valves may be indicated as beats on the monitor, thus doubling the rate.

Because monitors vary in the range of their response, one must know the specifics of the particular instrument used in her practice setting.

Direct Fetal Scalp Electrode. The most reliable technique for measuring fetal heart rate is a stainless steel spiral electrode that is inserted into the fetal scalp after the membranes have ruptured (either spontaneously or artificially). The electrical signal detected is the QRS complex, which denotes the passage of an electrical impulse through the heart. The machine computes the fetal heart rate on the basis of the time interval between each QRS complex.

MONITORING UTERINE CONTRACTIONS

The monitoring of fetal heart rate alone is sufficient. What is particularly significant is the relationship between fetal heart rate and uterine contractions. Like fetal heart rate, uterine contractions are also monitored externally or internally.

The External Tocotransducer

The external tocotransducer converts the force of each uterine contraction into an electrical signal that may then be displayed on a strip of paper. External monitoring is useful only in indicating the timing of contractions, not their intensity. In order to function properly, the external tocotransducer must be moved. External monitoring is also less comfortable for the patient.

Internal Measurement of Intrauterine Pressure

Changes in intrauterine pressure can be measured by inserting a small, open-ended plastic catheter that is filled with fluid through the cervix into the uterus. The catheter is attached to a strain gauge that sends out an electrical signal reflecting the pressure placed against it (Fig. 13–5). Through this internal system, one can monitor not only rate but baseline tone and intensity of contractions. This capability is particularly important if oxytocin is used to stimulate contractions (see below).

When using internal monitoring, remember that:

1. Any break in the system, such as an air bubble, a leak, or a meconium plug will impair accuracy.

2. The height of the strain gauge must match the height of the catheter tip.

Terms Describing Fetal Heart Rate and Uterine Contractions

A number of terms are used to describe fetal heart rate and uterine contractions.

FETAL E.C.G.   LEAD C

Figure 13–5 The placement of an electrode on the fetal scalp and a transcervical catheter to measure amniotic fluid pressure. (From Willis: *The Canadian Nurse*, Dec., 1970.)

AMPLI-FIER

Baseline fetal heart rate is the rate between contractions or between transient changes unrelated to contractions.

Baseline fetal heart rate variability refers to fluctuations in the baseline fetal heart rate (Fig. 13–6). Short-term variability occurs between successive pairs of heart beats. Long-term variability is related to fetal activity and averages 5 to 15 beats per minute when the fetus is active but may be suppressed when the fetus is asleep. The absence of short-term, beat-to-beat variability indicates a need for immediate

future evaluation of the fetus. It may be drug-related (narcotics, barbiturates, tranquilizers, anesthetics, atropine, or scopolamine) or due to fetal hypoxia and acidosis. A smooth baseline may precede the late decelerations described below as an indication of fetal hypoxia.

In small, premature infants absence of baseline variability reflects immaturity of the cardiac control mechanisms.

Fetal tachycardia is a fetal heart rate greater than 160 beats per minute. Prematurity, maternal fever, mild or

Figure 13–6 Fetal heart rate variability. *A*, Normal changes in rhythm; decreased beat-to-beat variability. *B*, Normal changes in rhythm and beat-to-beat variability. *C*, Decreased changes in rhythm and beat-to-beat variability. *D*, Decreased changes in rhythm; normal beat-to-beat variability. (After Yeh, Forsythe, and Hon: *Obstetrics and Gynecology*, 41:355, 1973.)

chronic hypoxia, intrauterine fetal infection, maternal anxiety, fetal activity, and drugs such as atropine, scopolamine, isoxsuprine (Vasodilan) and ritodrine are potential causes of fetal tachycardia.

Fetal bradycardia is a fetal heart rate less than 120 beats per minute. Hypoxia; maternal hypothermia; arrhythmias of the fetal heart; and drugs, including agents used for local anesthesia, are potential causes of fetal bradycardia. Fetal bradycardia does not always indicate severe fetal distress, but it should always be investigated.

Deceleration patterns, seen on the fetal monitoring strip, indicate the way in which fetal heart rate slows in a characteristic manner in response to certain stimuli. The timing and configuration of the deceleration in relation to the uterine contraction indicate certain factors about the fetus.

Acceleration patterns involve fetal heart rate acceleration above the baseline.

The Relationship between Fetal Heart Rate and Uterine Contractions

Deceleration patterns may be early, late, or variable. Some major characteristics of each type are summarized in Table 13–4 and Figure 13–7.

Early Deceleration. Compression of the descending fetal head during a uterine contraction elevates fetal intracranial pressure and thereby reduces the flow of blood to the fetal brain. Chemoreceptors in the brain are stimulated, and by reflex action fetal heart rate is slowed. This is the physiologic basis of early deceleration.

Although this sequence might appear threatening to the fetus, the transient hypoxia is apparently well tolerated by the fetus. Thus, early decelera-

tions are, in our present state of knowledge, benign.

Late Deceleration. When the flow of blood from the mother to the placenta is compromised and fetal Po_2 falls to 20 mm. Hg (normal is approximately 30 mm. Hg), fetal heart rate slows. The drop does not occur immediately at the time that the contraction begins. Rather it is progressive, dropping as the pressure of the uterine contraction increases and as the fetal oxygen stores (oxygen bound to fetal hemoglobin) decrease. Return to normal occurs following the contraction, as the flow of blood to the uterus increases.

Late decelerations and no beat-to-beat variability usually occur when the fetus is *chronically* asphyxiated and acidotic, resulting from chronic pathology involving the placenta or maternal-fetal exchange. One might expect such a pattern in some mothers with hypertensive disease, for example. The depressed fetal heart rate is due to the effect of hypoxia on the fetal myocardium.

Late decelerations with normal beat-to-beat variability and a normal baseline fetal heart rate usually indicate *acute* compromise of maternal-fetal exchange. The heart rate slows because of a reflex that is triggered by stimulation of the chemoreceptors within the brain, as in early deceleration. Because the stimulus is acute, intervention (e.g., administering oxygen, turning the mother to her side, see page 394) may often relieve this second cause of late deceleration.

Examples of the cause of late decelerations include maternal hypotension and uterine hyperactivity.

Often both chronic and acute conditions exist simultaneously. Careful evaluation will suggest which is the more significant at a particular moment in an individual woman's labor, and

Relation of Fetal Heart Rate to Uterine Contractions

Type of Deceleration	Configuration	Onset	Low Point	Return to Baseline	Comments	Mechanism
Early	U-shaped	Early in contraction cycle	Corresponds to peak of contraction	By end of contraction	The stronger the contraction, the greater the fetal heart rate; slowing rarely below 110–120 beats/minute. Occur in vertex presentation only. Appear after 6–7 cm. cervical dilatation	Compression of fetal head (see text)
Late	U-shaped	20–30 seconds or more after onset of contraction	After peak of contraction	After end of contraction	Degree of fetal heart rate slowing reflects intensity of contraction	Fetal hypoxia (see text)
Variable	Irregular	Variable relation of fetal heart rate to uterine contraction			Variable in every aspect including magnitude and occurrence with successive contractions	Umbilical cord compression
Prolonged	Wide U-shaped	Variable relation of fetal heart rate to uterine contraction			Cannot predict when or whether deceleration will end	Maternal hypotension Uterine hyperactivity Paracervical block Umbilical cord compression

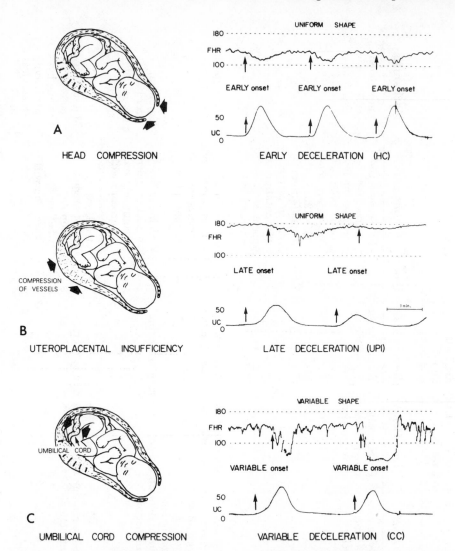

Figure 13–7   Patterns of fetal bradycardia. *A*, Early deceleration due to head compression (HC). UC is the tracing of uterine contraction. This is also known as a Type I dip. *B*, Late deceleration due to uteroplacental insufficiency (UPI). This is also known as a Type II dip. *C*, Variable deceleration due to cord compression (CC). (From Hon: *An Atlas of Fetal Heart Rate Patterns.* New Haven, Conn., Harty Press, Inc., 1968.)

thus the type of intervention most appropriate.

Variable Deceleration. Variable decelerations are also principally reflex in origin. Umbilical cord compression results in a lack of oxygen in the fetal blood from compression of the umbilical vein and in fetal hypertension from compression of the umbilical arteries.

Baroreceptors are activated by the former and chemoreceptors by the latter; as a result the vagus nerve is stimulated, and the fetal heart rate slows. The pattern is probably variable because the degree of cord compression changes from one contraction to another; cord compression may also occur between contractions.

Variable decelerations indicate fetal distress when (1) beat-to-beat variability is decreasing, or (2) baseline fetal heart rate is increasing.

Prolonged Deceleration. *Prolonged decelerations* are always a cause for concern; they may be due to maternal hypotension or to uterine hyperactivity or may follow a paracervical block. Nursing intervention includes administration of oxygen, maternal position change, and displacement of the uterus. Unless the cause is readily identified and corrected, delivery is indicated.

Acceleration Patterns. Acceleration in fetal heart rate above the baseline level between contractions usually indicates fetal well-being. Tactile stimulation, such as that during an examination, may cause fetal heart rate acceleration, as may the touch of the uterine lining during a contraction.

Acceleration may be a sign of danger when it occurs late in the contraction cycle and when beat-to-beat variability has been lost. This acceleration pattern may be a forerunner of a late deceleration pattern.

Recognition of Patterns. The recognition of fetal heart rate patterns is not always as straightforward as the examples described above. The reason may lie in the system itself (placement of the monitor or interference, for example) or in multiple factors affecting the fetal heart rate. Individuals with equal experience may interpret a pattern differently, just as some electrocardiogram (EKG) patterns in adults may be interpreted in more than one way. Nurses who care for laboring patients must constantly assess, improve, and evaluate their skills in this area.

Other Factors Affecting Fetal Heart Rate

Factors other than uterine contractions may affect fetal heart rate. Either bradycardia (a heart rate below 120 beats per minute) or tachycardia (a heart rate above 160 beats per minute) may occur in the baseline fetal heart rate for a number of reasons that are summarized in Table 13–5. Many of these factors are discussed in further detail in Chapters 14 and 15.

NURSING CARE DURING LABOR

Following the initial assessment, a plan of care for each mother is developed. The plan includes:

1. Facilitating the course of labor.
2. Protecting the mother and fetus.
3. Helping the mother cope with discomfort during labor.

Table 13–5   FACTORS AFFECTING BASELINE FETAL HEART RATE

Causes of Fetal Tachycardia (Rate > 160)	Causes of Fetal Bradycardia (Rate < 120)
Maternal hyperthermia	Fetal hypoxia (late sign)
Fetal hypoxia (early sign)	Response to vagal stimulus
Fetal sepsis	Maternal hypothermia
Maternal anxiety	Certain drugs
Fetal arrhythmia	Congenital heart block
Certain drugs	Idiopathic
Reaction to stimulus (transient)	
Idiopathic	

Nursing Intervention to Facilitate the Course of Labor

A number of measures may facilitate the course of labor. These include positioning the mother, avoiding a full bladder, and administering an enema.

Position

During early labor, it is not usually necessary for the mother to remain in bed (exceptions are noted below). When a woman is walking about or when she is sitting in a chair, gravity may enhance labor and make contractions more regular and efficient. Walking should not be carried to the point of fatigue, however. Contraindications to walking about include:

1. Rupture of the membranes when the head is not engaged, because of the danger of *prolapse* of the umbilical cord (Chapter 14).
2. Vaginal bleeding.
3. Abnormal presentation or position.
4. Administration of sedatives or narcotics.
5. Certain maternal conditions, such as heart disease.
6. Advanced labor.

In bed, a side-lying position is not only more comfortable for most mothers and important in avoiding hypotension (see above and below) but has been found to contribute to more efficient contractions, particularly during early labor. Not only are contractions more intense and coordinated, but they are less frequent, and thus there is more time for the uterus to relax between contractions.

When the woman is not lying on her side, the bed should be at a 30 to 40 degree angle.

The Urinary Bladder

Distention of the urinary bladder is not unusual during labor, but it is a condition that can and must be avoided for several reasons.

A full bladder may impede the descent of the baby's head (Fig. 13–8) and also, by reflex action, may inhibit uterine contractions. The possibility of trauma, and subsequent postpartum retention of urine, is increased when the bladder is allowed to become distended. Moreover, a full bladder is uncomfortable for the mother. By encouraging the mother to void every 2 hours during labor, distention can usually be avoided.

A   B

Figure 13–8   Notice how the full bladder (A) impedes the descent of the head. The empty bladder (B) is not a barrier. However, the full rectum (B) may be an impediment; contrast this with the empty rectum (A).

Because the bladder is anterior to the lower uterine segment during labor, it is usually easy to recognize distention both visually and by palpation (Fig. 13–9).

If distention occurs and if the mother is unable to void, catheterization is usually ordered. Special precautions important in catheterizing a woman during labor include:

1. Cleansing solutions must not enter the vagina.

2. A small flexible catheter is used to minimize discomfort and trauma.

3. The catheter is inserted between contractions, when the pressure of the fetal head against the urethra is not as great.

The Administration of an Enema

Just as a full bladder may interfere with the descent of the baby's head, so also may a full rectum. For this reason, an enema may be ordered for the mother shortly after she is admitted. In addition to its cleansing effect, a warm water enema often stimulates uterine contractions.

If the mother is not admitted until labor is advanced or if the head is well descended and pressing on the rectum, the enema may be omitted to avoid contamination of the sterile delivery field with liquid feces.

During early labor, the enema may be expelled in the toilet. If small amounts of fluid continue to be expelled, it is important to avoid contaminating the vagina and vulva with fecal material.

Fetal heart rate should be checked following the expulsion of the enema.

NURSING INTERVENTION TO PROTECT THE MOTHER AND FETUS

In addition to the hazards of the process of labor itself, there are potential dangers in the hospital environ-

Figure 13–9 A full bladder during labor can be recognized by the characteristic soft swelling suprapubically. (From Greenhill and Friedman: *Biological Principles and Modern Practice of Obstetrics.* Philadelphia, W. B. Saunders Co., 1974.)

ment. Protecting women from these hazards is also a part of the nursing care of mothers in labor. There are potential dangers related to: (1) medications, (2) infections, and (3) electrical equipment.

Dangers of Medications

The specific side effects, such as hypotension, of certain medications are discussed later in this chapter. In general, remember that medications given for the relief of pain may make the woman drowsy. She must be protected from falling by the use of side rails and should be accompanied if she is allowed out of bed.

The danger of explosion when oxygen and gases used for anesthesia are present in labor/delivery rooms must be remembered.

The Danger of Infection

Infection is a hazard to both mother and fetus. Even in excellent hospitals infection occasionally occurs, a circumstance that should be reviewed to determine the reason.

Nurses must help to develop and enforce policies that protect patients from infection. Standards for clothing, for the care of instruments and supplies, for the cleaning of rooms, and the like are helpful only if they are observed.

There is no reason to fear that fathers or other companions will be sources of infection (unless, of course, they are ill). Family members are usually eager to comply with requests about hand washing, dress, and the like—they know they are protecting their baby. Staff members are more likely to become casual.

Specific protection of the vaginal tract during preparation of the perineum, administration of enemas, and examination is described in appropriate sections.

Electric Hazards

More electrical equipment is used in the care of laboring women than ever before. A policy that insures frequent checking of this equipment by qualified people at designated intervals is essential. When a piece of equipment is checked, a label with the date should be attached. Only three-pronged plugs should be used. All equipment must be properly grounded. If even the slightest shock occurs, equipment should be unplugged.

NURSING INTERVENTION TO HELP THE MOTHER COPE WITH DISCOMFORT

The contractions of labor are hard work and cause discomfort. Factors influencing the degree of discomfort experienced by an individual woman have been discussed in Chapters 11 and 12. Nurses intervene (1) to assist the woman in coping with general discomfort, and (2) to help her cope with the discomfort of contractions.

Coping with General Discomfort

The physiologic process of labor results in bodily changes that can add, often considerably, to a mother's discomfort. Conversely, by attending to these needs, total comfort is enhanced. This supports the mother not only physically but emotionally because such attention demonstrates that her comfort is important to us.

Perspiration is common, as when any hard work is done, so that bathing of the face, hands, and back is comforting and relaxing. In a prolonged labor, a total bath is desirable. Gowns and clothes damp with perspiration must be changed as often as necessary.

Dryness of the lips and mouth is another discomfort during labor. The mother is allowed nothing by mouth. In addition the mouth-breathing techniques described in the section below contribute to dryness. Mothers who have attended childbirth preparation classes often bring lollipops, Vaseline, Chapstick or lip gloss with them to help relieve dryness. Ice chips and a clean, wet washcloth applied to the lips will help.

Discharge from the vagina may be in the form of mucus, blood, or amniotic fluid at various stages during labor, all of which add to a feeling of discomfort. The vulva must also be kept clean, with care that cleansing solutions do not enter the vagina.

Coping with the Discomfort of Contractions

There are many techniques that help mothers cope with the discomfort of labor, but they may be divided into two basic categories—coping without the use of medication and coping with the use of medication. For many women, a combination of these strategies is the most appropriate nursing intervention.

Coping without the Use of Medication

Many couples prepare for labor by attending classes in the Lamaze method, the Bradley method, or similar strategies for dealing with labor. There they acquire attitudes and tools to help them cope with labor. Unfortunately, many other women come to labor prepared with only "old wives' tales" and "horror" stories. They expect the worst, and their tension makes labor far more difficult for them than it might otherwise have been.

Although prior preparation is ideal, nurses who care for women in labor can use similar strategies to make labor a more positive experience for all women.

The basics of helping a mother cope with labor involve helping her to:

1. Find a comfortable position.
2. Listen to her own voice and to the voice of whoever is coaching her during labor.
3. Focus on some object to minimize distractions from breathing patterns.
4. Adjust her breathing patterns, which vary with the stage of labor.

There is no question that the woman who has practiced these techniques prior to labor has an advantage, at least partly because she *feels* prepared. Nevertheless, good nurse-coaching during labor itself can help the unprepared mother as well, in part because the close attention involved in the coaching will probably help her to be less tense and fearful.

A Comfortable Position

During early labor, sitting alternating with walking is the position of choice for many mothers. Walking is contraindicated if the membranes have ruptured and the head is not engaged (see above, below, and Chapter 14). We need to observe her for signs of fatigue during this period and encourage her to rest frequently.

During a contraction, the woman may stand and lean forward, supported by her husband or a nurse if she is walking at the time of onset.

In bed, for most women a side-lying position (Chapter 9) is far more comfortable than a back-lying position during labor. Traditionally, women have been asked to return to their backs during vaginal examination, but this should not always be necessary. Although it is true that the examiner may estimate dilatation as slightly less when the woman is on her side, this should present no major problem in evaluating the course of labor.

In addition to comfort, a side-lying position displaces the weight of the uterus from the inferior vena cava. When the mother is lying on her back, the weight of the uterus may cause *supine hypotensive syndrome*, i.e., hypotension because of interference with the flow of blood returning to the heart via the inferior vena cava. When this occurs, the woman is turned on her side and given oxygen. Alternatively, the uterus may be lifted off the vena cava.

Another position of comfort for some mothers during part of labor is the "pelvic rock" position (Fig. 13–10).

During the second stage, when the mother is pushing, she may wish to be at a 35 to 45 degree angle.

Listening

All of a mother's senses are heightened during labor. She will remember for many years the sights and sounds surrounding the birth of her baby. Her heightened sensorium can be helpful if she is "tuned in" to the sound of her own voice or the voice of her coach, usually her husband or nurse. If she has been prepared to use certain techniques, she can repeat to herself, or have her coach repeat, the instructions that she has practiced.

Focusing

Each of us has had some experience in which our attention is focused so intently on one matter that we are oblivious to other happenings around us. We may go to a movie with a headache and focus so intently on the film that the headache is completely forgotten, only to find when we leave the theater that the headache is still there after all. An athlete may be injured early in a football or basketball game but may feel no pain until the contest is over.

During labor, focusing accomplishes the same objective—attention is diverted from the uterine contraction to some other object. Nothing is more counterproductive for the laboring mother than to lie in bed wait-

Figure 13–10   Pelvic rocking on the hands and knees. The lower back is raised and the head lowered. (From Davis and Rubin: *De Lee's Obstetrics for Nurses*. 18th Ed. Philadelphia, W. B. Saunders Co., 1966.)

ing for a contraction to occur, with all her attention focused on the contraction. "Here it comes . . . boy, is this awful . . . I don't think I can stand it . . ." and so on.

Mothers may focus on their husband's face or on an object in the room, such as a picture or even a doorknob. If the mother brings an object from home, we should help her place it where she wishes.

It is essential that nurses, physicians, and whoever else enters the labor room *do not interrupt* the mother who is focusing. Wait until the contraction is over. If the husband is there and if he has been prepared for labor along with his wife, he can "run interference" for her, reminding others that his wife will answer their questions when the contraction is over. Mothers who attend classes in preparation for labor may be taught to ignore questions during contractions.

Breathing Techniques

Patterned breathing is a major technique used by mothers trained in prepared childbirth classes. The patterns vary slightly, depending upon the techniques taught in a particular community. However, most employ chest breathing and/or abdominal breathing, starting at a slow rate and progressing to a more rapid rate as labor progresses.

The particular techniques described here are related to the Lamaze method. It is most important for nurses to be familiar with the types of preparation offered in their own communities so that they can be supportive of the couples they care for. There is no evidence that one type of preparation is superior to another type for all mothers, although for an individual mother it is possible that one method may be more helpful. In smaller communities, of course, alternatives may not be available.

Why Is Patterned Breathing Effective? In Chapter 12 the relationship between tension and pain was noted (pain $\rightleftarrows$ tension). Another facet of tension is an increase in the rate of respiration; observe your own respiratory rate the next time you feel tense and anxious.

By consciously breathing slowly, one can aid relaxation and thus effectively relieve pain that is due to tension. Moreover, concentration on breathing gives one control over one's emotions. A woman is no longer helpless in the face of uncontrollable forces; she has tools that enable her to work along with her body, rather than against it.

A number of breathing techniques are taught in prepared childbirth classes. Different patterns are appropriate at different stages of labor.

THE CLEANSING BREATH. As each contraction beings, mothers are taught to take a *cleansing breath,* i.e., a deep breath that is blown out. The breath serves as a signal that a contraction is about to begin. A similar breath is taken at the end of the contraction.

SLOW CHEST BREATHING. Slow chest breathing is usually most helpful during that stage of labor at which contractions are about 3 to 5 minutes apart and are lasting 60 seconds; the cervix will usually be about 4 cm. dilated. It is a time when normal breathing patterns are no longer adequate to help the mother cope with contractions. This pattern can be described as the type of breath you would use to "fill a bra." If the woman holds her fingers over her ribs, she will feel them spread as she breathes. The initial rate is approximately 10 breaths per minute. As contractions intensify, the rate may increase to 12 to 18 breaths per minute and still be no faster than a normal breathing pattern.

Effleurage (Chapter 9) often accompanies slow chest breathing.

Later in labor, slow chest breathing may be helpful in aiding relaxation between contractions, although other patterns are more helpful for the contraction itself.

SHALLOW, LIGHT CHEST BREATHING. When slow breathing is no longer effective in helping a mother "keep on top of" her contractions, she may switch to a shallow, lighter breathing. This breathing should be as quiet and as low as possible; about one breath per second. Many women use shallow breathing during the middle of the first stage, from about 6 to 7 cm. dilatation, until the beginning of transition, about 8 cm.

Breathing during Transition. For many women, transition (the period during which the uterus dilates from 8 to 10 cm.) is the most difficult part of labor.

A combination of light, shallow breathing with a puff, as if to blow out a candle, (at one time called pant and blow) is helpful during this period. The rate is approximately one breath per second. The pattern is breath–breath–breath–breath–puff (4:1 ratio); the ratio can be 6:1 or 8:1. As the contraction becomes more intense, there is a tendency to breathe faster and faster; the woman can briefly halve the number of breaths she takes, with two, three, or four shallow breaths and a puff at the height of the contraction, returning to the former pattern as decrement begins. As in all breathing patterns, this pattern begins with a cleansing breath and ends with a breath to blow away the contraction.

This pattern requires considerable concentration on the part of the mother and her coach. The coach may need to hold the mother's face in his (her) hands to help her concentrate.

Sometimes the mother may have an urge to "push" during transition. However, it is important not to push until the cervix is fully dilated. To push prematurely is not only painful but also leads to soft tissue swelling and can prolong labor. Moreover, pushing at this stage leads to fatigue in an already tired mother.

Breathing patterns do not stop the urge to push; they just help the mother refrain from adding the force of her abdominal muscles to uterine forces. Mothers need to be reassured that breathing patterns that prevent pushing do not stop the movement of the baby through the passage. Breathing patterns that prevent pushing include: (1) slow, sustained exhalation; or (2) blowing, as if blowing out candles on a birthday cake.

Watch for signs of hyperventilation (below) when these techniques are used.

Breathing during the Second Stage. A colleague, Brenda McBride, R.N., tells the mothers in her childbirth preparation classes, "Pushing a baby out is the greatest work we will ever do." As the cervix becomes fully dilated and the second stage begins, the mother now has our permission, and our encouragement, to push with each contraction.

Although some mothers welcome our permission to push, others are reluctant. Pushing may hurt; this is especially true if the baby is in a posterior position (see below). The rectal pressure that accompanies pushing makes some mothers fear they will have a bowel movement in bed, and this makes them reluctant to push. The psychologic change from a prohibition against pushing to an encouragement to push is somewhat like changing horses in midstream; it takes some getting accustomed to, especially for some couples.

Mothers can, in most instances,

shorten labor by pushing effectively. How do we help them?

As mentioned above, a most effective position for pushing is a 35 degree angle. In traditional societies, pushing is often accomplished in a squatting position, also effective. Probably the least effective position for pushing is the position used in most American delivery rooms, in which the mother is lying on her back. This position is for the convenience of the birth attendant.

Pushing efforts should be directed toward the front of the woman's body, not the back. Thus, instructions such as "bear down as if you are having a bowel movement," heard frequently in delivery rooms, are not truly appropriate. (Babies are born through vaginas, not rectums.) Rectal pushing may also cause hemorrhoids. A better instruction is "pretend that you have a seat belt around your abdomen and try to break it with your abdominal muscles." Thus, effort will be concentrated in the abdomen.

Here is how we coach a mother to push:

1. Take one or two initial slow, cleansing breaths while you—
2. Wait for the contraction to build—
3. Take a breath that lowers the abdomen on the uterus, hold it as long as possible (about 20 seconds), and—
4. At the same time tighten abdominal muscles, pushing as described above, and—
5. Relax the vagina.

After about 20 seconds, the mother will need to take an additional breath, but she can keep her abdominal muscles tight.

If the second stage is moving too quickly, as it may be in a multipara, the mother may need to pant "like a puppy" in order to prevent pushing.

Hyperventilation. When breathing patterns become rapid with a longer period of expiration than inspiration, too much carbon dioxide is exhaled; this phenomenon is known as *hyperventilation.** Hyperventilation occurs more often in women who have not been prepared for labor, but it can occur in prepared women as well. Light, quiet, even breathing is a major deterrent to hyperventilation.

The signs are lightheadedness, dizziness, tingling of the fingers, and numbness around the lips. A woman may not say anything about her symptoms, but we may see her touching her lips, as if to test them, or rubbing her hands. We should then question her about her symptoms. A later symptom is cramping of the fingers; this indicates that the woman has been hyperventilating for some time.

A simple, effective method of relieving hyperventilation is breathing into a paper bag that is tightly sealed around the nose and chin. In this way, the woman will rebreathe her own carbon dioxide. Rebreathing should continue until symptoms disappear.

When the Fetus Is in a Posterior Position

When the fetus is in a posterior position (ROP, LOP, RSP, LSP, and so on), which may be as frequent as one in every four labors† (statistics vary from one study to another), labor is characterized by back pain that may be sufficiently intense that the discomfort of contractions seems very secondary.

---

*Hyperventilation, of course, can occur in individuals at many times other than labor.

†Although much of labor may be in the posterior position, the baby may rotate to an anterior position prior to delivery.

Back pain may also be significant in a breech presentation.

How can mothers with back pain be helped to cope with an often difficult labor? Such mothers can be assisted by providing emotional support, changing position, applying counterpressure, applying heat and cold, and encouraging conscious relaxation.

Emotional Support. When a mother realizes that her baby is in a posterior position (and she may recognize this before the position is confirmed by our examination), her first reaction may very well be, "Why me?" If her husband has been attending preparatory classes with her, he, too, may recognize that labor in a posterior position presents special needs and may share the feeling, "Why us?" We can let them know that it is all right to feel this way; they need to accept their feelings and then go on to cope with the special demands of a "back labor."

Position. In posterior labor, pain is centered in the lower back. The *most uncomfortable* position for a woman with posterior labor is lying on her back. With the possible exception of a brief period during which she is being examined, this woman should be off her back at all times. Why? It is the pressure of the baby's vertebral column against the mother's vertebral column that is causing the discomfort. Any position that takes the weight of the uterus off the mother's vertebrae will help. Frequent changes of position seem to be most helpful; several helpful positions are described below. The mother might assume one position for two or three contractions, then a second, then a third, and so on. For example, she may be on her left side for three contractions, assume a hand-knee position for one contraction, and then be on her right side for three contractions. She may then assume one of the sitting positions

for two or three contractions. The important point for us is to be flexible enough to allow her frequent changes, as she seeks the position most comfortable for her. The best position for an individual mother is the position that feels best for her.

Sitting positions: The mother leans forward with her legs through the side rails. A pillow on the side rails will make her more comfortable. Be sure the rail is secure. Or the mother may sit in a chair, western style, or in the bed, leaning forward.

Side lying: The side-lying position allows the uterus to lie on the bed rather than on the mother's backbone. It also allows counterpressure and applications of heat and/or cold to be applied to the back.

Hand-knee position: The mother assumes a position on her hands and knees in bed; she arches her back up as she exhales and comes down as she inhales. Mothers can be taught to "pretend you are a donkey pulling your tail between your legs" (Fig. 13–10).

Counterpressure. Counterpressure on the lower back can be helpful to the woman with posterior labor. Pressure can come from the heels of the husband's or the nurse's hands placed on each side of the lower spine. Even better, pressure may be obtained by using soup cans, adhesive tape cylinders, tennis balls tied in a stocking leg, or a rolling pin. The amount of pressure that feels good will vary from woman to woman, and from moment to moment in the same woman. She needs to guide her husband or nurse, saying "that's too hard," "push harder," or "that helps."

Back discomfort is almost constant during posterior labor; it does not occur only with contractions. Even if a husband is able to be with his wife, he will need periods of rest. Nurses who care for the mother will also need breaks. The bed should be at such a height that the coach (husband or nurse) does not have to bend over, a position that will lead to early fatigue and back pain for the coach. The pressure should come from the body of the coach, not the arms.

Heat and Cold. Warm, moist towels or ice packs, applied to the lower back, will feel comforting to many mothers. If heat is not helpful to a particular mother, try cold, and vice versa. Any time that heat is used, precautions against burning the skin are important.

Conscious Relaxation. Conscious relaxation of the area from 3 inches above the waist to the knees is important in a difficult labor, as in all labor.

PHARMACOLOGIC ASSISTANCE

In many instances, preparation reduces the need for medication during labor, but it does not necessarily eliminate that need. Even if every mother were ideally prepared, the circumstances of labor vary, pain thresholds vary, and a variety of needs make the use of medication a valuable help for some women. No woman should be made to feel that she has "failed" because medication was asked for or given.

Nurses have many responsibilities in relation to analgesia and anesthesia during labor. A thorough knowledge of each medication, the reason it is given, the advantages and disadvantages in relation to the mother and baby, and the progress of labor is essential both for the antepartal nurse who prepares couples for delivery and for the nurse who cares for families during labor. The nurse in the labor room must also recognize signs that indicate the presence of complications related to medications and must know how to quickly alleviate

problems that may arise. Each type of analgesia or anesthesia is associated with specific nursing needs.

Any medication used for analgesia or anesthesia during labor should be judged by the following criteria:

1. Neither the mother nor the baby should be endangered.

2. The efficiency of uterine contractions should not be decreased.

3. The woman should continue to be able to participate in her labor.

4. The method for giving the medication should be simple enough to avoid complications in administration.

It is apparent from Tables 13–6 and 13–7 that no medication currently used meets all of these criteria. Great care is essential when any medication is used.

Medications given during labor can be classified into six groups:

1. Sedatives and tranquilizers, which relieve apprehension and thus aid relaxation.

2. Amnesics, which erase the memory of pain.

3. Regional analgesics, which interrupt pain pathways.

4. General analgesics, which increase the tolerance of pain by approximately 50 per cent.

5. Local or regional anesthetics.

6. General anesthetics, which prevent perception of pain in the central nervous system (CNS).

Each group necessitates special care for the woman who receives one or more medications.

Sedatives

Barbiturates such as secobarbital, pentobarbital, and phenobarbital are the principal sedatives used in labor. For the woman in early labor who is very tense and anxious, sedatives are given to promote relaxation. They do not have any pain-relieving action, but

Table 13–6   PHARMACOLOGIC RELIEF OF PAIN DURING THE FIRST STAGE OF LABOR

Classification	Medication or Method	Standard Dose	Effect on Labor	Effect on Mother	Effect on Fetus
SEDATIVE	Pentobarbital (Nembutal)	100–200 mg. IM, 50 mg. IV	Large amounts impair uterine activity and prolong labor	CNS depressant Mother lethargic and sleepy Nausea, vomiting, decrease in blood pressure possible	Respiratory distress Drowsiness for 24–48 hours
	Secobarbital (Seconal) Phenobarbital (Luminal)	100–200 mg. IM, PO, 50 mg. IV 100 mg. IV, PO			
TRANQUILIZER	Diazepam (Valium)	2, 5, or 10 mg. IV, IM, PO	No recognized effect	Relief of apprehension	May cause delay in onset of respirations
	Promazine (Sparine)	25 mg. IM, PO		May cause maternal hypotension	
	Chlorpromazine (Thorazine)	25 mg. IM, PO			
	Promethazine (Phenergan)	25–50 mg. IM, PO			
	Hydroxyzine (Vistaril)	5–15 mg. IM, PO			
	Propiomazine (Largon)	20–40 mg. IM, PO			
AMNESIC	Hyoscine (scopolamine)	0.25–0.60 mg.		Woman may become excited and delirious Dryness of mouth and throat	

ANALGESIC				
Meperidine (Demerol)	25–100 mg. IM, q 3–4 h.	Minimal effect on contractions Relaxation may speed dilatation of cervix	Good analgesia; becomes most effective in 60–90 minutes; lasts 2–3 hours Side effects: facial flushing, dryness of mouth, decreased urinary output, diaphoresis, hypotension, nausea and vomiting	May cause serious respiratory depression if given 2–3 hours before delivery Minimum respiratory depression if given less than 1 hour before delivery
Morphine sulfate	8–15 mg. IM	Varies: may weaken or stop contractions May lead to more efficient contractions in irritable uterus	CNS depressant Mother lethargic and sleepy Side effects: facial flushing, dryness of mouth	May cause serious respiratory distress Peak action 1.5 hours after IM administration Administration within 3 hours of birth dangerous
Alphaprodine (Nisentil)	20–40 mg. IM, IV	No apparent effect on labor		

Table continued on following page

Table 13–6 PHARMACOLOGIC RELIEF OF PAIN DURING THE FIRST STAGE OF LABOR (*Continued*)

Classification	Medication or Method	Standard Dose	Effect on Labor	Effect on Mother	Effect on Fetus
INHALANTS	Self-administered by hand-held mask Methoxyflurane (Penthrane) Trichloroethylene (Trilene)			Analgesia during first stage of labor (may be used for analgesia or anesthesia during second stage) Too much Penthrane can cause maternal hypotension; slow and/or shallow respirations; too much Trilene can cause irregular pulse and rapid respirations; patient may experience numbness and/or dizziness	Possible hypoxia Possible CNS depression

REGIONAL ANESTHETIC	Paracervical block		Not predictable	Almost immediate relief (3–5 minutes) of pain of approximately 1–2 hours duration; may need to be repeated	Fetal bradycardia in 20–30%; in 5% bradycardia below 100
	Mepivacaine (Carbocaine)	10 ml. on each side	Some labors appear shortened; some appear inhibited	Transient numbness of lower extremities, maternal tachycardia, dizziness, euphoria, anxiety, hypotension reported	
	Lidocaine (Xylocaine)				
CONDUCTION ANESTHETIC	Caudal Epidural Procaine (Novocain) Dibucaine (Nupercaine) Lidocaine (Xylocaine) Tetracaine (Pontocaine) Mepivacaine (Carbocaine)		May slow labor if given too early or in too large a dose (obliterates bearing down reflex in second stage)	Begins to relieve pain in 5–10 minutes; effects last 45–60 minutes	Hypotension may lead to fetal hypoxia Behavioral differences in newborn in first days following delivery
				Potential hypotension; nausea, pallor, lightheadedness, abnormal vital signs are indications	

they do reduce the amount of analgesia needed when they are given in combination with analgesics.

When a mother is admitted with rupture of the membranes but without contractions, or when she has been in labor for a number of hours but contractions are weak and irregular, sedation may be given to allow her to nap. Mothers who have prepared for labor may resist this idea. However, we can explain that following a rest not only are contractions frequently more effective but she will be better able to work with her contractions when she has slept. The assurance that we will awaken her, if she does not awaken when regular contractions begin, is important.

Disadvantages. Sedatives may slow and prolong labor. In most women when pain is present, and in some women at any time, sedatives may have the opposite effect from that desired; the mother may become restless and even delirious rather than relaxed. Nausea, vomiting, and decreased blood pressure may occur.

Barbiturates may cause marked respiratory distress in the newborn and drowsiness for 24 to 48 hours following birth, because these drugs are metabolized more slowly by the infant than by the adult. Aside from the physiologic effect on the infant, the significance in terms of parent-infant interaction must be considered. For these reasons, barbiturates are never given when delivery is imminent. They are particularly dangerous in preterm deliveries.

Nursing Support. One factor concerning the effect of medication given during labor is the woman's expectation of the effect. Thus when a sedative or any medication is given, a comment such as, "This medicine will help you rest between contractions," or whatever

statement is appropriate, will actually help her to rest between contractions. It is also important to tell her how she is likely to feel, and when. For example, "You will begin to feel drowsy in a few minutes."

Once medication for sedation has been given, the room should be semidarkened and as quiet as possible. Certainly, the father, friend, or coach can remain with the mother, but they should understand the purpose of the medication and allow her to rest. Nursing assessment can be planned to allow periods of rest.

Tranquilizers

A variety of tranquilizing drugs (Table 13–6) may be given during early labor. Like sedatives, they are used chiefly during early labor to relieve apprehension. Because they potentiate the action of both barbiturates and analgesics, the doses of these other types of medications are reduced by half when they are given along with a tranquilizer.

Disadvantages. Both maternal hypotension and a delay in the onset of respirations in the infant are possible when tranquilizers are given. Tranquilizers are considered dangerous in preterm labor.

Nursing Support. The supportive care given a mother receiving barbiturate sedation is equally applicable to the mother receiving a tranquilizer.

Amnesics

Hyoscine (scopolamine) was formerly used as an amnesic. However, it is rarely used today. Women are no less aware of pain when it occurs but have no memory of pain afterward. They frequently sleep between contractions but are very restless and excited during the contraction. Because of this, women given scopolamine should not be left unattended. When used, scopolamine is given in conjunction with an analgesia to minimize restlessness during contractions.

Analgesics

Meperidine (Demerol) is the analgesic used most frequently during labor; morphine sulfate and alpha-prodine (Nisentil) are also used on occasion.

Demerol does not offer immediate or complete relief of pain. Within a few minutes, pain will be less sharp, but maximum effectiveness is not achieved for 60 to 90 minutes. At this point the woman's pain threshold will be increased by approximately 50 per cent. Effects last for 2 to 3 hours.

Disadvantages. Hypotension is the most serious side effect of Demerol. Other side effects may include facial flushing, dryness of the mouth, diaphoresis, decreased urinary output, and nausea and vomiting. Morphine may also cause facial flushing and oral dryness.

The biggest disadvantage of analgesia is respiratory depression in the infant. The degree of depression is related to the amount given, the time that the drug is given in relation to delivery, the infant's weight and gestational age, and the degree of trauma at the time of delivery. These drugs should not be given 2 to 3 hours prior to delivery. The danger is particularly great in preterm delivery. However, Demerol given with an hour of delivery does not appear to affect the initiation of breathing.

As little as 50 mg. of Demerol has been demonstrated to affect the infant's behavior during the first days of life, which in turn may affect interaction between parent and infant.

Naloxone hydrochloride (Narcan), .01 mg. per kg. of baby's weight, is the narcotic antagonist currently used to mitigate depression from narcotics. Given intramuscularly (IM) it begins to be effective in 2 to 3 minutes, acting by competing with the narcotic at binding sites. When naloxone is given, nurses who care for the baby following delivery must be informed; as the drug is metabolized, the baby may again become depressed.

The narcotic antagonists formerly used, nalorphine (Nalline) and levallorphan tartrate (Lorfan), reversed narcotic-induced respiratory depression in many instances but contributed to respiratory depression from other causes.

Nursing Support. Continuing assessment of both mother and fetus and reduction of environmental stimuli as described above are major areas of nursing support.

Self-administered Inhalant Analgesia

Methoxyflurane (Penthrane) and trichloroethylene (Trilene) are administered during the first stage of labor via a mask that the mother holds in her hand.

Disadvantages. These medications are potent anesthetics; they are sometimes given for anesthesia during the second stage of labor. For this reason, no one but the mother must hold the mask (see Nursing Support, below). Too much Penthrane can cause maternal hypotension and slow, shallow respirations. Too much Trilene can cause an irregular pulse and rapid respirations. Potential problems for the fetus/infant are hypoxia and central nervous system depression.

Nursing Support. A woman receiving inhalation anesthesia needs constant nursing supervision. As long as she hold the mask herself and does not prop the hand that is holding it, the mask will fall away if she loses consciousness. However, if anyone else holds the mask for her, she may become anesthetized. Vital signs are assessed frequently. Because Penthrane persists in the body between contractions, the dial on the inhaler may need to be adjusted downward after a period of use.

Any liquid remaining in the inhaler at the end of the day must be discarded; leftover medication may decompose.

Regional Anesthesia: Paracervical Nerve Block

A paracervical nerve block involves the administration of a local anesthetic into the pelvic plexus, those nerves located in the paracervical tissue that supply the uterus, vagina, bladder, and rectum. Five to 10 ml. of solution is injected on each side, at 3 o'clock and 9 o'clock or at 4 o'clock and 8 o'clock (Fig. 13–11). Because the pudendal nerve is not blocked, the perineum is not anesthetized.

Paracervical blocking is usual at from 4 to 6 cm. cervical dilatation. Relief of pain is almost immediate and lasts from 1 to 2 hours. When the block ceases to be effective, the return of pain is rapid. Depending on the progress of labor, the paracervical block may be repeated. When the fetal head reaches station +2 and when cervical dilatation reaches 8 cm., paracervical blocking becomes technically more difficult.

Disadvantages. Paracervical blocking is used only when the fetus is assessed to be healthy. In approximately 20 to 30 per cent of patients, there is transient fetal bradycardia; in 5 per cent the fetal heart rate drops below 100, possibly due to the depressant effect of the local anesthetic on the fetal myocardium. A paracervical block is not administered if delivery is expected within 30 minutes.

The effect on labor varies; labor appears to be inhibited in some women, while in others it appears to be shortened.

Maternal reactions may include hypotension, numbness of the lower extremities, tachycardia, dizziness, and euphoria.

Nursing Support. Fetal heart rate must be monitored very closely until it is stable; a fetal heart rate monitor is important if bradycardia is noted.

The mother's reaction to the anesthetic is also evaluated frequently.

Figure 13–11 Paracervical nerve block. The needle is introduced through a guide in the vagina into the mucosa for 6 to 12 mm. If there is no blood return, anesthetic solution is injected.

Regional Anesthesia: Pudendal Nerve Block

A pudendal nerve block involves the administration of a local anesthetic into the pudendal nerves on the right and left of the perineum (Figs. 13–12 and 13–13). The pudendal block anesthetizes only the perineum, relaxing perineal muscles and anesthetizing the area for episiotomy, delivery, and episiotomy repair. The pudendal nerve is blocked after dilatation is complete; the mother will usually be positioned for delivery. The mother can expect to feel pressure during the delivery even though she does not feel pain. Occasionally, a pudendal block fails to give relief of pain.

Disadvantages. Unless medication is injected into the pudendal artery by mistake, pudendal nerve block is safe for both mother and infant.

Figure 13–12 Pudendal block technique by the transvaginal approach, showing relationship of pudendal nerve to the ischial spine and sacrospinous ligament (inset) and the method by which the needle is guided by the fingers in the vagina and advanced through the sacrospinous ligament to block the nerve. (From Bonica: *Principles and Practice of Obstetrical Analgesia and Anesthesia.* Philadelphia, F. A. Davis Co., 1967.)

Figure 13–13 Blocking the pudendal nerve through the perineum (percutaneous transperineal pudendal nerve block). (After Oxorn and Foote: *Human Labor and Birth.* 3rd Ed.)

Nursing Support. Because the mother is usually draped for delivery at the time that the pudendal nerve is blocked, she may be anxious about what she cannot see. The idea of a needle through the perineum or vagina is not necessarily reassuring. We should explain how the injection will help and how she will feel. There may be some discomfort as the medication is injected; this will be brief.

Fetal heart rate and maternal vital signs are monitored each minute for 15 minutes following pudendal nerve block and then every 5 minutes until stable.

Peridural Anesthesia: Caudal and Lumbar Epidural

Peridural anesthesia involves the injection of an anesthetic into the extradural space. The anesthetic *does not* penetrate the dura or the spinal cord. There is no "spinal headache" because the basis of such headaches is the leaking of cerebrospinal fluid through the puncture hole in the dura. Only if the dura is accidentally penetrated should there be a problem of headache after peridural infiltration.

Peridural anesthesia may be administered into the caudal space within the sacrum or into the epidural space at the second, third, or fourth lumbar interspace (Fig. 13-14). A single injection may be made, or, frequently, a catheter may be threaded through the needle into the space to allow a continuous injection of medicine over a period of hours for anesthesia during both labor and delivery. Lumbar epidural anesthesia is the type most frequently used in many areas of the United States today.

Anesthesia is achieved because nerves supplying both the uterus and the perineum pass through the peridural space and are anesthetized by the solution that has been injected. Loss of sensation occurs in 5 to 30 minutes with caudal infiltration and in 5 to 10 minutes with epidural infiltration. Vasodilatation of the legs, which the mother reports as a "warm feeling," is usually the first sign that the block is effective. Anesthesia is effective from 45 minutes to an hour.

Caudal anesthesia is ineffective in about 15 per cent of the women to whom it is administered; the failure rate for lumbar epidural anesthesia is approximately 1.5 to 2 per cent.

Disadvantages. Started too early, peridural anesthesia may slow the course of labor; administration is therefore delayed until the cervix is more than 4 cm. dilated.

The major disadvantage is the pos-

Figure 13-14 Continuous caudal block anesthesia technique, showing needle in sacral canal (top), with plastic catheter threaded through it (middle) and with needle withdrawn (bottom), leaving the catheter in place for purposes of administering anesthetic solution. (From Bonica: *Principles and Practice of Obstetrical Analgesia and Anesthesia.* Philadelphia, F. A. Davis Co., 1967.)

sibility of severe maternal hypotension and resultant decreased blood flow to the fetus. Hypotension occurs because the interruption of sympathetic vasomotor innervation leads to decreased peripheral resistance and a decrease in venous return to the heart. Schifrin[22a] found that nearly 25 per cent of women who were given peridural anesthesia showed fetal heart rate patterns characteristic of uteroplacental insufficiency. The incidence of decreased uterine blood flow rose to 72 per cent when the woman was hypotensive. Because of this, constant monitoring of both the mother's vital signs and the fetal heart rate (preferably with a continuous fetal heart rate monitor) is essential.

The obliteration of both uterine and perineal sensations means that the mother does not have a desire to push during the second stage. The second stage may be lengthened, and forceps may be required for delivery. Coaching can alert her to the presence of a contraction and can encourage her to push at the most effective time.

Conduction anesthesia (both peridural and spinal, to be described below) interferes with the ability of the woman to void; frequent bladder observation and sometimes catheterization are necessary.

Infection is a potential hazard in any injection. Peridural anesthesia is not attempted if there is any evidence of infection at the puncture site. Excellent aseptic technique is essential in handling all equipment used for the injection of medication. Once contracted, infections of the epidural space are difficult to combat.

Nursing Support. Before the injection occurs, the mother needs to know how she will feel—her legs will feel weak and may shake briefly. This loss of control is frightening to some mothers if it is not anticipated.

It has already been emphasized that a nurse must remain with the mother to monitor her closely. If she complains of a metallic taste in her mouth, of dizziness or ringing in her ears, or appears confused or excited, it is possible that the anesthetic has entered the circulatory system through the epidural vessels.

Signs of hypotension that require immediate intervention include dizziness, pallor, nausea, and a change in vital signs in the mother and late decelerations (see below) in the fetus. Nursing intervention for hypotension has been described on page 394.

Following delivery, the mother who has had peridural anesthesia may be dizzy the first time she sits in bed. She should be prepared for this feeling so that she will not try to get up when she is alone.

Spinal Anesthesia

With the exception of low spinal anesthesia (see Saddle Block, below), spinal anesthesia is rarely used for vaginal delivery. Spinal infiltration is frequently used, however, for cesarean section. A local anesthetic is injected through the dura into the subarachnoid space at the level of the third or fourth lumbar interspace.

Disadvantages. As is true with other types of conduction anesthesia, hypotension is a potential problem. When hypotension occurs, uterine contractility is also diminished.

Because the dura is punctured, postspinal headache is possible. The mother will usually remain flat on her back for a period of time following delivery, a position that requires some planning in order to facilitate early interaction between the mother and baby.

Nursing Support. Nursing support is similar to that for a mother with an epidural anesthetic, in terms of hypotension.

Oxygen is given to the mother to maintain a good level of oxygenation at the level of the placenta. An intravenous infusion is started in the event that intravenous medication is needed.

Saddle Block (Low Spinal Anesthesia)

Injection of medication into the conus of the dural sac anesthetizes the area that would come in contact with a saddle when riding a horse, hence the term "saddle block."

A saddle block is given only when delivery is imminent; anesthesia of the perineum lasts for approximately 1 hour.

Disadvantages. The mother must sit for the injection of medication when a saddle block is used so that the medication will gravitate downward. At a time just prior to delivery, when the saddle block is instituted, this is a most difficult position, requiring not only physical assistance but a great deal of emotional encouragement and support. The mother remains sitting for approximately 30 seconds following infiltration and then is placed on her back with her neck flexed.

A saddle block has no apparent adverse effects on the mother or fetus.

The mother with a saddle block may occasionally have a postspinal headache.

Nursing Support. Nursing support for the mother with a saddle block is the same as for mothers with other types of conduction anesthesia (epidural, spinal).

THE EFFECT OF LOCAL AND REGIONAL ANESTHESIA ON THE NEWBORN INFANT'S BEHAVIOR. Although it has been recognized that various modes of analgesia/anesthesia affect the newborn infant's respiration, less attention has been paid to other possible effects of anesthesia. Studies by Standley and associates[24] and by Scanlon and associates[22] have noted differences in behavior.

Standley's group evaluated 60 first-born, healthy infants, 48 to 72 hours old, born to white, middle class mothers who had medically uneventful pregnancies and deliveries. Mothers had received commonly used analgesics (chiefly Demerol with Phenergan or Vistaril); anesthetic agents such as lidocaine, tetracaine, or mepivacaine via saddle block (42 of the 52 women receiving anesthesia); pudendal block; paracervical block; and so forth. Babies of mothers receiving anesthesia demonstrated decreased motor maturity and greater irritability when tested.

Scanlon's group tested 41 newborn infants during the first 8 hours of life. The 28 infants whose mothers had received continuous lumbar epidural blocks showed significantly lower scores on tests of muscle strength and tone and less vigorous rooting behavior (but no differences in sucking behavior).

Because the baby's early behavior is felt to be a significant factor in the early relationship between parents and infants (Chapter 15), this difference may prove to be an important one. It is also necessary to discover if there are differences at later periods, 1 week or 1 month, for example. Techniques for behavioral assessment (Chapter 16) have increased our capability of evaluating the effect of anesthesia on the newborn infant.

General Inhalation Anesthesia

General anesthesia is infrequently used for uncomplicated vaginal delivery today; the most common use is in an acute obstetric emergency.

Much of the care given to all

mothers during labor is directed toward the possibility that the mother may require a general inhalation anesthetic. She is allowed nothing by mouth (NPO), to prevent possible vomiting and aspiration. Antacids are frequently given so that if she does vomit and aspirate, the aspirate will be less acid. Nurses in the United States do not always realize that the practice of keeping women NPO during labor is by no means universal.

When inhalants are given to produce anesthesia (rather than analgesia), tracheal intubation is essential (below). Suction apparatus must be available and an intravenous infusion running.

One of several gases may be used. Each has specific advantages and disadvantages (Table 13–7).

Nursing Support. As with any patient who receives general anesthesia, vomiting is a danger for the mother in labor. She also presents special problems:

1. Unlike the surgical patient, she may have eaten a large meal shortly before she came to the hospital.

2. Stomach emptying is delayed during labor and may cease entirely. Thus, even if several hours have elapsed since she last ate, the potential for aspiration is still present.

Both during and after delivery, the woman who receives general anesthesia must be protected from aspiration.

In addition, the nursing assessment and support given to all patients who receive general anesthesia is also important for the mother.

On real disadvantage of general anesthesia is the barrier it raises to early maternal-infant interaction, as discussed below.

THE SECOND STAGE OF LABOR

As delivery becomes imminent, in most American hospitals the mother is moved to the delivery room. The exact stage at which the mother will be transferred varies with the individual. In a few hospitals, mothers now labor and deliver in a bed especially designed for both purposes, sometimes in the same

Table 13–7   GASES USED IN OBSTETRIC ANESTHESIA

Gas	Advantages	Disadvantages
Ether	Good muscle relaxation Does not interact with oxytocics Wide margin of safety	Flammable Takes effect slowly Causes nausea and vomiting Irritates respiratory tract
Methoxyflurane (Penthrane)	Nonflammable Nonirritating to respiratory tract	Too high a level leads to: 1. maternal hypotension 2. infant respiratory depression 3. maternal renal failure
Nitrous oxide (N_2O) and oxygen	Light anesthesia 25% N_2O can be eliminated from baby by ventilation after birth	High concentrations (above 75% N_2O) compromise oxygenation
Cyclopropane	Used chiefly in operative delivery	Highly explosive; not used intermittently for this reason

room and at other times in separate labor and delivery rooms. Such a system, which avoids transfer at a time when contractions are frequent and intense, has a great deal to recommend it.

The delivery room is a strange environment for both the mother and father. It is often cold (in temperature). While the mother is guided onto the delivery table, the father needs to be shown where he can sit at the head of the table close beside his wife's head, so that he can talk to her and support her. Both the mother and father will need our attention during the next hour as their labor draws to a climax.

Positioning on the delivery table involves placing of the legs in stirrups (both legs are elevated simultaneously) and showing the woman where she can place her hands in order to push more effectively. The mother is inevitably lying on her back in American delivery rooms, a position that is not really ideal. She is forced to push against gravity, which is one disadvantage. But perhaps the greatest problem is the danger of supine hypotensive syndrome, discussed above. A wedge, which is placed beneath the pad of the delivery table, will help to displace the uterus from the inferior vena cava. Supporting the mother's shoulders allows gravity to assist rather than to hinder delivery.

The vulva and surrounding area are cleansed with antiseptic solution, and the perineum is draped.

The area in which the baby will be received must also be warm and ready to receive the infant. All equipment for resuscitation should be available and ready for use (Chapter 18).

Perineal Lacerations

In a first degree perineal laceration, no muscles are involved. The muscles of the perineal body but not the rectal sphincter are involved in a second degree laceration. A third degree laceration extends to the rectal sphincter.

A major argument for episiotomy (below) is the prevention of perineal laceration.

Episiotomy

An *episiotomy* is an incision made in the perineum with a blunt scissors (Fig. 13–15). The vaginal opening is thus enlarged, and the likelihood of lacerations is decreased. As with many issues concerning birth, the need for episiotomy raises some controversy. In many hospitals, episiotomy is routine; others reserve episiotomy for those situations in which a perineal laceration seems likely.

Proponents of episiotomy argue that:

1. The straight, cleanly cut episiotomy incision heals more easily than a ragged laceration.

2. A laceration may involve adjacent structures, such as the rectum and/or anal sphincter; the direction of the episiotomy can be controlled.

3. Stretching and tearing of the perineum may predispose the mother to later perineal relaxation and to the possibility of cystocele and/or rectocele.

4. The second stage of labor is shortened.

5. The baby's head is not continually forced against the perineum.

An episiotomy is done far less frequently in Europe than in the United States. It has been suggested that one reason for the apparent necessity of episiotomy in the United States is the position in which women are placed on the delivery table (flat on their backs with legs in stirrups), which causes tension on the perineum and prevents a gradual stretching.

A technique termed "ironing out

Figure 13–15 Midline episiotomy. *A,* Muscles of the pelvic floor and perineum. The sites of median and mediolateral episiotomy are shown. *B,* Incision of the midline episiotomy. (From Oxorn and Foote: *Human Labor and Birth.* 3rd Ed., 1975. Courtesy of Appleton-Century-Crofts, Publishing Division of Prentice-Hall, Inc., Englewood Cliffs, N.J.)

the perineum," in which the perineum is stretched, is practiced by some midwives and physicians. There is a danger of separating the pelvic floor muscles, again leading to perineal relaxation.

Each mother should be evaluated individually. Although an episiotomy is probably not always indicated, it certainly would seem proper under certain circumstances.

Leboyer and the Second Stage of Labor

In 1975 the French obstetrician Frederick Leboyer published *Birth without Violence*, a book largely critical of traditional methods of delivery.[16] Leboyer's concepts rapidly became a major topic of discussion among many professional and lay men and women. Leboyer feels that infants suffer emotional trauma because of the violence of birth and that this trauma will affect the personality of the infant, not only at the time of birth but later in his life as well.

Unfortunately, much of the discussion of Leboyer's work has centered on questions such as "Should the baby be immersed in warm water following delivery?" and "Should the lights in the delivery room be dimmed?" while basic ideas are overlooked. We believe that the concepts of Leboyer described below are worthy of serious consideration.

1. The process of delivery should be gentle and controlled, with unnecessary intervention eliminated.

2. The baby should be handled gently, with head, neck, and sacrum supported.

3. The baby should not be overstimulated. He should be allowed to breathe spontaneously, without painful stimuli. Moderate suctioning is preferable to vigorous suctioning; overly vigorous suctioning may lead to reflex

bradycardia. Delayed cord clamping is advised. (Obviously, some babies do not breathe spontaneously and must be resuscitated, as described in Chapter 18.)

These concepts emphasize the "humanness" of the newly born infant; he is a being worthy of gentle handling. This principle is worthy of incorporation into our concept of care.

THE THIRD STAGE OF LABOR

The delivery of the infant ends the second stage of labor. Care is now divided between the newborn infant and the mother; adequate staff is essential to assure that neither is overlooked.

The mechanics of the third stage leading to the separation of the placenta have been described in Chapter 11. Separation usually occurs from 1 to 5 minutes after the baby is delivered. Evidence of placental separation includes:

1. The protrusion of the umbilical cord from the vagina.

2. A change in the shape (more globular), consistency (firmer), and position (higher in the abdomen) of the uterus.

3. A sudden gush of blood.

The fundus is not massaged before the placenta separates. Once separation occurs, the placenta must be expelled quickly and atraumatically. The mother is encouraged to push, just as she pushed her baby out. Unlike pushing at the time of delivery, when the mother was concentrating all of her attention on birthing her baby, she is now perhaps watching her baby or listening to his cry, a hundred thoughts rushing through her mind. She needs to be coached to push effectively.

If the mother is unable to push because of anesthesia, she must be assisted in expelling the placenta:

1. The fundus is palpated to be sure

that it is firm. If the uterus is not firm, it may become inverted when the placenta is expelled.

2. With one hand, exert downward pressure on the fundus; push the placenta out of the vagina.

After the placenta has separated, the fundus is massaged to facilitate contraction and thus to minimize blood loss. Accurate estimation of blood loss is essential. The average loss is approximately 250 to 300 ml.

If the placenta is not expelled, it must be manually removed. Manual removal is never a desirable situation; the risk of postpartal infection is increased and is still further increased in relation to the amount of time that elapses between birth and removal of the placenta.

The delivered placenta is always inspected; if it is not intact and fragments remain in the uterus, the chance for both postpartal hemorrhage (because the uterus cannot contract properly) and infection is heightened. Postpartal hemorrhage may be delayed for several days, occurring after the mother has returned to her home.

THE FOURTH STAGE OF LABOR

The first hour following the expulsion of the placenta, often called the fourth stage of labor, is a significant one for the family. It is a time for careful observation of both mother and baby from a physiologic perspective. Equally important, it is a time when attachment is facilitated between parents and their new infant.

The ideal environment during the fourth stage is a room in which mother, father, and baby can become acquainted. Mothers who have not been heavily medicated are often excited, aware, and "turned on" during the first hour after they deliver. Fathers are eager to be with the mother and baby. The baby of an unmedicated mother is usually alert and looking about for the first 30 to 45 minutes of life. If put to breast, he will suck, stimulating the secretion of oxytocin, which is the body's physiologic mechanism for contracting the uterus. Just the sight of her baby and the sound of his cry will also stimulate the mother's uterine contractions, through the mediation of the sympathetic nervous system.

Thus, if we consider maternal and infant behavior and physiology, the current practices of most hospitals in the United States appear designed in direct contradiction to the needs of infants and their parents.

Our current practices, as in the other stages of labor, evolved largely during the era of administering general anesthesia during birth. The first hour after birth, like the period following surgery, was one of recovery from anesthesia. The mother, asleep, was not aware of her baby. The baby slept as well. Immediate instillation of silver nitrate into his eyes for prophylaxis against ophthalmia neonatorum (Chapter 16) made the quiet, alert look of today's baby virtually unknown.

Perhaps the ideal situation is having both mother and baby together in a recovery bed with a warmer over the entire bed. Lacking such a warmer, the mother and baby can still be warmed with blankets; the heat of the mother's body also warms the baby. Adequately warmed, the mother and baby can touch skin-to-skin, whether the mother chooses to breast-feed or not (the significance of touch is discussed in Chapter 16). The father is with them, and the attachments of parents to baby and baby to parents begins.

Principal nursing goals for this period include:

1. Comfort for each member of the family.

2. Careful assessment of the mother.

3. Careful assessment of the baby.

4. Facilitation of attachment.

The assessment and immediate care of the baby is described in Chapter 16; the facilitation of attachment is discussed in Chapter 20.

Comfort

The father's comfort is enhanced by a comfortable chair beside the mother's bed, and often by a chance to go to the bathroom or have something to eat. A father who feels faint during or following delivery may be reacting to hunger, rather than to excitement.

A smooth, dry bed for the mother, a frequent change of perineal pads, a blanket because she may feel chilled all over or complain of cold feet—these are measures that provide comfort and thereby enhance bonding. If there is perineal discomfort, the application of an ice pack is frequently valuable in reducing edema and in providing relief.

Maternal Physiologic Assessment and Intervention

The major maternal danger during the fourth stage is postpartum hemorrhage. Thus, immediate physiologic assessment is directed toward those parameters that evaluate blood loss.

1. Is the fundus firm?

2. Where is the fundus in relation to the umbilicus?

3. Is there evidence of a perineal hematoma?

4. Does either maternal pulse (rapid, thready) or maternal blood pressure (falling) indicate abnormal bleeding?

5. Is the bladder full?

The Fundus. The uterus continues to contract and relax during the hour following delivery. When the uterus relaxes, bleeding from the vessels at the placental site occurs until thrombi form. Thus, it is important that the uterus be in a state of contraction.

The role of endogenous oxytocin (i.e., oxytocin produced in the mother's body) has been mentioned. Synthetic oxytocin is usually given to mother following delivery in the form of Pitocin, Methergine, or Ergotrate.

The firmness of the fundus is assessed every 15 minutes during the first hour (more frequently if the uterus does not remain contracted). Each time before the fundus is checked, the mother should be addressed, and if she is dozing, she should be alerted, with a statement such as, "Mrs. Yancy, I need to check your uterus to be sure it is firm." We need to recognize that this is not a comfortable procedure for the mother and to let her know that we realize this.

With the mother's legs flexed, the fundus is palpated by cupping one hand above the uterus and the other below (Figs. 13–16 and 13–17). The fundus should be felt in the midline at approximately the level of the umbilicus. The fundus is usually higher in multigravidas because the uterine muscles have been more stretched; factors such as polyhydramnios, multiple pregnancy, and a number of others will also affect uterine size and thus the position of the fundus after birth. If the fundus is not firm, it is gently massaged until it becomes firm.

The presence of blood and clots in the uterus is a barrier to contraction. Clots and blood are expressed by applying pressure for approximately 5 seconds, resting, and then reapplying pressure until all clots are removed. Hands are positioned for the expression of clots as they are for the assessment of the fundus.

Figure 13–16 Fundal massage, external view. While the left hand supports the bottom of the uterus, the right hand palpates the fundus and massages.

The same factors that affect the position of the fundus after delivery also predispose the mother to uterine *atony*, i.e., a lack of tone in the uterine muscles that makes it more difficult for them to remain contracted. In addition to hydramnios and multiple pregnancy, uterine atony or hypotonicity also is possible:

1. In any pregnancy in which the baby is large.

2. When labor has been very rapid or prolonged.

3. When the mother has preeclampsia and/or eclampsia.

4. When the mother has general anesthesia.

5. When the mother is a multipara.

The Perineum. Vaginal discharge following delivery is called *lochia*. The characteristics of lochia, which change during the days following birth, are described in Chapter 19. During the fourth stage, lochia is red (*ruber*) in color and contains blood, membrane fragments, decidua, lanugo, and vernix. Bright red blood in the lochia indicates fresh bleeding; this is *not* the expected color and requires immediate assessment to determine the source and intervention to control it. Lochia will smell like fresh blood, but it should not be foul smelling; foul-smelling lochia and/or mucus in the discharge indicates sepsis in the mother and potentially in the baby as well.

Lochia is partially absorbed by perineal pads; a record of the number of pads used, the degree to which they are saturated, and a description of clots provides an indication of excessive

Figure 13–17 Fundal massage, internal view. As in Figure 13–16, the left hand supports the uterus while the right hand palpates the fundus.

bleeding. When the pad is checked, the mother must be turned on her side so that lochia that may have pooled beneath the sacrum is not overlooked.

When the pad is checked, the perineum and surrounding skin should be gently washed; drying lochia is most uncomfortable.

Hematoma. Not only the amount and color of the lochia but the condition of the perineum itself should be assessed. The complaint of intense pain when the pad touches the perineum may indicate a hematoma, the result of tearing of a blood vessel and subsequent bleeding into the loose connective tissue. The skin over the area of hemorrhage is bluish-black. As bleeding continues, the hematoma may distend the perineum and dislocate the anus, rectum, and vagina. These subsequent symptoms are not usually evident until several hours after delivery, when pain may be reported in the vagina, rectum, or leg as well as in the perineum. However, early detection during the fourth stage may prevent a more extensive problem.

Aside from the intense discomfort, a hematoma may predispose to infection and, if bleeding is extensive, to anemia. Large hematomas are evacuated through the vaginal mucosa; the vaginal canal is then packed for 12 hours to assure hemostasis. Transfusion and antibiotics may be utilized if indicated. A small hematoma may be allowed to absorb; the mother should be carefully observed for signs of local or generalized infection.

A mother with intense pain is going to need particular help in enjoying her baby; this problem is discussed in Chapter 21.

Pulse and Blood Pressure. Usually blood pressure returns to normal prenatal levels shortly after delivery. Pulse rates are frequently somewhat slower than before pregnancy during the first 7 to 10 postpartal days.

Blood pressure and pulse are assessed every 15 minutes during the first hour, principally to ascertain excessive bleeding. However, changes in blood pressure and pulse may not occur until bleeding is already excessive; they are only one parameter by which bleeding is judged. When bleeding is so excessive that changes occur, a *rapid, thready pulse* usually precedes a drop in blood pressure. Thus, one cannot assume that an increase in pulse rate is insignificant if blood pressure remains normal.

Factors that may contribute to an elevated blood pressure during the fourth stage include excitement and certain medications, especially Ergotrate. Blood pressure is also affected by circadian rhythm (the 24 hour biologic cycle), being highest in the late afternoon and lowest in the middle of the night.

Sedation given during labor and certain types of anesthesia (caudal anesthesia, for example, or a saddle block) may lead to maternal hypotension in the hour following delivery.

The Urinary Bladder. A full urinary bladder inhibits contraction of the uterus and thus predisposes the mother to postpartal hemorrhage, both during the fourth stage and in the hours that follow.

Nursing evaluation of the fullness of the bladder is important because the effect of anesthesia may interfere with the mother's recognition of her need to void. A full bladder is felt above the symphysis pubis and below the fundus, which may be displaced upward and away from the midline.

EMERGENCY DELIVERY BY THE NURSE

Occasionally, a nurse finds herself caring for a mother for whom delivery is imminent, but there is no nurse-midwife or physician available. The mother may be in the hospital, but labor has progressed so rapidly that no one is prepared. Or she may be at home or in a public place.

It is not surprising that the mother and whoever is with her may be anxious to the point of near panic. We may feel equally anxious, but a major task for us is to assure her that most mothers can birth their babies with a minimum of difficulty. Nurse and parents work as a team with continuing communication.

The strict asepsis of the delivery room may not be possible outside of the hospital, but clean hands and a clean delivery area, covered with newspapers and/or clean linen of some type (towels, sheets), are usually possible.

1. The head will probably be crowning; encourage the mother to pant and *gently* control the progress of the head, particularly at the height of the contraction. Do not attempt to hold the head back. If possible, the head should be delivered between contractions to protect the baby's brain and the mother's perineum.

2. If the membranes have not ruptured when the head is delivered, rupture them immediately so the infant will not aspirate amniotic fluid when he breathes.

3. As the head is delivered, support it with one hand while you wipe away any blood or mucus on the face with the other.

4. In approximately 25 per cent of deliveries, one or more loops of cord are around the baby's neck. As soon as the head is delivered, feel around the neck to see if there are any loops of cord. A cord loosely wrapped about the neck may be slipped over the baby's head. If it is wrapped tightly, it will have to be clamped in two places and cut.

5. At the next contraction, help direct the anterior shoulder under the symphysis pubis with very gentle downward pressure on the side of the head. Supporting the baby, allow the birth of the posterior shoulder. The remainder of the body will follow easily.

6. Hold the baby so that the mucus will drain from his respiratory tract. Be sure there is no traction on the cord. The baby should cry; gently rubbing his back will help to stimulate that cry.

7. Dry the baby and place him on his mother's abdomen. Both of these acts help to keep him warm, which is vital (Chapter 15). He should be covered and positioned so that his head is dependent to facilitate further drainage of mucus.

8. The cord need not be cut right away. Cutting the cord with a dirty instrument is never the proper procedure. (This is obviously not a problem if the emergency delivery occurs in a labor room or somewhere else in the hospital but could be a major problem in a car or a shopping center.) Once the cord has stopped pulsating, it can be tied but left intact until the mother and baby can be taken to a hospital or until sterile equipment is available.

9. When it is apparent that the placenta has separated (above), ask the mother to bear down with the next contraction to deliver the placenta.

10. Putting the baby to breast following the delivery of the placenta stimulates the production of oxytocin, which in turn causes uterine contraction and prevents postpartal hemorrhage. As with all mothers, watch closely for postpartum hemorrhage. Massage the fundus if the uterus relaxes.

11. If the mother is not in the hospital, she and the baby should be transported to a hospital for further evaluation and care.

PLANNED HOME DELIVERY

The issue of home delivery was discussed in Chapter 4. A nurse who is participating in a planned home delivery (as opposed to an emergency home delivery) must be aware of the legal implications in her particular state.

In a planned home delivery, sterile equipment will usually have been prepared. Some plan in the event of an emergency for either the mother or the baby should be decided upon well in advance of the time of delivery.

SUMMARY

The number of hours of contact between parents and nurse during labor may be equal to or greater than the number of hours of contact during the entire prenatal period.

Nurses have much to offer families during these hours. By our careful assessment of the mother and fetus/infant, by planning and intervention that provides physical and emotional comfort and support, and by continuing evaluation of the care we give, we do provide the significant difference in childbearing for parents and their babies.

REFERENCES

1. Afriat, C., and Schifrin, B.: Sources of Error in Fetal Heart Rate Monitoring. *JOGN*, 5:11, 1976.
2. Barnes, A.: Prophylaxis in Labor and Delivery. *New England Journal of Medicine*: 294:1235, 1976.
3. Bing, E.: *Six Practical Lessons for An Easier Childbirth*. New York, Bantam Books, 1969.
4. Caldeyro-Barcia, R., Noriega-Guerra, L., Cibils, L., et al.: Effect of Position Changes on the Intensity and Frequency of Uterine Contractions During Labor. *American Journal of Obstetrics and Gynecology*, 80:285, August, 1960.
5. Chabon, I.: *Awake and Aware*. New York, Dell Publishing Co., 1966.
6. Dulock, H., and Herron, M.: Women's Response to Fetal Monitoring. *JOGN*, 5:68s, 1976.
7. Eiger, M., and Olds, S.: *The Complete Book of Breastfeeding*. New York, Bantam Books, 1973.

8. Ewy, E., and Ewy, G.: *Preparation for Childbirth*. New York, New American Library, 1972.
9. Grad, R. K., and Woodside, J.: Obstetrical Analgesics and Anesthesia: Methods of Relief for the Patient in Labor. *American Journal of Nursing*, 77:242, 1977.
10. Greenhill, J., and Friedman, E.: *Biological Principles and Modern Practice of Obstetrics*. Philadelphia, W. B. Saunders Co., 1974.
11. Hon, E.: *An Introduction to Fetal Heart Rate Monitoring*, 2nd Edition. Los Angeles, University of Southern California School of Medicine. Copyrighted by the author, 1975.
12. Huprich, P.: Assisting the Couple Through a Lamaze Labor and Delivery. *MCN* 2:245, 1977.
13. Karmel, M.: *Thank You, Dr. Lamaze*. Philadelphia, J. B. Lippincott Co., 1959.
14. Lamaze, F.: *Painless Childbirth: The Lamaze Method*. New York, Pocket Books, 1972.
15. Langhorne, F.: The Fetal Monitor: Friend or Foe. *MCN*, 1:313, 1976.
16. Leboyer, F.: *Birth Without Violence*. New York, Knopf-Random House, 1975.
17. Lowensohn, R. I.: Instrumentation for Fetal Heart Rate Monitoring. *JOGN*, 5:75, 1976.
18. Martin, C., and Gingerich, B.: Factors Affecting the Fetal Heart Rate: Genesis of FHR Patterns, *JOGN*, 5:305, 1976.
19. Miller, F. C., Petrue, R. H., Arce, J., et al.: Hyperventilation during Labor. *American Journal of Obstetrics and Gynecology*, 120:489, 1974.
20. Page, E., Villee, C., and Villee, D.: *Human Reproduction. The Core Content of Obstetrics, Gynecology and Perinatal Medicine*. 2nd Edition. Philadelphia, W. B. Saunders Co., 1976.
21. Parer, J.: Physiological Regulation of Fetal Heart Rate. *JOGN*, 5:265, 1976.
22. Scanlon, J., Brown, W., Weiss, J., et al.: Neurobehavioral Responses of Newborn Infants after Maternal Epidural Anesthesia. *Anesthesiology*, 40:121, 1974.
22a. Schifrin, B.: Fetal Heart Rate Monitoring during Labor. *Journal of the American Medical Association*, 221:992, 1972.
23. Scott, J. R., and Rose, N. B.: The Effect of Lamaze Preparation on Labor and Delivery. *New England Journal of Medicine*, 294:1205, 1976.
24. Standley, K., Soule, A., Copano, S., et al.: Local-Regional Anesthesia during Childbirth: Effect on Newborn Behaviors. *Science*, 186:634, 1974.
25. Wiley, J.: The Nurse's Legal Responsibility in Obstetric Monitoring. *JOGN*, 5:77s, 1976.
26. Yeh, S., Forsythe, A., and Hon, E.: Quantification of the Fetal Heart Beat-to-Beat Interval Differences. *Obstetrics and Gynecology*, 41:355, 1973.

Chapter 14

VARIATIONS IN LABOR

For many reasons, the course of labor may vary from the pattern described in Chapters 11 and 13. Some variations, such as those of presentation, have already been discussed.

Variations are related to:

1. A need to induce labor for specific reasons.
2. Failure of labor to progress.
3. Contractions that are too strong or too frequent.
4. Recognition of fetal distress.
5. Preterm labor.
6. Multiple gestation.
7. Emergencies that occur during the course of labor.
8. The needs of individual patients (the mother with heart disease, for example).

SUPPORTING THE PARENTS WHEN LABOR VARIES

When the course of labor varies from what parents have expected, it is understandable that the anxiety that all parents feel to some extent is compounded.

Nurses can help all parents during the prenatal period by emphasizing that there are many possible variations in labor and that by no means are all of them life-threatening or damaging to their baby.

When the unforeseen occurs during the course of labor, the mother and her companion should be told what is happening. No matter what we have to tell them, suspecting that something is not as it should be (and they will suspect this) and not being told the truth will make them even more anxious.

Although no mother should labor alone, the mother with a difficult labor is particularly in need of constant support. When staffing does not permit continuing attention to every mother (an unfortunate reality in most labor rooms), this mother has priority, not only for physiologic reasons but also because of her special emotional needs.

Keeping the mother continually informed will usually eliminate the necessity for abruptly presenting her with a dramatic change of plans—a sudden cesarean section, for example, which may cause total panic. Of course, there are instances in which sudden change occurs for which no one was prepared, such as a marked change in fetal heart rate. Nurse and physician must act rapidly to deal with the physical emergency, but at the same time the mother and her companion must also be informed.

When fathers were first allowed in labor rooms in increasing numbers in the late 1960's and the early 1970's, there were many questions about "what will we do with the father if there is some unexpected change in the mother's condition?" Nurses and physicians, barely comfortable with fathers during labor under the best of circumstances, often felt they could not cope with their presence during emergencies.

In many labor rooms, the atmosphere has changed. There is a recognition that fathers not only are able to cope with the unexpected but can help support the mother during an emergency or change of course in a way that professionals never could.

Obviously, this is not true for all fathers under all circumstances. Nor are all nurses or physicians as yet comfortable with parents in every situation. But the idea that fathers must immediately leave when complications are suspected is no longer practiced as a hard and fast rule.

INDUCTION

There are certain circumstances under which it is considered advisable not to wait for labor to occur spontaneously but to *induce* labor, i.e., to intervene to cause the labor to begin. Preeclampsia and premature rupture of the membranes are examples of medical indications for induction. Some physicians induce mothers to control the date of delivery, a practice termed *elective induction*, which is frequently debatable unless rather stringent criteria are met.

In prenatal classes, prospective parents often ask about induction. "Is it true that I can have my baby on a specific date"? Although the idea has a certain appeal to parents in terms of convenience, both elective induction and elective cesarean section (described below) may unnecessarily cause the birth of an immature infant. Tests for fetal maturity, for example, the lecithin/sphingomyelin (L/S) ratio, may one day become a prerequisite for elective induction.

Amniotomy

Amniotomy, the artificial rupture of the membranes, is used to initiate labor. However, labor does not always follow, and fetal infection becomes a risk, particularly if the membranes are ruptured more than 24 hours before delivery.

Oxytocic Agents

Oxytocic agents, such as Pitocin, are frequently used for the induction of labor as well as for other circumstances described in this chapter. Oxytocics are potent drugs. If the mother receiving a medication such as Pitocin is not very carefully and continually assessed, serious complications, including the possibility of fetal death or rupture of the uterus, may occur.

The most common method for administration of oxytocin is by intravenous drip. Buccal, sublingual, or transnasal routes are also used; taken orally, however, oxytocin is deactivated in the stomach. An infusion pump is used so that the rate of infusion will remain constant even when the mother changes position.

Initially 5 I.U. of oxytocin is added to 500 ml. of a 5 per cent dextrose in water solution and administered intravenously at a slow rate of approximately 6 to 8 drops per minute. Monitoring equipment should be used to assess contractions and fetal heart rate continually. The mother's pulse, respirations, and blood pressure are assessed every 15 minutes. If there is no evidence of fetal distress, the rate of infusion is increased approximately 4 drops per minute every 15 minutes until the rate is 16 to 20 drops per minute, with constant observation of the maternal and fetal signs described above. The rate of oxytocin is highly individualized; some mothers are sensitive to very small amounts. Desirable results are contractions lasting 45 to 60 seconds at 2 to 3 minute intervals, with complete relaxation between contractions. If contractions exceed 90 seconds in duration (a *tetanic* contraction) or if there is evidence of fetal hypoxia, the infusion is discontinued.

Tetanic contractions cause a marked decrease in uterine blood flow and subsequent fetal acidosis and bradycardia. If there is already a problem with placental perfusion, as in the mother with pre-eclampsia or hypotension, the problem is compounded.

Since the half-life of oxytocin is approximately 3 minutes, the amount in the blood drops rapidly when the infusion is discontinued. (This is the reason that intramuscular oxytocin is not used; circulating oxytocin is replenished by oxytocin in the muscles.)

Oxytocin has an antidiuretic effect; urine output will decrease during administration. If the woman reports that she has a headache and/or begins to vomit, she may have water intoxication.

THE FAILURE OF LABOR TO PROGRESS

Labor does not always progress in the manner described in Chapter 11. *Dystocia* is the term used to describe difficult labor. Dystocia may be due to a problem of powers, passage, or passenger (Table 14–1) or a problem in the interrelationship of one or more of these factors.

Assessing Failure to Progress

Continuing assessment of a woman's progress during labor is the basis by which failure to progress is recognized. Table 14–2 summarizes certain specific criteria that are useful in determining whether the course of labor is normal.

The Friedman curve (described in Chapter 11) is a simple method of recognizing abnormal patterns of labor. By plotting an individual woman's progress, patterns that vary from the norms may more quickly be recognized.

Prolonged Latent or Acceleration Phase. Figure 14–1 illustrates the *prolongation* of the *latent phase*. Too much analgesia given too early in labor is a common reason for such prolongation. Thus, an important aspect of nursing care during early labor is supporting the mother so that she will not require medication. If the cervix is not ready for labor ("unripe"), i.e., if it is thick, uneffaced, and undilated, efface-

Table 14–1 DYSTOCIA IN LABOR

Problem Area	Basis	Intervention
Powers	Dysfunctional contractions	Rest, possibly with sedation Possible oxytocin
Passage	Cephalopelvic disproportion (CPD)	Cesarean section
Passenger	Abnormal presentation Abnormal fetal development	Varies with specific cause

Table 14-2   A COMPARISON OF NORMAL AND ABNORMAL PATTERNS DURING LABOR

Type of Pattern	Assessment Criteria	Possible Cause
Normal		
Friedman curve	Duration: <20 hours primipara <14 hours multipara	
Hypoactive		
Prolonged latent phase Prolonged acceleration phase	Duration: >20 hours primipara >14 hours multipara	False labor Dysfunctional contractions Unprepared cervix Sedation given too early
Prolonged active phase	Dilatation: <1.2 cm./hr. primipara <1.5 cm./hr. multipara or No progress over a 2 hour period	Fetal malposition CPD Inefficient activity of uterine muscles
Prolonged deceleration	>3 hours primipara >1 hour multipara <1 cm./hr. primipara <2 cm./hr. multipara	Abnormal descent through the pelvis Fetal malposition Possible CPD
Slow descent of fetal head	No descent	
Hyperactive		

Tetanic contractions	Uterus does not relax between
	contractions
		Mechanical obstruction to descent,
		  including pathologic retraction
		  ring
		Overstimulation with oxytocics

Precipitate labor	Dilatation > 5 cm./hr.	Hyperactive contractions
Precipitate delivery	Unusually short second stage	
Irregular		
Irregular contractions	Intensity varies Duration varies No pattern	Etiology unclear

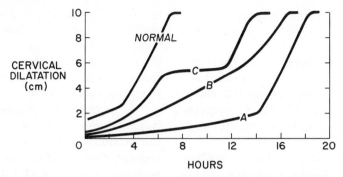

Figure 14-1 Major aberrant labor patterns. *A,* Prolonged latent phase; *B,* protracted active phase; and *C,* secondary arrest of dilatation. (From Page, Villee, and Villee: *Human Reproduction: The Core Content of Obstetrics, Gynecology and Perinatal Medicine.* 2nd Edition. Philadelphia, W. B. Saunders Co., 1976. Modified from Friedman.)

ment and dilatation will be slowed. About 10 per cent of the time, a prolonged latent phase may be due to ineffective contractions of the uterine muscles.

Allowing the mother to rest by giving her a sedative and/or a narcotic will usually result in: (1) cessation of contractions (indicating false labor) or (2) more effective contractions and active labor after the rest period. Should neither occur, oxytocin may be given.

Prolonged Active Phase. The prolongation of the active phase of labor may be primary, in that the entire course of labor is prolonged, or it may occur as a secondary arrest in a labor previously progressing in a normal fashion.

Primary dysfunctional labor is due to fetal malposition, cephalopelvic disproportion (CPD), or inefficient myometrial contractions, in that order. Excessive sedation or conduction anesthesia may cause a *secondary arrest* of labor; fetal malposition and CPD are also causes of secondary arrest.

The treatment of secondary arrest depends upon discovering the cause. Inefficient myometrial activity may be helped by rest and later by administer-ing oxytocin. Cesarean section will be necessary if CPD is the diagnosis (see below).

Nursing Intervention When Labor Fails to Progress

The discussion above has briefly indicated some types of medical intervention that are appropriate when labor fails to progress.

Nursing intervention may also alleviate the problem:

1. A change in position may lead to more effective contractions. Walking, if not contraindicated, may be helpful. A side-lying position is often more effective, producing more intense, although less frequent, contractions.

2. A distended bladder impedes descent of the fetal head. Frequent voiding and, if necessary, catheterization are therefore essential.

3. An enema, early in labor, eliminates feces as an impediment to descent and may also stimulate contractions.

OPERATIVE PROCEDURES

Medical intervention in difficult labor often involves operative procedures. The most common operative procedures are the use of forceps and cesarean section.

The Use of Forceps.   In their desire for a "natural" birth, some mothers fear the use of forceps in the delivery of their baby. Carefully and correctly used, forceps can assist in the safe delivery of a baby.

Most commonly, forceps are applied after the fetal head is crowning; this is called a *low forceps* or *outlet forceps* delivery (Fig. 14–2). The use of outlet

forceps is usually elective, i.e., the physician chooses to use forceps to better control the delivery, to protect the fetal head from "battering" against the perineum, and to minimize trauma to the perineal tissue.

A *midforceps* delivery, when the head is engaged but has not yet reached the perineal floor, is usually for a specific reason. That reason may be maternal (inability of the mother to push because of conduction anesthesia, insufficient uterine activity, eclampsia,

Figure 14–2   Low forceps delivery. *A,* The forceps are in place; the handles are separated with the left index finger and thumb; the pull is forward and downward with combined forces. *B,* Traction is continued, but with partial elevation of the head; the handles are separated to avoid compression of the fetal head. *C,* The head is delivered by further extension over the perineum. (From Greenhill and Friedman: *Biological Principles and Modern Practice of Obstetrics.* Philadelphia, W. B. Saunders Co., 1974.)

heart disease, or exhaustion, for example) or fetal (fetal bradycardia, meconium in the amniotic fluid, or fetal malposition, for example).

In all deliveries utilizing forceps:

1. The operator must be highly skilled (nurses do not apply forceps even in emergency deliveries; most nurse-midwives do not apply forceps).

2. Forceps are not used when there is cephalopelvic disproportion.

3. The head must be engaged.

4. The cervix must be completely effaced and dilated.

5. The exact presentation and position of the fetus must be known.

6. The presentation must be cephalic.

7. The membranes must be ruptured.

8 The bladder must be empty.

Anesthesia is given to the mother for a midforceps delivery in order to assure perineal relaxation.

Explanations to the mother, such as "the forceps will help guide the baby's head through the birth canal," are essential. Some mothers may wonder at the time about "forceps marks" on the baby and need to be reassured that they will be only temporary.

CESAREAN SECTION

Cesarean section is an operative procedure by which an infant is delivered through an incision in the abdominal and uterine walls. Approximately one baby in ten in the United States is delivered by cesarean section. The rate of cesarean delivery has been increasing steadily in the United States over the last 2 decades (Table 14–3). In some hospitals, the rate is greater than one of every five deliveries.

Because subsequent deliveries to women who have previously delivered by section are commonly also cesarean deliveries, one might suspect that "repeat sections" would be a major factor in this increase. However, both Hibbard[7] and Jones[8] in their separate studies found that repeat sections, which had accounted for approximately one-half of all sections in the 1960's, were responsible for one-third or less of all sections in the mid-1970's.

It is the number of *primary* or first sections that are responsible for the increase. Two probable factors are:

1. Difficult vaginal deliveries, including many breech presentations that might formerly have been attempted vaginally, are now delivered by section.

2. As a result of fetal monitorings, fetal distress and apparent fetal distress are recognized earlier, and labor is interruped by section rather than risking the possibility of further fetal compromise.

No one knows what the long-term effect of cesarean section is on infants;

Table 14–3   PERCENTAGE OF CESAREAN SECTIONS IN TWO HOSPITALS FROM 1969 TO 1975

California Hospital*		North Carolina Hospital†	
YEAR	PER CENT	YEAR	PER CENT
1969	6.0	1970	6.3
1970	9.4	1974	9.0
1974	9.1	1975	10.3
		(Jan.–June)	

*From Hibbard: *American Journal of Obstetrics and Gynecology*, 125:798, 1976.
†From Jones: *American Journal of Obstetrics and Gynecology*, 125:521, 1976.

the need for research in this area certainly grows as the number of sections increases. The perinatal death rate for infants delivered abdominally has decreased in the past decade.

A cesarean section may be an "elective" procedure or a response to factors that arise during the course of labor.

"Elective" cesarean section is not elective in the sense that the mother chooses to have the procedure, but rather that the decision for section is made prior to the onset of labor; the timing is thus elective. Indications include a previous section (although previous section does not always require subsequent section) or other surgery that has left a scar on the uterus. If pelvic measurement indicates a pelvis obviously inadequate for vaginal delivery, cesarean section is planned. The term cephalopelvic disproportion (CPD) is used to describe this situation. Mothers with diabetes mellitus are commonly delivered by section; mothers with pre-eclampsia or hypertension may also be.

Many indications for section arise during the course of labor. When the presentation is other than vertex, cesarean section is increasingly the method of delivery. Hibbard[7] states that the prevailing philosophy is abdominal delivery for breech presentations associated with one or more complicating obstetric factors, such as prematurity.

Signs of fetal distress, indicated by fetal monitoring and scalp sampling, have already been cited as a reason for intervention. Failure of labor to progress is an important indication. Maternal hemorrhage from abruptio placentae or from placenta previa unrecognized before delivery frequently leads to emergency sections.

Types of Cesarean Sections

Abdominal delivery may be accomplished by a *low segment cesarean section*, a *classic cesarean section*, or a *cesarean hysterectomy*.

Low Segment Cesarean Section. Low segment cesarean section is the most common type of abdominal delivery today. The incision is made in the lower part of the uterus, behind the bladder (Fig. 14-3). There is less hemorrhage because the incision is in an area of thin fibrous tissue. Vaginal delivery is usually possible in a subsequent pregnancy if the fundamental reason for the section no longer exists. (For example, abdominal delivery would still be necessary if the reason for the first section was a very small pelvis, but not if the reason was a breech presentation.) Jones noted in reviewing 2563 abdominal deliveries that in less than 3 per cent of succeeding pregnancies was there a cause for concern that the uterus might rupture at the site of the scar.[8] However, in actual practice, most obstetricians will continue to deliver a woman abdominally once she has had a section.

Fewer abdominal adhesions result from a low incision than from the other cesarean procedures.

Classic Cesarean Section. In the classic procedure, a midline incision is made in the abdomen between the umbilicus and the symphysis pubis. The baby is grasped by his feet and delivered through an opening in the uterus approximately 11 cm. long. Because the incision traverses the thick uterine muscle, there is a greater possibility of hemorrhage, of poorer healing and possible rupture, and of postoperative adhesions to the bowel and therefore of obstruction. Nurses caring for women following cesarean section must know the type of procedure used in order to make pertinent observations.

Under certain circumstances, such as a placenta previa (Chapter 10), a classic incision may be preferred by the obstetrician.

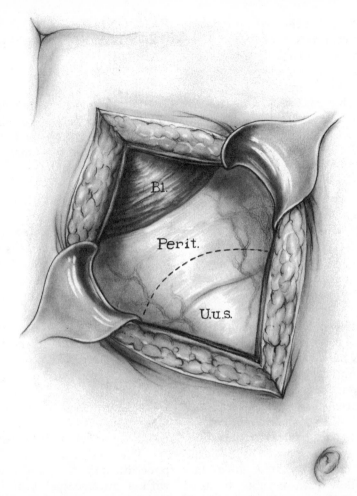

Figure 14–3 Low segment cesarean section. The abdomen has been exposed by a longitudinal incision, and the operative field is exposed. The dotted line shows the intended elliptical incision in the loose pubocervical peritoneum. *Bl.*, bladder, *Perit.*, peritoneum; and *U.u.s.*, upper uterine segment. The patient is oriented here so that her head is down and to the right. (From Greenhill and Friedman: *Biological Principles and Modern Practice of Obstetrics*. Philadelphia, W. B. Saunders Co., 1974.)

Cesarean Hysterectomy. In cesarean hysterectomy, the uterus is removed after the delivery of the baby. Possible reasons include uterine tumors, uterine rupture, and uncontrollable bleeding following delivery.

Nursing Support Following a Cesarean Section

The decision for cesarean section and the operative procedure itself are medical decisions in which neither nurse nor parents have a major role. However, the nursing role in other aspects of care for these mothers and their families is *significant*.

Consider the couple who have prepared for childbirth through reading, attendance at classes for expectant parents, or discussion with friends. The moment of birth often has come to have special meaning for them. They may have heard glowing descriptions of the joy of "pushing" their baby out and of the exhilaration of the moment of birth.

When they find that they will not have this experience, it is not surprising that some parents express a feeling of disappointment and loss, *if* they are given the opportunity to express that disappointment. They may feel "abnormal," different from other couples.

To compound their feelings of loss and abnormality, their baby may be treated differently. Because the incidence of respiratory distress is higher in infants delivered abdominally (Chapter 18) and because fetal distress, maternal diabetes, pre-eclampsia, or some other condition affecting the fetus may have necessitated the section, infants delivered by section are frequently placed in special care nurseries and separated from their parents for a longer period than are babies delivered vaginally. Thus hospital policies related to abdominal delivery may be a barrier to important early contact.

If the cesarean section is an elective procedure, preoperative preparation is similar to that for abdominal surgery. In addition to the physical preparation of the mother, the baby's heart rate should be checked. Time must be found to allow both parents to ask questions and to express their feelings about abdominal delivery.

Immediate physical postoperative care is again similar to that of a postoperative abdominal surgery care. Assessing the fundus is difficult because of abdominal dressings and tenderness, so that particularly careful attention must be paid to other signs that indicate bleeding, such as blood pressure and pulse rate. If the mother is awake (i.e., if she has had spinal anesthesia), she should have an early opportunity to see her infant.

Special infant needs will be related to specific problems, such as an infant with transient tachypnea, an infant of a diabetic mother, and so on (Chapter 18).

RECOGNITION OF FETAL DISTRESS: FETAL SCALP SAMPLING

Fetal bradycardia and/or a pattern of late deceleration or variable decelerations that do not respond to treatment indicate possible fetal distress. At the first indication of fetal distress, fetal scalp sampling is usually indicated. One reason is that although a "good" fetal heart rate pattern usually indicates a healthy fetus, a pattern of variable or late decelerations is not as reliable. In addition, the information from a series of fetal scalp samples is more valuable than the data from a single sample.

Laboratory values vary somewhat from one institution to another. A fetal scalp pH value of 7.25 or above is usually considered within normal limits. Values from 7.20 to 7.24 indicate a need for continuing assessment, while two or more values below 7.20 may indicate a need for immediate intervention.

The technique itself involves puncture of the fetal scalp (or buttocks) with a microscalpel that is inserted through a conical endoscope (Fig. 14–4). Following the collection of blood in a heparinized glass capillary tube, pressure is applied to the puncture site with a sponge throughout the next two contractions. The site is then observed during a third contraction; if no bleeding occurs, the endoscope is removed.

Continuing fetal distress that is not rapidly alleviated is an indication for medical intervention. Nurses are often the first to detect such distress and have a significant responsibility in communicating the exact nature of the distress to a physician immediately. A record of that communication should be in the mother's record for legal purposes. The importance of both the communica

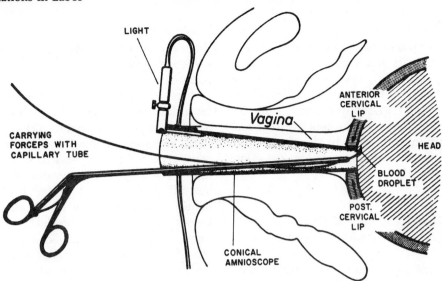

Figure 14–4 Diagram showing method of obtaining a fetal blood sample. (From Willis: *The Canadian Nurse*, Dec., 1970.)

ion and the record cannot be overemphasized.

PREMATURE LABOR

When a mother begins to have labor contractions prior to 38 weeks of gestation, she is understandably anxious for her baby's welfare. She also may feel guilty, wondering and asking "What did I do to cause this to happen?" (Chapter 22).

An attempt to stop labor with bed rest, sedation, and a pharmacologic agent such as intravenous alcohol may be attempted. Mothers receiving intravenous alcohol will often appear intoxicated; this can be very distressing to some families and should always be explained.

If it is at all possible, the mother should be admitted to a medical center that is equipped to care for a preterm baby. Transporting a fetus in utero presents far fewer hazards than transport-

ing an immature infant. Moreover, there are real advantages to having both mother and baby in the same hospital to facilitate bonding. Admittedly, that choice is not always available.

The delivery of a preterm infant (i.e., an infant delivered prior to 38 weeks, Chapter 18) must be even more gentle than a delivery at term. The cranial bones are poorly calcified and offer little protection to the brain; the danger of cerebral hemorrhage resulting in death or brain damage is a very real one. A large episiotomy and the very careful use of forceps are attempts to prevent injury to the baby's brain.

Little or no analgesia is used in order to prevent respiratory depression. Techniques of relaxation and breathing described in Chapter 9 are often very helpful to mothers during premature labor.

Because the baby may need resuscitation at birth and other medical attention and because he is at risk of hypothermia (Chapter 18), it is rarely possible for the mother and father to hold their baby during the time following birth. If at all possible, and especially if the baby is to be transferred to another hospital, they should have the opportunity to see and touch him. In addition, they must be kept aware of his condition and taken to the nursery to see him as soon as possible (see also Chapter 18).

LABOR IN A MULTIPLE GESTATION PREGNANCY

Just as the antepartal period may be complicated when there is more than one fetus (Chapter 10), so too may labor. Twins usually deliver prior to term, thus having the same problems of labor and premature delivery as those described above. The second twin, and the second and subsequent infants in other multiple deliveries, is particularly at risk.

The delivery of the first twin is similar to that of other preterm infants. The presentation and condition of the second infant is then evaluated; he may be delivered shortly after the first baby, or there may be a period of time that elapses before the second twin is ready for delivery. The presenting part may change several times before it is finally engaged and delivered.

Friedman and Little[4] report that second twins born between 2 1/2 and 15 minutes after the first twin fared best; mortality rates tripled if delivery was either sooner or later.

This is a most difficult time for parents. The first infant may be in poor condition, requiring resuscitation. The wait for the delivery of the second twin may seem far longer than the actual time involved. It is a time of "not knowing," which is always hard to cope with. Sometimes the professional staff is so involved in delivery and resuscitation that the anxious parents are overlooked. They need to know what is happening.

Not every multiple birth is equally hazardous. Recently our intensive care nursery was notified that a mother with twins and a second mother with triplets were expected to deliver within 2 or 3 hours. We prepared for five admissions but all of the triplets were healthy babies close to 5 pounds in weight who were able to be cared for in the full-term nursery and were discharged along with their mother when they were 4 days old. Only the preterm twins required intensive care.

The mother who delivers more than one infant usually has an overdistended uterus and is at risk of developing postpartum hemorrhage. Very careful observation during the fourth stage of labor and after she returns to the postpartal unit is essential.

COPING WITH EMERGENCIES DURING THE FOUR STAGES OF LABOR

Rupture of the Uterus

When labor does not progress for any of a variety of reasons mentioned in this chapter or when contractions are very intense, usually because of oxytocin infusion, rupture of the uterus may occur. Frequently, the baby is seriously damaged or dies; maternal mortality is from 5 to 10 per cent.

Uterine rupture is usually sudden, accompanied by a sharp abdominal pain. The mother has symptoms of shock. Both uterine contractions and fetal heart tones cease. Hemorrhage may be into the peritoneal cavity rather than into the vagina.

Immediate recognition and inter-

ention are essential; immediate hys-
erectomy is usually the course taken.

Prevention, by careful evaluation
f the mother throughout labor, and in-
ervention, when labor fails to progress,
an avert most instances of rupture of
he uterus.

rolapse of the Umbilical Cord

When the umbilical cord is at the
evel of the presenting part or below the
resenting part, the cord is said to be
rolapsed (Fig. 14–5). This is a serious
omplication because pressure on the
ord prevents the fetus from receiving
xygen and can cause serious brain
lamage or death if intervention is not
apid and successful. If the cord pro-
apses outside of the vagina, umbilical
vessels may constrict, also compromis-
ng fetal oxygen supply.

The risk of a prolapsed cord is
higher when certain circumstances
exist:

1. The membranes rupture before
the presenting part is engaged.

2. The presentation is breech or
transverse.

3. The infant is preterm.

4. The pregnancy is a multiple gestation.

5. Hydramnios is present.

A prolapse of the cord most commonly occurs following rupture of the
membranes. For this reason the mother
and fetus are carefully assessed at that
time. Observe the mother for protrusion
of the cord from the vagina (seen sometimes but not always), meconium staining of the amniotic fluid, or the passage
of meconium. (If the presentation is
breech, meconium does not necessarily
indicate fetal distress.)

Figure 14–5 Prolapse of the
umbilical cord. *A,* Occult prolapse.
Because the membranes are unrup-
tured, there is little pressure on the
cord. *B,* Forelying cord. There may
be pressure on the cord. *C,* Prolapsed
cord with a high risk of cord compression.

Fetal heart rate changes and variable decelerations on the fetal heart monitor are fetal indications of cord prolapse and compression.

Nursing Intervention. The goal of nursing intervention is to relieve pressure on the cord. At the same time, it is necessary to calm and support the mother so that she can cooperate in her own care. This mother must have constant nursing attendance; a second nurse must find the physician if one is not present in the delivery room.

Pressure on the cord is relieved by elevating the mother's hips on a pillow or by helping the mother to assume a knee-chest position (Figs. 14–6 and 14–7). Oxygen is given by mask to the mother in order to provide the highest possible level to the fetus. If the cord is protruding, it should be kept moist with sterile saline. Delivery should be as quick as possible by cesarean section.

Should a mother experience a prolapsed cord when she is not in the hospital (usually at the time of rupture of the membranes), she must be hospitalized as quickly as possible. In a car or ambulance, the same principles of care apply:

1. Elevate hips.

2. Give oxygen if available.

3. Apply a moist covering to the cord.

Amniotic Fluid Embolism

If amniotic fluid enters the mother's circulatory system, an embolus may form in the arterioles or capillaries of the pulmonary circulation, resulting in fetal and maternal death.

The mother receiving oxytocin who has rapid, intense contractions is most at risk; hence the careful monitoring of the mother receiving oxytocin is important. (This has been emphasized previously, but can hardly be overstressed.) A multipara with a large fetus is also at increased risk.

How does the amniotic fluid enter the mother's circulation? Potential pathways include:

1. Rupture of the membranes into the upper uterine segment, with entry through the site of the placenta.

2. Partial separation of the placenta, which exposes blood vessels in the myometrium.

3. Rupture of the uterus.

Figure 14–6 One approach to managing the prolapsed cord is the elevated Sims' position, whereby the pelvis is raised on pillows above the level of the uterine fundus. (From Greenhill and Friedman: *Biological Principles and Modern Practice of Obstetrics.* Philadelphia, W. B. Saunders Co., 1974.)

Figure 14–7 A useful method of displacing the head out of the pelvis to relieve cord compression by placing the patient in the knee-chest position. (From Greenhill and Friedman: *Biological Principles and Modern Practice of Obstetrics*. Philadelphia, W. B. Saunders Co., 1974.)

4. Entry through the endocervical veins.

When these conditions occur, very strong contractions may force amniotic fluid into the circulation. The mother will quickly become dyspneic and cyanotic. Immediate intervention is aimed at relieving respiratory distress by administration of oxygen and change of position and summoning assistance.

A side effect of amniotic fluid embolism is disseminated intravascular coagulation (DIC) (Chapter 10), related to the thromboplastic properties of amniotic fluid. Thus, the mother must be constantly evaluated for symptoms of hemorrhage and shock.

To be in labor and to suddenly find that you are unable to breathe is understandably overwhelming for the mother and whoever is with her. They should never be left alone for both physiologic and supportive reasons.

MATERNAL CONDITIONS REQUIRING MODIFICATION OF CARE DURING LABOR

Care during labor is modified for mothers with particular problems. The most common conditions are pre-eclampsia, diabetes, and heart disease.

The Mother with Pre-eclampsia or Eclampsia

When a mother has severe pre-eclampsia or eclampsia (Chapter 10), her care is directed toward: (1) improving her condition, and (2) determining the maturity and condition of the fetus.

The aim of her care is to control the manifestations of her disease until the fetus shows evidence of being sufficiently mature for extrauterine existence (Chapter 13).

Once he is believed to be mature, labor is induced by amniotomy and oxytocin infusion (see above). Mother and fetus are carefully monitored, watching especially for symptoms of pre-eclampsia–eclampsia in the mother and for fetal distress. The fetus is at risk because the blood supply to the placenta is often compromised.

Induction is not always possible. It may have been attempted and failed. The cervix may not appear ready ("ripe"). For these and other reasons, cesarean section may be necessary.

Regardless of the type of delivery, there is the possibility of a high risk infant; adequate personnel and equipment must be ready to care for a sick baby.

Following delivery, the mother with eclampsia continues to need especially careful observation. She is at risk of seizures until she has started to diurese, which may be as late as 48 hours after the birth of her baby. If she remains in an obstetric intensive care unit and if her baby is in an intensive care nursery, it may be difficult to provide contact between mother and baby. Any action that can promote her attachment—a Polaroid picture of her baby or a careful description of his condition and care—is very important.

Once diuresis occurs, blood pressure usually returns to prepregnancy levels, edema disappears, and the mother is no longer at risk.

The Mother with Diabetes

Labor and Delivery. The last 3 to 4 weeks of pregnancy are particularly hazardous to the fetus of a diabetic mother; mortality is high, possibly because of inadequate placental function.

When the fetus is judged mature on the basis of the tests described in Chapter 10, or when his status is obviously deteriorating, he is delivered. A large number of babies of diabetic mothers are delivered by cesarean section, although labor, monitored to assess fetal well-being, may be permitted. Regular insulin and intravenous glucose are given to the mother on the day of delivery, when she is allowed nothing by mouth.

Perinatal mortality statistics indicate that no diabetic mother should be allowed to continue her pregnancy beyond the expected date of delivery.

Following Delivery. When the placenta is delivered, a major source of insulin-antagonism is removed very suddenly from the mother's body. Insulin needs drop dramatically; less insulin may be required than prior to pregnancy. Some mothers require no insulin during the first 24 to 48 hours after delivery. The mother will need both close monitoring of her serum glucose and support during this period of reregulation of her diet and insulin.

Because her baby may be in an intensive care nursery during the first hours and perhaps days after birth (Chapter 18), she will also need supportive nursing care to help her deal with her fears and other feelings about the baby (Chapter 22).

About 6 to 9 months following delivery, insulin requirements will probably be at prepregnancy levels. This means that long-term follow-up will be necessary for mothers with diabetes. The single check-up at 4 to 6 weeks is not appropriate. Contraceptive instruction prior to discharge from the hospital is also important; a pregnancy immediately following delivery would not be advisable.

The Mother with Heart Disease

Mothers with heart disease are normally delivered vaginally. Cesarean section is performed only if there is an obstetric reason, such as cephalopelvic disproportion. Cardiac disease, per se, is not an indication for cesarean section.

During labor, as during pregnancy the goal is to decrease cardiac load. The amount of work done by the woman herself is minimized. This mother labors in the semi-Fowler's position and at times on her side. Supine hypotensive syndrome (Chapter 13) is particularly dangerous for her, so she should never lie flat on her back.

Several specific measures are important in protecting the mother with heart disease during labor. This mother should be very closely supervised, not just by mechanical monitoring, although this will probably be a part of ner care, but also by close nursing observation. Her vital signs, particularly pulse, respirations, and blood pressure, must be checked and recorded more frequently than those of an apparently healthy mother.

If she is receiving intravenous fluids, the rate is closely monitored to prevent fluid overload and subsequent congestive failure. A pulse rate over 100 and/or a respiratory rate over 28 strongly suggest the possibility of congestive heart failure. Should heart failure occur, the treatment is medical: morphine, oxygen by mask, intravenous digitalis, and a diuretic such as furosemide (Lasix).

Every effort is made to reduce the levels of anxiety and of pain, which may in themselves lead to heart failure. Although this should be the goal for every mother, special effort must be made for the mother with cardiac disease. Continuous caudal or epidural anesthesia may be used for this purpose; spinal anesthesia is not used for mothers with cardiac disease because of the effect on the cardiovascular system (Chapter 13).

Antibiotics may be given to prevent the possibility of endocarditis.

The mother with heart disease should not "push" during the second stage. Frequently she is anesthetized to prevent pushing. If there is no progress after 30 to 60 minutes, the delivery may be assisted with forceps.

The position for delivery is the semi-Fowler's position, with the legs supported at the level of the heart or below.

During the third stage of labor (1) fluid moves from the extravascular space to the vascular tree, and (2) blood from the lower extremities flows unobstructed toward the heart with the emptying of the uterus and the removal of pressure on the vena cava. Thus during the third and fourth stages mothers must be observed very carefully for signs of heart failure.

SUMMARY

Mothers with a labor that varies from normal need both emotional support to help them cope with the unexpected variations and the anxiety and fear that accompany the unknown and careful, knowledgeable attention to the physiologic aspects of their care. Families must not be excluded in the care of these mothers.

REFERENCES

1. Freeman, R. K.: Intrapartum Management of the Pregnant Patient with Heart Disease. *Clinical Obstetrics and Gynecology*, 18(3):75, 1975.
2. Friedman, E.: *Labor: Clinical Evaluation and Management*. New York, Appleton-Century-Crofts, 1967.
3. Friedman, E. A., Hunt, H. B., and Sachtleben, M. R.: Disordered Labor: Simplified Method for Recognition. *OB/GYN Digest*, 17:12, 1975.
4. Friedman, E. A., and Little, W. A.: An Evaluation of the Management of Twin Delivery. *Bulletin of Sloane Hospital*, 4:39, 1958.
5. Greenhill, J., and Friedman, E.: *Biological Principles and Modern Practice of Obstetrics*. Philadelphia, W. B. Saunders, Co., 1974.
6. Harrison, E., and Roschke, E. J.: Pregnancy in Patients with Cardiac Valve Prostheses. *Clinical Obstetrics and Gynecology*, 18(3):107, 1975.
7. Hibbard, L.: Changing Trends in Cesarean Section. *American Journal of Obstetrics and Gynecology, 125*:798, 1976.
8. Jones, O. J.: Cesarean Section in Present-Day Obstetrics. *American Journal of Obstetrics and Gynecology, 125*:521, 1976.
9. Manning, P., Mestman, J., and Lau, F.: Management of the Pregnant Patient with Mitral Stenosis. *Clinical Obstetrics and Gynecology, 18*(3):99, 1975.
10. Oxorn, H., and Foote, W.: *Human Labor and Birth*. New York, Appleton-Century-Crofts, 1975.
11. Page, E., Villee, C., and Villee, D.: *Human Reproduction. The Core Content of Obstetrics, Gynecology and Perinatal Medicine*. 2nd Edition. Philadelphia, W. B. Saunders Co., 1976.
12. Ziegel, E., and Van Blarcom, C.: *Obstetric Nursing*. 6th Edition. New York, The Macmillan Company, 1972.

Chapter 15

TRANSITION TO EXTRAUTERINE LIFE

Probably no other 24 hour period in an individual's history is as momentous as the first. Even mere survival is significant; approximately half of the neonatal deaths (i.e., deaths during the first 28 days of life) occur within these first 24 hours, largely, but not entirely, due to prematurity.

Consider the changes that the newborn must face. Externally his environment could hardly be more different. Formerly warm, dark, and totally liquid, it is now chilly, filled with glaring light, and dry. Strange sounds, sights, touches, and tastes surround him.

Changes in his internal environment are equally dramatic. He must, almost instantly, convert to a different mode of respiration and circulation. Blood vessels carrying blood high in oxygen content prior to birth will now carry blood with lower oxygen content. Liver and kidney functions alter, and a number of metabolic processes must reorganize for a new way of life.

Equally significant are the beginning relationships between the baby and his parents that develop during the first day.

NURSING GOALS

The goals of nursing care during these first 24 hours are basically three:

1. Utilizing careful observation to detect any sign or behavior that indicates abnormality is essential. Since changes in newborn infants occur in a very short period of time, their detection is dependent upon the nurses who are with the baby.

2. Meeting the basic physiologic needs of the baby, achieved through the interaction of parents and nurses.

3. Facilitating the relationship between the baby and his parents.

Each goal is equally important, and we plan to achieve them simultaneously. Even in a life-threatening situation, for example, when an infant and his parents may need to be separated, we can facilitate their relationship by our own relationship with his mother and father (Chapter 22).

In order to achieve these goals, nurses must know:

1. What the newborn is like during the first 24 hours of transition.

2. What physiologic changes normally take place.

3. What his immediate needs are and how they can best be met.

4. What the significance of parent-baby contact is during the first 24 hours and how we can best facilitate it.

SPECIFIC PERIODS DURING THE TRANSITION

Close observation shows that both the vital signs and the clinical appearance of a newly born baby vary within the first 24 hours. The initial transition includes an immediate period of reactivity, an interval during which the baby is relatively unresponsive and inactive, and then a second, more active period. The transition usually is complete in the healthy full-term newborn by about 6 hours of age.

The initial period of reactivity lasts for approximately 15 to 30 minutes after birth and is characterized by activity in many body systems. The heart beats rapidly, muscle tone is increased, and the baby is alert and exploring. He may have tremors of his extremities or chin and sudden outcries that stop as suddenly as they began. He sucks, swallows, grimaces, and moves his head from side to side.

If the mother has not been anesthetized, the baby is generally alert during this period and will look at his mother and father attentively. This period seems designed by nature for the attachment of parents and baby. Then, for approximately an hour and a half, he becomes much more quiet and relatively unresponsive. His color improves as his muscle tone returns to normal. Heart and respiratory rates decline. Both external and internal stimuli bring little response.

A second period of reactivity completes the transition. Specific differences in these three periods are compared in Table 15–1. By comparing the activities of healthy infants with these norms, nurses can come to recognize more readily what is usual and unusual during this significant time.

PHYSIOLOGIC CHANGES

The physiologic functioning of the infant differs from that of the fetus in several important respects.

Respiratory Changes

At approximately 24 weeks' gestation, alveolar cells begin to produce *surfactant*, a lipid substance essential in preventing alveolar collapse after birth. By 26 to 28 weeks, pulmonary alveoli proliferate, and capillaries multiply in very close proximity to them, two additional antecedents necessary for post-delivery respiration.

Throughout fetal life, the lungs are filled with lung fluid, which keeps them partially expanded so that it will not be as difficult for them to expand at the time of delivery.* What happens to this fluid? In a vertex delivery the pressure of the birth canal on the fetal thorax literally "squeezes" part of the fluid from the lungs and out through the baby's nose and mouth. The remaining fluid is picked up by the blood vessels and lymphatics surrounding the lungs, a process greatly facilitated by the changes in pulmonary vasculature described below (see circulatory changes).

When the baby is delivered in a presentation other than vertex, by cesarean section or by breech presentation, for example, this fluid is not as easily expelled from the lungs. The lungs are

---

*Consider how much easier it is to blow up a balloon that has been previously filled with water or air than a brand new one that has never been expanded.

Table 15–1   THE TRANSITION TO EXTRAUTERINE LIFE IN THE HEALTHY TERM NEWBORN

	Initial Period of Reactivity (First 15 to 30 Minutes)	Period of Relative Inactivity (30 Minutes to 2 Hours)	Second Period of Reactivity (2 to 6 Hours)
Respirations	Irregular; peak at 60–90 per minute; transient rales; grunting, nasal flaring, thoracic retractions; sternal retractions not unusual; brief apnea	Respiratory rate declines: periods of rapid respirations with dyspnea; shallow, synchronous breathing with barreling of chest	Brief periods of rapid respirations; periods of irregular respirations with apneic pauses
Heart rate	Tachycardia; mean peak 180 beats per minute at 3 minutes	Heart rate declines; 120–140 beats per minute	Labile; wide swings from bradycardia to tachycardia
Color	Brief cyanosis; acrocyanosis	Color improves; flushing when crying	Abrupt color changes
Body temperature	Drops	Low	Begins to rise
Bowel sounds	Absent initially; present after 15 minutes	Present	Bowel cleared of meconium
Oral mucus	May be visible	Small amounts watery mucus	Prominent; may have gagging and vomiting
Activity	Alert, exploratory, intensely active	Sleeps; quiet activity	
Response to stimuli	Vigorous	Relatively unresponsive to external and internal stimuli	More responsive
Signs of possible illness	Rapid, shallow breathing; signs of cerebral hemorrhage: twitching, apnea, full fontanel, opisthotonos	Signs of respiratory distress: grunting, tachypnea	Persistence of subnormal temperature; hypoglycemia; apnea, cyanosis; lethargy

stiff, and the baby breathes rapidly for several days, a condition termed *transient tachypnea* of the newborn (Chapter 16).

A combination of factors appears to cause the baby to take his first breath (below). Within 10 minutes after birth the volume of air remaining in the lungs at end expiration is the same as it is at 5 days of age. Vital capacity reaches values proportional to those of an adult within 8 to 12 hours after birth.

Circulatory Changes

Fetal circulation is illustrated in Figure 15–1. The establishment and maintenance of good respiration influence the changes that occur in the cardiovascular system at the time of birth (Fig. 15–2). Within moments following delivery:

1. Oxygen enters the lungs, and pulmonary alveoli expand.

2. The oxygen lowers resistance in the pulmonary vessels, allowing blood to flow more freely to and from the lungs. (In the fetus, no more than 10 per cent of the total circulating blood flowed through the lungs.)

3. Pressure in the right atrium decreases because of the increased flow of blood to the lungs.

4. Pressure in the left atrium increases because of the increased flow of blood from the lungs.

5. With oxygenation, the ductus arteriosus begins to constrict, becoming functionally closed during the first 24 hours. (If the Pao_2 is low or becomes low during the first days of life, the ductus arteriosus has the capacity to remain open or to reopen.)

6. The umbilical vessels, already clamped in the delivery process, contract.

7. As pressure in the left side of the heart begins to exceed that in the right side (due to the activation of pulmonary circulation described above), the valve of the foramen ovale becomes "plastered" against the septum secundum, thus functionally closing the foramen ovale.

Although functional changes in circulation take place very shortly after birth, structural changes occur over a period of many months (Table 15–2).

Changes in Kidney Function

Prior to birth the kidney is apparently not essential to life, although it forms urine that becomes part of the amniotic fluid from about the twelfth gestational week. Even a fetus with total renal agenesis may exist intact, because the placenta carries on the necessary regulatory functions. At birth, however, the kidney must immediately begin to function; the infant totally lacking kidneys cannot survive.

Just as pulmonary vascular resistance decreases, allowing more blood to flow to and from the lungs, so also does the vascular resistance of the renal vessels decrease, allowing increased blood flow to the kidneys with a marked improvement in kidney function within a few days.

Kidney function, however, remains immature for many months. The glomerular filtration rate is low, a factor particularly significant in the sick baby because the excretion of drugs by the kidney is limited. Acid-base balance is labile because the bicarbonate threshold is low. (In adults no bicarbonate is spilled into the urine until serum levels reach 24 to 26 milliequivalents per liter [mEq./L]; term newborns lose bicarbonate when serum levels reach 21 to 22 mEq./L and preterm babies at levels of 19 to 20 mEq./L.) Newly born infants also retain hydrogen ion, another factor in acid-base metabolism.

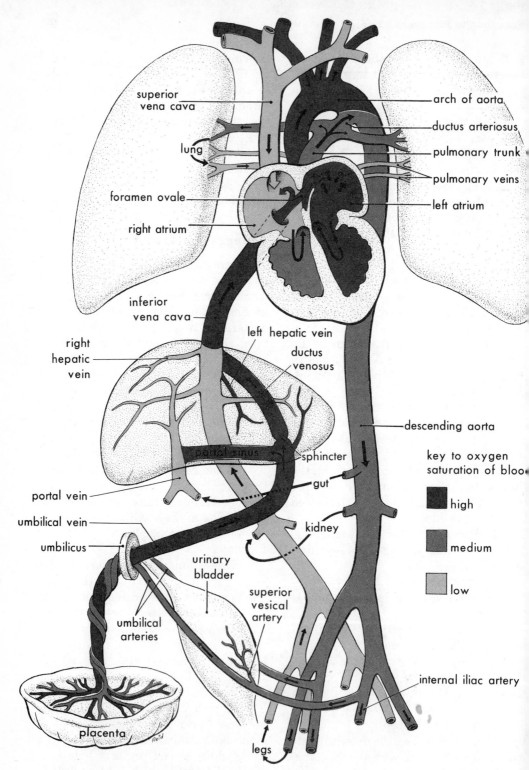

Figure 15–1 A simplified scheme of the fetal circulation. The darkened areas indicate the oxygen saturation of the blood and the arrows show the course of the fetal circulation. The organs are not drawn to scale. (From Moore: *The Developing Human: Clinically Oriented Embryology.* 1st Edition. Philadelphia, W. B. Saunders Co., 1973.)

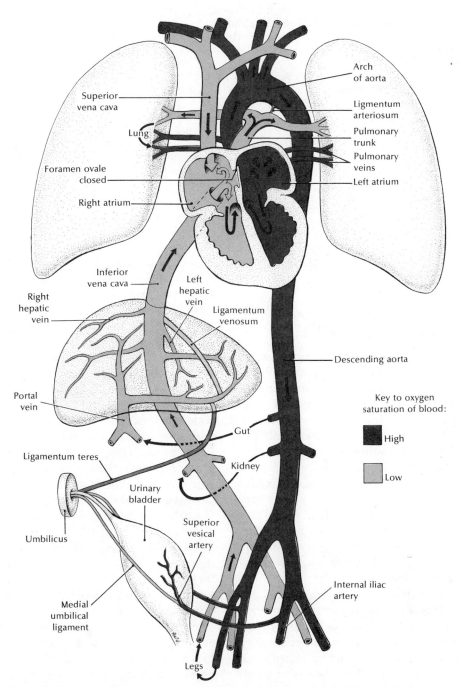

Figure 15–2 A simplified representation of the circulation after birth. The adult derivatives of the fetal vessels and structures that become nonfunctional at birth are also shown. The arrows indicate the course of the neonatal circulation. The organs are not drawn to scale. (From Moore: *The Developing Human: Clinically Oriented Embryology.* 1st Edition. Philadelphia, W. B. Saunders Co., 1973.)

Table 15–2   STRUCTURAL CHANGES FROM FETAL TO INFANT CIRCULATION*

Structures in Fetal Circulation	Approx. Time of Anatomic Obliteration	Resulting Structures
Foramen ovale	1 year	Fossa ovalis
Ductus arteriosus	1 month	Ligamentum arteriosum
Ductus venosus	2 months	Ligamentum venosum of the liver
Umbilical arteries	2–3 months	Distal portion: lateral umbilical ligaments Proximal portion: internal iliac arteries, which function throughout life
Umbilical vein	2–3 months	Ligamentum teres of the liver

*From Moore: *The Newborn and the Nurse.* Philadelphia, W. B. Saunders Co., 1972.

Because the loop of Henle is short, newborns have a limited ability to concentrate their urine.

Changes in Liver Function

In the fetus the liver is the chief organ of blood formation from the third to the sixth months and continues to produce some cells into the first postnatal week.

Some functions that were handled by the placenta during fetal life must now be undertaken by the liver, such as the excretion of bilirubin. Placental excretion of bilirubin would seem to explain why there is usually minimal rise of serum bilirubin levels in cord blood in newborn infants with erythroblastosis (Chapter 18), but a rapid increase within a few hours after birth.

Glucuronyl transferase, the enzyme necessary for the conversion of indirect bilirubin to water-soluble direct bilirubin that can then be excreted by the kidneys, is less active during the first days of life. Thus even the small degree of hemolysis that normally occurs in the newborn can cause a pronounced degree of hyperbilirubinemia and subsequent jaundice.

Prothrombin and blood clotting Factors VII (proconvertin), IX (plasma thromboplastin component), and X (Stuart-Prower) are synthesized in the liver. The prothrombin level is low in cord blood. Prothrombin time, which measures the activity of Factors VII and X,* may be within a normal range or low at birth, but will become most prolonged at 3 to 4 days of life and will continue at abnormally prolonged levels for 2 to 3 additional days. About 75 per cent of term infants and an even greater number of preterm infants show this drop in clotting factors. These changes are related to the inability of the baby to synthesize and utilize vitamin K; they mean that the infant has a greater risk of hemorrhage than those infants who have no drop in clotting factors.

In most nurseries 1.0 mg. of vitamin K is given to every newborn shortly after birth. This practice has virtually eliminated hemorrhagic disease of the newborn. Larger amounts of vitamin K do not enhance its therapeutic value;

---

*Factor V (proaccelerin) is also measured in prothrombin times, but is at normal levels in the newborn.

oreover, larger doses predispose the aby to hyperbilirubinemia and kernicerus. Giving vitamin K to the mother uring labor, rather than to the baby, as been found to be less dependable. atural vitamin K preparations (e.g., quaMephyton, Konakion) act more apidly than synthetic preparations .g., Hykinone, Synkamin) and are nsidered a better choice for that reason.

Infants of low gestational age have n even more limited ability to synthesize clotting factors, even in the presence of large amounts of vitamin K.

hanges in the Blood

By the sixth month of fetal life the one marrow has become the chief site f blood formation. At the time of birth is highly active, with most of the marw space involved in red cell producon. This means that there is little 1arrow reserve to increase red cell production if any excess hemolysis occurs. s mentioned above, the liver may connue to produce red blood cells during 1e first week of life because of this lack f marrow reserve; the spleen is an additional site of extramedullary ematopoiesis.

Hemoconcentration appears to be a 1ajor characteristic of the first hours of fe. Hemoglobin concentration rises by s much as 17 to 20 per cent during the rst 2 hours, then drops slightly, but till remains elevated until some time etween the first and third weeks. Iemoglobin levels in the term newborn ange from 17 to 22 grams per 100 ml. nd from 15 to 17 grams per 100 ml. in 1e preterm baby. Decreasing hemoglon levels during the first week indicate ed cell destruction or blood loss. Iematocrit values also rise abruptly uring the first hours of life and then ecline slowly; values at 1 week of age

are close to values in cord blood (57 to 58 per cent for term newborns; 45 to 55 per cent for preterm infants) (Appendix A).

Red blood cells increase during the first hours, so that the level of cells is more than 500,000 per cu. mm. higher than the level of cells in cord blood. The red blood cells of the newborn infant are usually larger than those of an older infant; by the end of the second month cells are close to adult size in infants born at term. Most studies seem to indicate that the lifespan of red blood cells of term infants is the same or only slightly shorter than that of a normal adult, while that of preterm infants is definitely shorter. There is no universal agreement about this, however.

A small increase in the white cell count likewise occurs at the time of birth, possibly also due to hemoconcentration. Following this initial peak, the white cell count drops, and leukocytes become markedly less efficient at phagocytosis after the first 24 hours and throughout the first month. One study reports the mean number of leukocytes as 18,000 at birth, 12,200 at 7 days, and 11,400 at 14 days.[1] (See also Appendix A.) This decrease in number and activity of leukocytes is one factor in the newborn's lowered resistance to infection (Chapter 17). White cell counts vary widely from infant to infant and even within the same infant from day to day for no apparent reason. Thus a single elevated white cell count is of little value; two or more tests are needed when sepsis is suspected.

When comparing blood values during the first hours and days of life, it is important to remember that capillary samples, usually obtained from the heel or toe, have higher concentrations than venous samples. It is believed that this is because of the relatively sluggish circulation in the peripheral blood vessels, which in turn leads to transudation of the plasma. Warming the area by wrapping it with a warm towel for a few minutes before the sample is obtained and also discarding the first few drops of the sample minimize these differences. Even then, capillary samples should not be compared with venous or arterial samples.

Acid-Base Balance

All newborn infants are to some degree acidotic at the time of birth. In infants with normal lungs and ventilation, the acidosis corrects itself within the first hour (Table 15–3). Infants who have had a period of apnea or a delay in the onset of respirations will be more acidotic, with pH values falling below 7.0.

Values will vary according to the site from which the sample was obtained. There is considerably less oxygen and slightly more carbon dioxide in venous blood. If the sample is obtained from a heel stick and the heel is not warmed adequately, the blood obtained may be venous blood. The pH and Pco_2 values will vary slightly, but the Po_2 of venous blood is normally 40 mm. Hg while the Po_2 of arterial blood is normally 90 to 100 mm. Hg. Thus in high risk babies who need close monitoring an umbilical artery catheter is usually inserted shortly after delivery (Chapter 18).

Metabolic Changes

Because plasma glucose and calcium are regulated by the placenta during fetal life, even a healthy newborn shows immaturity in glucose and calcium metabolism during his first days It is from 1 to 2 weeks before homeostasis is obtained. Babies who are preterm, who develop postnatal illness, or who are infants of diabetic mothers or mothers with hyperparathyroidism may have their metabolism severely taxed. See hypoglycemia and hypocalcemia (Chapter 18).

THE DELIVERY ROOM: MEETING IMMEDIATE NEEDS

In the moments following birth the baby needs both warmth and established respirations. An initial physical assessment must be made. He should be protected from ophthalmia neonatorum and must also be properly identified Parents should have some opportunity to see and hold their child.

The Need for Warmth

The temperature of the newborn infant at the moment prior to delivery is about 3/4 of a degree higher than that of his mother. The need of the newborn baby for warmth is therefore his first priority. We place it ahead of the establ

Table 15–3   NEONATAL ACID-BASE BALANCE

	pH	Po_2	Pco_2	HCO_3 (Bicarbonate)
Cord blood	7.2	16–32*	60–70	23
Arterial blood at 1 hour	7.32	90–100	35–40	20

*Values vary considerably, even in vigorous newborns, from as low as 0 to as high as 96 mm. Hg in a number of studies. Mean Po_2, if from cord blood, varied from 16 to 32 mm. Hg in several reports.

lishment of respirations in this text (although for practical purposes attention to the two is virtually simultaneous) because when resuscitation is necessary, body temperature must be maintained during any attempt at resuscitation, or these efforts will be hampered.

The Baby's Attempts to Maintain Warmth. Delivery rooms in the United States are usually cold, chilly places—about 15 degrees colder than the environmental temperature in the uterus. For those who are wrapped in sterile gowns and working under hot lights, this is comfortable. But for even a normal newborn infant, wet with amniotic fluid and naked, this cold is highly undesirable. (Who among us enjoys walking into an air-conditioned room directly from a swimming pool?) A term baby can compensate for a certain amount of cold stress because of stores of glucose and brown fat. For a baby prior to term, stress from cold can truly be the difference between life and death.

The chief reason why cold is so threatening is that cold increases oxygen consumption.* The baby becomes unable to meet his oxygen needs from room air and switches to anaerobic metabolism, causing an accumulation of lactate with the subsequent development of metabolic acidosis. Chilling may also lead to vasoconstriction and, in turn, to tissue hypoxia, and may result in an earlier predisposition to kernicterus (Chapter 18).

Energy expenditure is also increased. A newborn infant can lose as

*Knowing that hypothermia is used in surgery to reduce oxygen consumption, the question quite naturally is why chilling should increase oxygen consumption in the baby. The distinction must be made between the true, deep hypothermia in a controlled situation, which lowers the metabolic rate, and chilling, which increases metabolism.

many as 200 calories per kilogram per minute in the delivery room through four separate mechanisms: evaporation, convection, radiation, and conduction. If we realize that an adult who is fully able to compensate for heat loss generates only 90 calories per kilogram per minute, we can appreciate how severe this heat loss is.

Like the older child or adult, the baby does attempt to maintain his body temperature by retaining and producing heat. *Vasoconstriction* is the principal means of heat retention. Vasoconstriction is more difficult for those babies whose mothers have been treated with magnesium sulfate for toxemia of pregnancy. *Insulation,* a significant means of heat conservation in older individuals, is limited in a newborn because of both the small amount of subcutaneous fat and the large surface area in relation to body weight. (The surface area to body mass ratio is also important in fluid balance.) The smaller the infant, the more deficient his insulation; infants weighing less than 2500 grams have virtually no subcutaneous fat. *Assumption of the fetal position* is a further attempt to conserve heat.

Heat production in newborns is accomplished principally by increasing the metabolic rate, thus causing the increase in oxygen consumption. This is termed *nonshivering thermogenesis*, in contrast to the shivering thermogenesis of older humans.

Brown fat, which accounts for approximately 2 to 6 per cent of the total body weight in term babies, is one of two energy sources required for increasing this metabolic rate (glucose is the other). Brown fat is found chiefly at the base of the neck, in the mediastinum, and surrounding the kidneys. When temperature receptors perceive cold, norepinephrine acts upon brown fat to release free fatty acids as energy sources for increased metabolism.

Meeting the Needs of the Baby for Warmth. Ideally, a baby should be placed in a *thermoneutral environment* as quickly as possible after birth. A thermoneutral environment is one that enables the baby to maintain a body temperature of 36.5°C. (97.7°F.), plus or minus 0.5°C., with the minimum use of energy. The younger and smaller a baby, the higher the thermoneutral environment must be. Older, larger newborns have a wider tolerance of cold than smaller infants, but not the tolerance of a baby 1 to 2 months old.

Every delivery room should be equipped with a means of warming the baby without restricting the care that is given to him. Both the warmer and the blanket in which the baby is to be wrapped should be heated in anticipation of the delivery so that the baby is immediately placed in a warm environment. In this way heat loss by radiation and conduction is minimized. Without such warming, the baby would radiate heat in an attempt to raise the temperature of the entire delivery room—rather like trying to raise the temperature of an entire building with a single fireplace.

Conductive heat loss is eliminated by laying the baby on a warm, dry towel or blanket. The single act of drying the baby reduces heat loss from evaporation by 50 per cent. By avoiding the possibility that a current of cool air might blow across the baby, convective heat loss is also controlled.

In our justifiable concern for keeping the baby warm, it is easy to overlook the desire and need for parents to touch and hold their baby immediately following birth. In addition, an increasing number of mothers are asking to breast-feed at this time. Celeste Phillips, a California nurse, has done some interesting research in this area which is discussed on page 466.[19]

One final note on warming: *hyperthermia*, as well as hypothermia, also increases oxygen consumption and thereby compromises the baby. Hyperthermia occurs far less often in our cold delivery rooms; it is more a possibility in a nursery in which the room or incubator temperature is not well regulated or in which the infants are placed too near sunshine or heating ducts (Fig. 15–3).

The Establishment of Respirations

What causes the newborn to take his first breath? Multiple stimuli—thermal, tactile, chemical, and reflex—are probably all important. *Thermal* stimulation is inevitable; the contrast between the 37°C. temperature of the uterus and the roughly 23°C temperature of the average delivery room provides more than the needed difference. Further chilling, as discussed above, is highly undesirable.

Tactile stimuli should be gentle; the traditional "spank" is neither necessary nor advisable. The handling of the baby that is involved in the delivery process will usually be adequate. A light flick to the soles of the feet may be an additional help.

How *chemical* stimulation affects the initiation of breathing is unclear. As already mentioned, the infant is normally acidotic at birth, with acid-base balance restored within the first hour of life.

Reflex stimulation may be due to receptors in the airway. Their location and their role in the initiation of respiration is not clear.

The initial force necessary to aerate the lungs for the first breath is 10 to 20 times greater than that needed for the second and subsequent breaths, an im-

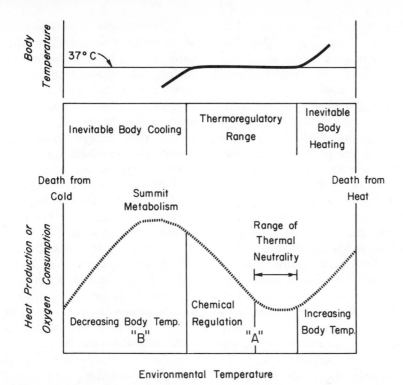

Figure 15-3 Effect of environmental temperature on oxygen consumption and body temperature. (From Klaus and Fanaroff: *Care of the High-Risk Neonate.* Philadelphia, W. B. Saunders Co., 1973. Adapted from Merenstein and Blackmon.)

portant factor if resuscitation is necessary.

Facilitating the Establishment of Respirations. For over 90 per cent of newborns, clearing fluid and mucus from the air passages by gentle suction with a bulb syringe and gravity is all that is necessary to facilitate respirations. The baby is placed in the warmer in a *head down* position, preferably on his side, so that any additional fluid can drain from his respiratory tract and will not be aspirated. Resuscitation of those infants who do not breathe spontaneously is discussed in Chapter 18.

Prevention of Ophthalmia Neonatorum

Prior to the use of silver nitrate prophylaxis, 25 per cent of the children in schools for the blind in the United States were blind because of ophthalmia neonatorum, a gonococcal infection of the eye contracted during labor and delivery by direct contact with gonococcal organisms in the cervix. Occasionally the infection occurs during the first days of life, possibly by contamination from the mother's fingers.

The occurrence of ophthalmia neonatorum dropped dramatically both in the United States and in Europe as Credé prophylaxis with silver nitrate, and later antibiotic prophylaxis to a lesser extent, became legally mandatory in many areas. In the United States, silver nitrate must be used in 15 states; silver nitrate or an "other equally effective agent" is specified in the laws or regulations of 33 other states and the District of Columbia.* However, as the worldwide incidence of gonorrhea has increased to epidemic levels, so too has the incidence of ophthalmia neonatorum increased.

Careful instillation of prophylactic silver nitrate in the eyes of each infant within the first hour following birth is therefore extremely important. Because silver nitrate is irritating and causes the baby to shut his eyes, we prefer to delay instillation until after the initial meeting of parents and baby.

The packaging of silver nitrate in wax ampules, which prevent both evaporation and overconcentration, has virtually eliminated serious chemical eye injury. Chemical irritation does occur, however; a mild chemical conjunctivitis *should* result if prophylaxis is properly performed. This is a transient condition with no permanent sequelae.

An antibiotic ointment as an alternative to silver nitrate has been used in those states so permitted by law, largely because of the chemical irritation caused by the silver nitrate. However, it is currently believed that:

1. Antibiotic preparations offer no better prevention.

2. Penicillin may lead to sensitivity or untoward reaction.

3. There is an increase in the number of gonococci that are resistant to penicillin.

4. Antibiotics could encourage the colonization of antibiotic-resistant organisms in babies in the nursery.

Prophylaxis does not always prevent gonococcal infections. There are a number of possible reasons why this is so, several of which are directly related to nursing care.

*A summary of the laws and regulations requiring use of a prophylactic for the prevention of ophthalmia neonatorum in effect as of August 1968 is available from the National Society for the Prevention of Blindness, Inc., 79 Madison Avenue, New York, New York 10016.

The medication may have been inadvertently overlooked. Perhaps the baby was in severe distress and was rushed immediately to an intensive care nursery, with total attention being focused on lifesaving procedures. Or perhaps the mother needed unusual attention from delivery room personnel. In each obstetric-neonatal system there must be checks against overlooking such an important facet of care.

The medication may have been improperly administered. One drop should be placed in each conjunctival sac. The lids must be separated so that the medication touches the cornea. If it touches only the lids and lid margins, instillation should be repeated. After the first drop is administered, there may be severe blepharospasm, which makes it difficult to place the drop in the second eye. Wait to be sure that both drops are effectively instilled. The Committee on Ophthalmia Neonatorum of the National Society for the Prevention of Blindness *does not recommend irrigating the eye* following silver nitrate prophylaxis.

In addition to those factors related to the procedure itself, prophylaxis may fail because the disease has become established before birth, by premature rupture of the maternal membranes, or was acquired by the baby subsequent to prophylaxis, by contamination from the hands of the mother or hospital personnel. Silver nitrate will not prevent other types of newborn conjunctivitis caused by other infectious agents.

Recognition of the symptoms of ophthalmia neonatorum and its treatment are discussed in Chapter 16.

IMMEDIATE PHYSICAL ASSESSMENT

Immediate physical assessment of the newborn at the time of delivery includes Apgar scoring at 1 and 5 minutes after birth, estimation of the state of maturity, and a screening examination for congenital anomalies and neonatal disease.

Apgar Scoring

Apgar scoring has been termed an "instant physical." It is valuable because it quickly assesses cardiopulmonary and neurologic function and also communicates a picture of the baby's condition, not only to those present at the time of delivery but to those who will care for the baby in the days that follow. Moreover, researchers in years to come can understand from an accurate Apgar rating a great deal about the baby's condition in those first minutes of life.

Although the system developed by Dr. Virginia Apgar has been in use for approximately 2 decades, a 1970 study by the American College of Obstetricians and Gynecologists found that the system was not used at all in 36 per cent of the American hospitals surveyed. In addition, of those hospitals using Apgar scoring, only 46 per cent scored infants at both 1 and 5 minutes. The 1 minute time was chosen after a large series of observations, because it was found to be the point at which the lowest score was likely to be obtained. The second scoring at 5 minutes indicates the baby's recovery and prognosis. Both mortality and morbidity have been shown to be related to 1 and 5 minute scores, with low 5 minute scores more highly correlated with both mortality and neurologic defects.

The method of scoring is summarized in Table 15-4. Although all items scored are numerically equivalent, a score of 9 obtained because the heart rate is less than 100 beats per minute is obviously more significant than a score of 9 obtained because the extremities are blue, the latter occurring in about 85 per cent of normal, healthy newborns. However, because low scores in heart rate and respiratory effort are usually accompanied by low scores in other areas as well, such problems in evaluation of total scores usually do not arise.

A baby with an Apgar score of 0 to 2 is severely asphyxiated; a score of 3 to 6 represents mild to moderate asphyxia. Infants with scores of 7, 8, 9, or 10 rarely need resuscitation and have low rates of mortality and morbidity.

The Components of Apgar Scoring. *Heart rate* is the most important of the five signs. If a slow heart rate (less than 100 beats per minute) can be cor-

Table 15-4   THE APGAR SCORING METHOD*

Sign	0	1	2
Heart rate	Absent	Below 100	Over 100
Respiratory effort	Absent	Minimal; weak cry	Good; strong cry
Muscle tone	Limp	Some flexion of extremities	Active motion; extremities well flexed
Reflex irritability (response to stimulation on sole of foot)	No response	Grimace	Cry
Color	Blue or pale	Body pink; extremities blue	Pink

*From Apgar: *Anesthesia and Analgesia,* 32:260, 1953. Apgar, et al.: *J. American Medical Association,* 168:1985, 1958.

rected, respirations will probably follow. (A heart rate greater than 170 beats per minute may also indicate moderate asphyxia, although it is not a part of Apgar scoring and is not as significant as the severe asphyxia related to bradycardia.) Heart rate is most accurately obtained by using a stethoscope. The rate can be visually observed at the junction of the umbilical cord and the skin. Score 2 points for heart rates over 100 beats per minute, 1 point for those under 100 beats per minute, and 0 for the absence of heart rate on auscultation.

Respiratory effort is second in importance. Untreated apnea leads to respiratory and metabolic acidosis and death if successful intervention does not occur. Vigorous respirations score 2 points; irregular and ineffective (but present) respirations score 1 point; and apnea scores 0.

Muscle tone in the just-born baby means good motion of all extremities and active flexion of arms and legs with resistance to extension. Such behavior scores 2 points. Less tone scores 1 point, while a limp, flaccid baby receives a score of 0.

Reflex irritability refers to some form of stimulation. After pharyngeal suction, the tip of the catheter is placed just inside the nares. If the baby coughs or sneezes, the score is 2 points, with 1 point for a grimace, and 0 for no response. When there is a delay in clamping the umbilical cord, this procedure has been found unsatisfactory, and the flicking of the sole of a foot may be substituted, with a score of 2 points for a cry in response, 1 point for a grimace, and 0 for no response.[3]

Color is the most obvious and least significant of the Apgar criteria. Only 15 per cent of infants are pink all over at 1 minute and thus score 2 points; more common is the pink baby with blue hands and feet who scores 1 point. A baby totally blue or pale scores 0. Because blue hands and feet are so common in newborns, some neonatologist feel that an Apgar rating of 10 is an unlikely finding.

Estimation of Gestational Age

The gestational age of a baby is the number of completed weeks that have elapsed from the first day of his mother's last normal menstrual period to the time of birth. Accurate estimation of gestational age is important in planning the care for each newborn that best meets his needs. Until relatively recently, maternal history, obstetric evaluation, and the weight of the new born baby have been the principal criteria for estimating the gestational age of an infant. But many mothers are unsure of menstrual dates or have irregular periods. Some have first trimester bleeding, which may be mistaken for a period. The obstetric evaluation of the height of the fundus is only a rough estimate of gestational age, because it assumes normal fetal growth. When mothers receive no prenatal care, parameters such as the height of the fundus and fetal heart tones are obviously not available. The baby's weight can be misleading, as some babies weigh less than might be expected for their age while others are large in size yet deliver before term.

A *term* infant has a gestational age of from 38 weeks to 41 weeks, 6 days. An infant born prior to 38 weeks is called preterm; an infant of 42 or more weeks' gestation is called postterm. When estimated gestational age is compared with birth weight, preterm, term, and postterm babies are classified as small for gestational age (SGA), appropriate for gestational age (AGA), or large for gestational age (LGA). SGA infants may be intrauterine growth retarded (IGR). These concepts are discussed more fully below.

Because babies within every combination of age and weight have particular characteristics and needs during the first 24 hours, as well as later, an immediate assessment of age is highly important. In more and more nurseries, nurses are assuming this responsibility.

The accurate assessment of gestational age is based upon the fact that a number of physical characteristics and neurologic signs vary with the gestational age of the baby. However, it has been recognized that estimating age on the basis of one or two characteristics (ear cartilage and breast tissue, for example) is not sufficiently accurate because of individual variations. But when a number of criteria are scored, the total score is a reasonably reliable index of the infant's gestational age. Criteria from Farr and colleagues' scoring of physical characteristics[7]and from Dubowitz and colleagues' neuromuscular assessment[6] are shown in Table 15–5 and Figure 15–4, scored in Figure 15–5, and described below.

Scoring should be done as soon as possible after birth. Skin criteria are not accurate after 24 hours; if assessment is delayed beyond that time a more accurate estimate is obtained by eliminating the external criteria and doubling the neurologic score. Scoring can usually be done regardless of the baby's state, i.e., awake or asleep, hungry or recently fed, and so on.

External Physical Characteristics. The lower the gestational age, the thinner the infant's *skin* will be. Because of the thinness of the skin, blood vessels are closer to the surface in the preterm infant. Veins and venules are distinctly seen, particularly on the abdomen, and the skin is much redder than in the term baby. With each suc-

cessive week the skin becomes thicker and paler and abdominal veins are less clearly seen.

Prior to 28 weeks, *lanugo,* a fine, downy hair, covers the entire body. In each subsequent week until term, some of the lanugo disappears, first from the face and later from other areas of the body. At term it is slight, if present at all.

Transverse creases on the sole of the infant's foot are absent prior to 32 weeks. From 32 to 36 weeks, approximately, the creases are found only on the anterior one-third of the foot; two-thirds of the foot are covered by 38 weeks. By 40 weeks the entire sole is a series of complex crisscrosses (Fig. 15–6).

There is usually no *breast nodule* before 33 weeks. Until 36 weeks the nodule will usually be no larger than 3 mm.; at term the nodule is from 4 to 10 mm., surrounded by a full areolar area.

Because ear cartilage is not developed before 36 weeks, the pinna of the ear is flat and stays folded. Term babies have a firm ear that recoils when folded (Figs. 15–7 and 15–8).

In both males and females the genitals continue to develop during the last weeks of gestation. Prior to 28 weeks the testes are undescended, and no rugae are present on the scrotum. From 28 to 36 weeks the testes normally are descending and are found first high in the inguinal canal and subsequently lower in the canal. Rugae also develop during these weeks, so that by approximately 36 weeks the testes are in the scrotum, which has well-developed rugae. Testes remain undescended in approximately 3 per cent of term infants, illustrating why no one criterion is adequate in determining gestational age.

In female infants the relative size of the labia majora and labia minora

Table 15–5 SCORING SYSTEM OF EXTERNAL PHYSICAL CHARACTERISTICS*

External Sign	Score†				
	0	1	2	3	4
Edema	Obvious edema of hands and feet; pitting over tibia	No obvious edema of hands and feet; pitting over tibia	No edema		
Skin texture	Very thin, gelatinous	Thin and smooth	Smooth; medium thickness. Rash or superficial peeling	Slight thickening. Superficial cracking and peeling, especially of hands and feet	Thick and parchment-like; superficial or deep cracking
Skin color	Dark red	Uniformly pink	Pale pink; variable over body	Pale; only pink over ears, lips, palms, or soles	
Skin opacity (trunk)	Numerous veins and venules clearly seen, especially over abdomen	Veins and tributaries seen	A few large vessels clearly seen over abdomen	A few large vessels seen indistinctly over abdomen	No blood vessels seen
Lanugo (over back)	No lanugo	Abundant; long and thick over whole back	Hair thinning especially over lower back	Small amount of lanugo and bald areas	At least ½ of back devoid of lanugo
Plantar creases	No skin creases	Faint red marks over anterior half of sole	Definite red marks over > anterior ½; indentations over < anterior ⅓	Indentations over > anterior ⅓	Definite deep indentations over > anterior ⅓

Nipple formation	Nipple barely visible; no areola	Nipple well defined; areola smooth and flat, diameter < 0.75 cm.	Areola stippled, edge not raised, diameter < 0.75 cm.	Areola stippled, edge raised, diameter > 0.75 cm.
Breast size	No breast tissue palpable	Breast tissue on one or both sides, < 0.5 cm. diameter	Breast tissue both sides; one or both 0.5 to 1.0 cm.	Breast tissue both sides; one or both > 1 cm.
Ear form	Pinna flat and shapeless, little or no incurving of edge	Incurving of part of edge of pinna	Partial incurving whole of upper pinna	Well-defined incurving whole of upper pinna
Ear firmness	Pinna soft, easily folded, no recoil	Pinna soft, easily folded, slow recoil	Cartilage to edge of pinna, but soft in places, ready recoil	Pinna firm, cartilage to edge; instant recoil
Genitals: Male	Neither testis in scrotum	At least one testis high in scrotum	At least one testis right down	
Genitals: Female (with hips ½ abducted)	Labia majora widely separated, labia minora protruding	Labia majora almost cover labia minora	Labia majora completely cover labia minora	

*Adapted by Dubowitz, Dubowitz, and Goldberg: *J. Pediatrics*, 77:1, 1970 from Farr, Mitchell, Neligan, et al.: *Developmental Medicine and Child Neurology*, 8:507, 1966.

†If score differs on two sides, take the mean.

NEUROLOGICAL SIGN	SCORE					
	0	1	2	3	4	5
POSTURE						
SQUARE WINDOW	90°	60°	45°	30°	0°	
ANKLE DORSIFLEXION	90°	75°	45°	20°	0°	
ARM RECOIL	180°	90–180°	<90°			
LEG RECOIL	180°	90–180°	<90°			
POPLITEAL ANGLE	180	160°	130°	110°	90°	<90°
HEEL TO EAR						
SCARF SIGN						
HEAD LAG						
VENTRAL SUSPENSION						

Figure 15–4 Scoring system for neurologic criteria. (From Dubowitz, Dubowitz, and Goldberg: *J. of Pediatrics*, 77:1, 1970.)

changes as the fetus becomes more mature. Before 28 weeks the clitoris and labia minora are prominent. In the weeks that follow, the labia majora grow, covering the labia minora by 36 to 38 weeks (Figs. 15–9 to 15–11).

Signs of Neuromuscular Maturity. Muscle tone is flaccid at 28 weeks, accounting for many of the criteria associated with neuromuscular maturity. *Posture* should be observed with the baby lying quietly on his back. Flexor muscle tone increases as the baby approaches term and is strong in an infant of 40 weeks' gestation (Figs. 15–12 to 15–16).

The *square window* refers to the angle at the wrist when the infant's hand is flexed (Fig. 15–17). The examiner's thumb is placed on the dorsal aspect of the baby's hand, with the examiner's index and third fingers on the dorsal aspect of the baby's forearm. As the baby increases in gestational

Score   Units

	0	1	2	3	4	5	6	7	8	9
0						26.0	26.0	26.5	26.5	27.0
10	27.0	27.5	27.5	28.0	28.0	28.5	29.0	29.0	29.5	29.5
20	30.0	30.0	30.5	30.5	31.0	31.0	31.5	31.5	32.0	32.0
30	32.5	33.0	33.0	33.5	33.5	34.0	34.0	34.5	34.5	35.0
40	35.0	35.5	35.5	36.0	36.0	36.5	36.5	37.0	37.5	37.5
50	38.0	38.0	38.5	38.5	39.0	39.0	39.5	39.5	40.0	40.0
60	40.5	40.5	41.0	41.0	41.5	42.0	42.0	42.5	42.5	43.0
70	43.0									

Figure 15–5 To determine gestational age in weeks, take score from examination, find on chart, and read off value in weeks. For example, for a score of 44, find 40 in the far left column. Then read across to the column headed by 4. The gestational age is 36.0 weeks. (From Dubowitz, Dubowitz, and Goldberg: *J. of Pediatrics*, 77:1, 1970.)

A   B   C

Figure 15–6 Plantar aspect of the foot in infants of varying gestational ages. *A,* Thirty-six weeks' gestation. Note the transverse creases on the anterior third only. *B,* Thirty-eight weeks' gestation. Note that the transverse creases extend to the heel. *C,* Forty weeks' gestation. Note transverse crease over entirety of sole, and additional wrinkling. (From Klaus and Fanaroff: *Care of the High-Risk Neonate.* Philadelphia, W. B. Saunders Co., 1973.)

Figure 15–7 Immature ear. (From Lubchenco: *The High Risk Infant*. Philadelphia, W. B. Saunders Co., 1976.)

Figure 15–9 Very immature female genitalia, 28 weeks' gestation. (From Lubchenco: *The High Risk Infant*. Philadelphia, W. B. Saunders Co., 1976.)

Figure 15–8 Mature ear at term. (From Lubchenco: *The High Risk Infant*. Philadelphia, W. B. Saunders Co., 1976.)

Figure 15–10 Immature female genitalia, 35 weeks' gestation. (From Lubchenco: *The High Risk Infant*. Philadelphia, W. B. Saunders Co., 1976.)

Figure 15–11 Term female genitalia. (From Lubchenco: *The High Risk Infant*. Philadelphia, W. B. Saunders Co., 1976.)

age, the angle at the wrist decreases to 0.

Like the wrist joint evaluated in the square window, the *ankle dorsiflexion* (Fig. 15–18) evaluates the flexibility of the joints. Early in gestation the joints are relatively stiff; they become more relaxed closer to term, an accommodation that allows the larger infant to mold himself into the small space available to him within the uterus.

Arm recoil is measured with the baby lying supine. The arms are extended by pulling on the hands. The angle of the elbow is measured after the release of the hands.

Leg recoil is also measured with the baby supine. The hips and knees are fully flexed for 5 seconds, then extended by traction on the feet, and then released.

Figure 15–12 Hypotonia, less than 28 weeks. (From Lubchenco: *The High Risk Infant*. Philadelphia, W. B. Saunders Co., 1976.)

Figure 15–13 Beginning hip flexion, 32 weeks. (From Lubchenco: *The High Risk Infant*. Philadelphia, W. B. Saunders Co., 1976.)

Figure 15–14 Froglike position, extended arms, 34 weeks. (From Lubchenco: *The High Risk Infant*. Philadelphia, W. B. Saunders Co., 1976.)

Figure 15–15 Flexion, arms and legs, loose, 36 weeks. (From Lubchenco: *The High Risk Infant*. Philadelphia, W. B. Saunders Co., 1976.)

Figure 15–16 Tight flexion, all extremities, 38 to 40 weeks. (From Lubchenco: *The High Risk Infant*. Philadelphia, W. B. Saunders Co., 1976.)

Figure 15–17 Technique for square window. (From Dubowitz, Dubowitz, and Goldberg: *J. of Pediatrics, 77*:1, 1970.)

The *popliteal* angle is also measured with the infant supine and the pelvis flat on the examining table. The baby's thigh is held in the knee-chest position by the examiner's left index finger and thumb. The leg is then extended by gentle pressure applied behind the ankle from the examiner's right index finger, and the popliteal angle is measured.

Assessment using the *scarf sign* is based on the position of the elbow when the baby's hand is drawn across his body to the other shoulder, as far as it will go without resistance.

In the *heel-to-ear maneuver* the baby's foot is drawn toward his head, and the distance from his foot to his ear is assessed. The knee is left free; it will fall alongside of the abdomen.

Head lag is measured with the infant supine. Grasp each forearm just above the wrist and gently pull the baby to a sitting position. To what extent does he support his head? This is a measure of active muscle tone, which increases with gestational age.

The position of the infant when he is held in *ventral suspension* is another measure of active tone. Hold the baby with his chest in the palm of your hand. Note the increasing muscle tone, as shown in Figures 15–19 to 15–21.

Comparing Gestational Age and Body Measurements

Either before or after gestational age is ascertained, the baby is weighed and length and head circumference are measured. Using the Colorado Growth

Figure 15–18 Technique for dorsiflexion of foot. (From Dubowitz, Dubowitz, and Goldberg: *J. of Pediatrics, 77*:1, 1970.)

Figure 15–19 Ventral suspension, 35 weeks. (From Lubchenco: *The High Risk Infant.* Philadelphia, W. B. Saunders Co., 1976.)

Figure 15–20 Ventral suspension, 38 weeks. (From Lubchenco: *The High Risk Infant.* Philadelphia, W. B. Saunders Co., 1976.)

Figure 15–21 Ventral suspension, 42 weeks. (From Lubchenco: *The High Risk Infant.* Philadelphia, W. B. Saunders Co., 1976.)

Charts (Fig. 15–22), the baby's measurements can then be compared with the norms of the chart. (Although the Denver norms may not be totally accurate for all parts of the country—babies born at sea level are somewhat larger—they are considered the best standard of reference currently available).

If length, weight, and head circum-ference are all below the tenth percentile* on the Colorado Growth Charts the baby is considered both small for gestational age and intrauterine growth retarded. The insult to these babies probably occurred early in pregnancy, perhaps caused by an early viral

*Tenth percentile means that 90 per cent of the babies of that gestational age are larger.

Illness. The long-term prognosis for normal development of these babies is usually poor.

When length and weight are less than the tenth percentile for the baby's gestational age, but head size is normal (approximately the fiftieth percentile), the baby's growth was probably affected during the third trimester. Common causes are maternal toxemia, hypertension, long-term malnutrition in the mother, and maternal vascular disease. These babies are small for gestational age and are more at risk than babies who are appropriate for gestational age, but they usually have a brighter future than those infants with intrauterine growth retardation.

Babies whose weight, length, and head circumference fall between the tenth and ninetieth percentiles are appropriate for gestational age. At every age these infants have a better chance for survival than babies of the same age who are either SGA or LGA infants.

A baby with measurements above the ninetieth percentile is large for gestational age. The special problems of in-

Figure 15–22   Colorado Growth Charts. (From Lubchenco, Hansman, and Boyd: *Pediatrics, 37*:403, 1966.)

fants in each of these groups are discussed in Chapter 18.

Physical Screening

In addition to Apgar scoring, measurement, and estimation of gestational age, additional physical screening is also important in planning the baby's care. Although some variations from normal are obvious (a meningocele, for example), others are more subtle and may be overlooked if each baby is not evaluated systematically. The scope of this brief screening is summarized in Table 15–6 and is discussed in detail in Chapter 16 in relation to the more extensive examination of the baby in the nursery.

In addition to the baby, the placenta should also be examined, as described in Chapter 13.

Identification

Before either mother or baby leaves the delivery room, the baby must be identified. Identification bands for mother and infant, with matching numbers as well as names, are one means of identification. The bands should include the name of the mother and the sex of the baby and should be checked each time the baby is removed from his crib or taken from the nursery, as well as the time of discharge.

Footprinting is another widely used means of identification, but unless it is done properly, it is worthless. In a study by the Chicago Board of Health, policemen who were accustomed to interpreting fingerprints found that 98 per cent of the footprints submitted by Chicago hospitals were valueless and could not be used as a means of identification. However, 2 minutes of instruction to the hospital personnel responsible for taking footprints produced prints from which positive identification could be made in 99 per cent of the cases.[10]

The following steps are suggested in order to produce footprints that are reliable and useful:

1. Use a disposable footprinter ink plate and a smooth, high gloss paper.
2. Wipe the baby's foot immediately after birth so that the vernix will not dry on

Table 15–6   INITIAL ASSESSMENT

	Within Normal Limits	Needs Further Investigation
Skin	Covered with vernix	Absence of vernix
	Acrocyanosis, perioral cyanosis	Generalized cyanosis
	Petechiae of head and neck-breech presentation	Generalized petechiae Pallor Meconium staining
Cry	Lusty	Weak or absent
Head	Molding	Tense or rigid anterior fontanel
Respirations		Dyspnea
		Subcostal, substernal retractions
Cord	Two arteries, one vein	Single umbilical artery
	Unstained	Stained
Motor activity	Symmetrical	
Moro reflex	Present	Absent
	Symmetrical	Absent on one side

t. This will make the foot easier to clean when the footprint is made.

3. Before making the print be sure the baby's foot is clean and dry. Cleaning should be gentle, so that the skin of the baby's foot will not peel.

4. Be sure that there is not too much ink on the pad.

5. Flex the baby's knee so that his leg is close to his body; grasp the ankle between the thumb and middle finger, with the index finger pressing on the upper surface of the foot just behind the baby's toes to prevent the toes from curling.

6. Press the footprinter firmly to the baby's foot.

7. Touch the baby's foot gently to the footprint chart, which should be attached to a hard surface such as a clipboard. Place the heel on the paper first and "walk" the foot gently onto the chart with a heel-to-toe motion. Then lift the foot off the chart; do not slide it off. The foot should not be rolled back and forth, either on the inking pad or on the footprint chart. It is particularly important to get a good impression of the ball of the foot, since the best identification can be made from the friction ridges in that area.

8. Before the baby leaves the delivery room, check the print for legible friction ridges, preferably with a magnifying glass. If the ridges are not clear, take another print.

After a satisfactory print is made, the excess ink is wiped from the baby's foot. Commonly the mother's fingerprints are placed on the same sheet as the baby's footprint. As in every other aspect of newborn care, it is most important that the baby not be chilled during the process.

An alternate means of identification has been suggested by Shepard,[20, 21] which involves writing a name or code on the infant's chest with a pen or pencil treated with silver nitrate. The method is rapid and can easily be carried out under the warming cradle. The silver nitrate leaves an indelible tattoo that lasts for 3 to 4 weeks and eventually disappears completely.

THE BABY AND HIS PARENTS IN THE DELIVERY ROOM

The baby born in many American delivery rooms today becomes an instant occupant of a highly technical world. Often (but not always) his father is excluded from his world, or is only tolerated as an unnecessary onlooker. His mother may get only the briefest glimpse before her new baby becomes "the property" of nurses and hospital regulations. Many parents have started to question practices that separate them from their infants during the first moments and days of life. As nurses, we must look carefully at the assumptions on which such practices are based.

First we must differentiate the care that is given the full-term, apparently healthy newborn and that which is necessary for the survival of a small or sick infant. An 800 gram (less than 2 pound) baby or one with an Apgar score of 3 or lower needs specialized care from the moment of birth. No parent would wish anything but the very best of medical attention for such a child. We can support these parents by our honesty about the baby's problem, close communication about his progress, and acceptance of their grief and other feelings (Chapter 22). But these babies in most institutions represent less than 10 per cent of all deliveries.

What about the remaining 90 per cent of babies, born at term and apparently healthy? Can we provide opportunities for very early parent-baby interaction in the delivery room and/or recovery room for these families? Is it important that we do so?

The Concept of a Critical Period

The concept of birth as a critical period in the development of a mother-infant bond suggests that later maternal behavior is highly dependent upon what happens in the period immediately following delivery. The validity of this concept has been demonstrated in a number of animal species, such as goats, sheep, cattle, mice, rats, and monkeys. Subsequent mothering behavior is disturbed when mothers and their young are separated shortly after birth. Similar periods of separation several days later do not have the same influence on the mother's behavior.

We do not know for a certainty that a similar critical period exists for human infants. It has been well documented that more extensive separation, such as the separation that a preterm baby may have from his mother for a period of weeks, does apparently interfere with mothering (Chapter 22). Moreover, Klaus and Kennell[15a] have demonstrated in a group of 14 mothers that those with extended early contact with their infants showed an increased level of caretaking and mothering. Behavior of these mothers, compared with a control group, continued to differ when the babies were a year old and again at 2 years after birth. These studies suggest that it may very well be that the time a mother and father spend with their baby in the first hour or so after delivery may have some significance for that baby's long-range development.

Although most research has concentrated on mothers, one study done in Sweden[15c] suggests that fathers who had extended contact with their newborn sons and daughters were more likely to interact with them as they grew older.

Physiologic and Psychologic Needs: A Conflict?

If a mother, and perhaps a father as well, is allowed to touch and hold the newborn infant in the delivery roon will the baby's physiologic needs fo warmth and the observation of his prog ress be compromised? A greater amoun of research in this area is very muc needed. An excellent example of th contribution that nursing can make t such research is the work of Phillips, who hypothesized that term newborr who were well dried (to prevent hea loss from evaporation) and covered (t prevent heat loss from convection) coul be held by their mothers on the deliver table for 15 minutes without significan loss of body temperature. All of the 11 infants in the study weighed over pounds, had 1 minute Apgar scores of or higher, and were delivered vaginall. Neither mother nor baby had any majo complications.

The infants' temperatures were re corded at both 5 and 15 minutes afte delivery. Note in Figure 15–23 that at minutes postdelivery the mother-hel babies had higher temperatures tha those babies in heated beds. Tempera tures of the mother-held infants drop ped more at 15 minutes than those of th babies in the heated cribs, but remaine well above 97.0°F. (36.1°C.).

An interesting additional findin that infants' temperatures droppe more in 72.0°F. (22.0°C.) delivery roon than in 75.0°F. (24.0°C.) delivery roon indicates that further study of optimur delivery room temperature might b useful.

Nursing observations and care the baby need not be hindered becaus the baby is lying in his mother's arm. The reason for the care need only b explained to the parents.

Breast-feeding in the Delivery Room

An increasing number of mothe are asking to return to the centuries ol custom of putting their baby to breas shortly after delivery. Physiological

Figure 15–23 *A,* Mean rectal temperature (°F) of 51 newborns put into heated beds (——) and of 33 newborns given to their mothers to hold (--------) while room temperature was maintained at 72° F. *B,* Mean rectal temperatures (°F) of 14 newborns put into heated beds (——) and of 17 newborns given to their mothers to hold (--------) while room temperature was maintained at 75° F. (From Phillips: *JOGN,* 3:11, 1974.)

this is the way mothers' bodies are designed. Oxytocin, released from the posterior pituitary when the breast is suckled, causes the smooth muscle of the uterus to contract and aids in the prevention of postpartum hemorrhage. However, we have replaced this physiologic process with an injection in most contemporary delivery rooms.

Very early nursing also assures rapid drainage of the colostrum that is in the duct system of the mother's breast and allows the milk, as it forms, to move through the ducts to the milk reservoirs. Colostrum may also aid the peristalsis of meconium, which is in the baby's intestinal tract at the time of birth.

Not every mother, or couple, wishes or is ready to participate in the kinds of experiences described here. A mother groggy from medication or anesthesia will probably be unable to hold her baby. Heavy medication also interferes with early breast-feeding, not only because of the mother's level of consciousness but because the baby may suck poorly, owing to the effects of drugs that have crossed the placenta. However, we believe that for many families interaction between parents and infants in the delivery room need not compromise physiologic well-being.

CONTINUING PHYSIOLOGIC NEEDS

At some time in the hour following his birth, the baby will be transferred either to a central nursery or perhaps to a room with his mother. As already noted, during the first hour or so most babies sleep. Physiologically they begin to stabilize. Nursing responsibilities include monitoring and maintaining temperature and administering vitamin K to prevent hemorrhage, discussed above. Skin and cord care are important nursing functions during the transition period. Protection from infection, an immediate and continuing need, is discussed in Chapter 17.

Monitoring and Maintaining Body Temperature

Taking the initial body temperature rectally shortly after birth accomplishes the dual purpose of checking for an imperforate anus and for temperature. Subsequent temperature checks may be taken in the axilla to eliminate the danger of irritating and/or perforating the rectum. An axillary temperature of 96.0°F. (35.5°C.) to 99.0°F. (37.2°C.) is considered within normal limits, although a temperature above 96.8°F. (37.0°C.) is desirable. Heavier infants tend to have higher body temperatures.

The need for a thermoneutral temperature continues in the hours and days that follow birth. During the first hours a term newborn who is healthy will probably maintain temperature

adequately with blankets and perhaps a hot water bottle, the latter filled halfway at a temperature of 105° (checked by thermometer at each filling). Air should be expressed from the hot water bag, and the bag should be completely covered and placed outside the blanket in which the baby is wrapped. Radiant warmers have replaced hot water bottles in many nurseries. A baby under a warmer should not be clothed. In both instances the infant's temperature should be rechecked frequently.

A nursery temperature of approximately 75.0°F. (24.0°C.) is considered adequate for the term baby to maintain temperature. (See Chapter 18 for variations in preterm and postterm infants.)

Initial and Subsequent Skin Care

In 1953 Wolfenstein pointed out that many infant and child care practices follow trends that are as much or more related to the belief that new ideas are better than old ones as they are to new scientific knowledge.[24] As a basis for her study, she examined the widely distributed government publication *Infant Care* for its advice on common matters such as breast-feeding, toilet training, and thumb sucking.

The skin care that is given to new infants is one aspect of nursery care that in many ways appears to follow somewhat cyclic trends. Recognizing that such cycles, or swings of a pendulum, may occur is not merely a curious and interesting sidelight of nursing care. Awareness of such trends should (hopefully) make us more perceptive in our evaluation of new ideas. Then perhaps we will be able to balance the tendency of some to reject new ideas simply because they are new with the equally strong predilection of others to see all new ideas as better than old ways.

Much of the advice given student

nurses and mothers in the first decade of the twentieth century, a time of home delivery and no central heating, was not a great deal different from our ideas today.

. . .We must remember that the newborn baby is a very tender object, exceedingly susceptible to the influence of cold, and with a very delicate skin. Indeed, in the case of children weakly at birth the physician often forbids any washing whatever until the vitality has increased. In giving a bath it is consequently necessary to guard most carefully against draughts. The doors and windows must be closed, and the child should be protected still further by placing a folding screen around the nurse's chair and the tub, and by doing the bathing before a fire unless the weather be very hot.

The washing and drying should be done thoroughly, rapidly, and yet with the greatest gentleness. . . .[12]

It was considered important to remove the vernix caseosa, and oil was used for that purpose.

The new-born baby is more or less covered with a whitish, waxy substance which must be removed entirely, especially from all the folds and hollows of the body, such as the armpits, hollows of the knees, groins, and ears, as otherwise irritation of the skin is apt to be set up. As the cleansing is not easily accomplished by ordinary washing, it is necessary first to rub the skin all over with olive oil or with purified white vaseline. This is much better than lard unless the latter has been carefully freed from salt by washing. . . .[12]

We may be amused by some of the 1907 statements, but has our practice changed all that much? For example,

The first washing of the baby is the business of the monthly nurse, and the mother has no share in it.[12]

An initial oil bath was still advised nearly half a century later in an obstetric nursing text.

The baby's first bath is usually an oil bath to remove the vernix caseosa. This also prevents unnecessary evaporation from the skin and chilling of the body. The oil (sweet oil, mineral oil or some special preparation used by the hospital) for this purpose should be poured into a container which is placed in hot water and allowed to stand until it is thoroughly warm. The nurse should apply the oil gently but rapidly all over the parts where the baby has much vernix . . . In some hospitals this initial oil bath is followed by a soap-and-water bath with only the daily oil bath thereafter. In others the initial oil bath is followed by the daily soap-and-water bath. In still others the bath is omitted altogether until the day of discharge, at which time a soap-and-water bath is given.[25]

Subsequently, questions arose about the possible value of the vernix as a barrier to infection, and for a time it was recommended that the vernix be left undisturbed.

In 1963 Gluck advised that the bathing of all infants in the nursery with a hexachlorophene preparation each day would virtually eliminate staphylococcal infections.[11] This practice spread widely in the United States. However, in late 1971 warnings were issued by the Food and Drug Administration after both animal and human studies demonstrated absorption of hexachlorophene into the bloodstream. Most hospitals discontinued the use of hexachlorophene for infant bathing, although they continued to use it for personnel handwashing. During this period it was felt that the vernix might encourage infection, and it was thoroughly removed.

Current Recommendations for Skin Care

In 1975 the American Academy of Pediatrics made the following recommendations for the skin care of newborns. These recommendations have been endorsed by the executive board of the American College of Obstetricians and Gynecologists.

1. Cleansing of the newly born infant's skin should be delayed until the

infant's temperature has stabilized after the cold stress of delivery.

2. Cotton sponges (not gauze) soaked with sterile water are used to remove blood from the face and head and meconium from the perianal area. As an alternative, a mild nonmedicated soap can be used, with careful water rinsing. Potential bacterial contamination of bar and liquid soaps should be remembered.

3. The remainder of the skin should be untouched unless grossly soiled. There is evidence to indicate that the vernix caseosa may serve a protective function, some evidence to indicate that it has no effect, and no evidence to indicate that it is harmful.

4. For the remainder of the infant's stay in the hospital nursery, the buttocks and perianal region should be cleansed with sterile water and cotton. As an alternative, a mild soap with water rinsing may be used as required at diaper changes and more often as indicated.

Such a regimen, termed dry skin care, is felt to diminish skin trauma and to avoid the risk of exposing newborn babies to agents with known or unknown side effects.

Cord Care

Because the stump of the umbilical cord is a potential portal of entry for septic organisms, observation and care of the cord is an important nursing responsibility. No single method of cord care has been proved to totally eliminate colonization and disease. Alcohol, iodophor preparations, and triple dye are probably the three substances used most frequently, either alone or in combination. Mothers are instructed to continue cord care at home until the stump drops off, which may be as early as 5 to 7 days or as late as 2 weeks after delivery.

SUMMARY

In this chapter the major changes of the transition to extrauterine life have been discussed. Immediate needs were considered, together with the ways in which nursing can best meet those needs in the light of our current knowledge. In the chapter that follows we will examine the term newborn more closely in order to differentiate appearance and behavior that are within the range of normal from appearance and behavior that need special attention.

REFERENCES

1. Altman, P. L., and Dittmer, D. S.: Blood and Other Body Fluids. Washington, D.C., Federation of American Societies for Experimental Biology, 1961.
2. Apgar, V.: Proposal for a New Method of Evaluation of the Newborn Infant. Anesthesia and Analgesia, 32:260, 1953.
3. Apgar, V., Holaday, D. A., James, L. S., et al.: Evaluation of the Newborn Infant: Second Report. Journal of the American Medical Association, 168:1985, 1958.
4. Dargassies, S.: Neurological Maturation of the Premature Infant of 28 to 41 Weeks' Gestational Age. In Falkner, F. (ed.): Human Development, Philadelphia, W. B. Saunders Co., 1966.
5. Dubowitz, L. M. S., and Dubowitz, V.: Assessment of Gestational Age. Nursing Mirror, Aug. 13, 1971.
6. Dubowitz, L. M. S., Dubowitz, V., and Goldberg, C.: Clinical Assessment of Gestational Age in the Newborn Infant. Journal of Pediatrics, 77:1, 1970.
7. Farr, V., Kerridge, D. F., and Mitchell, R. G.: The Value of Some External Characteristics in the Assessment of Gestational Age at Birth. Developmental Medicine and Child Neurology, 8:657, 1966.
8. Farr, V., Mitchell, R. G., Neligan, G. A., et al.: The Definition of Some External Characteristics Used in the Assessment of Gestational Age in the Newborn Infant. Developmental Medicine and Child Neurology, 8:507, 1966.
9. Fisher, D., and Behrman, R.: Resuscitation of the Newborn Infant. In Klaus, M. H., and Fanaroff, A. A. (eds.): Care of the High Risk Neonate. Philadelphia, W. B. Saunders Co., 1973.

10. Gleason, D.: Footprinting for Identification of Infants. *Pediatrics*, *44*:302, 1969.

11. Gluck, L., and Wood, H. F.: Staphylococcal Colonization in Newborn Infants With and Without Antiseptic Skin Care. *New England Journal of Medicine*, *268*:1265, 1963.

12. Griffith, J. P.: *The Care of the Baby: A Manual for Mothers and Nurses*, Philadelphia: W. B. Saunders Co., 1907.

13. *Hospital Care of Newborn Infants*. Evanston, Ill., American Academy of Pediatrics, 1971.

14. Johnson, R. W.: The Case of the Nearly Mixed-up Babies. *RN*, Oct. 1974.

15. Klaus, M. H., and Fanaroff, A. A. (eds.): *Care of the High Risk Neonate*. Philadelphia, W. B. Saunders Co., 1973.

15a. Klaus, M., and Kennell, J.: *Maternal-Infant Bonding*. St. Louis, The C. V. Mosby Co., 1976.

15b. Klaus, M., Jerauld, R., Kreger, N., et al.: Maternal attachment: importance of the first post-partum days. *New England Journal of Medicine*, *286*:460, 1972.

15c. Lind, J.: Personal communication cited in Klaus, M., and Kennell, J.: *Maternal-Infant Bonding*. St. Louis, The C. V. Mosby Co., 1976.

16. Lubchenco, L. O.: Assessment of Gestational Age and Development at Birth. *Pediatric Clinics of North America, 17*:125, 1970.

17. Moya, F., and Lehr, D.: Drug Therapy. *In* Abramson, H. (ed.): *Resuscitation of the Newborn Infant*. St. Louis, The C. V. Mosby Co., 1966.

18. Oski, F., and Naiman, J.: *Hematologic Problems in the Newborn*. 2nd Edition. Philadelphia, W. B. Saunders Co., 1972.

19. Phillips, C. R.: Neonatal Heat Loss in Heated Cribs vs. Mothers' Arms. *JOGN, 3*(6):11, 1974.

19a. Ringler, N., Kennell, J., Jarvella, R., et al.: Mother to infant speech at two years— effects of early postnatal contact. *Journal of Pediatrics, 86*:141, 1975.

20. Shepard, K. S.: *Care of the Well Baby*. Philadelphia, J. B. Lippincott Co., 1968.

21. Shepard, K. S.: Further on Footprinting. *Pediatrics, 43*:639, 1969.

22. Statement of the Committee on Fetus and Newborn, American Academy of Pediatrics: Skin Care of Newborns, *Pediatrics, 54*:December, 1974.

23. Sweet, A. Y.: Classification of the Low-Birth-Weight Infant. *In* Klaus, M. H., and Fanaroff, A. A. (eds.): *Care of the High Risk Neonate*, Philadelphia, W. B. Saunders Co., 1973.

24. Wolfenstein, M.: Trends in Infant Care. *American Journal of Orthopsychiatry, 33*:120, 1953.

25. Zabriskie, L., and Eastman, N.: *Nurses Handbook of Obstetrics*, Philadelphia, J. B. Lippincott Co., 1952.

Chapter 16

THE TERM NEWBORN: PHYSICAL AND BEHAVIORAL ASSESSMENT

As nurses, we need to be thoroughly familiar with the normal variations in a newborn infant's appearance and behavior for two equally important reasons. First, because the condition of a newborn changes rapidly, nurses are usually the first to suspect that some change may be outside the range of normal and in need of special attention. Moreover, parents most frequently query nurses about their baby. Mothers and fathers often have an unrealistic image of how their baby will look—an image that more closely resembles a child of several months than a just-born infant. And so to many parents a "molded" head looks misshapen, and *milia* (tiny cysts) may seem to be blemishes on their baby's skin. Our explanation and reassurance can help them accept their baby as he is at this time in his life, laying a foundation for the acceptance of each subsequent stage of development in its turn.

Observation of the newborn is a unique skill and one that can be learned. Although babies are limited to nonverbal communication, their signal system, once understood, tells a great deal about them. The position in which they lie in their bassinet, the color of their skin, their cry, and the way they root and suck—these signs and many others indicate health or illness.

The characteristics described in this chapter are for term newborns; characteristics of preterm and postterm infants are described in Chapter 18.

TYPES OF ASSESSMENT

Newborn infants may be assessed by a variety of parameters, each designed to give specific kinds of information. *Assessment of gestational age* was described in Chapter 15. This examination evaluates both physical and neurologic characteristics.

A *general physical* assessement is a part of each baby's care. An initial assessment is made following delivery. Daily assessments are also essential because of the rapid changes a baby undergoes during the first days after birth.

472

An assessment of interactive behavior, developed by Brazelton,[2] is not a part of the assessment of every infant. However, a basic understanding of the Brazelton assessment offers considerable insight into the world of the newborn infant.

States of Consciousness

Brazelton has demonstrated that babies are not just awake or asleep but exist in six distinct states. Four of these are waking states; two are states of sleep. Since a baby's state at a given moment influences assessment (from cardiac and respiratory rate to alertness and feeding behavior), nurses must be aware of these states.

Sleep States:

State 1. The baby is deeply sleeping. His eyes are closed, and there are no eye movements. At regular intervals, however, one may observe startles or jerky movements.

State 2. The baby is sleeping lightly; his lids are closed, but one can observe rapid eye movements (REM). Respirations are irregular; there are occasional sucking movements. Random movements and startles can be observed.

Awake States:

State 3. The baby is drowsy; his eyes may be opened or closed. He reacts to sensory stimuli (e.g., light, sound), but his reactions may be slow.

State 4. This is called the quiet, alert state; the baby has a "bright-eyed" look. He focuses his attention on a sight or sound. Motor activity is minimal (Fig. 16–1).

State 5. The baby is awake and very active; his arms and legs are moving.

State 6. The baby is crying intensely; it is difficult to catch his attention with visual and auditory stimuli.

VITAL SIGNS IN NEWBORNS

Within Normal Limits

Temperature: 97.4–98.6°F. (36.3–37.0°C.); mean: 98.0°F. (36.7°C.)

Heart rate: 90 to 180 beats per minute (average: 120 to 140)

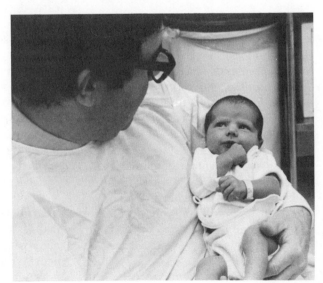

Figure 16–1 In the quiet, alert state, Sharon intently examines Dr. Robert Dillard's face.

Respiratory rate: 30 to 60 respirations per minute (average: 40)
Transient tachypnea of the newborn
Diaphragmatic and abdominal breathing
Blood pressure: systolic: 70–75 mm. Hg; diastolic: 30–40 mm. Hg

In Need of Special Attention

Wide variation in temperature (greater than 2°) from one reading to the next
Weak pulse
Absence of femoral pulses
Heart sounds on the right side of the chest
Intercostal retractions; retractions of the xiphoid
Grunting on expiration
Flared nostrils

VITAL SIGNS IN NEWBORNS

Body temperature in newborns is measured in the axilla for 2 to 3 minutes. As noted in Chapter 15, frequent taking of rectal temperatures could harm the rectal mucosa. It would seem preferable for mothers to use the axilla also if they need to check the baby's temperature at home during his first weeks.

Infant temperatures normally range from approximately 97.4°F. (36.3°C.) to 98.6°F. (37.0°C.). The problems associated with a temperature that is too low were discussed in Chapter 15. An elevated temperature in a newborn is not necessarily a sign of infection, as it often is in an older child; it is just as likely to indicate a reaction to a room that is too warm, too much clothing or too many covers, or dehydration. In babies who are not fed or who do not feed well, dehydration is not uncommon on the second or third day of life. With adequate hydration, temperatures become normal.

Instability of temperature, with temperature swings of more than 2°F. from one reading to the next or with subnormal temperatures, is often the first sign of illness in a baby. Here again, however, changes in environmental temperature that the baby reflects may be the culprit. For example, if the baby is in such a position in the nursery that the sun shines on his bed for part of the day, his temperature may rise, and then fall as the sun moves on.

Heart Rate

Heart rate may not be checked routinely on healthy term newborns after the initial transition period. Pulse does tend to vary normally within rather wide limits; a baby may have a rate as low as 70 beats per minute when sleeping and as high as 180 beats per minute when vigorously active. Pulse rates also tend to vary with respiratory rates. Heart disease in newborns is caused by congenital anomaly, with cyanosis, tachypnea, respiratory distress, hepatosplenomegaly, and weak pulses the major symptoms, rather than altered heart rate (Chapter 18). A weak pulse should be noted, since it may indicate decreased cardiac output. Both femoral pulses should be checked each day; absence of femoral pulsation suggests coarctation of the aorta.

Heart sounds should be most audible on the left side of the chest between the sternum and the nipple. Heart sounds originating on the right side of the chest may be due to *dextrocardia*, not an immediate threat in itself, or to a *diaphragmatic hernia*, a condition in which a portion of the abdominal organs enters the thoracic cavity through a defect in the diaphragm. The defect is usually, but not always, on the left. In a baby with a diaphragmatic hernia, the heart is pushed to the right, the left lung may not expand, and the baby is often in severe respiratory distress. A diaphragmatic hernia is a true surgical emergency. Prompt recognition is very important.

Pneumothorax is another life-threatening cause of heart sounds heard on the right.

Heart murmurs heard during the first days of life, with no other symptoms of heart disease, are often benign and will disappear; the absence of a murmer in a baby with other symptoms of heart disease is considered serious (Chapter 18).

Respiration

Normal respiration in newborn infants differs from respiration in older infants and adults in several distinct ways. The difference is even more marked in preterm infants. One of the more obvious of these differences is rate. Respiratory rate should always be measured when the baby is quiet. If checking cardiac rate and temperature at the same time that respiration is being evaluated, respiratory rate should be measured first. This is because the baby may become active or may cry when the thermometer is inserted or when he is touched with the stethoscope. Average respiratory rate during the first 2 weeks of life is approximately 40 respirations per minute, although apparently healthy babies may show momentary extremes ranging from 20 to 100 respirations per minute under normal resting conditions. The infant's position has been shown to affect respiratory rates very slightly. More important than the rate at any given moment is the trend in rate over a period of time.

The increased respiratory rate in infants in comparison with the rate in older individuals is due to the infant's metabolic need to move much more air per minute in proportion to his body weight because of his proportionally larger area of skin surface.

In many hospitals, the rate of respiration is not routinely checked on new infants. Such a check during the first 6 hours, once each hour for low risk infants and once each 30 minutes for high risk infants (Chapter 18), would be a helpful screening procedure. Rates over 60 respirations per minute or rates that show an increasing trend merit further investigation. In addition to checking rate, it is important to listen for good breath sounds on both sides.

Although respiratory rates in transient tachypnea of the newborn may exceed the usual range of normal, the condition is not considered pathologic. Transient tachypnea may follow delivery by cesarean section or breech presentation. Air exchange is usually good in transient tachypnea. The baby's only problem is that he must be fed carefully to avoid aspiration during these first days. Transient tachypnea is differentiated from more serious respiratory problems in that there are no retractions, cyanosis, or respiratory grunts, nor are the blood gases abnormal. Oxygen may be required.

Neonatal breathing is diaphragmatic and abdominal; movement of the chest and abdomen should be synchronized. A lag on inspiration or alternating "seesaw" movements of the chest and abdomen are signs of respiratory distress (Fig. 16-2).

If intercostal muscles are being used to any extent or if retractions are visible in the xiphoid area, there is respiratory distress. A respiratory grunt is still another sign of distress. The grunt occurs when the baby closes his glottis to slow down expiration, nature's way of compensating for a low carbon dioxide. Although marked nasal flaring indicates respiratory distress, occasional flaring is seen in many newborns.

	UPPER CHEST	LOWER CHEST	XIPHOID RETRACT.	NARES DILAT.	EXPIR. GRUNT
GRADE 0	SYNCHRONIZED	NO RETRACT.	NONE	NONE	NONE
GRADE 1	LAG ON INSP.	JUST VISIBLE	JUST VISIBLE	MINIMAL	STETHOS. ONLY
GRADE 2	SEE-SAW	MARKED	MARKED	MARKED	NAKED EAR

Figure 16–2 This index is designed to provide a continued evaluation of the infant's respiratory status. An index of respiratory distress is determined by grading each of five arbitrary criteria: chest lag, intercostal retraction, xiphoid retraction, nares dilatation, and expiratory grunt. The "retraction score" is computed by adding the values (0, 1, or 2) assigned to each factor that best describes the infant's manifestation at the time of a single observation. A score of 0 indicates no respiratory distress; a score of 10 indicates severe respiratory distress. (From Silverman and Anderson: *Pediatrics, 17*:1, 1956.)

Respiratory rates below 30 or very shallow respirations may reflect analgesia (particularly Demerol) given to the mother during labor. The baby of a toxemic mother who received large amounts of magnesium sulfate prior to delivery may have rapid, shallow respirations due to hypermagnesemia.

Blood Pressure

Blood pressure is not routinely checked on the healthy term neonate in most nurseries. Blood pressure monitoring of sick infants is discussed in Chapter 18.

SIZE

Mean weight: 6.2–9.1 pounds (approximately 2800–4115 grams)
Mean length: 18.8–21.0 inches (47.6–53.3 cm.)
Head circumference: 13–14 inches (33–35.5 cm.)
Chest circumference: 12–13 inches (30.5–33.0 cm.)

SIZE

Weight

Ninety-five per cent of term infants weigh between 5.5 pounds (2.5 kg.) and 10 pounds (4.6 kg.). The mean is approximately 7.5 pounds for boys and 7.4 pounds for girls. Nonwhite babies tend to weigh slightly less than white infants of the same gestational age. The various reasons for birth weights that fall outside these ranges and the special problems entailed in the care of these babies are discussed in Chapter 18.

All babies lose some of their birth weight during the first days of life. The loss averages about 7 per cent of initial weight, with the range normally falling between 5 and 10 per cent. Why this loss of weight? The passage of meconium from the intestines is one factor. A second is the consumption of fat, protein, glycogen, and glucose in the production of energy by the baby. The third reason is a loss of more fluid from the body, both in urine and in insensible water loss, than is taken in. Since water constitutes approximately 35 per cent of body weight at the time of birth, the baby is not harmed by negative water balance within normal limits.

Weight gain begins from 3 to 5 days after birth; most infants have attained their birth weight by the time they are 10 days old. Birth weight normally doubles at 4 to 5 months and triples by the baby's first birthday.

Length

The average length of a term infant is 20 inches (50.8 cm.), with the mean for girls being slightly less than for boys. Measuring length is somewhat difficult because of the strong tendency of the baby's legs to flex; however, accuracy is important. If the baby is placed so that the top of his head is parallel with the end of the mattress and if a mark is placed at the point to which his heel reaches, the distance, rather than the squirmy baby, can be measured. The significance of an error of just 1 inch is clear when we realize that a baby measuring 20 inches is at the fiftieth percentile while a baby measuring 19 inches is very close to the tenth percentile. Length increases about 4 inches (10 cm.) during the first 3 months, 2 additional inches (5 cm.) by 6 months, and a total of 10 to 12 inches (25 to 30 cm.) during the first year (Appendix B).

Head and Chest Circumference

Head circumference is measured at the level of the occiput and the supraorbital ridges. At birth it is approximately 13 to 14 inches (33 to 35.5 cm.). The size of the head is even less affected by intrauterine growth retardation than is length, so here again percentile tables can be useful in evaluating what has happened to the baby in utero.

An accurate record of head circumference at birth is also important in evaluating head growth. The head should increase about 2 inches during the first 4 months and a total of 4 inches during the first year. If head circumference is above the ninety-seventh percentile at birth and continues to exceed normal measurements, or if it remains below the third percentile, medical evaluation is necessary.

Chest circumference, measured at the level of the nipples, is approximately 1 inch smaller than head circumference, about 12 to 13 inches (30.5 to 33.0 cm.) at birth. The chest grows slightly more rapidly than the head in the first months. In babies whose head and chest size are above the fiftieth percentile, chest size may exceed head size by 6 months of age. In small infants (below the tenth percentile), head size remains larger until 15 to 18 months of age. If the head exceeds the chest by more than one inch (2.5 cm) at three months or, at the other extreme, if the head is smaller than the chest in the early months, medical evaluation of the baby is important.

NEUROMUSCULAR
DEVELOPMENT

Within Normal Limits

Strong flexor muscle tone
Symmetrical posture and movement
Brief tremors or twitching

In Need of Special Attention

Hypotonicity or hypertonicity
Lack of movement on one or both sides
Weak, random movements
Prolonged tremors or convulsions

NEUROMUSCULAR DEVELOPMENT

Normally a term newborn assumes a characteristic position. When lying on his abdomen, his knees are drawn up, raising his pelvis. On his back he rolls to one side or the other. Whatever his position, his arms and legs are strongly flexed and his alignment is basically symmetrical. These two characteristics—symmetry and flexion—are significant indicators of normality. However, certain exceptions, related to the mode of delivery, are not considered abnormal. The baby born in the breech position with his legs extended will usually continue to have extended legs during the newborn period. Babies who present face first during delivery lie in a position resembling *opisthotonos*, an arched position of the body. Unlike the baby with true opisthotonos, these infants have normal muscle tone.

Both "floppiness" (hypotonicity) and rigidity (hypertonicity) in a term baby are abnormal findings. (By contrast, preterm infants have far less muscle tone, the degree of the tone being a strong indicator of gestational age.) (See Chapter 15.) A variety of central nervous system problems, neuromuscular and connective tissue disorders, infection, dehydration, and other types of illness may be the cause of both hypotonicity and hypertonicity.

A fractured clavicle or an injury to the brachial plexus is a common reason for lack of movement on one or both sides. With these conditions the *Moro reflex* (below) will also be unilateral. Both of these conditions are treated as soon as they are discovered.

The arm and shoulder of a baby with a fractured clavicle are immobilized, usually with a stockinette bandage that holds the arm against the chest with the hand across the chest. Fractures of the clavicle heal with no deformity. Occasionally the clavicle may be fractured without the loss of movement; a knot felt along the clavicle from 3 to 4 days to about 1 week after birth is the only symptom. The knot, or callus, is gradually absorbed.

Injury to the nerve fibers of the brachial plexus may occur during delivery if there is traction on the head during the delivery of the shoulder. Such an injury can lead to paralysis of part of the arm or even of the entire arm. Most common is Erb-Duchenne paralysis of the upper arm resulting from injury to the fifth and sixth cervical nerves. The affected arm lies immobile at the baby's side (Fig. 16–3). Treatment involves positioning of the arm and physical therapy. Even during bathing and dressing the baby, the arm should be positioned at shoulder level. This means that the mother, in order to feel confident, must have the opportunity to care for her infant while they are both in the hospital (Chapter 22). The degree of nerve injury is the principal factor in recovery. If nerves are intact, muscle function will generally return in a few months. If nerve fibers are lacerated, neuroplasty may bring about partial recovery.

Although brief tremors or twitchings are not unusual in normal newborns, they must be differentiated from somewhat more prolonged tremors and from seizures, which may indicate a variety of pathologic conditions such as hypoglycemia, hypocalcemia, infection, or neurologic damage (Chapter 18).

Because of the immaturity of the newborn infant's cerebrum, seizure behavior is different that that of an older child or adult. Neonatal seizures may consist of no more than chewing or swallowing movements, deviation of the eyes, rigidity or flaccidity, or pallor or

Figure 16–3 Brachial palsy of the left arm (asymmetric Moro reflex). (From Nelson, Vaughan, and McKay: *Textbook of Pediatrics.* 9th Edition. Philadelphia, W. B. Saunders Co., 1969.)

lushing. Rarely will the classic grand mal, petit mal, or jacksonian types of seizures be seen.

During a seizure a baby must be watched carefully for any sign of regurgitation. Charting should include the duration of seizure activity, the time at which it occurred, and the areas of the body involved. The baby's behavior and cry before and after the seizure should be recorded.

Neonatal seizures do not automatically suggest permanent brain damage. In one study by Rose and Lombroso[20] it was found that newborns with seizures but with a *normal electroencephalogram (EEG)* had an 86 per cent chance of normal development at the age of 4 years.

Reflexes

Evaluation of reflexes in the term infant is important in recognizing neurologic abnormalities and, by evaluating certain reflexes, recognizing such problems as brachial plexus injury or fracture of the clavicle. In the preterm baby reflex evaluation is an additional help in estimating gestational age (Chapter 15). As the baby matures and becomes able to respond in other ways, newborn reflexes disappear. Persistence of these reflexes beyond the time at which they should no longer normally be present suggests central nervous system pathology.

Table 16–1 and Figures 16–4 to 16–7 summarize significant information about major reflexes of newborn infants.

THE SENSES

An interest in the newborn's sensory system is not a matter of academic curiosity. Our understanding of how the baby perceives the world influences our behavior toward him and his needs.

Touch

Of all the senses, touch appears to be the most significant in the infant's first weeks of life. A term newborn has approximately 25,000 square cm. of skin surface, by far the largest organ system in the body. Through his skin—his fingertips, his lips, and his total body—he first experiences the world and becomes aware of it. Cutaneous stimulation has been shown to be absolutely essential for life in a variety

Table 16–1 NEONATAL REFLEXES

Reflex	Manner of Eliciting	Gestational Age When Consistently Present	Age When Disappears	Comments
Moro	A hand clap or slap on the mattress. The baby should respond with extension of the trunk and extension and adduction of the limbs, followed by flexion and adduction of the limbs (as if to embrace) (Fig. 16–4).	32 weeks	From 1 to 3 or 4 months	A sudden noise or sudden motion may also elicit response. Consistent absence suggests brain damage Absence on one side may indicate brain damage, fractured clavicle or injury to the brachial plexus.
Tonic neck reflex	When the baby is supine and the head is turned to one side, the arm and leg the baby is facing extend while the opposite arm and leg flex in a "fencing" position (Fig. 16–5).	Incomplete at birth in normal term infant; often more definite in leg than arm.	During the first year, although a partial response may remain until the second or third year.	Both persistent asymmetry and a full response easily obtained suggest a cerebral lesion.
Stepping	When held erect and body supported under the arms with soles flat on table top and trunk inclined forward, baby takes regular, alternating steps	May "tip-toe" at 32 weeks; heel-to-toe motion at 40 weeks.	7 to 8 months	Failure to step on several different occasions suggests neurologic abnormality; stepping with one foot only indicates a unilateral problem.

Placing	When held erect with dorsum of foot drawn against under-edge of table top, foot is lifted and placed atop table.	37 weeks	7 to 8 months	Failure to place, or unilateral placing, suggests neurologic abnormality, as does persistent extension or scissoring of legs.
Grasp reflex	Pressing the examiner's finger into the baby's metacarpal phalangeal groove causes the baby to grasp the finger.	Finger grasp is present as early as 28 weeks, but it is approximately 36 weeks before the baby can lift himself off the mattress (Fig. 16–7).	4 to 5 months	
Rooting reflex	Stroking the upper or lower lip or the side of the cheek causes the baby to turn his mouth and face toward the stimulus and to open his mouth.	Fairly good by 32 weeks; complete at 34 weeks	3 to 4 months when baby awake; 7 to 8 months when baby asleep	May be difficult to elicit immediately after feeding.
Sucking reflex	Stroking the lips produces sucking	Excellent by 34 weeks; reasonably strong at 32 weeks	12 months	May be difficult to elicit in recently fed baby; weak or absent in baby with brain damage. Utilize both rooting and sucking reflexes when putting baby to breast or offering a bottle.

Figure 16-4   Moro reflex. (From Davis and Rubin: *De Lee's Obstetrics for Nurses.* 18th Edition. Philadelphia, W. B. Saunders Co., 1966.)

Figure 16-5 The tonic neck reflex in a week old baby.

of animal species. Other studies suggest that it may be equally significant in the relationship between human parents and their babies. As our knowledge of the significance of touch increases, many of our current practices that keep mothers and infants separated for long hours of the day so that the baby is "untouched" need to be re-evaluated.

Vision

Like the brain, the eye achieves a greater proportion of total growth before birth than does the rest of the body. And so at the time of birth the eye is ready for limited vision. The eye is considered anatomically mature at 3 years and visually mature by the sixth year.

The principal evidence of functional vision is the ability to fix upon an object and to follow it with the eyes. Greenman found that 95 per cent of one group of 127 healthy term infants showed visual following one or more times in the first 19 hours of life.[10] Some alert preterm neonates will also follow an object with their eyes. However, most babies are 6 to 8 weeks old before fixing and following are consistently reliable.

Figure 16–6 Stepping reflex. (From Davis and Rubin: *De Lee's Obstetrics for Nurses*. 18th Edition. Philadelphia, W. B. Saunders Co., 1966.)

Various studies indicate that visual acuity in the newborn baby may be as good as 20/150, with some degree of color discrimination and pattern vision.

Figure 16–7 Grasp reflex. (From Davis and Rubin: *De Lee's Obstetrics for Nurses*. 18th Edition. Philadelphia, W. B. Saunders Co., 1966.)

Both Fantz[8] and Hershenson and colleagues[11] demonstrated a baby's preference for a patterned or a more complicated figure over a plain or more simple one.

Visual attention plays an important part in parent-child interaction. Listen to mothers when a sleeping baby is brought to them. "I've never seen his eyes," they tell you in disappointment. "When will he open them"? Visual attention from their baby gives obvious pleasure to both parents, who will then hold and cuddle him to get more visual attention.

Korner and Grobstein[14] suggest still another relationship between maternal attention and visual alertness. They found that when a baby cried and was picked up and placed on the shoulder, the infant not only ceased crying but frequently became alert and began to scan the environment (Fig. 16–8). Thus it would appear that the baby who is picked up frequently would have many more opportunities to scan his world. What this might mean in terms of infant learning we can only imagine at this time.

Consider the Aivilik Eskimo infant, who during his early months sees the world from every possible angle while strapped to his mother's back. Aivilik adults demonstrate superior mechanical ability, repairing equipment that American mechanics have abandoned in despair. The Aivilik need not turn a book "properly" to look at an illustration; such is his visual orientation that he sees the picture right side up even if it is held in a horizontal or upside down position.[3] The possible correlation of these adult characteristics with care and visual experiences during early infancy seems a promising area for future research. Do other infants who spend much of their early months on their mothers' backs have similar abilities? Will the increasing practice of

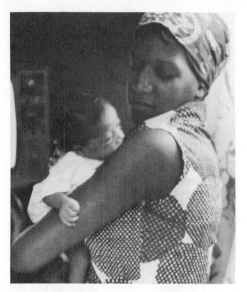

Figure 16–8 A baby held at the mother's shoulder frequently becomes alert and scans the environment.

"backpacking" American infants change their visual-spatial orientation?

Hearing

A newborn infant should be able to hear sounds and respond to them. Hearing defects can be detected as early as the first day of life by the use of an audiometer with an intensity level set at 90 decibels. Shimek reports that the ideal time for testing is midway between feedings.[22] The just-fed infant is often too content to respond, while the hungry infant may be too overactive. Light sleep is the best pretest state.

In the Shimek study, neonates most frequently responded to the audiometer tone with a general restless movement. If the baby was already active when the sound was heard, cessation of activity was the response. Limb movement, eye blink, and eye movement were also observed.

By 3 weeks a baby may open his eyes or squint in response to sound.

Taste

In early fetal life taste buds are distributed throughout the mouth and throat, but prior to term they begin to disappear from all areas but the tongue. Jensen[12] demonstrated that newborn infants do discriminate between water, acid, glucose, various concentrations of a salt solution, and milk. Discrimination was tested by linking a special feeding bottle to a manometer that measured sucking responses to various substances and recorded them on a polygraph.

Smell

A sense of smell, that is, a response to olfactory stimuli, is present at birth and appears to increase over the next several days. Published studies in this area include those of Engen and coworkers[6, 7] and Lipsitt and coworkers.[16]

SKIN

Within Normal Limits

Lanugo
Vernix caseosa
Milia
Mongolian spots
Erythema toxicum
"Stork's beak mark"

In Need of Special Attention

Impetigo
Cracked or peeling skin
Hemangiomas

SKIN

The softness of newborn skin is heralded in advertisements for a variety of cosmetic preparations. In the first day or so after birth, however, sensitive infant skin does not often resemble that of the baby of television or magazine illustrations. Mothers and fathers can be disappointed if we don't help them understand what is normal during the first week or so of life.

Both the fine downy hair called lanugo and vernix caseosa have been discussed in the preceding chapter. Vernix, which is a mixture of water and oil and contains sebum, skin cells, and other materials, protects fetal skin from maceration by amniotic fluid prior to delivery.

Milia are tiny cysts frequently found across the bridge of the nose or on the chin. They disappear without treatment within a few weeks after birth.

Mongolian spots, seen most commonly on the sacrum or buttocks of some black babies, may appear at first glance to be bruises. They also disappear spontaneously within a few weeks to several months.

Differentiation of the lesions of the very common *erythema toxicum* (Fig. 16–9) (also called urticaria neonatorum or "flea-bite rash," although fleas are in no way involved) from that of the far more serious *impetigo* (Fig. 16–10) is highly important. From 30 to 70 per cent of normal term infants will develop toxic erythema, but it is rare in preterm babies. Although most commonly occurring during the first 4 days of life, the rash may be seen at any time during the initial 2 weeks. Papules appear on the first day, look worse on the second, and are often entirely gone within 72 hours. The baby's trunk and diaper area are usually affected.

Unlike toxic erythema, which almost never requires treatment, impetigo is a bacterial infection (caused by group A beta hemolytic streptococci or by *Staphylococcus aureus*) that can lead to a generalized infection, always serious in a newborn. The pustular vesicles rupture to produce a thick, moist, yellow crust that must be soaked off, and antibiotic ointment must be applied to the area. Everyone who comes in contact with the baby must wash very carefully to avoid infecting other infants in the nursery. Special care must also be taken with the baby's linen and other items involved in his care.

Cracked or peeling skin may be seen in the baby who is small for gestational age.

"Birth Marks"

Any large, discolored area of the skin, even when it is not a threat to the baby's physical well-being, is highly distressing to the baby's parents because it is so obvious. To the extent that birth markings affect the way parents feel about their baby and the way in which they treat him, they can have far-reaching significance.

At first glance a "stork's beak mark" may appear to be a nevus flammeus or a port wine stain (see below). However, the affected area, which is usually on the occiput, the eyelids, or the glabella (the smooth space between the eyebrows above the nose) blanches on pressure and is often lighter in color than a nevus flammeus or a port wine stain. These marks disappear completely before the end of the first year.

A port wine stain is a flat, purple or dark red lesion, consisting of mature capillaries, which is present at birth (Fig. 16–11). Port wine hemangiomas located above the bridge of the nose tend to fade; others do not, but since they are level with the surface of the skin, they can be covered with a cosmetic preparation such as Covermark.

Strawberry hemangiomas (nevus vasculosus) are elevated areas consist-

Figure 16–9 Irritative rashes that were evident at birth. Such lesions are not contagious and ordinarily do not become secondarily infected. (From Davis and Rubin: *De Lee's Obstetrics for Nurses.* 18th Edition. Philadelphia, W. B. Saunders Co., 1966.)

Figure 16–10 Impetigo of the newborn. (From Davis and Rubin: *De Lee's Obstetrics for Nurses.* 18th Edition. Philadelphia, W. B. Saunders Co., 1966.)

ing of immature capillaries and endothelial cells. They may be present at birth or may appear during the first 2 weeks following birth, and continue to enlarge for 6 months to a year. After the baby's first birthday they begin to regress, the process of involution taking as long as 10 years (Fig. 16–12). One-half to three-fourths of strawberry hemangiomas disappear by the time the child is 7 years old, leaving virtually no physical evidence that they ever existed. The end result seems to be better if the hemangioma is untreated, unless it interferes with normal function-

ing because of its location. Helping parents to accept both their child and the concept that no treatment is the best treatment is a major challenge. A series of illustrations showing regression of similar marks in other children may help parents through the years of waiting.

A third type of lesion, the cavernous hemangioma, consists of dilated vascular spaces with thick walls that are lined with endothelium (Fig. 16–13). The overlying skin is not involved. Enlargement may precede regression, which occurs only in some instances.

Figure 16–11 Port wine stain, present from birth, does not usually fade but can be covered with a cosmetic preparation. (From Moschella, Pillsbury, and Sturley: *Dermatology*. Philadelphia, W. B. Saunders Co., 1975.)

SKIN COLOR

Within Normal Limits

Red
Cyanosis of the lips, fingernails, toenails, hands, and feet (acrocyanosis)
Cyanosis of the presenting part
Jaundice after 36 to 48 hours
Harlequin sign

In Need of Special Attention

Pale or gray color
Generalized cyanosis
Jaundice during the first 24 hours
Mottled skin

SKIN COLOR

The very red color of a just-born baby's skin is due to both the high concentration of red blood cells in the vessels and the thin layer of subcutaneous fat that causes the blood vessels to be closer to the surface of the skin.

Artificial lighting in a hospital nursery may make it difficult to evaluate slight changes in a baby's color. A periodic check of the baby's color in natural light coming from a window helps to detect these changes. Hospital nurseries should be painted a cream color to allow better observation of color changes.

Figure 16–12 Vascular nevus (strawberry type), showing spontaneous, progressive involution in male infant. A, Age 6 weeks; B, age 8 months; C, age 2 years. (From Nelson, Vaughan, and McKay: *Textbook of Pediatrics.* 10th Edition. Philadelphia, W. B. Saunders Co., 1975.)

Figure 16–13 A cavernous hemangioma. (From Moschella, Pillsbury, and Hurley: *Dermatology.* Philadelphia, W. B. Saunders Co., 1975.)

Cyanosis

It is not unusual for a newborn infant to have localized cyanosis caused by either immature peripheral circulation in the lips, hands, and feet, or by stasis, which tends to produce cyanosis in the part presenting at delivery. (Stasis leads to cyanosis because the very slow passage of blood through the tissues causes an increased amount of oxygen to be released from hemoglobin.)

Generalized cyanosis, however, is a cause for concern. Sometimes generalized cyanosis is so slight that the baby must be compared with an infant who has obviously good color in order to detect its presence. The need for such a comparison is indicated when the baby is having other symptoms of respiratory distress and the possibility of cyanosis is raised. In babies with dark skin, cyanosis can often be best observed in the mucosal lining of the mouth.

The relationship between cyanosis and crying is an important observation. The baby may be cyanotic except when he cries vigorously and thereby raises his intake of oxygen. The baby with atelectasis is one such example. Other babies are cyanotic chiefly when they cry, a sign that may warn of the later, more persistent cyanosis of some types of congenital heart disease.

Cyanosis related to apnea can usually be terminated by provoking the baby to cry, by gently flicking either the soles of his feet or his buttocks.

Cyanosis is one of a number of nonspecific signs associated with hypoglycemia and hypocalcemia, both of which have a particularly high incidence in the infants of diabetic mothers.

Babies with bilateral choanal atresia (occlusion of the posterior nares by either bone or membrane) will be cyanotic, for infants are obligate nose breathers; they breathe through their mouth only with great difficulty. Diagnosis is made by holding a wisp of cotton in front of each nostril; the air movements of respiration can then be readily observed.

Babies with choanal atresia require surgery, because, as just mentioned, all babies are obligate nose breathers. Until surgery is arranged, they can breathe through their mouth if a nipple with a large hole in it is taped in place, or an airway is inserted.

Sudden cyanosis and apnea in a baby who apparently has been doing well may be due to excessive, thick mucus obstructing the upper respiratory tract. For this reason a bulb syringe should be kept in each baby's bed, and a suction machine with a supply of catheters should be available for nasal suction. Lowering the baby's head will aid in draining the mucus, a technique that can easily be shown to mothers. Once the obstructing mucus is removed, the baby becomes pink and immediately resumes respirations.

Damage to the central nervous system, either because of developmental abnormalities or because of trauma during delivery, is another reason for cyanosis. This baby is likely to have very irregular breathing and may have some other signs of central nervous system damage, such as a high-pitched cry, muscle tone that is either very floppy or rigid, or the absence of a Moro reflex. As is true of infants who are cyanotic because of respiratory distress, crying and oxygen tend to improve color.

Babies who are cyanotic because of cardiac anomalies are rarely helped by oxygen and generally appear worse when they cry. At first these newborns may be only briefly pale or cyanotic during feeding or following an injection. Babies with markedly decreased cardiac output and/or in heart failure will have arms and legs (not just hands and feet) that are cool to the touch. Babies who are pink in the upper half of their body, but cyanotic in the lower trunk and legs, probably have a patent ductus arteriosus, with blood shunted from right to left through the ductus (i.e., returning to the body without going to the lungs to be perfused with oxygen). (See also Chapter 18.)

Pallor

Pallor may be due to anemia, hemorrhage, hemolysis of red blood cells, or shock. Loss of blood may have occurred through fetal-maternal transfusion before the cord was clamped. Sometimes when twins share a single placenta, there is a transfusion from one twin to the other. If there is no visible source of external hemorrhage, such as from the umbilical cord, a pale baby must be watched for signs of internal bleeding in the vomitus or stool. Babies with intracranial damage are often pale because of shock. Gray color is also associated with infection and with chloramphenicol intoxication. Either pallor or cyanosis confined to one extremity is a sign of interference with local circulation.

Jaundice

About 40 to 60 per cent of term infants (and a higher percentage of preterm babies) are jaundiced on the second to third day of life. Because there is no discernible pathologic reason for this jaundice, such as a hemolytic anemia or sepsis, the jaundice is termed physiologic, which is perhaps a misnomer since it obiously does not occur in every infant.

By definition, jaundice that is termed physiologic never occurs during the first 24 hours, does not cause levels of indirect bilirubin that rise above 10 to 12 mg. per 100 ml., and rarely lasts past the first week of life, the exception occurring occasionally in breast-fed infants.

The yellow color of the jaundice in these babies, as in individuals of any age, is due to high levels of bilirubin; the source of bilirubin is the breakdown of red blood cells.

Both globin, which is a protein, and iron are reused by the body. Indirect bilirubin, which is fat soluble and cannot be excreted by the kidneys, is converted to direct bilirubin, which is water soluble and can be excreted by the kidneys, by the hepatic enzyme glucuronyl transferase.

There is no universal agreement concerning the cause of physiologic jaundice. Production of bilirubin by the newborn (at rates of 6 to 8 mg. per kg. per 24 hours) is approximately two and one half times that of an adult, at least partially due to the fact that the lifespan of red blood cells in newborns is 90 days, compared with the 120 day lifespan of adult erythrocytes. Less blood goes to the liver in some infants because the ductus venosus remains open, and thus some blood, which would otherwise do so, does not circulate in the liver.

A deficiency of glucuronyl transferase has been considered a factor in neonatal jaundice, but this has been questioned by one study.[5] The decreased amount of Y and Z carrier proteins in the cells of the liver is now considered a more likely answer.

As long as the bilirubin remains within the circulatory system, no jaundice is visible because the red of the hemoglobin obscures the yellow of the bilirubin. But when the indirect bilirubin level rises above 7 mg. per 100 ml. in term infants, bilirubin moves outside the vascular space and is then visible. It often takes higher levels of bilirubin to bring about visible jaundice in low birth weight babies because the capillary bed lies closer to the skin surface since there is less subcutaneous fat. The red of the hemoglobin is thus reflected on the skin surface, obscuring the yellow of the jaundice. Jaundice can be visualized, however, by blanching the skin with the thumb.

Some breast-fed infants may have a jaundice that develops on the third day of life and lasts beyond the first week.

This is believed to be due to the presence of pregnanediol in breast milk, which depresses the action of the glucuronyl transferase enzyme. Most of the babies can continue to breast-feed, with frequent checks of indirect bilirubin levels. Occasionally breast-feedings are withheld for a brief period until the bilirubin level drops, after which breast-feeding can usually be resumed with no further difficulty. During the interim, if the baby is fed by dropper and the mother's breast is pumped, breast-feeding can be resumed with little difficulty. The baby should not be bottle-fed. Sucking from a bottle is different from sucking at breast, and the baby may reject the breast.

Rarely is treatment necessary for physiologic jaundice in an otherwise healthy baby. There is serious danger of kernicterus (Chapter 18) to an infant whose level of indirect bilirubin rises to 20 mg. per 100 ml. or more, but in physiologic jaundice (by definition) bilirubin levels do not exceed 12 mg. per 100 ml. and are usually lower. Phototherapy is used occasionally to treat the baby with physiologic jaundice, but since its chief use is with babies of low birth weight, this treatment is discussed in Chapter 18. Jaundice other than physiologic is also discussed in Chapter 18.

THE HEAD

Because the head is the most obvious of all the body areas, head contour is a particular source of concern to many parents. Those variations that most concern mothers and fathers are likely to be the more common ones, which are usually within normal limits. We must be aware of other variations that suggest possible illness.

THE HEAD

Within Normal Limits

A large head in proportion to the rest of the body
Anterior fontanel: diamond-shaped; approximately 2 to 3 cm. wide
Posterior fontanel: triangular; approximately 0 to 1 cm. wide
Molding
Craniotabes
Caput succedaneum
Cephalhematoma

In Need of Special Attention

Microcephalus
Hydrocephalus
Anencephalus
Fontanels that are depressed or bulging

A newborn's head is large in proportion to the rest of his body, about one-third the size it will be when he reaches adulthood. His brain weighs approximately 400 grams; it will be more than doubled, weighing 1000 grams, by his first birthday.

The measurement of head circumference has already been described. Head circumference is measured during the initial examination in the nursery not only to identify present abnormalities but to record a baseline measurement for the evaluation of future growth. Although head measurement is not the only indication of conditions such as hydrocephalus and microcephalus, it is one valuable factor in the assessment of head growth and in the early identification of problems. *Hydrocephalus*, in which an excessive amount of cerebrospinal fluid leads to rapid head growth, may be present at birth or may even be predicted during antenatal examination. More commonly it is recognized in the early weeks and months of life. *Micro-cephalus* occurs when brain growth is arrested and the skull does not grow. Possible causes include infection, injury, and genetic maternal irradiation during early pregnancy.

If the anterior end of the neural tube fails to close (Chapter 6), the cranial vault will be mainly absent, a condition termed *anencephalus*. An anencephalic baby will not survive for long, although rarely he will live for days or even weeks. Our concern for these families is to help them cope with a devastating experience (Chapter 22).

The fontanels, and especially the anterior fontanel because of its larger size, have been the substance for folk beliefs for many generations. Some mothers are still afraid to touch the baby's head; we see babies who are a few weeks old with varying degrees of skin problems because the mother has not shampooed the baby's head for fear of damaging his brain. We need to anticipate such a possibility by explaining the function of the open fontanel both as protection of the head during delivery by allowing for molding (see below) and as a provision for further brain growth over the next 18 months. Reassurance that the brain is well protected by the tough membrane that covers it and needs no special handling and encouragement to wash the baby's head at each bath are also important.

A closed anterior fontanel is usually related to microcephaly and is a matter of serious concern. The posterior fontanel, however, may be closed in a normal newborn. Both a bulging fontanel, which may indicate intracranial hemorrhage or infection, and a depressed fontanel, which indicates dehydration, are abnormal. The fontanels should be inspected each day when the baby is bathed.

Molding describes the process by which the bones of the head accommodate themselves to the vaginal canal in order to facilitate delivery. The baby's head may look misshapen to the parents, but we can assure them that it will be well rounded within a few days.

Craniotabes refers to the softening of localized areas in the cranial bones. These areas are easily indented by the pressure of a fingertip, but resume their shape when the pressure is removed. The cause of craniotabes is unknown, and there is no treatment. Although the condition may persist for a number of months, it eventually disappears completely.

A *caput succedaneum* is edema of the superficial tissues that overlie the bone of the part of the head presenting first during delivery. It is caused by the pressure of the cervix on the tissues involved, the cervix acting as a tourniquet with resultant venous congestion, edema, and extravasation of blood. There may be some discoloration of the skin. A caput succedaneum presents no physical problem to the baby but may be a source of worry to the parents. It is visible immediately after birth and is usually absorbed within a few days (Fig. 16–14).

Another common condition in newborns, *cephalhematoma*, takes several weeks or even months to be completely absorbed. In a cephalhematoma blood collects between a cranial bone and the overlying periosteum (Fig. 16–14*B*). Because of this, the cephalhematoma is confined to areas between suture lines, although a baby may have more than one. By contrast, a caput succedaneum, because only the soft tissue is involved, crosses suture lines. Neither a caput nor a cephalhematoma requires treatment; the fluid is never aspirated. To do so would risk infection.

Figure 16–14 *A*, Edema and hemorrhage in caput succedaneum. *B*, Location of swelling in cephalhematoma; note that the swelling does not cross the suture lines. *C*, A baby with a large caput succedaneum. (Reprinted with permission of Daniel J. Pachman, M.D., of the University of Illinois Pediatric Department. *A* and *C* appeared in *Pediatrics*, Vol. 29, 1962.)

EYES

Eye-to-eye contact is one of the significant steps in bonding a mother and father to their infant. Although neonates tend to keep their eyes shut rather tightly during the first days of life, it is important that we, as well as the parents, have an opportunity to observe them. Tilting the head gently backward may cause the baby to open his eyes. Never try to force the lids apart with the fingertips.

EYES

Within Normal Limits

Transient strabismus
Subconjunctival hemorrhage
Swelling and watery discharge following the administration of silver nitrate (chemical conjunctivitis)
Swelling following forceps delivery

In Need of Special Attention

Constant and fixed strabismus
Discharge beginning after the first 24 hours or lasting more than 3 days
Purulent discharge
Opacity of the pupil
Large cornea; corneas of unequal size
Epicanthic folds in nonoriental babies

The gray-blue color of a newborn baby's eyes is actually an absence of pigmentation, which will develop throughout the first year. Eye color is usually distinguishable by 3 months. Although the lacrimal gland is small, it is capable of producing tears. The absence of tears is not unusual in the first weeks of life, however.

Because convergence of the eyes is not fully developed until about 3 months, newborns at times appear "cross-eyed," a matter of some concern to their parents. This apparent strabismus is normal and transient; it is 3 to 4 months before eye movements are consistently coordinated. However, constant strabismus, even in these early weeks, needs medical evaluation.

Pupils should react equally to light from the time of birth.

A red ring around the cornea, or a small patch of red, indicates subconjunctival hemorrhage, which is due to changes in vascular pressure during delivery. The hemorrhage absorbs in 2 to 3 weeks without treatment and apparently without complication.

Ophthalmia Neonatorum

Prophylaxis against ophthalmia neonatorum, the gonococcal infection of the newborn's eyes, has already been discussed (Chapter 15). Although preventive treatment radically reduces the incidence of this serious condition, it does not entirely eliminate the possibility that it may occur. Recognition of ophthalmia neonatorum is further complicated by the fact that the earliest symptoms, conjunctivitis and a watery discharge, resemble a reaction to the silver nitrate that is given for its prevention. Drug-related conjunctivitis, however, rarely lasts longer than 24 hours; any conjunctivitis that lasts longer than 3 days is considered due to infection. Because of an incubation period of 1 to 3 days, conjunctivitis due to ophthalmia neonatorum will occur at a later period of time than that related to silver nitrate administration and will be followed in approximately 24 hours first by a watery discharge and subsequently by a thick, purulent exudate. The cornea becomes dull and ulcerates rapidly. A gelatinous exudate appears in the anterior chamber of the eye. This exudate is under great pressure; everyone who handles the baby should do so carefully and should protect their own eyes.

Once ophthalmia neonatorum is suspected, samples of the exudate are examined. Because the disease progresses rapidly to ocular perforation and blindness, parenteral penicillin therapy is begun as soon as the causative organism is identified as being gram positive (the group in which the gonorrhea bacteria belong). A single large dose (150,000 units of aqueous penicillin) is given, because peak blood level rather than total dose is the critical factor. Local treatment includes saline eyewashes and topical antibiotics. Great care is taken to protect the uninvolved eye; it may be taped shut.

Response to treatment is usually dramatic. The baby is significantly improved within 24 hours and is no longer considered infective. Treatment continues, however, for 2 to 5 days. If there is no response within 24 to 48 hours, the possibility of a resistant organism is considered.

Congenital Disorders

An opaque pupil indicates *congenital cataract* (Fig. 16–15), a condition that may, but does not always, cause major visual problems. Surgery is the treatment if there is significant visual difficulty that cannot be corrected by glasses, but results are often not as satisfactory as those in adult cataract surgery. When maternal rubella is the cause (and this is the most frequent cause), surgery should be delayed until after the second birthday, in order not to activate the virus.

A baby with an unusually large cornea (the corneas may be of unequal size) is likely to have congenital

Figure 16–15 Congenital cataract. The opaque lens stands out sharply. (From the collection of Dr. Arnall Patz. *In* Schaffer and Avery *Diseases of the Newborn.* 4th Edition. Philadelphia W. B. Saunders Co., 1977.)

glaucoma, a condition that requires immediate treatment if the baby's vision is not to be permanently damaged. The cornea may also be hazy or cloudy. Confirmation of glaucoma is made by measuring intraocular tension. The treatment is immediate surgery.

A fold of skin across the inner angle of the eye (epicanthic fold) is normal in oriental babies, and not necessarily abnormal in other infants. But since epicanthic folds in nonoriental babies are sometimes associated with Down's syndrome and certain other congenital abnormalities, they should be noted on the baby's record for proper follow-up.

EARS

The normal position of the newborn's ears is with the upper part on the same plane as the angle of the eye. Ears that are set lower may be associated with a congenital renal disorder or an autosomal chromosomal abnormality (Fig. 16–16). Sinus tracts in front of the ears and preauricular skin tags should be noted.

Figure 16–16 The normal position of the newborn's ears *(A)* contrasted with low set ears *(B)*.

B

MOUUTH AND JAWS

MOUTH AND JAWS

Within Normal Limits

Sucking pads
Epithelial "pearls"
Labial tubercle
Large tongue with short frenulum
Some mucus

In Need of Special Attention

Cleft lip and palate
Thrush
Excessive frothy mucus
Corners of the mouth that don't
move when the baby cries
Micrognathia

MOUTH AND JAW

The mouth of a newly born baby is uniquely designed for its principal function—sucking. Stimulating the baby to cry will make him open his mouth so that the inside can be inspected. Note the pads of fat in the cheeks (sucking pads) that prevent collapse of the cheeks, which would make sucking difficult. Occasionally a newborn will already have one or more teeth; these teeth are usually pulled to facilitate sucking.

Epithelial "pearls" (also called Epstein's pearls and Bohn's nodules) are raised white areas of epithelial cells that are not infrequently found on the hard palate or gums. They present no problem (except possible concern to the parents) and will shortly disappear. Epithelial pearls should not be confused with thrush (see below).

The labial tubercle is also of occasional concern to parents because it looks like a blister and is frequently termed a "sucking blister." It occurs in the center of the upper lip, is of no known significance, and needs no care.

For a day or so after birth, some babies have a fairly large amount of mucus, which can usually be aspirated with a bulb syringe. Continued excessive mucus that is frothy, as if the baby were "blowing bubbles," suggests a tracheoesophageal fistula. This calls for an immediate examination of the baby, during which an attempt is made to pass a catheter through the esophagus into the stomach. If the catheter curls up or will not pass, the baby must not be fed until further testing is done.

Although a cleft lip and a large cleft of the hard and soft palate are immediately visible, smaller clefts may not be noticed unless we are careful to inspect each baby's mouth for evidence (Fig. 16–17). Even small clefts are important; the baby is at higher risk of infection, speech may be affected, and proper dentition is made difficult.

Figure 16–17 Large midline cleft in the posterior half of the palate. (From the files of Harriet Lane Home. *In* Schaffer and Avery: *Diseases of the Newborn.* 4th Edition. Philadelphia, W. B. Saunders Co. 1977.)

Monilia (Thrush)

Thrush, an infection caused by the fungus *Candida albicans*, is unfortunately common in some nurseries. Numerous small white and gray patches on the tongue and in the mouth (Fig. 16–18) are the indications of thrush. In addition to distinguishing

Figure 16–18 Numerous small white and gray patches on the tongue and palate are an indication of thrush. (From Pillsbury, Shelley, and Kligman: *A Manual of Cutaneous Medicine.* Philadelphia, W. B. Saunders Co., 1961.)

hrush from epithelial patches, we must lso not mistake milk curds for thrush.

Babies with thrush will usually be oor eaters. Although there are many ther more serious reasons for failure of baby to feed well—heart defects, inction, and central nervous system amage, for example—any baby who is ating poorly should be given a thorugh examination of the mouth. Babies eceiving oral antibiotics are particularly susceptible. Most healthy neworns who acquire thrush do so in the elivery process, being infected by Canida in the mother's vagina.

Treatment usually includes the dministration of a nystatin solution iven orally every 6 hours. The solution hould be administered slowly and ently so that it will be widely distribted throughout the oral cavity before c is swallowed. Individual lesions are ometimes painted with a 1 per cent soution of aqueous gentian violet. Excess mounts of gentian violet should not be sed because the solution may be irtating if the baby swallows it. After entian violet is used, the baby should e placed face downward so that saliva ontaining the solution will drain out of he mouth. A paste of sodium bicarboate can be used to remove gentian violet stains from clothing and bedding. 'reatment is continued for at least 3 ays after all visible evidence of thrush gone to assure that the fungus itself is radicated.

Limited Facial Movement

Movement on one side of the face nly when the baby cries is due to injury a facial nerve, either because of presure in utero or injury during delivery. Vhen the baby cries, the mouth is rawn to that side. Occasionally such aralysis is congenital and unrelated to rauma. Outcome depends upon the ex-

tent of the injury to the nerve fibers. If the nerves are only slightly injured, improvement usually occurs within a few weeks without treatment. If the nerve fibers have been torn and paralysis persists, neuroplasty may be necessary. If the baby is unable to close his eye on the affected side, eye care is also essential.

An abnormally small jaw, *micrognathia,* may cause respiratory distress because the tongue falls back into the pharnyx. This can be partially relieved by keeping the baby on his stomach so that the tongue falls forward. Sometimes the tongue is temporarily sutured in place until the jaw grows. Many babies with micrognathia have a cleft palate as well.

TRUNK

Within Normal Limits

Breast engorgement
Bluish-white umbilical cord
Cutis navel
Granulation tissue in navel

In Need of Special Attention

Knot on clavicle
Bleeding from or around the cord
Yellow discoloration of the cord at the time of birth
Exudate at the cord site
Cord with one artery and one vein
Distended, "shiny" abdomen
Scaphoid abdomen
Umbilical hernia
Mass in the abdomen

TRUNK

A knot on the clavicle indicates a fracture, which will heal without difficulty.

Breast engorgement is often a concern to a mother when she examines her baby. During pregnancy, maternal hormones cross the placental barrier and enter the fetal circulation. When these hormones are withdrawn at the time of birth, the breasts enlarge and may even secrete fluid resembling colostrum or milk, referred to as "witches milk" by some mothers. The enlargement lasts from a few days to as long as several weeks. Mothers need to know that this enlargement is perfectly normal. The breasts should not be handled other than in routine bathing. No attempt should ever be made to express the fluid in the breasts; to do so is to risk mastitis.

The Umbilical Area and Cord

The umbilical area and cord also cause many parental questions. Bluish-white at birth, the cord begins to dry right away and usually separates in 6 to 8 days, with the umbilicus healing in about 2 weeks. Because mothers and their term babies often stay in the hospital only 3 to 4 days, and many times even less, cord care quickly becomes the mother's responsibility. It is generally recommended that the cord and the umbilicus be cleaned each day with a cotton ball dipped in alcohol and that submerging the baby's body in his bathtub be delayed until after the area has healed.

The cord should be checked initially for the presence of a single umbilical artery; normally there are two arteries and one vein. The single artery occurs in about 1 per cent of all newborns, more frequently in white infants. For some reason the single artery is associated with an increased incidence of various congenital anomalies and with higher perinatal mortality. It is probably a part of a complex of malformations, rather than the cause of those malformations. For those infants with a

single artery who survive the perinatal period, there is no apparent differenc in mortality and morbidity (other tha a higher incidence of hernia), an impor tant fact for reassuring parents abou this infant and for future genetic coun seling.

Yellow discoloration of the cord a the time of birth is an indication c hemolytic disease; these babies nee careful observation and evaluatio (Chapter 18). Exudate around the cor usually signifies infection, although baby may have an umbilical infectio serious enough to cause generalize sepsis with no local signs at all. A weep ing cord should be cleaned with alcoho several times a day. Cord bleeding ma be due to inadequate tying, or it may b a symptom of a bleeding disorder.

Cutis navel describes an umbilica cord that projects beyond the skin. I looks at first glance as if the baby migh have an umbilical hernia, but a herni can be returned to the abdomen while cutis navel cannot. In addition, herni become more pronounced when th baby cries. No special treatment of cuti navel is required; the navel will slowl invaginate.

Umbilical hernia is more commo in black newborns than in infants c other races. The hernia is due to weakness or imperfect closure of th umbilical ring. Most umbilical herni that occur in small infants disappea spontaneously by the baby's first birth day. Possibly because there is no gen eral agreement on how, or even if, um bilical hernias should be treated, "folk remedies abound. A silver dollar may b found strapped to the baby's abdome when he comes for a check-up, or vari ous forms of binders may be wrappe around him. Studies have produce conflicting evidence about the value o "strapping" the hernia. Surgery is usu ally avoided unless the hernia persist

Figure 16–19 Large omphalocele. Note covering of the sac and its relationship to the umbilicus, which extrudes from the lower portion. (From Avery: *Neonatology: Pathophysiology and Management of the Newborn*. Philadelphia, J. B. Lippincott Co., 1975.)

until the child is 3 to 5 years old or unless it creates problems for the baby or becomes progressively larger after the baby is a year old.

Abdominal Wall Defects

A central defect in the peritoneal, muscular, and ectodermal layers of the abdominal wall is termed an *omphalocele*. The defect is covered by a translucent membrane that covers both bowel and solid viscera (Fig. 16–19). An omphalocele may vary in size from a small hernia to a huge mass that contains all the abdominal viscera.

Gastroschisis (Fig. 16–20) differs from an omphalocele in that the abdominal wall is developed, but a defect remains at the base of the umbilical stalk.

Prior to surgery, every effort is made to keep the viscera sterile by

Figure 16–20 Patient with gastroschisis. Note edematous, matted bowel, the result of the intestines floating freely in the amniotic fluid. Remarkably, these distorted viscera will ultimately fit back into the abdominal cavity and will finally assume a normal appearance and function. (From Avery: *Neonatology: Pathophysiology and Management of the Newborn*. Philadelphia, J. B. Lippincott Co., 1975.)

covering them with moist sterile saline sponges or gauze and sterile plastic. The viscera are only partially replaced during initial surgery; an envelope is created over the remainder, a little more bowel being returned to the abdomen each day in order to keep respiratory distress at a minimum. An alternative procedure involves suturing the skin over the abdominal contents and deferring their return to the abdomen until both baby and abdomen have grown larger.

Abdominal Distention

Although the abdomen is moderately protuberant in all babies, a distended abdomen, which may appear shiny because the skin is stretched, is definitely abnormal. An overly distended abdomen may be related to several conditions. An infant with the type of tracheoesophageal fistula in which there is an opening between the trachea and the stomach will become distended from the continual entry of air. Distention is also an early sign of infection. Congenital obstructions of the gastrointestinal tract and congenital megacolon are also conditions causing distention in newborns. It is important to know whether distention is increasing or decreasing. Marking the area of the distention with a waxed pencil makes this easier to detect.

The opposite of distention, a scaphoid abdomen, suggests the possibility of a diaphragmatic hernia (Chapter 18).

Visible peristaltic waves may move from left to right, as in pyloric stenosis (seen usually in the 2 to 4 week old infant rather than immediately after birth) or from right to left, as in small bowel obstruction. Most prominent during and after feeding, peristaltic waves may be more easily visualized by focus-

ing a light on the baby's abdomen while he is being fed.

Any solid mass in the abdomen that can be palpated is abnormal.

GENITALIA

Within Normal Limits: Female

Red and swollen
Vaginal discharge
Vaginal bleeding
Hymenal tag

Within Normal Limits: Male

Scrotal swelling

In Need of Special Attention

Excessive vaginal bleeding
Undescended testicles in a term baby
Hypospadias, epispadias
Ambiguous genitalia

GENITALIA

Edema of the genitalia is not uncommon in either male or female babies. It is especially noticeable in babies delivered from the breech position. Such edema disappears within a few days.

A vaginal discharge of thick, white mucus is passed by all baby girls in the first week of life. Occasionally the mucus is blood tinged about the third or fourth day, staining the diaper. This pseudomenstruation, like breast engorgement described previously, is due to the withdrawal of maternal hormones. Excessive vaginal bleeding is not normal; it may be due to a blood coagulation defect.

A hymenal or vaginal tag may be distressing to the mother, but it will drop off within a few weeks.

Undescended Testicles

Normally, testicles descend into the scrotum in the eighth month of fetal life. It is possible that a baby boy with undescended testicles is of a younger gestational age than originally suspected. Gestational age should be evaluated as described in Chapter 15.

Hypospadias and Epispadias

Hypospadias is a condition in which the urethra opens on the ventral surface of the penis (Fig. 16–21). Surgical correction is usually made by the time the boy is 2 years old and should always be made before he starts school, so that he will be able to urinate in the same way as the other boys in his class. These babies should *not* be circumcised because the foreskin is used in the surgical repair.

Epispadias is the opening of the urethra on the dorsal aspect of the penis. Epispadias is far less common than hypospadias and is also surgically corrected.

Ambiguous Genitalia

When the anatomy of the genitalia is such that there is doubt about the sex of the baby, further study is necessary as soon as possible. As discussed in Chapter 5, almost all parents tend to treat boys differently than girls, even those parents who consciously would not do so. Mistaken beliefs about a baby's sex can obviously lead to long-term problems.

THE EXTREMITIES

Within Normal Limits

Flexion of arms and legs
Extension of legs in a baby born in breech position

Figure 16–21 Anomalies of the human genitalia. *A*, Hypospadias, showing in one drawing a composite of the different locations. *B*, Hypospadias of a severe degree in a false male hermaphrodite. *C*, Epispadias. (From Arey: *Developmental Anatomy: A Textbook and Laboratory Manual of Embryology*. Revised 7th Edition. Philadelphia, W. B. Saunders Co., 1974.)

In Need of Special Attention

Abnormal position or posture of an extremity
  Polydactyly
  Syndactyly
  Single transverse palmar crease (Simian crease)
  Talipes equinovarus
  Talipes calcaneovalgus
  Inability to abduct thigh

Figure 16–23 Syndactyly involving webbing of the third and fourth fingers. (From Swenson: *Pediatric Surgery*. 1958. Courtesy of Appleton-Century-Crofts, Publishing Division of Prentice-Hall Inc., Englewood Cliffs, N.J.)

THE EXTREMITIES

The flexed position of the baby's arms and legs has already been mentioned. Ordinarily extension of the extremities is abnormal, but it is not unusual in a baby born with his legs extended in the breech position.

Abnormal positioning of an arm may be due to brachial plexus injury or to a fractured clavicle, discussed above, or, rarely, to a fractured humerus.

An extra finger or toe, polydactyly (Fig. 16–22), or webbing of the fingers or toes, syndactyly (Fig. 16–23), may be a familial trait or may be associated

Figure 16–22 Polydactyly, showing a supernumerary finger. (From Swenson: *Pediatric Surgery*. 1958. Courtesy of Appleton-Century-Crofts, Publishing Division of Prentice-Hall, Inc., Englewood Cliffs, N.J.)

with other anomalies. When the extra finger or toe is little more than a skin tag, it may be tied off shortly after birth. When surgery is indicated, it is usually delayed for 2 to 3 years in polydactyly and even longer in syndactyly.

A single transverse crease in the palm of the hand (simian crease) is often associated with Down's syndrome, but also occurs in normal, healthy babies.

About 95 per cent of clubfoot deformities are *talipes equinovarus* (Fig. 16–24), in which the foot is turned downward and inward (medially), somewhat like the hoof of a horse (hence the name). The force required to return the foot to normal position gives some indication of the severity of the problem. With treatment started even before the baby is discharged from the nursery, good results are likely. Such treatment usually involves a series of casts that gradually change the position of the foot until it is overcorrected. In *talipes calcaneovalgus* (Fig. 16–25), the foot is flexed and deviates laterally. Often passive exercise is the only treatment required, although casts may also be used.

Inability to Abduct Thigh

Early recognition of congenital hip dysplasia is very important in successful treatment. With the baby lying on

Figure 16–24 Congenital clubfeet. (From Miller: *J. of Pediatrics, 51*:527, 1957.)

Figure 16–25 Calcaneovalgus deformity. *A*, Feet at rest. *B*, Same feet under test. (From Miller: *J. of Pediatrics, 51*:527, 1957.)

his back, the thighs are flexed, one at a time, outward and then downward to touch the table or bed (Fig. 16–26). When one thigh does not abduct easily, the diagnosis is quite probable. Other indications include a consistent sharp click heard on the affected side during abduction and higher or extra creases on the buttock of the affected side when the baby is observed lying prone.

VOMITING

Within Normal Limits

Mild regurgitation

In Need of Special Attention

Persistent vomiting
Bloody emesis
Bile-stained emesis
Projectile vomiting

VOMITING

Mild regurgitation is not at all unusual in newborns and is due principally to two factors, swallowed air and a certain amount of immaturity of the cardiac sphincter.

Vomiting is quite another matter. Vomiting that occurs shortly after birth or within the first 24 hours is likely to be due to obstruction of the upper digestive tract or to increased intracranial pressure. After the first day, vomiting may still be related to these causes, but it can also be a sign of many other conditions including septicemia, overfeeding, pyloric stenosis, milk allergy, and adrenal insufficiency.

Blood in the vomitus of a breast-fed baby, unless copious, is very possibly from fissures in the mother's nipple. Maternal blood swallowed during delivery is also a common cause of blood appearing in the vomitus of the newborn in the first 2 or 3 days of life. An *Apt test* differentiates maternal blood from fetal blood, based on the fact that fetal hemoglobin is much more alkali resistant than adult-type hemoglobin.

Bloody emesis accompanied by marked abdominal distention and sudden distress may indicate gastric perforation.

Dark green vomitus indicates an obstruction of the gastrointestinal tract (Chapter 18).

Whether or not vomiting is pro-

Figure 16–26 Infant with subluxation of left hip. The nurse is able to abduct the right thigh down to the level of the table, but not the left. (From Pray: *Pediatrics, 9*:94, 1952.)

ectile is always a significant observation. Projectile vomiting in the first week is often related to intestinal obstruction; beginning in the second week the cause may be pyloric stenosis.

STOOLS

Within Normal Limits

Meconium stools for 3 to 4 days
Transitional stools
Stools that vary with type of feeding
Darkened stools in the baby receiving iron
Faint purple stools in the baby treated with gentian violet
Bright green stools in the baby under phototherapy lights (Chapter 18)

In Need of Special Attention

Failure to stool
Meconium stool but no feces
Thick, putty-like meconium
Small, putty-like stool
Diarrhea
Bloody stools

STOOLS

The consistency, color, and odor of stools are all important in evaluating a baby's general condition. Because color changes can occur shortly after defecation, evaluation has to be made right away if it is to have meaning.

Stool consistency and color vary during the first days according to both age and type of feeding. The first stools are of *meconium*, an odorless, viscid material that is dark green to black in color. Meconium stools may last from 3 to 4 days.

Meconium stools are followed by greenish-brown to yellow transitional stools. In breast-fed infants, the next stools will be golden to mustard colored. Stools of breast-fed infants are less frequent than those of bottle-fed babies; there may be as few as one, or even no stools, in some 24 hour periods. The stools of bottle-fed babies are pale yellow in color. They tend to be more formed, more frequent, and more regular than those of breast-fed infants.

No stool passed with 48 hours after delivery usually suggests intestinal obstruction. If meconium is passed initially, but then no feces are passed, the obstruction is in the ileum. Thick, putty-like meconium is the initial symptom of meconium ileus, the neonatal symptom of cystic fibrosis. A small, putty-like stool may be due to stenosis or to atresia somewhere in the bowel.

Diarrhea

Diarrhea is a somewhat nonspecific symptom in newborns. It may simply be the result of overfeeding, although "starvation stools" are probably a more common cause. Some babies will have diarrhea from formulas that will have no adverse effects on other infants. Diarrhea due to enteric infection (Chapter 17) can spread rapidly through a nursery if the ill baby is not immediately isolated.

Aside from the danger of sepsis, diarrhea is extremely serious in newborns because of the baby's very labile water balance. The extent of water loss can be estimated by measuring the water margin around the stool if the baby has not voided in the diaper. Because infant stools are acid and the intestinal membranes of newborns are delicate, bloody diarrhea is not as unusual at this age as it is in older patients.

A baby may also have flecks of

blood in his stool from an anal fissure. A stool with either bright red or old blood is usually a sign of intestinal bleeding. As with blood in the vomitus, a distinction must be made between fetal and maternal blood.

URINE

Within Normal Limits

Peach-colored crystals

In Need of Special Attention

Failure to void
Bloody urine

URINE

The peach-colored discoloration of the diaper of a newborn is due to crystals of uric acid, which are not pathologic at this age.

It is exceedingly important that the occurrence of voiding be noted on the baby's chart during his hospitalization. Failure to void may be due to decreased production of urine or to a mechanical obstruction to voiding. The most common cause of failure to void in the newborn period is dehydration; babies who are small for gestational age are particularly susceptible. Other causes of decreased urine production include hypotension, severe asphyxia, and renal anomalies such as the absence of one or both kidneys or polycystic kidneys.

It is not unusual for an infant to fail to void in the first 12 hours following birth. He may not void until the second or even the third day, depending upon his fluid intake, the environmental temperature, and the condition of his digestive and nervous systems.

Bloody urine suggests renal injury. The cause may be birth asphyxia, renal vein thrombosis, or an infection.

EDEMA

It is not always easy to recognize generalized edema in a newborn. Normally a baby should have very fine wrinkles over the knuckles of his hands and feet. If these wrinkles are not evident, generalized edema may be present. Severe generalized edema at the time of birth may indicate erythroblastosis fetalis, heart failure because of congenital heart disease, or electrolyte imbalance. Firm, sustained pressure is necessary to demonstrate pitting edema in a newborn, because of the limited amount of subcutaneous tissue.

On the other hand, edema of the presenting part is not unusual or a cause for concern. Some preterm babies have a transient edema for no discernible reason. Although infants of diabetic mothers may appear edematous, their excess weight is due to fat rather than to accumulated fluid.

BEHAVIOR

Within Normal Limits

Strong, vigorous cry
General alertness and responsiveness
Spontaneous activity
Sleeps 65 to 70 per cent of the time

In Need of Special Attention

Shrill or hoarse cry
Absence of a cry
Hyperirritability
"Sleepy" baby

BEHAVIOR

The crying of a healthy term infant is strong and vigorous; he may cry for as long as 2 hours in each 24 hour period. Listening to the cries of infants will enable us to become more skilled in recognizing an abnormal cry, such as the high-pitched, shrill cry or the excessive, irritable crying of the baby with an infection or brain damage or the baby of a drug-addicted mother. A total absence of crying also suggests brain damage. If the crying sounds very hoarse, there may be partial paralysis of the vocal cords. Crying because of hunger will usually be accompanied by rooting and sucking. Even a tiny baby may also cry because of a desire to be held. Such a desire is really a need; *babies truly need to be touched and held*. Meeting such a need is in no way "spoiling" a baby. Excellent nursing care involves being able to recognize that need, just as we now recognize the need for feeding, and taking the baby to his mother for "loving" or, if this is not possible at a particular moment, taking time to hold the baby ourselves. (See also Consolability, below.)

A shrill, high-pitched cry suggests some type of central nervous system damage, such as hemorrhage or infection. A shrill cry may also be the first sign of kernicterus (Chapter 18). If you cringe when the baby cries, there is probably something wrong.

A hoarse cry is usually related to congenital laryngeal malformation or to an injury of the larynx during birth. A laryngoscopic examination is usually necessary to determine the exact cause, which may range from a mild problem that requires no treatment to a life-threatening condition.

Sleep

The concept of sleep *states* was discussed at the beginning of this chapter.

Careful observation indicates that newborns do not sleep as much as we may have believed at one time. Even during the first 3 days of life, a healthy term infant may be awake for brief periods that total 7 to 8 hours, roughly 30 per cent of the 24 hour span. Part of the waking time will be spent in crying (state 6), as noted above. From 2 to 3 hours will be feeding time. Periods of light sleep (state 2) will be interspersed with times when the baby is alert and responsive (state 4).

Many parents seem to expect their baby to sleep most of the time. Unless they are aware that a certain amount of wakefulness, sometimes accompanied by fussiness, is normal, they may feel that something is wrong. Although extreme hyperirritability in an infant is abnormal, the drowsy, "sleepy" baby who is rarely awake needs to be evaluated as well.

Assessment of Interactional Behavior

It is frequently stated that each newborn infant is an individual. Yet to a large extent we persist in treating infants as if they were all alike.

The Brazelton assessment emphasizes the individual personality of each newborn. It is not possible to assess an intact newborn infant using the Brazelton scale and ever again to believe that all newborns are all alike or that newborns function on a subcortical, reflex level. During the months in utero, the personality has been shaped, but there has not been a systematic way to evaluate personality.

The items evaluated in the Brazelton assessment are listed in Table 16–2. A detailed description of each item and the scoring of the response are beyond the scope of this book. The assessment process is described in detail in *Clinics in Developmental Medicine*, No. 50,[2] and

Table 16–2   THE BRAZELTON ASSESSMENT*

Environment: Quiet, semidarkened room; temperature of room 72°–80°F.

Infant: Asleep, covered, dressed, midway between feedings

Observe for 2 minutes—note state
Response decrement to flashlight
Response decrement to rattle
Response decrement to bell
Uncover infant; note reaction
Response decrement to light pinprick
Speed of state change
Test ankle clonus, foot grasp, Babinski response
Undress infant
Pull to sit
Standing
Walking
Placing
Incurvation
Body tone when held across hand
Crawling—prone responses
Pick up and hold
Glabella reflex
Spin
Orientation (inanimate and animate); visual, auditory, and visual and auditory
Cloth on face
Tonic neck response
Moro response

*Adapted from Brazelton: *Clinics in Developmental Medicine. No. 50.* Philadelphia, J. Lippincott Co., 1973.

in a series of three films (see Appendix H).

Brazelton emphasizes that repeated assessments are of far more value than a single assessment.

Because the total assessment takes approximately 30 minutes, there are few, if any, nurseries that can screen every baby using the Brazelton scale.

However, we would like to describe several ways in which items of the Brazelton scale are of value in better understanding the baby and in helping his parents to understand him better.

Response Decrement to Inanimate Visual and Auditory Stimuli. A flashlight, a rattle, and a bell are used as stimuli. When a baby is first presented with a stimulus, such as a light flashing in his eyes, he responds with a grimace and with body movements;

perhaps he awakens. But as the stimulus is presented again and again he normally begins to ignore it and eventually has little or no response. This process, called habituation, is one measure of central nervous system integration. The baby who consistently fails to habituate to stimuli should have careful follow-up during the neonatal and postneonatal periods. His failure may be related to a transient problem such as a high level of medication that crossed the placenta barrier during labor, or to a more serious central nervous system problem.

These responses are measured in sleep state 1, 2, or 3, described at the beginning of this chapter.

Orientation Response to Visual and Auditory Stimuli. Most infants will focus their attention on a bright red ball and follow it briefly when they are in the quiet-alert state (state 4) or will shift their eyes and turn their head toward the sound of a rattle or bell in state 4 or 5.

Even more entrancing to most babies is the human face, which the baby may follow from right to left and up and down. When the examiner moves her face from the baby's line of sight and talks to him from one side in soft, continuous, high-pitched tones, many babies will become alert, turn their head toward the stimulus, and search for the sound with their eyes (Fig. 16–27).

Demonstrating this behavior to parents is one way of helping them recognize their baby's capabilities. Many parents believe that playing with a newborn baby—talking to him or looking at him—will either spoil him or is a game that is fun for them but means little to the baby because he can't see or hear. As they see us interact with their baby and begin to interact with him themselves, and as he responds to them, both bonding and a pattern of caretaking that will provide for sensory stimulation are facilitated.

Cuddliness. Infants respond in various ways to being held. In the Brazelton assessment, cuddliness is assessed with the infant held against the examiner's chest (see Fig. 16–1) or up on the examiner's shoulder (state 4 or 5).

Some babies resist being held; they stiffen or thrash or push away. Others are passive, neither resisting nor participating. Still others relax and mold themselves to the body of the holder, nestling their head in her (his) arm. If held to the shoulder, a cuddly baby molds to the holder's body and nestles his head against the holder's shoulder.

The baby who is *consistently* irritable when held and never "cuddles" may be brain damaged. However, normal infants vary markedly in how cuddly they are. Schaeffer and Emerson[21] followed 37 mother-infant pairs throughout the first 18 months of the infants' lives. Nine babies were evaluated as noncuddlers, nineteen as cuddlers, and nine

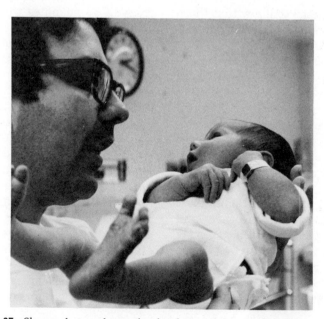

Figure 16–27 Sharon alerts and turns her head toward the sound of the doctor's voice.

as intermediate between the other two groups. Cuddlers enjoyed, accepted, and even sought physical contact. Noncuddlers were highly intolerant of physical restraint; they were active and restless. The noncuddlers tended to have accelerated motor development, while the cuddlers were more placid, slept more, and formed earlier and more intense attachments.

It is interesting that Schaeffer and Emerson found no consistent differences in mother-child interaction between cuddlers and noncuddlers, suggesting that the baby's behavior was indeed an expression of his personality. They also suggest that cuddlers may be more affected by a lack of physical contact than noncuddlers, and thus this kind of deprivation will affect some infants more than others.

From the standpoint of anticipatory guidance, helping parents assess the relative cuddliness or noncuddliness of their baby could be significant. Some parents feel that they must be doing something wrong if their baby does not cuddle to them. They can feel rejected. They need to know that there is a wide range of variability in perfectly normal babies.

Consolability. When the baby is actively crying (state 6), how easily is he consoled? A few babies may be consoled by face alone, or by seeing a face and hearing a voice. Others require (in progressive order) a hand on their abdomen, restraint of one or both arms, holding, rocking, dressing, and a pacifier or finger to suck.

What kind of intervention is most soothing to neonates? Korner and Thoman[15] explored the efficacy of body contact in comparison with vestibular stimulation (i.e., picking the baby up and moving him). They found that vestibular stimulation was more effective,

both in soothing the infant and in bringing him to an alert state, than was body contact and suggest that such stimulation is often overlooked with the prevailing emphasis on the importance of body contact.

Self-consolation. Infants console themselves in a variety of ways—by attempting to place a hand in the mouth, by sucking a fist or the tongue, or sometimes by gazing at an object or listening to a sound. Here again, normal infants vary considerably in their ability. These differences can make a marked difference in the way the new baby adjusts during the first weeks of life—both in how much he is able to comfort himself and to what extent his mother, father, or others must intervene to console him. Korner[13] also suggests that the strength of the oral drive and the baby's ability to comfort himself may also influence the intensity with which weaning is experienced.

Part of becoming acquainted with a baby is the recognition of the way in which an individual baby responds to various kinds of soothing. In one small study of 35 neonates who were 2 to 3 days old, Birns and her coworkers found that babies easily soothed by one stimulus were easily soothed by all stimuli, while others were difficult to soothe in any manner. It is not hard to imagine how mothers of those babies easily soothed may begin to feel competent rather quickly, while the mother of a baby who cries a great deal, no matter what she does, may begin to doubt her ability to ever become a good mother. Just why some babies are difficult to console (other than those who are brain damaged or ill) is not clear. Freedman and Freedman[9] compared 24 Chinese-American neonates with 24 European-American newborns. Although there was no significant difference in the amount of crying in the two groups of babies, the Chinese infants stopped crying in a "dramatically immediate" period of time when they were picked up.

Behavioral Assessment and Nursing Practice and Research

One need not systematically assess each baby by using a Brazelton scale to utilize the concept of behavior assessment in practice. Each time a baby is picked up, his cuddliness may be assessed. His response to face and voice can be noted when he is alert. His ability to console or quiet himself is usually apparent. All of these cues can help us guide his parents in recognizing their baby's individuality and needs as distinct from the needs of other babies (including any siblings) and as distinct from their own needs and ideas of how a baby should be nurtured. Brazelton's book *Infants and Mothers*[1a] describes infant individuality in an "average" baby, a "quiet" baby, and an "active" baby as they develop during the first year of life. This book is written for parents (parents with a high school education or greater); we recommend it to many families.

The potential value of newborn behavioral assessment in nursing research seems almost unlimited. Some examples, from other researchers, have been indicated above. Brazelton assessments have indicated differences in the behavior of infants receiving certain local-regional anesthetics (Chapter 13). Systematic crosscultural evaluations are also possible.

SUMMARY

Newborns as a group are unique. What is normal in terms of appearance and behavior at this special time of life differs in many ways from the norms of any other period.

Because the newborn infant's condition can change so rapidly, nurses are the primary observers of each baby's condition. A combination of knowledge and experience ensures good care for each baby in our nurseries.

REFERENCES

1. Birns, B., Blank, M., and Bridger, W.: The effectiveness of various soothing techniques on human neonates. *Psychosomatic Medicine, 28*:316, 1966.
1a. Brazelton, T. B.: *Infants and Mothers: Differences in Development.* New York, Dell Publishing Co., 1969.
2. Brazelton, T. B.: Neonatal Behavioral Assessment Scale. *Clinics in Developmental Medicine. No. 50.* Philadelphia, J. B. Lippincott Co., 1973.
3. Carpenter, E.: Space Concepts of Aivilik Eskimos. *Explorations Five*, June, 1955.
4. Craig, W. S.: *Care of the Newly Born Infant.* Baltimore, The Williams and Wilkins Co., 1969.
5. DiToro, R., Lupi, L., and Ansanelli, V.: Glucuronation of the Liver in Premature Babies. *Nature, 219*:265, 1968.
6. Engen, T., and Lipsitt, L. P.: Decrement and Recovery of Responses to Olfactory Stimuli in the Human Neonate. *Journal of Comparative Physiology Psychology, 59*:312, 1965.
7. Engen, E., Lipsitt, L. P., and Kaye, H.: Olfactory Response and Adaptation in the Human Neonate. *Journal of Comparative Physiology Psychology, 56*:73, 1963.
8. Fantz, R. L.: Pattern Vision in Newborn Infants. *Science, 140*:296, April 19, 1963.
9. Freedman, N. C., and Freedman, D. G.: Behavioral Differences Between Chinese-American and European-American Newborns. *Nature, 244*:1227, 1969.
10. Greenman, G. W.: Visual Behavior of Newborn Infants. *In* Solnit, A. J., and Provence, S. A. (eds.): *Modern Perspectives in Child Development.* New York, International University Press, 1963.
11. Hershenson, M. R., Munsinger, H., and Kessen, W., et al.: Preference for Shapes of Intermediate Variability in the Newborn Human. *Science, 147*:630, February 5, 1965.

12. Jensen, K.: Differential Reactions to Taste and Temperature Stimuli in Newborn Infants. *Genetic Psychology Monographs*, *12*:361, 1932.

13. Korner, A.: Individual Differences at Birth: Implications for Early Experience and Later Development. *American Journal of Orthopsychiatry*, *41*:608, 1971.

14. Korner, A., and Grobstein, R.: Visual Alertness as Related to Soothing in Neonates: Implications for Maternal Stimulation and Early Deprivation. *Child Development*, *37*:867, 1966.

15. Korner, A., and Thoman, E.: Visual Alertness in Neonates as Evoked by Maternal Care. *Journal of Experimental Child Psychology*, *10*:67, 1970.

16. Lipsitt, L. P., Engen, T., and Kaye, H.: Developmental Changes in the Olfactory Threshold of the Neonate. *Child Development*, *34*:371, 1963.

17. McKay, J.: The Fetus and Newborn Infant. *In* Vaughan, V. C., and McKay, R. J. (eds.): *Nelson Textbook of Pediatrics*. 10th Edition. Philadelphia, W. B. Saunders Co., 1975.

18. Montagu, A.: *Touching: The Human Sig-*

nificance of the Skin. New York, Harper and Row Perennial Library, 1972.

19. Peiper, A.: *Cerebral Function in Infancy and Childhood*. Nagler, B., and Nagler, H (translators) New York, Consultants Bureau, 1963.

20. Rose, A., and Lombroso, C.: Neonatal Seizure States: A Study of Clinical, Pathological and Electroencephalographic Feature in 137 Full-term Babies with a Long Term Follow-Up. *Pediatrics*, *45*:404 1970.

21. Schaeffer, H., and Emerson, P.: Patterns of Response to Physical Contact in Early Human Development. *Journal of Child Psychology and Psychiatry*, *5*:1, 1964.

22. Shimek, M.: Screening Newborns for Hearing Loss. *Nursing Outlook*, *19*:115, February, 1971.

23. Spears, W. C., and Hohle, R. H.: Sensory and Perceptual Processes in Infants. *In* Brackbill, Y. (ed.): *Infancy and Early Childhood*. New York, The Free Press 1967.

24. Vulliamy, D. C.: *The Newborn Child*. Boston Little, Brown and Co., 1967.

Chapter 17

THE TERM NEWBORN: NEEDS AND RESPONSES TO NEEDS

What does the newborn baby need—not just to sustain life in the first days and weeks—but to build a foundation for growing both biologically and emotionally in the months and years that follow?

It is impossible to separate biologic needs from emotional needs. For example, food intake is an obvious biologic need—a certain quantity of fluid, carbohydrate, protein, and so on is required. But studies demonstrate that merely providing the proper nutrients is not sufficient: babies appear to have a real need for being held and touched while they are being fed.

What are the newborn's needs? How can they best be met? How do we communicate this information to his parents? This chapter will explore needs relating to warmth, cleanliness, nutrition, and protection from infection. In Chapter 20, the need for parenting and the ways that we can guide parents in meeting the emotional needs of their babies will be discussed.

THE NEED FOR WARMTH

The significance of warmth for each newborn infant from the moment of birth was emphasized in Chapter 15. Once the transition period is over, term newborns who are healthy usually have no difficulty maintaining satisfactory body temperature in the hospital. But what happens when the baby goes home? Commonly, babies are overdressed and overwrapped at home and are too warm rather than too cool. Mothers and grandmothers mistakenly interpret the cool hands and feet that are common to newborns (because of their immature peripheral circulation) as a sign that the baby is chilled and needs additional clothing and wrapping. Thus babies return for periodic check-ups on a midsummer's day wrapped like a polar Eskimo, and even in winter newborns may show signs of heat rash.

In most homes with central heating, in which a thermostat maintains temperature at about 70°F., the baby will be warm and comfortable in a diaper and shirt with a covering of one or two lightweight blankets. The home temperature may be increased for a brief period prior to and during bathing, when the baby will be undressed and wet. Cotton clothing, which allows evaporation, is more useful and com-

515

fortable than garments of synthetic fibers, which hold moisture and heat close to the body.

In those homes without modern heating, in which the house may not be as warm in the winter, additional clothing may be necessary. Two or three layers of clothing, part of which can be easily removed if the baby appears too warm, are better than one very heavy garment.

THE NEED FOR BATHING

Bathing as a part of nursery care has been discussed in Chapter 15. Our concern here is what we teach mothers about bathing. In many hospitals the "baby-bath demonstration" is the central focus of teaching. Perhaps we make it seem too important at times. We certainly miss the point if we so emphasize a certain procedure that as a result mothers feel more inadequate rather than more knowledgeable.

Bathing serves three main purposes. The obvious one is cleanliness, important in protection from both infection and irritation. A second purpose is the opportunity for observation. We have already noted that the initial bath in the hospital gives us a chance to carefully observe many of the baby's characteristics. Subsequent bathing, both in the hospital and at home, may alert the mother to the first signs of eczema or heat rash or to any one of a multitude of signs that do not seem quite normal.

Perhaps the most important purpose of all is the opportunity that bathing provides for interaction between mother or father and baby. Although a tiny baby does not particularly seem to enjoy bath time and appears happiest at the end, when he is out of the water and snugly wrapped in a warm towel, before many weeks bath time can become a real pleasure for everyone involved.

We need to teach mothers how to bathe their babies in a manner that is as uncomplicated as possible. Few mothers have someone to help them once they go home from the hospital, after only 3 or 4 days following delivery. Baby nurses who work in homes, once common, are practically nonexistent. Grandmothers may live hundreds of miles away, and many are busy with their own lives. Neither of these changes is necessarily bad. The presence of someone who seems to know "everything" about babies can make young parents feel inadequate.

No elaborate equipment is needed for bathing the baby. A kitchen sink with a counter beside it serves well. Or a plastic dishpan makes an excellent tub if a separate container is preferred. Provide a mild soap, washcloth, and towel. Cotton balls and alcohol are necessary to cleanse the umbilicus during the first 2 weeks. If a circumcision is not healed, Vaseline and gauze pads will protect the penis if the diaper appears to be rubbing, and certainly this is necessary during the first 24 hours at home. (Some babies are circumcised shortly before discharge.) Baby powder is really not necessary and probably not advisable. For those mothers who feel they are neglecting their babies unless they powder them, cornstarch is a more acceptable substitute. It should be used only on the baby's bottom.

Until the baby's umbilicus is healed, a sponge bath is suggested. Immersing the baby might risk infection through the umbilical portal of entry.

A basic regimen for infant bathing is described in Table 17–1. Mothers, and fathers too, should have as many opportunities to bathe their baby in the hospital as possible. A second bath in the evening will not harm the baby if the father would like such an opportunity. Parents don't gain confidence by watching nurses bathe babies, either by ob-

Table 17–1   BABY'S BATH AT HOME

Sponge Bath	Complete Bath
1. Gather equipment, including baby's clean clothes, so that you won't have to leave the baby once the bath begins.	
2. Fill basin, sink, or tub with water that feels comfortable to your elbow. (Hands accustomed to hot water used in dishwashing are not as good indicators as sensitive elbow skin.)	
3. Wash each eye from the nose outward, using a clean section of washcloth for the second eye. Do not wash across the bridge of the nose; infection, if present, could be transferred.	
4. Soap the baby's head with bath soap. Holding the baby securely in a football position, rinse the head with water. Dry with a towel.*	
5. Wash the baby's face with soap; rinse and dry.	
6. Soap trunk, arms, and legs with hands; turn baby to abdomen to wash back. Wash genital area last.†	
7. Rinse with washcloth and clear water, rinsing genital area last.	7. Immerse baby in tub for rinsing.
8. Pat baby dry. Check to be sure that creases, such as the neck folds and inguinal area, are dry and clean.	
9. Clean the area around the umbilicus with alcohol until it is healed, at about 2 weeks of age.	9. Cleaning umbilical area no longer required.
10. Dress the baby, and brush his hair.	

*Because of the open fontanel, many mothers are afraid to wash the baby's head, and subsequent scalp infections are not uncommon at check-up time. This therefore becomes an important part of teaching.

†In girls, the labia are gently separated, and the genitalia are cleansed from front to back. In boys, the folds of the scrotum are cleansed; the foreskin is not retracted. A Vaseline dressing covers the penis during the first 24 hours following circumcision. Soap will be irritating to the circumcision area for several days; the area is best rinsed with clear water until it heals. Normally the circumcision will be healed earlier than the umbilicus and thus prior to the time the baby has a tub bath.

serving through the nursery window or in a classroom or even at the mother's bedside. Our "efficiency" and expertise may only overwhelm them, making them feel even less adequate. Parents gain confidence by caring for their own baby *as much as possible*, and our responsibility is to give them as much opportunity as they desire. This is possible even in hospitals that do not formally practice "rooming-in." Instead of bringing the baby to his mother dressed and "bundled" in the morning, the baby can be brought to his mother's room for his bath.

Bath time could just as easily be in the evening as in the morning. It might vary from family to family, depending on individual needs and desires. This kind of flexibility is valuable not only during the brief hospital period, but, perhaps even more important, it conveys to parents a "permission" to be flexible and adaptive in baby care at home. Some previous generations of mothers, and some mothers still, felt that a daily bath before the 10 A.M. feeding was a binding rule. The "to the minute scheduling" of some maternity units may reinforce this kind of rigidity. Mothers should know that babies may be bathed at a time that best fits the schedule of both parents and infants. For example, nearly every baby has a "fussy" period during his first weeks, a time when he is neither hungry nor sleepy but seems at somewhat of a loss as to what he wants—probably some companionship and loving. The time of day varies from one baby to another but is remarkably consistent in an individual infant. In many instances this time is a good one for bathing.

There will also be some days when a bath seems more than a mother can manage, particularly when she is still recovering from pregnancy and delivery. Mothers need to know that an occasional missed bath is all right too. A sponge bath can be substituted for a tub bath—just a quick wipe with the washcloth to be sure that there is no milk in the neck folds and that the baby's bottom is well washed.

THE NEED FOR NUTRITION

If animal mothers could listen and reflect upon the many discussions and arguments of humans about the subject of infant nutrition, they would probably be amused. Feeding their young must seem a simple matter. But because we are reasoning beings who are as influenced by our culture as by our biologic heritage, issues concerning infant feeding have become complex and need thorough review.

We are coming to recognize the lifelong significance of feeding during the first weeks and months of life. Not only is undernutrition a real hazard during the time of rapid brain and body growth, but overnutrition during infancy may contribute to adult obesity and to all the problems associated with obesity. Moreover, the emotional context in which food is offered probably has long-term meaning.

THE NUTRITIONAL NEEDS OF THE BABY

As a biologic organism, an infant needs water, protein, carbohydrate, fat, vitamins, and minerals, just as we all do, although proportionately his needs will vary from ours. The discussion in this section describes the requirements of normal, term newborns. The nutritional needs of preterm infants and others with special problems are discussed in Chapter 18.

A baby's diet must enable him to grow and meet his need for energy. By the analysis of data from several sources, Fomon has demonstrated that in the baby's first 4 months of life (during which most babies double their birthweight) nearly one-third of caloric intake is used for growth.[8] During the subsequent 8 months of the first year, both growth rate and the percentage of calories required for growth decline appreciably (Table 17–2). By the time a baby is 2 to 3 years old, only 1 per cent of his caloric intake is used for growth, the remainder is required to meet the energy needs of a very active toddler.

Table 17–2 WEIGHT GAIN AND CALORIES USED FOR GROWTH DURING THE FIRST YEAR

	0–4 Months	4–12 Months
Percent calories used for growth	32.8	7.4
Approximate weight gain (kg.)	3.5	3.5
Approximate weight gain (pounds)	7.7	7.7

The Need for Water

The need of a newborn baby for water is proportionately higher than that of an older child or an adult for several reasons:

1. The percentage of water in relation to total body mass is greater than at any other period of life, a total of 70 to 75 per cent. About 30 to 35 per cent of total body weight in the newborn is extracellular water, compared with 25 per cent in the older infant and an average of 20 per cent in the adult. Because of this, the infant has proportionately less fluid reserve. Loss of fluid or lack of intake will deplete his extracellular fluid very rapidly. In a 24 hour period an infant replaces about 50 per cent of his extracellular water; by contrast an adult replaces only 14 per cent of his extracellular water in the same period. A large part of the difference in weight between a newborn and an older infant disappears by the time the baby is 10 days old, because the loss of the excess extracellular water accounts for much of the weight loss that occurs during the first days of life.

2. The larger surface area of the newborn in relation to his body mass means a higher ratio of water loss through evaporation, the rate of loss per kg. being twice that of an adult. Thus the newborn's fluid balance is much more susceptible to environmental temperature and humidity. Water loss can be very high in a high temperature-low humidity environment, both in the hospital or at home.

3. Metabolic rates are higher in newborn infants. A newborn produces 45 to 50 calories per kg. of body weight every 24 hours. The basal metabolic level for adults during the same period is from 25 to 30 calories per kg. Since metabolism uses water, a higher rate of metabolism utilizes a proportionately greater quantity of water.

4. The kidneys of a newborn have about half the concentrating ability of the kidneys of a normal adult. Although this is quite adequate for the baby's needs under normal conditions, newborn kidneys are less able to conserve fluid if the baby is stressed. In an older person, scanty urine is a fairly reliable sign of dehydration, but because of this limited ability to conserve water, newborns may not have decreased urinary output until severely dehydrated. Normally high r levels of phosphate and potassium in the blood of newborns are also related to renal immaturity.

How much fluid does a newborn need? The amount is in proportion to body weight, with larger babies having an increased need. During the first 10 days of life, the need is approximately 80 to 100 ml. of fluid per kg. of body weight. Thus a baby weighing 3 kg. (6.6 pounds) would need approximately 240 to 300 ml. of fluid in 24 hours, or roughly 40 to 50 ml. at each of six feedings (Table 17–3).

By the end of the first week, amounts are increased to about 2.5 oz. per feeding in average-sized babies (those weighing 3.4–3.5 kg.; about 7.5 pounds) in order to meet increased caloric needs. Babies rarely take the exact amount of milk at each feeding, a concern to some mothers. We can reas-

Table 17–3 FLUID INTAKE REQUIREMENTS—FIRST 10 DAYS

Baby Weighs	24 Hour Intake	Average Feeding × 6
3 kg. (6.5 pounds)	240–300 ml.	40–50 ml. (< 2 oz.)
5 kg. (10.5 pounds)	400–500 ml.	65–80 ml. (< 3 oz.)

sure them that as long as their baby has an adequate intake over 24 hours, the somewhat varying amounts taken at a single feeding are of no concern. One advantage of breast-feeding is that these small variations are not obvious.

Unless the baby seems particularly thirsty or his surroundings are so hot and dry that his insensible water loss is very high, additional water is not necessary, although he may certainly have some if he wants it. Some infants seem to like occasional water, while many others are uninterested.

The Need for Calories

How many calories does an infant need for energy and for growth? Fomon[8] observed the caloric intakes of normal term babies and suggests that the average requirements are probably no greater than those shown in Table 17–4. (They may be less.) The lower figure is based on the intake of girls at the 50 percentile in Fomon's study; the higher figure is for boys at the 50 percentile.

Consider what this means for a baby weighing 3 kg. (6.6 pounds) in the second week of life. During the first 2 weeks the average need would be approximately 336 calories per day (112 calories per kg. × 3 kg.). Most term newborns receive formulas containing 20 calories per kg. Thus the baby would need about 17 ounces of formula during a 24 hour period. If divided among six feedings, this would mean slightly less than 3 ounces per feeding.

Although it is important to be aware of caloric needs, it is also important not to be so fascinated with numbers that our view of infant feeding becomes highly rigid. One of the real advantages of breast-feeding is that we do not know just how much milk a baby takes during a particular feeding or during a particular day. When the baby appears satisfied, he is allowed to stop eating. The bottle-fed baby should have the same privilege, assuming he is a normal, healthy infant. Consistent failure to feed well, if adequate time is allowed at a feeding, may indicate illness. It is, for example, often an early sign of congenital heart disease (Chapter 18).

We know that bottle-fed infants gain weight more rapidly than breast-fed babies (Fig. 17–1). At one time this was thought to represent an advantage of formula-feeding over breast-feeding, but recent concerns about infant feeding and adult obesity have forced us to reconsider this supposition. It is believed that a high caloric intake during the first weeks and months of life leads to cellular mitosis in the fat cells. The result is an increased number of fat cells and consequent hyperplasia of fat tissue. Once these fat cells are present, the possibility of fat cell hyperplasia, with subsequent hypertrophy, may be continuously present. Even if the fat cells "shrink" during a weight reduction program, they continue to be present in fatty tissue with the potential to hypertrophy again.

Are formula-fed infants overfed? Weight gains far in excess of the gains of a healthy, breast-fed baby could be con-

Table 17–4   CALORIC REQUIREMENTS

	Age in Days					
	8–13	14–27	28–41	42–55	56–83	84–111
Calories per kg. per day	111–113	117–121	111–116	108	97–100	94–96

Figure 17–1 Comparison of weight gain and length. Heavy lines indicate formula-fed infants and haded areas cover values for breast-fed infants. (From Fomon, et al.: *Acta Paediatr. Scand.* (Suppl. 223), 971.)

idered excessive and could present potential problems for the obese baby in ater years.

The Need for Protein

Considering the rapid rate of growth during a baby's first year, it should not be surprising that protein is highly important in newborn nutrition. A dietary intake of approximately 9 grams of protein per day is necessary to provide for growth and to cover protein osses from the skin and in the urine. Recommended intakes are usually calculated at the slightly higher level of 14 grams per day during the first month, 5 grams per day for the second month, and 16 grams per day from the fourth month through the remainder of the first year. (Although infants in the later months of the first year need an increased amount of protein for maintenance, their rate of growth decreases, and thus their overall protein need remains stable.)

The principal protein in human milk is lactalbumin; casein is the primary protein in cow milk. Lactalbumin contains a higher percentage of essential amino acids. Casein in raw, unprocessed cow milk is a tough, rubbery substance that tends to make the cow milk curd difficult to digest. However, modern processing softens the curd and eliminates the major cause of its indigestibility.

Mothers with limited incomes sometimes try to stretch formula by making it more dilute and by offering sugar water at some feedings, obviously compromising protein as well as other nutrients. Our role in such instances is not to chastise, but to help mothers understand the importance of proper feeding and especially to help them find the milk their infants need for adequate growth.

The Need for Carbohydrate

Thirty-seven per cent of the calories in human milk come from carbohydrate. In commercially prepared formulas the percentage of carbohydrate varies from 32 to 51 per cent, with the majority of preparations falling in the 40 to 45 per cent range. When the proportion of calories from carbohydrate in a formula is too low, (below 20 per cent), babies are not able to tolerate the high levels of protein and fat that would then make up their formula. If carbohydrate is in excess of 50 per cent, the baby may have loose stools because of his inability to hydrolyze disaccharides, resulting in impaired growth and development.

The carbohydrate of milk is lactose. The lactose content of human milk is proportionately higher than that of milk of any other species. Babies with galactosemia, an autosomal recessive disorder, lack the enzyme (galactose-1-phosphate uridylyltransferase that is necessary to metabolize lactose. They must be fed nonmilk formulas.

The Need for Fat

Free fatty acids are now considered the most important source of energy for the young infant. Studies in rats indicate that when fat intake is too low, cerebral function is affected. This is important because myelinization of the human brain takes place over the first 3 years of life.

A formula providing 1 per cent of the caloric intake from two of the essential fatty acids, linoleic acid and arachidonic acid, is apparently sufficient for healthy development. But such a formula would be so high in protein that the renal solute load (see below) would be excessive, and the carbohydrate would be so high that diarrhea would result. Those formulas that derive 30 to 35 per cent of their calories from fat are generally the most acceptable.

Although the fat content of cow milk is higher than that of human milk,

the proportion of fatty acids varies. Fat is the main source of calories in human milk. The fat of human milk is more easily digested than the fat of cow milk. In addition, human milk contains the enzyme lipase, essential to the digestion of fats. Because of lipase, free fatty acids become available to the baby in large proportion even before digestion can begin in the intestine.

Skim milk has no place in infant diet and is not advised for children under the age of 2 years. There are three major reasons for this:

1. The calories in skim milk appear to be inadequate to meet needs for growth and energy. Body stores of fat are used to fulfill energy requirements. As fat stores are depleted, any illness that interferes with food intake could then become life-threatening.

2. Protein intake is very high in skim milk diets.

3. Essential fatty acids may be inadequate in skim milk diets.

The Need for Vitamins

The need for vitamins is met somewhat differently in breast-fed babies than in babies receiving formulas.

Human milk satisfies all of the baby's vitamin requirements except for that of vitamin D, *if the mother's vitamin intake is adequate*. Adequate maternal intake is particularly important in relation to vitamin C, which must be included in the mother's diet each day. The vitamin C content of human milk is in the range of 40 mg. per liter. The vitamin D content of breast milk is less than 100 I.U. per quart, about one-fourth the recommended daily intake, and thus supplementation is necessary.

Cow milk is deficient in both vitamin C and vitamin D. Levels of B vitamins are probably adequate. The folic acid content, although apparently sufficient for infants weighing more than 2500 grams (5.5 pounds), may be inadequate for low birth weight babies. Limited folic acid intake leads to megaloblastic anemia, so called because the primordial erythrocyte does not mature past the megaloblastic stage, by a process outlined in the following diagram.

Folates
|
(necessary for)
↓
Synthesis of purine and pyrimidine compounds
↓
(utilized in)
↓
Formation of nucleoproteins
|
(necessary for)
↓
Maturation of primordial erythrocytes (precursors of mature red blood cells)

Megaloblastic anemia is sometimes masked in infancy because of the more common iron deficiency anemia.

Hypervitaminosis A, rather than a vitamin A deficiency, is the more likely risk for babies on many formulas. About 600 I.U. of vitamin A per day is considered an adequate intake; many commercial formulas contain from 1500 to more than 2700 I.U. of vitamin A per liter. Babies receiving skim milk formulas and those with chronic steatorrhea (fatty stools) do need to receive supplementary vitamin A in a water-miscible preparation.

The possibility of toxicity from excessive vitamin D has been suggested but is unproven at this time. In the United States, evaporated milk, most commercial formulas, and most fresh whole milk is fortified at the level of 400 I.U. of vitamin D per quart, the recommended daily intake. If the formula contains less than this amount or if, as noted above, the baby is breast-fed, supplementation will be necessary.

Relatively little is known about the role of vitamin E in newborn nutrition, although there is some indication that a vitamin E dependent anemia may exist in some preterm babies.

The importance of vitamin K was discussed in Chapter 15. The vitamin K content of cow milk is generally higher than that of human milk. By the second week of life, the healthy baby's intestinal flora will have sufficiently developed to supply all of the baby's needs for vitamin K. In the interim a single injection of vitamin K is given to the baby to prevent possible hemorrhage.

Obviously, the need for vitamin supplementation is highly individualized. In some commercial formulas, vitamins are included in the preparations themselves. Often these formulas are prescribed to protect the baby, on the theory that even the best mothers may forget to give extra vitamins at least part of the time. The cost of "complete" formulas is higher than standard formulas, however, which may present problems for some families. There is also a difference in the cost of dry preparations, which the mother mixes with water, in comparison with the same but higher priced formula, which is already mixed. Mothers are often not aware of this; in our daily practice we find mothers on the verge of destitution feeding their infants the more expensive ready-to-use products. By keeping ourselves up to date on the relative costs of the formulas prescribed in our communities and by teaching mothers to prepare the less costly milk products, we can make a real contribution to infant nutrition.

The Need for Minerals

A number of minerals play a role in newborn nutrition, but the need for most of them is apparently met with little difficulty. The most frequent exception to this is iron. Studies have shown that the incidence of iron deficiency anemia (defined as a hemoglobin concentration of 10 grams per 100 ml. or less) ranges from 25 to 76 per cent in infants over 6 months of age from economically deprived areas and from 1 to 2 per cent in babies from more affluent families.

Iron requirements during the first year of life equal the difference between the level of iron at birth and the amount of iron required for growth and hemoglobin production between birth and the first birthday. Twins and premature and low birth weight infants accumulate limited stores of iron in utero, as do babies of iron-deficient mothers. Bleeding after birth, from the cord or circumcision or internally, and clamping of the umbilical cord before pulsation has stopped are additional factors in depleting iron stores.

Formulas fortified with iron are frequently given to babies with a high risk of iron deficiency anemia. Human milk does not supply adequate amounts of iron. Term infants, whose mothers had adequate iron intake during pregnancy, will have a store of iron sufficient for the first 3 to 4 months, after which time iron must be added to the diet. If cereals fortified with iron are offered by age 3 months and continue to be used throughout the first year, the occurrence of iron deficiency anemia can be reduced considerably. Egg yolk and meat, which are added to babies' diets during the first year, also contribute iron. The *term* baby most at risk of developing iron deficiency anemia (that is, the baby whose mother was herself anemic) is often the baby whose mother can least afford the baby meat and egg yolk and tends to switch him from the more expensive, iron fortified cereals as

soon as possible. This baby may also receive less well-baby care and hemoglobin monitoring.

Calcium absorption and metabolism are more efficient with human milk consumption, largely eliminating the risk of hypocalcemia in the breast-fed neonate. Not only the total amount of calcium present but also the ratio of calcium to phosphorus is significant. When phosphorus levels increase in the blood, calcium is eliminated. Pure cow milk, given to newborns, may overload the body with phosphorus and lead to hypocalcemia.

Some research suggests that high levels of *sodium chloride* ingested during the early months may lead to adult hypertension.

Renal Solute Load

Renal solute load refers to the amount of urea and electrolytes excreted in the urine. If a preparation with a high concentration of solutes is ingested, increased water must be excreted to eliminate the waste products of that preparation.

The renal solute load of cow milk, even when it is diluted with water and carbohydrate, is considerably higher than that of human milk. The renal solute load of commercially prepared formulas varies. In the healthy term infant renal solute load is of limited concern, but it becomes important if the baby has a high level of insensitive water loss (due to fever, for example) or lives in a hot environment.

MEETING NUTRITIONAL NEEDS: INFANT FEEDING

A healthy term infant's needs can be met by breast- or bottle-feeding. The decision as to how she will feed her baby should be made by the mother, after disussion with her husband (an important consideration sometimes overlooked). Our role, as nurses, is to support the family's decision, whatever it may be, and to help prepare parents to feed their baby in the manner that they have selected. It is equally inappropriate to "force" breast-feeding on the mother who, for whatever reason, does not wish to do so as it is to fail to help the mother who truly desires to breast-feed.

Differences in Breast Milk and Formula

Table 17–5 summarizes some major differences between breast milk and formulas, which have already been discussed in the preceding section. An additional difference is the role of colostrum and breast milk in maintaining resistance to infection. Traditionally, it has been recognized that breast-fed babies have a lower incidence of infection than those who are bottle-fed. To some extent this may be attributed to a lack of contamination of the milk itself, but this is not the only factor.

Colostrum, the fluid in the breasts prior to delivery and during the first 24 to 72 hours postpartum, contains very high levels of the immunoglobulin IgA, which offers protection against *Escherichia coli*, one of the major newborn pathogens (p. 579). When mothers have a high level of antibody to poliomyelitis, some transfer of immunity has been found in their babies. Antibodies for mumps, vaccinia, influenza, and Japanese B encephalitis have also been found in human milk, but it is not known to what extent these antibodies protect the baby.

The intestinal flora (another factor in maintaining resistance to infection) of the breast-fed baby differs from the flora of the bottle-fed baby. The flora of the breast-fed baby has been shown to protect against certain additional organisms, as well as those organisms that the flora of the bottle-fed baby protects against.

Other antimicrobial factors found in human breast milk include lysozyme, which is bacteriolytic against Grampositive bacteria; complement C3, which is important in the lysis of bacteria; lymphocytes, which can synthe-

Table 17–5 COMPARISON OF BREAST MILK AND FORMULA

	Breast Milk	Formula
Protein	1.1 gm./100 ml. Lactalbumin predominates	Casein predominates
Carbohydrate	Represents 37% calories	Represents 32–51% calories
Fats	More easily digested Contains lipase, which makes free fatty acids available	
Vitamins	Contains all but vitamin D, which must be supplemented	Requires vitamin supplementation. Some formulas have added vitamins.
Minerals	Iron inadequate	Iron inadequate (some formulas fortified)
	More efficient calcium absorption Physiologic calcium-to-phosphorus ratio	
Renal solute load	Lower in breast milk	

size immunoglobulin IgA; and macrophages, which are capable of ingesting bacteria. Macrophages may be particularly valuable in the prevention of necrotizing enterocolitis, a hazard to preterm and other high risk newborns, which is described in Chapter 18.

HELPING THE MOTHER WHO CHOOSES TO BREAST-FEED

In contemporary Western society it is highly unrealistic to suppose that mothers who wish to breast-feed will automatically be able to do so. In tribal villages and in traditional societies, and in the Western world of several generations ago, many women lived close to one another in extended families. Consequently, a girl grew to adulthood with many opportunities to observe mothers and infants together and could thus learn of breast-feeding gradually, through the years. But few mothers in the Western world today have such opportunities. Many have never seen an infant fed at breast. Female relatives are usually fewer in number and are often separated by many miles.

Assistance in breast-feeding—advice, counsel, and emotional support—comes chiefly from two groups. The first is composed of professionals, nurses and physicians. The second is made up of mothers who have themselves successfully breast-fed. The latter group provides assistance through a more formal structure such as the La Leche League or informally as neighbors and friends. Perspectives about breast-feeding vary somewhat between these two groups. Knafl,[16] in a small study that is part of a larger investigation, reports that in the second group both La Leche literature and mothers stress breast-feeding as an integral part of total mothering. Factors

such as convenience and nutritional superiority appear less important, although not necessarily unimportant, to this group. However, the nurses whom Knafl interviewed (the staff from two hospitals and the nurse faculty from a university school) thought of breast-feeding in terms of better nutrition and temporary immunity for the baby and maternal convenience and health after discharge from the hospital. Only 8 of 19 nurses (42.1 per cent) mentioned mother-infant interaction as a benefit.

Knafl's findings support our own observations and what we hear in discussions with nurses. Some mothers have intense feelings about breast-feeding that are not shared by staff members. The staff may feel hostile toward these mothers for their "unrealistic expectations." The mother, in turn, may feel that staff members have more concern for "routine" than for mothers and their infants. Such tension is detrimental to successful breast-feeding (see below) and can be a long-lasting source of disappointment to mothers.

Dealing with such conflict, or potential conflict, is as much a nursing responsibility as is the physical care of mothers and babies. Joint meetings between mothers, La Leche leaders, and staff nurses and physicians can afford an opportunity to deal with specific points of conflict, such as breast-feeding in the delivery room, feeding on demand, and supplemental feedings between times at breast. Nurses might attend La Leche meetings, not to espouse their own point of view, but to better understand the feelings of breast-feeding mothers and to show our genuine concern for these feelings.

Even with open communication, there will be occasional problems between individual mothers and staff. But if these conflicts can be recognized as individual idiosyncracies, rather than being used to label all breast-feeding mothers as "fanatics," they can be resolved in helpful ways. The goal of both professionals and volunteers is the same—the start of an interaction between mother and baby that is mentally and physically sound.

Support for the mother who chooses breast-feeding should begin in the prenatal period, as soon as the decision to breast-feed is made. Following delivery, previous learning can be reinforced and supplemented. (See Chapters 19 and 20 for further discussions of breast-feeding.)

HELPING THE MOTHER WHO CHOOSES TO BOTTLE-FEED

Because more mothers in the United States bottle-feed than breast-feed, because "failure to thrive" in the early weeks of life is often related to poor feeding technique, and because inadequate nutrition in the first months following birth may compromise the baby's long-term potential, our nursing role in helping mothers who choose to bottle-feed is significant. It is no more realistic to expect a mother to "instinctively" know how to bottle-feed her baby than it is to expect a mother to intuitively know how to breast-feed. The mother who plans to bottle-feed needs to know how to prepare feedings and when, how much, and how to feed her baby.

Formula Preparation

The preparation of formulas has been greatly simplified in recent years. Some of the simplifications, such as ready-to-feed formula and disposable bottles, add considerable expense to infant care, with only a very small advantage in ease of preparation and saving of time.

In the simplest method of formula preparation, the *single bottle method*, each bottle is prepared individually at the time that it is to be used. Bottles, caps, and nipples are washed in hot, soapy water and are rinsed thoroughly. Tap water is mixed with either a powder or a concentrated liquid formula preparation. When there is any question about the safety of the water supply, the water should be boiled for 5 minutes prior to use. Some pediatricians would prefer that all water be boiled during the first months of life.

When the single bottle method is used, the bottle should be given to the baby immediately after preparation. It will not need to be warmed, since the water used is at room temperature. Even cold formula is not harmful to babies, although some may not care for it. Any formula that remains in the bottle after a feeding must be discarded. Following feeding, the bottle and nipple are rinsed in cold water, so that they will be easier to clean later.

The single bottle method eliminates a great deal of relatively costly equipment that also takes up space in small kitchens. No refrigeration is required, other than that for a single can of concentrated formula, and none at all is necessary if a powder preparation is used. This method is also valuable for the breast-feeding mother when she needs a supplementary feeding.

A second method still in use is *terminal sterilization*. A day's supply of bottles is prepared; the bottles are placed in a large pan in 3 to 4 inches of water and are sterilized for 25 minutes, with timing started when the water boils. The pan is cooled until it can be comfortably touched; the bottles are then refrigerated until feeding time. Many mothers warm these refrigerated bottles before feeding the baby, but this is not essential.

A third method, the *aseptic method*,

involves boiling both equipment and ingredients and then combining them under aseptic technique. Prepared bottles are then refrigerated. The aseptic method is little used in the United States today, as newer, less time-consuming methods have proved to be safe.

Formula preparation involves not only cleanliness but also proper combination of the necessary ingredients. Mothers on limited budgets may try to "stretch" expensive milk products by adding more water than called for. Or, misunderstanding directions, they may not add sufficient water, giving the baby a very highly concentrated preparation as a result. Nurses must help mothers understand not only how to prepare formula but also why accuracy is important in measuring ingredients.

When to Feed

Lactation is facilitated when breast-fed babies are fed "on demand," that is, when they are awake and show they are hungry by rooting and sucking. Bottle-fed babies also need to be fed when they are hungry. The length of time between feedings will vary. At first many babies seem to want to eat every 3 hours, even though in the majority of hospitals that do not have "rooming-in," babies may be allowed to eat only every 4 hours. Hospital rigidity may convey the impression to new mothers that the every 4 hour schedule is the only "right" way to feed an infant, an unfortunate idea. There may be one period during the day when a baby will wait as long as 5 hours, interspersed between shorter intervals. When a baby seems consistently hungry less than 3 hours after each feeding, he probably needs to be offered more formula. By the time a baby is a few weeks old, he will probably have developed a pattern of feeding and

sleeping that is fairly consistent from day to day.

How Much Formula?

In the review of fluid and calori needs earlier in this chapter, it wa noted that six feedings of approximatel 3 ounces would meet the requirement of a baby weighing 6.5 pounds. Offerin 3 ounce feedings after 24 to 48 hours o age is a good beginning. Amounts ar increased as the baby shows that he i still hungry when the bottle is finishe (wide awake, sucking, and searching fo more). Twenty-four hour intake shoul not exceed 1 quart, however.

Mothers should know that babies appetites vary from one feeding to th next, so that they will not become overl concerned when the baby takes les formula. Consistent failure to feed wel however, is often a first sign of illness.

Techniques of Bottle-feeding

The bottle-feeding mother, like th breast-feeding mother, needs to be com fortable and relaxed before she begins t feed her baby. Feeding will take from 2 to 30 minutes (many mothers don' realize that this much time is neces sary), and the mother may tire befor her baby has finished if she is "dan gling" on the side of her bed o "perched" on the edge of a chair.

Encouraging the mother to wasl her hands before she holds and feeds he baby during the time that she is in th hospital may help to establish a habi that will carry over when she is home.

No one, not even a tiny baby, ca swallow well lying flat on his back; th baby should be held in a semi-erect posi tion. The bottle is held so that the nippl is filled with milk. The baby needs fre quent opportunities to "burp" at leas once midfeeding and again at the end o feeding (below).

Mothers who are bottle-feeding must be encouraged to hold their babies throughout each feeding. Skin-to-skin contact is possible and important for these mothers and their babies, just as it is for mothers and their breast-fed babies.

One advantage of bottle-feeding is the opportunity it gives fathers to have an important role in caring for their baby.

At least once or twice during the mother's hospital stay, we can talk with her while she is feeding the baby in order to observe to process and also to answer questions that arise during feeding that she may forget later. Plans for subsequent teaching and referral are based on observations made at this time.

CARE FOLLOWING FEEDING

Whether they are fed at breast or by bottle, babies swallow air along with their milk. Following feeding, a baby needs to be "bubbled" or "burped." This may be effectively accomplished in several ways. The traditional posture of holding the baby against the mother's shoulder and gently rubbing his back is certainly satisfactory. An alternate method is to hold the baby in a sitting position, supporting his head and chest with one hand and gently rubbing his back with the other.

Some babies do not easily bring up an air bubble. Efforts to make the baby burp should not be so vigorous that a sleeping baby is awakened, since sleep after feeding is a normal physiologic pattern. Putting the baby to bed on his stomach or on his right side will allow him to bring up air within a few minutes.

Because it is normal for the baby to sleep after feeding, his care should be planned so that baths and other care are given prior to feeding, rather than afterward.

NUTRITIONAL DEPRIVATION DURING THE FIRST WEEKS OF LIFE

What happens when nutrition is not adequate during the newborn period? Obvious effects may be inadequate growth in length and failure to gain weight. It is strongly suspected that nutritional deficiency may affect the central nervous system as well. The effects of nutritional deficiencies on the central nervous systems of very young animals have been demonstrated in a succession of studies over nearly 50 years. Rats with inadequate caloric intake during the period of most rapid postnatal brain growth exhibited marked retardation.[30] Severe undernutrition has been shown to influence the chemical composition of the brains of infant pigs, so that their brains resemble those of considerably younger pigs.[8]

Even more important than a lack of calories is a lack of protein. A number of animal studies have examined protein deficiency in the presence of adequate caloric intake. In a London study, weanling rats, piglets, and puppies born of well-nourished mothers were fed diets adequate in calories but severely deficient in protein. The animals showed signs of degenerative changes in their nerve cells. Electroencephalograms (EEG's) were abnormal; one researcher noted certain resemblances between the EEG's of pigs in the study and those of children with kwashiorkor, a condition involving severe protein deficiency.[20]

The animal studies showed that the time at which nutritional restriction occurs is significant. Food restriction prior to weaning was associated with permanent changes in the size and chemical composition of the brains in rats. Food restriction for an equal period of time, but imposed at the time of weaning, also led to brain alterations, but these later alterations disappeared during a subsequent period of adequate nutrition.[35]

Evidence from another study supports this concept. Abnormalities in the myelination of the nervous systems of rats, brought about by undernutrition from the period after weaning (age 3 weeks) until 11 weeks of age, were corrected by normal diet between 11 and 19 weeks of age.[8]

Lack of specific vitamins and minerals also led to deformities in animals studied.

In human infants rapid development of the brain occurs after birth. Head circumference increases from approximately 34 cm. at birth to 46 cm. by the first birthday and then at a rate of roughly 0.5 cm. each succeeding year until the adult size of 52 cm. is reached. Similarly, the weight of the brain, about 400 grams at birth, more than doubles during the first year, to 1000 grams, and continues to grow for many years. Brain mass increases until about 25 years of age.

In addition to these changes in size, a major change in brain structure occurs during the first years of life. At birth, the infant brain contains most of the 10 billion neurons that it will have during the individual's lifetime. But neurons are packed very densely in the small infant skull. The neurons enlarge and the connecting links between them increase in number and complexity very rapidly until 4 years of age and then more slowly until 12 years of age. Because of this, it is believed that when nutritional deficiencies, particularly protein deficiencies, are severe enough to limit height and weight gains during the first years of life, brain development and the related motor, language, and

adaptive behaviors are also likely to b affected. The earlier the period of depr vation, the more serious the conse quences. In studies of children wit kwashiorkor, rates of progress in behav ioral development were related to th age at which the children were admitte to the hospital. Relatively little prog ress was made by children who ha kwashiorkor at the age of 3 to 6 month; there was better development in chi dren who were 15 to 29 months old a the time they were admitted. Childre who were 37 to 41 months of age at th time of admission demonstrated th best rate of behavior development.[8]

Maternal Deprivation or Undernutrition?

Whitten has proposed that under nutrition may not always be recognize for what it is.[36] Studies in the 1940 suggested that emotional deprivation i an infant or young child could be di rectly responsible for the child's failur to grow and thrive.[12, 31, 32] Whitte points out that none of these psychologi studies determined the babies' calori intakes. His own study involved 1 maternally deprived infants, 11 c whom gained weight at an accelerate rate when they were fed adequately in hospital environment that deliberatel simulated their home situations; i.e they were confined in windowless room and were neither talked to or smiled a nor held for feeding. The two babies wh did not gain remained anorectic. Both c them had a history of repeated attempt by the mother to force-feed them. It wa reported that one father, reacting to hi baby's poor intake, had tried to "ram hamburger down the infant's throat."

In a second group of seven infant; all seven gained rapidly in their ow homes when they were fed an adequat diet in the presence of a public healt nurse acting as an observer. Whitten believes that there was no improvement in home environment that could account for the increase in weight. For example, one infant, who was visited 42 times by the nurse (3 times a day for 14 days), was found alone in a crib in a back room on every occasion. Forty-one times the baby was returned to the back room before the nurse left. Yet during the 14 day period the baby gained 26 ounces.

A second infant gained 22 ounces during an 8 day feeding program in spite of the fact that during that period his family was evicted for nonpayment of rent and he had been physically abused by his father.

When the mothers were questioned prior to the period of the observed feedings, most of them claimed that their babies ate adequately. During supervised home feedings, however, some mothers began to realize that their babies actually had been underfed.

There is no question that maternal deprivation can seriously affect the development of an infant or child. We suggest here, however, that inadequate knowledge of nutritional needs also is a factor in "failure to thrive."

THE NEED FOR PROTECTION FROM INFECTION

In centuries gone by, and in parts of the world today, infection claimed, and claims, the lives of many, many newborns. One of the major advances of modern maternity care has been the reduction of deaths by infection, a highly significant achievement. But in reducing infection we have often erected barriers to a comfortable relationship between parents and their babies. In meeting one need, protection from infection, we have subverted an equally important one—the need of parents to

become acquainted with their baby—to hold and care for him—and the need of their baby for that care. Because of this, the issue of infection in newborn infants needs to be examined carefully, so that we plan nursing care based on *all* the needs of the infant and his family. The discussion below relates chiefly to the apparently healthy term infant. The prevention of infection in newborns with special kinds of problems is discussed in Chapter 18.

Why Are Newborns Prone to Infection?

The body's response to infection is both cellular and immunologic. In both types of response, newborns differ from older children and adults.

Cellular Factors. White blood cells and lymphocytes are the cells that enable all of us to resist infection. The white blood cells important in newborn resistance are the polymorphonuclear leukocytes (called polys) and the monocytes (called macrophages when they are in tissue).

The action of polys in newborns (and even more so in preterm infants) is not as efficient as in older children and adults. This is because in order to ingest bacteria the poly must first travel to the site of the infection, a process dependent upon complements C3 and C5. Newborns have only 50 per cent of the C3 and C5 complement of older individuals. Like polys, monocytes also participate in the phagocytosis of bacteria. In addition, monocytes play a role in the initiation of antibody formation.

Lymphocytes produce antibody and govern cell-mediated immunity; they function adequately in newborns. However, because there has normally been no previous contact with an antigen (bacteria), there is no pre-existing antibody.

Immunologic Factors. A second response of the body to infection involves immunoglobulins, which are synthesized by plasma cells and which react specifically with the antigens that stimulate their formation. Immunoglobulins are classified into five groups: IgG, IgM, IgA, IgD, and IgE.

IgG crosses the placental barrier, and the baby will thus be passively immune to certain infections (e.g., diphtheria, tetanus, measles, rubella, mumps, and diseases caused by certain group A streptococci) *if* his mother is immune to them. Because much of the IgG crosses the placenta during the third trimester, levels are lower in preterm infants. The preterm baby partially compensates by producing IgG more rapidly than the term baby following delivery. Note that pertussis is not among the diseases against which the infant is protected; immunization is usually started at 4 to 6 weeks following delivery to give the baby protection against pertussis.

IgM is the first immunoglobulin made by the baby after birth; it does not cross the placenta (the molecule is too large). If IgM is found in cord blood, intrauterine infection is suspected. The absence of IgM does not rule out infection, however. Since the immunoglobulins against Gram-negative bacteria are chiefly IgM molecules, this *may* be one reason why Gram-negative sepsis is the more common bacterial infection in newborns. (It would not seem to be the only factor; at one time Gram-positive organisms were the chief offenders.)

IgA is the primary immunoglobulin of colostrum. The IgA of colostrum is somewhat different from the IgA in blood; it is more stable against oral acids. IgA is the immunoglobulin for Gram-negative rods such as *E. coli,* which probably explains the protection against *E. coli* diarrhea afforded b breast milk.

Little is known about IgD at thi time. IgE is the antibody involved i allergic reactions and is not presentl believed to be significant during th newborn period.

Potential Portals of Entry

A third factor in the increased ris of infection in newborns is the relativel large number of potential portals of er try: the umbilical vessels, circumc sions, and skin breaks from forceps, fc example. Delicate infant skin break down easily. Low gestational age an many types of congenital anomalies ir crease the risk of infection still furthe (Chapter 18).

Newborn Defense Mechanisms

The newborn is not totally defense less against infection. In addition to th mechanisms described above, he ha certain unique characteristics.

Gastric acid levels in the baby ar very high on the first day of life. This i probably protective, in that the bab may swallow Gram-negative organism at the time of the first breath; however the organisms may be destroyed by th high level of acid. Gastric acid level drop on the second day, when colostrun with its protective immunoglobulin i available to the infant, one more exam ple of the physiologic interaction be tween mother and baby.

Shortly after delivery the baby be gins to develop intestinal flora. Thi bacterial flora, commonly alpha hemolytic streptococci, protects th baby from invasion by pathogenic bac teria. If the baby is given antibiotics fo some reason, the normal flora is de stroyed, allowing the invasion of mor virulent bacteria.

Sources of Infection

Even prior to birth the newborn is at risk of postnatal infection, particularly if:

1. The mother has had an infection or a temperature elevation in the week prior to delivery.

2. The mother has an infectious disease such as syphilis, gonorrhea, tuberculosis, residual rubella, vaccinia, poliomyelitis, salmonellosis, cytomegalic inclusion disease, toxoplasmosis, or herpes.

3. The mother's membranes, a barrier to infection, have been ruptured more than 24 hours.

4. Labor is prolonged.

5. There is excessive manipulation during labor.

6. Amniotic fluid is purulent or foul smelling.

If the baby requires resuscitation following birth, the risk of infection increases. In delivery rooms and nurseries, possible sources of infection include personnel, other infants, and equipment.

Prevention of Infection

Proper handwashing is the most important single factor in protecting newborn infants from infection. Brushes for scrubbing, particularly scrubbing for several minutes, have been found to be neither necessary nor desirable in the nursery. Hands and arms (to the elbows) should be washed with a hexachlorophene or iodophor preparation for 2 to 3 minutes on entering the nursery and rewashed for a shorter period of time if any equipment considered "contaminated" is touched. Contaminated surfaces include pens and pencils, telephones, charts—anything that is not specifically designed for the baby. Touching one's face or nose also contaminates one's hands.

Hands should, of course, be washed after caring for one baby before touching another infant or any equipment belonging to another infant.

Because iodophor preparations are active against both Gram-negative and Gram-positive organisms, they are considered superior to hexachlorophene preparations, which are active against only Gram-positive bacteria. Some individuals, however, are sensitive to the iodophor preparations, so it is recommended that both be available. The containers for handwashing preparations must be sterilized at regular intervals.

Mothers and fathers should wash their hands well each time they hold their baby, a pattern that not only helps to prevent infection in the hospital but suggests an important habit for baby care at home.

Neither parents nor personnel should care for a baby if they have an infectious illness—a fever of undetermined origin, a cold, vomiting or diarrhea, an open skin lesion, a herpes infection, or a communicable disease. If a mother must be isolated from her baby because of infection, it is a major part of our nursing responsibility to maintain other contacts between the family and their infant, such as frequent opportunities to see the baby and to talk with us about him.

Visitors other than the father (who should not really be considered a visitor) and possibly other children in the family (see page 649) do not seem necessary on obstetric units. Limiting visitors not only reduces the chance of infection but also gives the mother more time for rest and for her baby.

Babies must also be protected from other babies with infections by isolating the affected infant.

Proper care of the furnishings and equipment and of the nursery itself is still another way of preventing newborn infection. Any equipment that becomes wet during use must be cleaned and sterilized each 24 hours. Special attention is also important for areas such as sinks and sink drains, which are continually wet, and for floors, walls, windowsills, and countertops.

Each individual baby's unit should be thoroughly cleaned before a new infant is admitted. This cleaning includes the walls of the unit and the drawers and shelves, as well as the baby's mattress and bassinet. Some institutions use a disposable bassinet of heavy cardboard with its own mattress, which the mother may then take home with her at the time of discharge and use as a baby bed during the first weeks of life.

The physical set-up of the nursery may help to prevent infection. An ideal arrangement is that of small, multiple nurseries of four to six infants to which no new infants are admitted until all previous babies are discharged and the entire nursery is cleaned. Such a system is called a "cohort" system.

Since the baby will spend at least part of each day in his mother's room, these rooms must also be scrupulously clean for the protection of both baby and mother. Coats and packages should never be placed on the mother's bed, nor should visitors be allowed to sit on the bed. A diaper placed between the baby and the bedclothes is an added protection. Wrapping the baby in a blanket and discouraging the mother from unwrapping him is not justified as a prevention against infection. Most mothers will ignore such prescriptions in their very natural and necessary desire to inspect their baby.

Rooming-in and Infection

The original rationale for the separation of mothers and babies in hospitals, in an era when infant mortality was far higher than it is today, was the protection of the baby from infection. It is legitimate to wonder if putting mothers and babies back together for either part or all of the day, as in "rooming-in" (Chapter 20) might lead to an increased incidence of infection. More than 20 years of experience have not shown this to be a problem. The precautions of careful handwashing and eliminating contact with individuals who have infections are, as discussed above, important in rooming-in.

REFERENCES

1. Applebaum, R. M.: The Modern Management of Successful Breast Feeding *Pediatric Clinics of North America* 17:203, 1970.
2. Brazelton, T. B.: *Infants and Mothers: Differences in Development.* New York, Del Publishing Co., 1969.
3. Brazelton, T. B.: Neonatal Behavioral Assessment Scale. *Clinics in Developmental Medicine. No. 50.* Philadelphia, J. B Lippincott Co., 1973.
4. Brazelton, T. B.: *Does the Neonate Shape His Environment? Perinatal Reprint Series* White Plains, N.Y., National Foundation/March of Dimes, 1974.
5. Brown, J., and Helper, R.: Stimulation—A Corollary to Physical Care. *American Journal of Nursing,* 76:578, 1976.
6. Eid, E. E.: Follow-up Study of Physical Growth of Children Who Had Excessive Weight Gain in the First Six Months o Life. *British Medical Journal,* 2:74, 1970
7. Fantz, R.: Pattern Vision in Newborn Infants *Science,* 140:296, 1963.
8. Fomon, S. J.: *Infant Nutrition.* 2nd Edition Philadelphia, W. B. Saunders Co., 1974
9. Fomon, S. J.: What Are Infants Fed in the United States? *Pediatrics,* 56:350, 1975
10. Fomon, S. J., and Anderson, T. (eds.): *Practices of Low Income Families in Feeding Infants and Small Children.* Washington, D.C., MCH Service, U.S. Department of Health, Education, and Welfare 1972.
11. Fomon, S. J., Filer, L. J., Thomas, L. N., et al Growth and Serum Chemical Values o Normal Breastfed Infants. *Acta Paediatrica Scandinavica,* (Suppl. 202), 1970.
12. Fried, R., and Mayer, M.: Socio-emotional Factors Accounting for Growth Failure in Children Living in an Institution *Journal of Pediatrics,* 33:444, 1948.

13. Hammar, S. L., Campbell, M., Campbell, V., Moores, N., et al.: An Interdisciplinary Study of Adolescent Obesity. *Journal of Pediatrics, 80*:373, 1972.

14. Johnson, N.: Breast-Feeding at One Hour of Age. *MCN, 1*:12, Jan/Feb., 1976.

15. Kanaaneh, H.: Detrimental Effects of Bottle Feeding. *New England Journal of Medicine, 286*:791, 1972.

16. Knafi, K.: Conflicting Perspectives on Breast Feeding. *American Journal of Nursing, 74*:1848, 1974.

17. Korner, A.: Individual Differences at Birth: Implications for Early Experience and Later Development. *American Journal of Orthopsychiatry, 41*:608, 1971.

18. Korner, A., and Thoman, E.: Visual Alertness in Neonates as Evoked by Maternal Care. *Journal of Experimental Child Psychology, 10*:67, 1970.

19. Naismith, D.: Bottle Feeding Makes Fat Mamas—and Fat Babies, Too. *Medical Opinion, 3*:38, November, 1974.

20. Nelson, G., and Dean, R.: The Electroencephalogram in African Children: Effects of Kwashiorkor and a Note on the Newborn. *Bulletin of the World Health Organization, 21*:799, 1959.

21. Newton, M., and Newton, N.: The Normal Course and Management of Lactation. *Child and Family, 9*:102, 1970.

22. Newton, N.: Decline of Breast Feeding, 1: Psychological Implications. *Nursing Times*, September 22, 1967a, p. 1267.

23. Newton, N.: Decline of Breast Feeding, 2: Social Aspects of Breast Feeding. *Nursing Times*, September 29, 1967b, p. 1320.

24. Newton, N.: Decline of Breast Feeding, 3: Psychophysical Regulating Mechanisms. *Nursing Times*, October 6, 1967c, p. 1346.

25. Newton, N.: Trebly Sensuous Woman. *Psychology Today*, July, 1971, p. 68.

26. Newton, N., and Newton, M.: Psychological Aspects of Lactation. *The New England Journal of Medicine, 277*:1179, 1967.

27. Ravelli, G., Stein, Z., and Susser, M.: Obesity in Young Men After Famine Exposure in Utero and Early Infancy. *New England Journal of Medicine, 295*:349, 1976.

28. Schaeffer, H., and Emerson, P.: Patterns of Response to Physical Contact in Early Human Development. *Journal of Child Psychology and Psychiatry, 5*:1, 1964.

29. Schmidt, M. H.: Superiority of Breast Feeding: Fact or Fancy. *American Journal of Nursing, 70*:1488, 1970.

30. Scrimshaw, N.: Infant Malnutrition and Adult Learning. *Saturday Review, 16*:64, March, 1968.

31. Spitz, R.: Hospitalism: An Inquiry Into the Genesis of Psychiatric Conditions in Early Childhood. *Psychoanalytic Study of the Child, 1*:53, 1945.

32. Talbot, N. B.: Dwarfism in Healthy Children: Its Possible Relation to Emotional, Nutritional and Endocrine Disturbances. *New England Journal of Medicine, 236*:783, 1947.

33. Tronick, E., and Brazelton, T. B.: Clinical Uses of the Brazelton Neonatal Behavioral Assessment. *In* Friedlander, B. Z., et al. (eds.): *Exceptional Infant, 3: Assessment and Intervention*. New York, Brunner/Mazel, 1975.

34. Wenick, M.: Malnutrition and Brain Development. *Journal of Pediatrics, 74*:667, 1969.

35. Wenick, M., and Noble, A.: Cellular Response During Malnutrition at Various Ages. *Journal of Nutrition, 89*:300, 1966.

36. Whitten, C., Pettit, M., and Fischhoff, J.: Evidence that Growth Failure from Maternal Deprivation is Secondary to Undereating. *Journal of the American Medical Association, 209*:1675, 1969.

Chapter 18

CARING FOR THE NEWBORN WITH SPECIAL PROBLEMS

No area of maternal and child health has changed, or continues to change, more rapidly than that involving the care of high risk newborn infants, those babies who differ from "normal" because of their gestational age, their weight, or because of some congenital or acquired abnormality. Care of these babies involves careful attention to physiologic, emotional, and developmental needs. It should take place in a nursery that involves parents in planning and giving care and should be provided by personnel who are as sensitive to the needs of these parents as they are to the needs of high risk babies.

A general textbook concerned with the care of mothers and infants cannot cover in detail all that a nurse needs to know in order to give highly specialized newborn intensive care. We have chosen in this chapter to look at those concepts of high risk care that we feel should be a part of the basic knowledge of all nurses who care for mothers and infants. These concepts include:

1. A philosophy of care for high risk newborns.

2. Early recognition of the baby who is at risk.

3. Resuscitation of the baby wh[o] fails to breathe spontaneously.

4. Identification and care of th[e] most common problems occurring dur[-]ing the first days of life.

5. Transportation of the high ris[k] newborn.

Chapter 22 discusses the needs o[f] the parents of high risk babies and th[e] ways in which we can help them cop[e] with those needs.

A PHILOSOPHY OF CARE

As technology has enabled us t[o] sustain life at an earlier gestationa[l] age—first at 36 weeks, then at 3[4] weeks, and now at even less than 3[0] weeks—there has been a growing con[-]cern about the quality of the life that i[s] given to the tiny babies who surviv[e] these first weeks. Physiologically, th[e] single most important factor in th[e] quality of these babies' lives is an intac[t] central nervous system. As perinata[l] mortality drops, this is an appropriat[e] focus for our concern.

Lubchenco studied infants weigh[-]ing less than 1500 grams who were bor[n] in the years 1949 to 1953, when inten[-]

536

sive care nurseries as we know them today had not yet been developed.[38] She found that over half of these low birth weight babies had some central nervous system impairment (Table 18–1) and scored less than 90 (considered the lower limit of normal) on intelligence tests. Others, although of average intelligence, were clumsy and had poor hand-to-eye coordination and other perceptual motor problems, indicating a failure of central integration. Note that 66 per cent had retrolental fibroplasia (RLF) (see below), a finding that disappears almost completely in later studies.

The preventability of many of the other serious sequelae of preterm or high risk births seems obvious in later studies, in which the incidence of serious defects drops to far lower levels. However, the incidence of minimal brain dysfunction has not dropped in the studies currently available. Because of the time lag between the date of giving care and the dates at which sequelae can be evaluated, we cannot yet know the effect of the care we give in the 1970's.

Central Nervous System Development

If a major goal of high risk newborn care is an intact central nervous system, knowledge of central nervous system development in utero and in the period following birth is a foundation for such care.

Neuronal development peaks at 12 to 18 weeks of gestational age (Fig. 18–1). Insults during the period of rapid neuronal development lead to a decreased number of neurons and to mental retardation, which is often severe. Examples of such insults are viral diseases (rubella, cytomegalic inclusion disease) and radiation. Nothing that we

now know reverses the effects of these insults; they must be prevented.

The cerebellum reaches its peak of development during the first days after birth. If the baby fails to receive cerebellar nutrition (oxygen, glucose, maintenance of acid-base balance) in the first days following birth, problems in cerebellar development will result in perceptual motor difficulty. The child may be clumsy and lacking in fine coordination, even though his intelligence may be normal.

The cells of the brain stem and of the cerebral cortex grow more slowly than those of the cerebellum, developing during the months and years following birth. Their development is dependent upon continued support during these months, rather than being dependent upon support for a period of a few critical days. Thus a child may be intelligent (a function mediated by the cerebral cortex) and still have perceptual motor difficulty (which is mediated by the cerebellum).

A great deal of the myelinization of the neurons also takes place following birth. Myelin is a cholesterol substance that acts as "insulation" for the neurons. Without myelinization, when neurons "fire," messages go off in all directions. Thus a newborn, with normally incomplete myelinization, reacts to a stimulus with his whole body. As a child grows older, his movements normally become less general and more specific, and he is able to accomplish finer coordination. When myelinization is incomplete, this finer coordination is never achieved.

How can we use this knowledge of central nervous system development to plan better care for mothers and babies? First, it seems obvious that we must have a concept of care that embraces the entire perinatal period, beginning at conception and not merely at birth. This

Table 18–1 INCIDENCE OF CENTRAL NERVOUS SYSTEM IMPAIRMENT AND RETROLENTAL FIBROPLASIA IN LOW BIRTH WEIGHT INFANTS

Study	Number of Infants	Birth Weight	Time Neonatal Care Delivered	Length of Follow-up	Number of Infants with Subsequent Defects		
					Retrolental Fibroplasia (RLF)	Neurologic Defect or Low Developmental Score	Other Defects
Rawlings, 1971 (London)[48]	68	1500 grams	1966–1969	4 years	—	5 abnormal (7%) 4 doubtful (6%)	—
Lubchenco, 1972 (Denver)[38]	91	1500 grams	1949–1953	10 years	60 (66%)	45 moderate to severe (50%)	14–mild RLE and mild splastic diplegia 18–severe RLF, IQ score: 80–89 28–blend, IQ score: 80

Dweck, 1973 (Birmingham)[15a]	14	960–1100 grams	Born after July, 1968	Up to 33½ months	—	1 (14%)	1–IQ score: 90 (Cattell Infant Intelligence Scale)
Fitzhardinge, 1975 (Montreal)[20]	67	33 weeks' gestational age	Born after September, 1970	12 months	—	2 (13%)	8–IQ score: 95 (Griffiths Mental Development Scale)
Fitzhardinge and Ramsey, 1973 (Montreal)[22]	32	1250 grams	1960–1966	5 years	—	13 (41%) IQ less than 90 2 (6%) major neurologic abnormalities 9 (28%) minimal brain dysfunction	—
Reynolds, 1974 (London)[49]	164	1000 grams (RDS—mechanically ventilated)	1967–1972	7 years	—	1 (2%)	—

HUMAN WHOLE BRAIN

Figure 18–1 DNA accumulation is an indication of cell number (neurons). Cholesterol content measures the deposition of myelin. (From Räihä: *Pediatrics, 53*:147, 1974.)

care begins with the early recognition of the mother who has a potential for delivering a high risk baby, together with the assurance that she receives the kind of care she needs (Chapter 10).

RECOGNITION OF THE BABY AT RISK

A baby is considered at high risk because of gestational age (less than 37 weeks or more than 42 weeks) and/or because of weight (less than 2500 grams). Obviously, within these parameters there are varying degrees of risk; the prognosis for a baby weighing more than 2000 grams is far different than for a baby weighing less than 1250 grams, other factors being equal (such as the presence of congenital malformations and so on). Babies may also be at high risk because of congenital malformations, birth injury, sepsis, respiratory distress, metabolic disorders, or hematologic problems. Many high risk newborns have two or more simultane-

ous problems. Many preterm babies have respiratory distress, hypoglycemia, hyperbilirubinemia, and sepsis, for example.

Signs of difficulty may be obvious immediately following birth, or they may not appear for several hours or days. Still other types of difficulties may not appear for weeks or months (some types of congenital heart defects, for example). In certain genetic disorders, although the potential is present at the time of birth, the disease itself may not appear until later in life. Examples are Huntington's chorea and certain muscular dystrophies.

THE BABY AT RISK IN THE DELIVERY ROOM

THE BABY WHO DOES NOT BREATHE SPONTANEOUSLY

Resuscitation of the newborn baby who does not breathe spontaneously is a major emergency. Not only do we hope to save the infant's life, but we also hope to prevent brain damage (which may manifest itself in major problems such as seizures, cerebral palsy, and developmental retardation, as well as in learning disorders and other more subtle difficulties).

The goal of resuscitation is a healthy baby who retains his maximum potential for growth and development. This goal is accomplished by:

1. Providing oxygen and removing carbon dioxide.

2. Providing alkali for buffering the excess acid that is produced during anaerobic metabolism.

3. Maintaining circulation.

What is the role of the nurse in the resuscitation of a distressed newborn? In 69 per cent of the hospitals surveyed in the *National Study of Maternity Care*,[42] the attending physician was responsible for both the mother and the newborn infant in distress. Obviously in these hospitals the delivery room nurse must also be highly knowledgeable about newborn resuscitation, for the physician's attention is necessarily divided. In an additional 10 per cent of the hospitals in the same study, the delivery room nurse was listed as *the individual responsible* for a distressed newborn. Only in 20 per cent of the hospitals surveyed was someone else (anesthesia staff, house staff, or pediatrician, for example) available to direct and/or carry out resuscitation for the baby who did not breathe quickly and easily.

The ideal situation is, of course, the one last described. When one considers what it must be like for a mother, lying on the delivery table, aware that she has not heard her baby's cry, aware from seeing worried faces that something is amiss, it is not hard to imagine that a major nursing responsibility is support for the mother, and for the father, as well, if he is present. Unfor-

tunately, in the hurry of the average delivery, this is the responsibility that seems most often overlooked.

If regionalization of maternity care (Chapter 10) brings a majority of mothers whose babies are at risk to adequately equipped and staffed centers for delivery, this ideal may be achieved. In the meantime we must be prepared to give the very best care within the framework of our current practice.

Preparation of Equipment for Resuscitation

Before *every* delivery, equipment for resuscitation of the baby should be ready. Not every instance of respiratory distress can be anticipated from the maternal history or from the course of labor. Basic equipment includes:

1. A bulb syringe for suctioning.

2. A DeLee glass bulb with catheter for aspiration of mucus.

3. A laryngoscope with small blades (size 0 and size 1).

4. Small endotracheal tubes with obturators (sizes 10 to 18F; size 8F is too small to permit the passage of a suction catheter; some physicians do not use obturators).

5. A resuscitation bag with the proper adapters to connect it to the endotracheal tubes or mask.

6. Oxygen and suction equipment.

7. Syringes and needles.

8. Umbilical vessel catheters.

9. Drugs, including sodium bicarbonate, 10 per cent dextrose in water, epinephrine 1:10,000, and narcotic antagonists.

Resuscitation Technique

1. The baby's head should be slightly dependent and turned to the side to facilitate drainage of the fluid in

the trachea. This fluid, which amounts to approximately 30 cc. per kg. of body weight, is not amniotic fluid, but arises from the alveolar cells.

2. The airway must be cleared. Suctioning with a bulb syringe may be all that is necessary. A longer suction catheter used during the first 5 minutes following delivery may stimulate the vocal cords and lead to laryngospasm, with subsequent apnea and cyanosis. Be sure that the baby's tongue is not obstructing his airway. Pulling the baby's chin forward and up will relieve obstruction by the tongue. A small airway may also be useful.

3. Tactile stimulation, such as "flicking the heel," may initiate respiration. Vigorous stimulation, such as back slapping or immersion in cold water, is more dangerous than helpful.

These steps will be all that is necessary for many babies. If the infant still fails to breathe:

4. Oxygen may be given by bag and mask at the rate of 20 to 30 breaths per minute. This rate is, of course, half the baby's normal respiratory rate. The reason for the slow rate is that although normal breathing involves negative pressure in the thoracic cavity, which augments venous return to the heart, the bag transmits positive pressure to the thoracic cavity, which decreases cardiac filling. (Later, *in the nursery,* for a baby with established respirations, 30 to 40 breaths per minute may be necessary to keep ventilation in phase with

the baby.) Pressure on the bag must be light, or the infant's lungs will be overexpanded. Watch for chest expansion, and, if possible, listen with a stethoscope to determine whether air is entering the lungs. A baby with primary apnea* or one who is gasping when resuscitation begins and infants with Apgar scores of 3 to 6 will usually respond within 15 to 20 seconds to suction and oxygen by face mask (Table 18–2).

5. Mouth-to-mouth breathing is an alternative to bag and mask ventilation. This method uses only the amount of air in the breather's mouth, not the total volume of air in the lungs, again to avoid overexpansion. Oxygen may flow from a tube into the blower's mouth to increase the oxygen concentration of air blown into the baby's lungs.

6. If heart rate does not increase immediately, intubation will be necessary. When the baby is totally unresponsive at birth (the rag-doll, Apgar 1 baby), intubation is generally the initial step. Immediate intubation is also recommended for the baby born through septic amniotic fluid and for the baby delivered in the vertex position through "pea-soup" meconium. If these babies are bagged before they are intubated and suctioned, meconium or septic fluid will be forced into their lungs. A

---

*Primary apnea is defined as apnea during which spontaneous respirations can be induced by appropriate sensory stimuli; secondary apnea is apnea in which respirations cannot be induced by sensory stimuli.[19]

Table 18–2   RESUSCITATION IN RELATION TO APGAR SCORING

Apgar Score	Level of Asphyxia	Probable Treatment
0–2	Considered asphyxiated until proved otherwise	Intubation
3–6	Mild to moderate	Suction; oxygen by bag and mask
7–10		Rarely will need resuscitation

stillborn baby who, by accurate fetal monitoring, has been known to be dead for less than 10 minutes prior to delivery may also be immediately intubated. Brain damage would be too severe to resuscitate a baby dead for a longer period.

The baby's head is slightly extended, and a laryngoscope is inserted by someone *experienced* in its use (Figs. 18–2 and 18–3). Mucus and blood are quickly aspirated. Prolonged suction not only wastes time but may cause reflex bradycardia. An endotracheal tube is inserted, and mouth-to-tube or bag-to-tube ventilation is begun. The baby's inspiratory phase should be slightly less than half the time of the ventilation cycle, so that adequate time is allowed for passive expiration. As in other forms of resuscitation, the baby's chest should be monitored by observation and auscultation.

Pulmonary infection is a risk in both mouth-to-mouth and mouth-to-tube resuscitation; pneumothorax and pneumomediastinum can occur from too vigorous ventilation by any route.

7. The heavy use of narcotics during labor, so popular only a few years ago, has now decreased markedly in most delivery rooms. Morphine and meperidine (Demerol) are still used, however. Much of the respiratory depression caused by morphine and Demerol can be overcome by the use of naloxone (Narcan), which acts by competing with the narcotics at receptor sites. Narcan is given intramuscularly in a dose of 0.01 mg. per kg. The nursery personnel *must be told* that the baby has received Narcan, because the baby may have respiratory depression again in the hours following delivery and may require an additional dose.

8. Accurate records of treatment of the baby must be kept.

Figure 18–2 Note the positioning of the head for intubation with chin up and shoulders slightly elevated. The laryngoscope is held in the left hand, and the fourth and fifth fingers can help control the position of the head. When held properly, the blade should be easy to control and soft tissue injury avoided. (From Klaus and Fanaroff: *Care of the High-Risk Neonate.* Philadelphia, W. B. Saunders Co., 1973.)

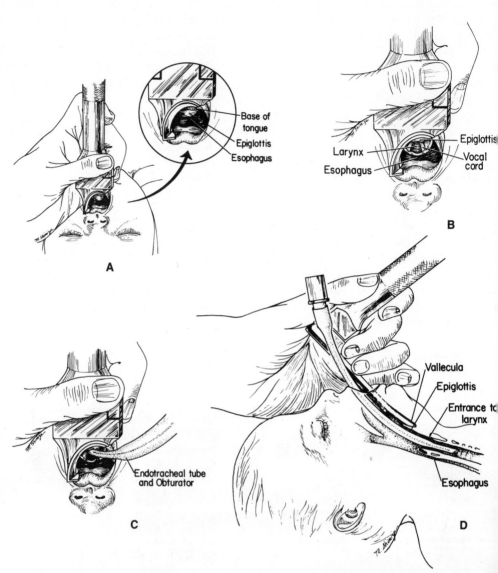

Figure 18–3 Technique of endotracheal intubation. The Miller blade should be inserted near the midline and moved to the left side of the mouth, gently deflecting the tongue. As it is advanced, the base of the tongue and epiglottis are visualized. The blade should be advanced in the same plane of movement into the vallecula (see *D*); as the blade is gently raised, the epiglottis swings anteriorly, revealing the opening of the larynx. If secretions or meconium are noted, gentle suctioning should be done before insertion of the endotracheal tube. On certain occasions when the epiglottis is not adequately raised, the blade tip may be placed posterior to the epiglottis, which can then be gently raised to expose the vocal cords. The endotracheal tube is advanced from the right corner of the mouth and inserted while maintaining direct visualization. The laryngoscope blade is then carefully withdrawn while the position of the tube is maintained by the right hand on the infant's face. Note the tip of the blade in the vallecula. (From Klaus and Fanaroff: *Care of the High-Risk Neonate.* Philadelphia, W. B. Saunders Co., 1973.)

Combating Acidosis

A baby who is not breathing converts from the aerobic metabolism (i.e., metabolism using oxygen) of glucose to anaerobic metabolism (metabolism without oxygen). Lactate accumulates during anaerobic metabolism, and very quickly the baby develops *metabolic acidosis*. In addition, carbon dioxide levels rise rapidly, so that the baby has a *respiratory acidosis* as well. Sodium bicarbonate (2 to 3 mEq. per kg.), diluted with an equal volume of water, is given slowly through an umbilical catheter to combat acidosis. It is important to recognize that for each 4.4 mEq. per kg. of sodium bicarbonate that is given, the baby produces 40 to 60 cc. of carbon dioxide; he must ventilate or be ventilated to get rid of this carbon dioxide.

Establishing and/or Maintaining Circulation

If the heart rate continues to be depressed once ventilation is established and sodium bicarbonate is administered, closed cardiac massage is started at the rate of 80 to 100 compressions per minute, so that vital areas such as heart muscle and brain tissue will be oxygenated. This rate, slower than the desirable rate for the baby, allows the heart to fill after massage. The baby must lie on a firm surface during massage, which is accomplished by depressing the sternum at the junction of the middle and lower third with the tip of the thumbs (Fig. 18–4). Ventilation must be maintained during cardiac massage at a ratio of five massages to each breath. Massage is discontinued briefly each 30 seconds to check for a spontaneous heartbeat, and is stopped once a rhythmic beat occurs.

How Long Can the Neonate Tolerate Asphyxia?

In adults asphyxia of 4 minutes or longer leads to irreversible brain damage. The length of time a just-born infant can tolerate asphyxia is unknown, but apparently it is a somewhat longer period. This is probably due to a lower metabolic rate in certain key areas, such as the brain, and to the availability of glucose and other substances for anaerobic metabolism.

Maintenance of circulation is important in assisting the baby's survival of asphyxia, in part because it may help to distribute the lactate resulting from anaerobic metabolism to tissues with a lower hydrogen ion concentration.

If hypoxia continues, these protective mechanisms will be overcome, with brain damage and death resulting.

WEIGHT AND GESTATIONAL AGE AS FACTORS IN HIGH RISK

Until recently infants were classified as full-term or "premature" largely on the basis of whether they

Figure 18–4 External cardiac massage. The correct position for the thumbs is on the sternum with the fingertips on the back. EKG electrodes permit continuous monitoring of heart rate. (From Avery: *Neonatology: Pathophysiology and Management of the Newborn.* Philadelphia, J. B. Lippincott Co., 1975.)

weighed more or less than 2500 grams (5 pounds, 8 ounces) at birth. Such designations are still used in the statistics of many nations. As noted in Chapter 15, it is now considered more useful to group infants as post-term (greater than 42 weeks' gestational age), term (38 to 41 weeks, 6 days' gestational age) and preterm (less than 38 weeks' gestational age). Post-term, term, and preterm infants may be small for gestational age (SGA), appropriate for gestational age (AGA), or large for gestational age (LGA). Table 18–3 summarizes major potential problems in each of nine categories. The criteria for placing infants in one of these categories are described in Chapter 15.

THE PRETERM INFANT

The baby born prior to 38 weeks' gestation has a number of problems specifically related to his immaturity.

The younger the baby's gestational age, the more severe these problems are likely to be. In addition, serious congenital malformations may lead to early labor and thus preterm infants may have an increased incidence of malformations.

Major problems of preterm infants include respiratory distress, hypoglycemia and other nutritional problems, hyperbilirubinemia, anemia, and hypothermia. A number of secondary problems, such as sepsis, are also common. Because treatment for physical problems often leads to a separation of mothers and babies, there is a possibility of disturbed family relationships (Chapter 22).

THERMOREGULATION IN THE PRETERM INFANT

Basic problems of thermoregulation for newborns were discussed in Chapter 15. These problems are mag-

Table 18–3   POTENTIAL PROBLEMS OF INFANTS IN RELATION TO SIZE AND GESTATIONAL AGE

	Preterm		Term	Post-Term	

SGA	Anemia
	Hypoglycemia
	Intrauterine
	  infection
	Major malformations
		Hypoglycemia
		Hypothermia
		Respiratory
		  distress syndrome (RDS)
		Hyperbilirubinemia
		Anemia
			Polycythemia
			Hypoglycemia
			Intrauterine
			  infection
			Major malformations
				Polycythemia
				Hypoglycemia
				Intrauterine
				  infection
				Major malformations
					Neonatal
					  asphyxia
					Meconium
					  aspiration

AGA		Hypoglycemia
		Hypothermia
		RDS
		Hyperbilirubinemia
		Anemia
					Neonatal
					  asphyxia
					Meconium
					  aspiration

LGA		Hypoglycemia
		Hypothermia
		RDS
		Hyperbilirubinemia
		Anemia
			Hypoglycemia	Hypoglycemia	Neonatal
					  asphyxia
					Meconium
					  aspiration

nified in the preterm infant, who is unable to maintain thermoneutral temperature unless his environment is warmer than that of standard room temperature. Table 18–4 gives the approximate environmental temperature necessary to maintain thermoneutral temperature.

In many intensive care and premature nurseries, an open bed with a radiant warmer is now preferred to an isolette, particularly for the sickest babies. The open bed has several advantages.

1. In terms of thermoregulation per se, the baby's temperature is maintained at a constant level by a servomechanism, which is taped to the baby's abdomen. Like the thermostat of a furnace, the warmer turns on when the baby's own temperature falls below the desired level of thermoneutrality (36.5°C.; 97.8°F.). If the warmer is functioning properly, temperature lability caused by the warmer should not be a problem. The baby's axillary temperature should also be monitored at regular, frequent intervals as a check of the monitor.

2. Because the baby is in an open bed, he is more easily accessible for care. Moreover, care does not interfere with thermoregulation, as it may in an isolette. Each time the "portholes" of the isolette are opened, environmental temperature within the isolette drops to some extent. If the baby requires prolonged attention (the starting of in-travenous fluids, for example), he can become hypothermic.

3. Another advantage of an open bed with radiant heat is the removal of a barrier between the baby and his parents. The importance of early touching of the baby by his parents is widely recognized (Chapter 18). Yet many parents are hesitant to reach into the "box" (isolette). They seem less reluctant to hold the baby's hand or to stroke him in the open bed.

There are also disadvantages to care in an open bed. One involves infection control. There is sometimes a tendency to touch the baby without the proper preliminary handwashing, particularly for personnel who are not working in the nursery continuously. This can be overcome with proper teaching.

A second and more difficult problem involves the recognition of those times when the baby is unable to maintain his temperature. Temperature instability is often an early sign of sepsis. In an isolette with a servomechanism, the baby's temperature may remain the same, but the fluctuation in isolette temperature will indicate temperature variability. For this reason isolette temperature should be recorded each and every time that the baby's own temperature is charted. However, no such monitoring is currently available for the baby in an open bed warmed by radiant heat.

Isolettes continue to be satisfactory

Table 18–4 APPROXIMATE ENVIRONMENTAL TEMPERATURES TO MAINTAIN INFANT TEMPERATURE AT 97.8°F. (36.5°C.)

Temperature (F.)	Temperature (C.)	Weight of Baby (Grams)
95.0°	35.0°	1000
90.0°	32.2°	2000
85.0°	29.4°	3000

for many less critically ill infants. Many babies "graduate" from open beds with radiant warmers to isolettes, and subsequently to open beds without radiant heat. When the baby can maintain a temperature of 97.6°F. (36.4°C.) in an 87.0°F. (30.5°C.) environment, he is ready for an open bed. If parents initially become acquainted with their baby in an open bed, the isolette may seem less of a barrier. However, we will need to both observe and talk with parents about their feelings throughout the course of their baby's hospitalization (Chapter 22).

RESPIRATORY DISTRESS SYNDROME (RDS)

More than 25,000 deaths each year (roughly 500 a week) in the United States alone are caused by respiratory distress syndrome, also called hyaline membrane disease.* Preterm infants are particularly at risk of RDS. Statistically, male infants are more likely to have RDS, but this difference may be more apparent than real because at every stage of development boys tend to weigh more than girls. Thus a boy weighing 4 pounds may be 1 or 2 weeks younger than a 4 pound girl; we may be comparing younger boys with somewhat older girls if we use weight as our sole basis of comparison.

Respiratory distress syndrome is also found more often in infants of diabetic mothers (see below). Although respiratory distress syndrome is found more often in the baby delivered by cesarean section, the increase is related to the reason for the section itself. When a previous section is the only reason for performing a subsequent cesarean, the likelihood of RDS is not increased. A

---

*The hyaline membrane is a pathologist's diagnosis; it is seen only at autopsy.

section for abruptio placentae, on the other hand, increases the likelihood of respiratory distress by eight to nine times. Any condition that leads to fetal anoxia may interfere with surfactant production (below) and increase the risk of RDS.

Physiology of Respiratory Distress Syndrome

During fetal life the lungs develop more slowly than many other organ systems. The alveoli, the tiny air sacs at the terminal end of the respiratory system through which oxygen and carbon dioxide are exchanged, are not developed until 26 to 28 weeks of age. Alveolar capillaries, necessary for gas exchange between the alveolus and blood, develop at 28 weeks.

Lining the alveoli are Type I and Type II cells. In the Type II cells a fatty "soap-like" substance called *surfactant* (actually a name given collectively to several compounds) is produced. Surfactant compounds enable the alveoli to remain open during exhalation, when the amount of air pressure in the lungs is decreased. Lecithin is the most abundant of these compounds, accounting for 50 to 70 per cent of surfactant. Lecithin production begins about the twenty-second to twenty-fourth week of gestation. (The monitoring of lecithin and another compound, sphingomyelin, in the fetus was described in Chapter 10.)

In respiratory distress syndrome the production of surfactant is impaired. When the baby exhales, alveoli collapse. Each breath the baby takes must again open the alveoli, just as the first breath taken at delivery opened them. Such an effort increases the work of breathing tremendously. Moreover, there is little or no gas exchange in the collapsed alveoli. The Po_2 drops because the baby's bloodstream is unable to pick up the oxygen it needs from the collapsed alveoli. The P_{CO_2} begins to rise because of inadequate gas exchange in the alveoli; resulting in respiratory acidosis. As the cells of the body become hypoxic and change to anaerobic metabolism, lactic acid is produced, resulting in metabolic acidosis. Acidosis results in the destruction of certain enzyme systems in the baby's body. Understanding this sequence is fundamental to understanding both the symptoms of respiratory distress syndrome and the care that these babies must receive.

Symptoms

The onset of RDS may occur in the delivery room or at any time within the first 8 hours following birth. Every nurse who cares for newborn infants should be thoroughly familiar with the symptoms of RDS. The principal symptoms are:

1. Cyanosis
2. Grunting.
3. Retractions.
4. Nasal flaring.
5. Increased respiratory rate.
6. Very rapid, regular heart rate.
7. Low blood pressure.
8. A "frog-like" position.

Cyanosis is a primary symptom. The baby is unable to oxygenate properly in room air. For some babies with RDS, oxygen for a period of 3 to 5 days is the only treatment necessary. An *audible grunt* results from nature's attempt to keep alveoli from collapsing. The glottis closes to prolong expiration and thus to allow a better diffusion of the inspired oxygen across the alveolar membrane.

Marked *retractions* (intercostal, suprasternal, substernal, and sternal) demonstrate intense respiratory effort, necessary because of the collapsed alveoli.

Respiratory rates above 60 respirations per minute and heart rates greater than 150 to 160 beats per minute are considered elevated.

The frequency of blood pressure *monitoring* has increased in high risk nurseries in the last few years. When blood pressure is too low, there is inadequate perfusion of vital organs. Blood pressure is commonly measured with an infant cuff and a Doppler device. In very small babies, blood pressure is best measured in the leg at the popliteal artery, because the cuff will be too large in relation to the size of the arm. Just as in a larger person, a cuff of the wrong size will give a false reading. When blood pressure is recorded, record the site as well, e.g., left arm (L. A.) and so on. Table 18–5 gives approximate blood pressure values for babies of varying weights. Pulse pressure (the difference between systolic and diastolic pressures) is also significant in newborns. A wide pulse pressure is often associated with patent ductus arteriosus (page 583).

Chest X-rays of babies with RDS show a characteristic "ground glass" appearance, the white areas representing collapsed, nonfunctioning alveoli.

Care

The care of a baby with RDS is basically aimed at *respiratory support* until the baby is able to produce lecithin at a rate sufficient to prevent alveolar collapse. Such care includes provision of a thermoneutral environment, maintenance of adequate respiration, initiation of alkali therapy to combat acidosis, and provision of fluids and nutrition. The baby must be closely observed and carefully cared for by nurses throughout this critical period. Nor must we forget his parents, who often feel shut out of the highly specialized world of the intensive care nursery, worried, and very much alone.

We emphasize that it is difficult to

Table 18–5   APPROXIMATE BLOOD PRESSURES IN NEWBORN INFANTS

Weight (Grams)	Approximate Blood Pressure (Systolic/Diastolic)
800	46–48/20–22
1000	50/25
2000	60/36
3000	70/35

care for these babies properly in a small community hospital. Their care involves skilled nursing care around the clock, 24 hour X-ray facilities, 24 hour laboratory facilities that permit close monitoring of blood gases, and specialized respiratory equipment that is usually available only in medical centers. Babies with RDS should be transferred to such a center when early signs of difficulty appear; waiting to see if they will improve on their own may cost an infant his life or leave him severely impaired. Prompt recognition of early symptoms by nurses can be the critical difference between a healthy life and mortality or neurologic damage.

Oxygen is a second essential. Although neither oxygen nor any form of assisted ventilation is a cure for RDS, treatment may enable the baby to survive until he is able to begin surfactant production on his own. The amount of oxygen given to the baby (the FiO_2 or fraction of inspired oxygen) is dependent upon the arterial oxygen concentration (Po_2) of the baby. If the Po_2 is greater than 90 to 100, there is a risk of retrolental fibroplasia and/or pulmonary oxygen toxicity (see below). At Po_2 levels of less than 50, pulmonary blood vessels constrict, further hindering gas exchange in the alveoli. Brain damage may occur at Po_2 levels below 40. The level of FiO_2 necessary to maintain Po_2 levels between 50 and 90 will vary not only from baby to baby but from hour to hour within the same baby. Oxygen therapy is a risky proposition in hospi-

tals that cannot monitor oxygen levels in the blood, preferably through an umbilical artery catheter. (Even using the umbilical artery, we are not measuring the oxygen at the level of the lungs researchers are constantly trying to find more precise methods that are practical as well).

Oxygen given to a baby (or to any patient) must be delivered in combination with humidity and with warmth *Humidity* is necessary to prevent oxygen from drying out the respiratory mucosa. This leads to mucosal crusting which impedes the normal function of the respiratory cilia and not only makes suctioning the baby difficult but increases the chance of airway obstruction. Moreover, the crusted mucus affords a medium for bacterial growth.

The need for humidity is one reason that heat is so important. Warm air holds more moisture than cold air. In order to give warm, moist oxygen to the baby, the gas must be heated to 101 or 102°F. (38.3 or 38.8°C.) at the oxygen source. Cooling occurs in the tubing carrying the oxygen to the baby, and, as a consequence, condensation occurs and water is seen in the tubing. Cold gas robs the body of water, in addition to being an additional source of chilling.

Currently the most common means of delivering oxygen to babies with respiratory distress are the head hood continuous positive airway pressure (CPAP), and mechanical ventilation with end expiratory pressure.

Oxygen by Hood. If the baby'

eed is simply to breathe air with a
higher concentration of oxygen, FiO_2
levels of from 80 to 90 per cent can be
achieved with a head hood (Fig. 18–5).
The hood does not correct carbon dioxide
levels, nor does it assist ventilation in
any way. Oxygen concentrations in the
hood should be checked and charted
every 30 minutes, as well as frequent
checking and charting of blood gases.
Temperature within the hood should
also be monitored every 30 minutes; the
area can become quite warm. Constant
observations of the baby's respiratory
effort are essential. The symptoms described above as the initial symptoms of
RDS are those with which we are par-
icularly concerned.

***Continuous Positive Airway Pres-
sure (CPAP).*** Remembering that the
basic problem in RDS is the tendency of

Figure 18–5 A preterm infant receiving oxygen by hood. The wires are a part of the heart and
respiratory monitor. The dressing on the baby's
right side holds the thermistor from the radiant
warmer in place. Note the nipple cover used for a
urine receptable and the cord clamp.

the alveoli to collapse on expiration, it is
logical that some form of therapy that
prevents this collapse would be of value.
This is the principle of CPAP. Positive
pressure on both inspiration and expiration prevents alveolar collapse and
enables oxygen to diffuse into the
bloodstream. CPAP has no effect on the
elimination of carbon dioxide. If Pco_2
levels are high (as determined by blood
gas measurement), periodic bag and
mask ventilation may be ordered to
eliminate excess carbon dioxide.

CPAP may be administered
through nasal prongs or the baby may
be intubated (Figs. 18–6, 18–7, 18–8). In
either case the baby continues to
breathe for himself. His respirations are
less labored, however, because he is not
working against collapsed alveoli.

CPAP is ordered both in terms of
pressure (usually from 1 to 10 mm. Hg)
and of FiO_2. As already noted, the baby's
respiratory effectiveness is closely monitored by determining blood gas values.
If nasal CPAP is used, the prongs must
be adjusted so that they do not lie on the
baby's lip; the tender skin beneath
can easily necrose. A cortisone ointment may be ordered for the nostrils to
prevent inflammation. This is a routine
order in some hospitals. As in an older
patient receiving oxygen, mouth care
with lemon and glycerin is helpful. A
newborn's secretions are acid and
should be wiped from his cheeks and
neck.

Babies on both CPAP and on ventilators (see below) should be turned
and suctioned every 1 to 2 hours. If the
baby has been intubated, careful sterile
technique should be employed in suctioning. Sterile saline (0.2 cc.) may be
placed in the tube prior to suction to
help liquefy secretions. A sterile suction
catheter should be used and replaced
after each suction period. Suction
should be applied only on the withdrawal of the catheter. The catheter

Figure 18–6 Nasal prongs for the administration of CPAP. (From Klaus and Fanaroff: *Care of the High-Risk Neonate:* Philadelphia, W. B. Saunders Co., 1973.)

should be inserted quickly (remember that the baby has no oxygen while the suction catheter is in the tube) and withdrawn quickly with a slight rotation of the catheter.

Physical therapy to the chest, the light percussing of the chest with the fingers prior to suction, will loosen secretions.

Mechanical Ventilation with End Expiratory Pressure. If the baby is unable to breathe for himself, a mechanical ventilator may assist him. Unlike the two modalities discussed above, mechanical ventilation controls levels of carbon dioxide as well as of oxygen.

Most mechanical ventilators used with newborn infants have settings for three possible breathing patterns: assist, assist-control, and control.

On the *assist* setting the baby initiates every breath himself. The *assist control* pattern, probably the one most frequently used, allows the baby to initiate his own breathing as often as he is able; if he stops breathing, the ventilator will give him a programmed number of breaths per minute. On the *control* setting, the baby has no role in his own respiration; the ventilator breathes for him.

Positive end expiratory pressure

Figure 18–7 Nasal CPAP. Notice the position of the baby's head, slightly extended, in a "sniffing position."

PEEP) is frequently used in connection with ventilators. PEEP serves the same function as CPAP; it prevents alveolar collapse on expiration by maintaining positive pressure in the airway.

Although the technical aspects of caring for a baby on a ventilator are a nursing responsibility in many hospitals, these details are beyond the scope of an introductory text. Nurses are re-

Figure 18–8 System for applying CPAP. *A,* Gas flow; *B,* oxygen sampling port; *C,* normal elbow (modified T piece); *D,* endotracheal tube connector; *E,* endotracheal tube; *F,* Sommers T piece; *G,* corrugated anesthesia hose; *H,* reservoir bag (500 ml.) with open tail piece; *I,* screw clamp; *J,* aneroid pressure manometer; *K,* plastic T connector; *L,* plastic tubing (1 cm. internal diameter); and *M,* underwater "pop-off." Arrows indicate direction of gas flow. (Adapted from Gregory, Kitterman, Phibbs, et al.: *New England J. of Medicine,* 284:1333, 1971. *In* Klaus and Fanaroff: *Care of the High-Risk Neonate.* Philadelphia, W. B. Saunders Co., 1973.)

ferred to the literature that accompanies the machines used in their own institutions and to respiratory therapy texts.

Negative Pressure (NEG). A fourth modality for treating RDS, involving negative pressure outside the chest wall rather than positive pressure in the airway, is not in wide use at the time of writing. The negative pressure chamber limits access to the baby. Moreover, each time the "seal" is broken, pressure is lost. The tight cuff around the baby's neck often leads to abrasion. One advantage of the negative pressure concept is the elimination of the tube, always a potential source of infection. It is our understanding that further research is now underway to make the negative pressure concept more practical.

WEANING FROM MECHANICAL VENTILATION. It is not particularly difficult to initiate mechanical ventilation for a baby. It is often far more difficult to wean a baby from the ventilator. Historically, infants have died because they could not be weaned from respiratory assistance.

Weaning involves reduction in end expiratory pressure and in oxygen concentration. Sometimes these are decreased simultaneously; sometimes first one and then the other is lowered. The weaning is monitored by blood gas determinations; oxygen and/or pressure is reduced, and values are checked within 30 minutes to see if the baby is able to tolerate the lower levels. Careful nursing observations to check for retractions and cyanosis are equally important.

Endotracheal tubes should not be left in place once the baby is "disconnected" from mechanical ventilation. A baby can no more breathe through an endotracheal tube without assistance than we can breathe through a straw. The resistance of the tube makes adequate air exchange impossible.

Another consideration during weaning is the way in which oxygen concentration is decreased. A very rapid drop will cause reflex constriction of the pulmonary arteries with a subsequent decrease in blood flow to the lungs, cyanosis, and other signs of respiratory distress. This behavior is sometimes termed the "flip-flop phenomenon."

Weaning usually involves first a transition from assisted ventilation to CPAP and then to the head hood.

Hazards of Oxygen Therapy

The two chief hazards of oxygen therapy, as noted previously, are retrolental fibroplasia and pulmonary oxygen toxicity (bronchopulmonary dysplasia). Pneumothorax and/or pneumopericardium and/or pneumomediastinum may occur when oxygen is given under pressure (CPAP or ventilator).

Retrolental Fibroplasia. Prior to 1940 *retrolental fibroplasia* was virtually unknown. By 1950 it had become the greatest single cause of blindness in children in the United States, greater than all of the other causes combined. The fact that almost all of the cases occurred in the better-equipped medical centers while the condition was virtually unknown in small towns and rural areas was a mystery until 1953, when it was shown that high oxygen concentrations were to blame. The large centers with the newest equipment were able to deliver the oxygen so much more efficiently.

As oxygen was monitored more closely, the incidence of retrolental fibroplasia dropped. There is concern that there may be a resurgence if arterial oxygen is not closely monitored, as we save more and more infants of earier gestational age by the use of high oncentrations of oxygen.

The basis of retrolental fibroplasia s in the development of the blood sup-ly of the retina. Until the fourth month f gestation no retinal vessels are pres-nt; vascularization of the retina is not omplete until after the eighth month. baby born at 30 weeks of gestation, for xample, has no blood vessels in much of is retina (Fig. 18–9). It is the incom-letely vascularized retina that is sus-eptible to oxygen damage. Once the essels are completely developed, they re not damaged by oxygen.

Since newborn puppies and kittens lso have incomplete retrolental vas-ularization, it is relatively easy to dem-nstrate the sequence of events when xygen is given. The initial effect is the mmediate and almost total constriction f retinal vessels. This can happen within 5 minutes after oxygen is given at concentrations of 70 to 80 per cent. It as been suggested that a careful examination of the fundus is one means f determining the level of oxygen con-entration to be used, the finding of vasoconstriction indicating an im-mediate need to lower oxygen concen-ration. This is rarely done, however.

After about 10 minutes of sustained

oxygen, arterioles and capillaries re-open and remain dilated for the next several hours. New blood vessels appear in the retina. Leakage of fluid and blood from these newly formed vessels and in-vasion by fibroblasts eventually lead to retinal detachment in the weeks that follow.

A second or cicatricial stage, during which the retrolental membrane is formed, occurs several weeks later. The extent of the damage done in the second stage depends upon the severity of the acute stage and is related to:

1. The concentration of oxygen.
2. The length of time during which oxygen is administered.
3. The degree of immaturity of the eye.

There is no cure for a fully de-veloped case of retrolental fibroplasia (Fig. 18–10).

It is believed that by keeping Po_2 levels within the supposedly safe limits of 50 to 90 mm. Hg the danger of retro-lental fibroplasia will be minimal. The danger cannot be totally eliminated, be-cause for some babies there appears to be a danger at any oxygen level above that of room air. It is important to rec-ognize that arterial oxygen levels in the baby can suddenly change without a

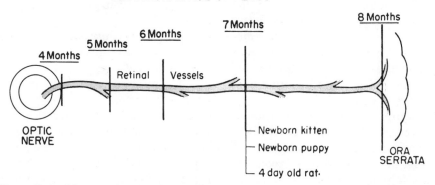

GESTATIONAL AGE OF FETUS

Figure 18–9 Schematic drawing showing the chronology of the development of the blood supply of ie retina in the human fetus. (From Patz: *Pediatrics*, *19*:508, 1957.)

Figure 18–10 Terminal stage of retrolental fibroplasia. The child is totally blind. (From Patz: *Pediatrics, 19*:508, 1957.)

change in oxygen concentration if the baby's ability to ventilate improves.

The American Academy of Pediatrics recommends the following for oxygen therapy in newborns:

1. Oxygen tension of arterial blood should not exceed 100 mm. Hg and should be maintained between 60 and 80 mm. Hg.

2. Inspired oxygen may be needed in relatively high concentrations to maintain the arterial oxygen in the normal range.

3. If blood gas measurements are not available, a mature infant who is not apneic but who has generalized cyanosis may be given oxygen in a concentration just high enough to abolish the cyanosis. However, if supplemental oxygen is necessary for an immature infant, he should be taken to a center at which inspired oxygen concentration can be regulated by blood gas measurements.

4. The ideal sampling sites for arterial oxygen tension studies are the radial or temporal arteries. In most circumstances, however, a sample from the descending aorta through an indwelling umbilical arterial catheter is satisfactory.

5. Equipment for the regulation of oxygen concentration (as provided by some incubators and respirators) and devices for mixing oxygen and room air may not function properly. Therefore, when an infant is placed in an oxygen-enriched environment, the concentra-

tion of oxygen must be measured with an oxygen analyzer at least every 2 hours. The performance of the oxygen analyzer must be checked daily by calibration with room air and 100 per cent oxygen.

6. A person experienced in recognizing retrolental fibroplasia should examine the eyes of all infants born at less than 36 weeks' gestation or weighing less than 2000 grams (4.2 pounds) who have received oxygen therapy. This examination should be made before the baby is discharged from the nursery and again at 3 to 6 months of age.

Pulmonary Oxygen Toxicity (POT). This disorder, also termed bronchopulmonary dysplasia, refers to a second condition that may occur in newborns exposed to high concentrations of oxygen. It has been recognized even more recently than retrolental fibroplasia, being first described by Northway and associates[42a] in 1967.

Pulmonary oxygen toxicity is related to:

1. The concentration of oxygen.

2. The amount of pressure in the oxygen delivery system.

3. The length of time during which oxygen is given.

If oxygen levels above 70 per cent are given for longer than 4 to 5 days, severe pulmonary disease may result. Concentrations of 100 per cent oxygen for 36 hours can lead to pulmonary changes. The principal changes occur in the alveolar epithelium and in the endothelium of the blood vessels around the alveoli. As a result there is progressive thickening of the blood-air barrier. In some babies these changes appear to reverse themselves over a period of 2 to 3 months. Other babies do not recover and eventually die.

Pneumothorax. A third complication is not related to oxygen, per se, but is often caused by the pressures of ventilation, either manual or mechanical. This is *pneumothorax* (air in the thoracic cavity). Related conditions that may or may not also occur are *pneumomediastinum* (air in the mediastinum) and *pneumopericardium* (air in the pericardial sac). Pneumothorax may also occur spontaneously at the time of birth. It is estimated that in approximately 7 per cent of all babies some degree of pneumothorax is present, but it is not always symptomatic.

The cause of pneumothorax is rupture of the alveoli from pressures that are too high, with escape of air into the pleural space. As more and more air escapes, breathing becomes more and more difficult. Nurses caring for babies with respiratory distress need to be alert for signs of possible pneumothorax, which often appear as *sudden* respiratory distress. Listening through a stethoscope for air exchange on both sides of the chest should be routine when pulse and respiration are checked.

Kuhns has described the use of a high intensity transilluminating light to detect pneumothorax and pneumomediastinum.[34] After the overhead lights in the nursery are turned out, a high intensity transilluminating light is placed against the baby's chest, first in an area superior to the nipple and then inferior to the nipple on both sides.

If an area around the sternum appears translucent, or if either side of the chest transilluminates more than the other, several other spots at varying distances from the sternum on either side are transilluminated.[34]

It would seem very useful for nurses to become familiar with this rapid, noninvasive means of observation. Figure 18–11 compares the transilluminated chest of a baby with a massive pneumothorax with X-rays of the same baby's chest.

Needle aspiration of air and/or placement of a chest tube is the treatment for pneumothorax. Transillumination is also being used to guide needle and tube placement.

NUTRITION FOR PRETERM INFANTS

In writing about nutrition for the preterm infant and other newborns who require intensive care, Rickard and Gresham say:

There is perhaps no other time when nutrition will be as important in influencing the quality of the infant's subsequent life . . . an acceptable nutritional program (is) an essential part of the comprehensive medical care these infants require.[50]

Major nutritional problems of preterm babies are summarized in Table 18–6. Because nurses have such a central role in meeting the nutritional needs of infants, we need to examine each of these problems in some detail.

Early Provision of Adequate Calories

Calories are needed both for energy and for growth. Failure to provide adequate calories results not only in inadequate growth but in starvation and in increased incidence of hypoglycemia and hyperbilirubinemia.

Figure 18–11 Transillumination to detect pneumothorax. *A,* Corona of light around the thorax; n pneumothorax indicated. *B,* Entire thoracic cage transilluminates; suggests large pneumothorax. *C* and *D* Chest X-ray showing massive right pneumothorax. (From Kuhns: *Pediatrics, 56*:355, 1975.)

Energy is stored by the human body as glycogen and fat. The preterm baby has very little fat, and glycogen stores are practically nonexistent. Moreover, because of a higher metabolic rate in relation to body weight (in comparison to even the term newborn as well as to older children and adults), the energy needs of the preterm baby are relatively higher. Any metabolic or surgical stress (including the very common respiratory distress syndrome discussed above) still further increases energy needs.

How many calories does the preterm baby need for energy and growth? Recent studies suggest that the pattern of weight loss that follows the birth of a term baby, with no apparent resultant problems, may not be appropriate for a preterm baby, particularly one who is very small and/or very young in gestational age. If is felt that preterm babies should not lose more than 5 to 8 per cent of their birth weight, with smaller babies losing no more than 5 per cent. When you consider that 5 per cent of 1500 grams is 75 grams (approximately 2½ ounces) and 5 per cent of 1000 grams is 50 grams (less than 2 ounces), this is a very tiny weight loss.

Lubchenco's studies show that a *fetus in utero* gains approximately 1

Table 18–6 NUTRITION FOR THE PRETERM INFANT

Problems	Needs
Small energy stores; relatively higher energy needs	Early provision of adequate calories
Glucose intolerance: Hypoglycemia Hyperglycemia	Careful monitoring of blood glucose and glucose intake
Immature gastrointestinal system: Impaired lactose tolerance Relative inability to digest fats Increased nitrogen catabolism with respiratory distress syndrome	Feedings adjusted to the special needs of the preterm baby
Immature sucking and swallowing reflexes	Alternate routes of feeding

rams of weight per day from 28 to 32 weeks' gestation and 38 grams per day from 32 to 36 weeks' gestation.[35] It has been suggested that similar gains may be appropriate for the baby of the same gestational age, but at the time of writing, a formula that would provide the nutrients for such a weight gain in a properly balanced form does not exist.

Approximately 120 calories per kg. per day is the rough estimate currently in use, although the requirements of some preterm babies may be considerably higher. Weight gain is an important clue to the adequacy of caloric intake. For very small preterm babies, the best type of feeding is really unknown at the time of writing.

Glucose Intolerance

It has been recognized since the 1960's that hypoglycemia is a major danger to perterm babies because of inadequate glycogen storage and the increased demands upon the body for energy, as mentioned above. (Hypoglycemia in the infant of a diabetic mother and in the baby who is small for gestational age is discussed later in this chapter.)

During the first 3 days of life, hypoglycemia is defined as a blood glucose level below 20 mg. per 100 ml. in a preterm baby and below 30 mg. per 100 ml. in a term infant on two successive samples obtained at least 1 hour apart. After 3 days a blood glucose level below 40 mg. per 100 ml. is considered hypoglycemic. It has been suggested that levels below 40 mg. per 100 ml. should be corrected.

Hypoglycemia can lead to brain damage and lifelong impairment. To be consistent with a philosophy of giving parents a baby with an intact central nervous system, hypoglycemia is best noted by careful monitoring of blood glucose levels in the nursery, a nursing responsibility in many hospitals.

Hypoglycemia is treated with glucose. Intravenous administration is considered the best route. Babies who are to be transferred from community hospitals to medical centers should receive intravenous glucose on route if they are hypoglycemic (checked by Dextrostix).

When babies are receiving intravenous glucose, hyperglycemia also becomes a potential hazard. Hyperglycemia causes diuresis as the body attempts to rid itself of excess sugar, and in small babies very rapid dehydration may follow. Monitoring blood glucose levels and carefully maintaining the desired rate of flow of intravenous glucose are the best ways of preventing hyperglycemia.

Immaturity of the Gastrointestinal Tract

The immature digestive system of the preterm baby makes certain dietary adjustments necessary. Not only must the type of carbohydrate, fat, and protein be adaptable to the special needs of the preterm baby but factors such as renal solute load must be considered.

Lactose is the carbohydrate of human milk and of several commercially prepared formulas. The enzyme *lactase* is necessary for lactose digestion. Since lactase enzymes do not attain maximal activity until 9 months after birth, preterm infants may have impaired lactose tolerance. Because breast milk has a higher lactose concentration than prepared formulas, some nutritionists feel that breast milk will be less well tolerated by preterm infants. (On the other hand, the possible role of breast milk in the prevention of necrotizing enterocolitis and other possible benefits of breast milk for the preterm baby are currently under investigation.)

Fats, even those digested rather easily by term infants (the fats in human milk, for example), are not believed to be well assimilated by preterm babies. Medium chain fatty acids are readily absorbed into the blood, however. Medium chain triglyceride (MCT) is an example of a fat often added to preterm infant formulas. In addition to providing essential fatty acids, added fats provide 9 calories per gram of formula in contrast to the 4 calories per gram provided by proteins and carbohydrates, making them a valuable source of energy.

Protein breakdown is very high in preterm infants with respiratory distress syndrome, occurring at a time when the body has great need for protein for brain development.

Provision of minerals is also a major problem. Lack of calcium can lead to undermineralization of the skeleton; however, it is not clear whether calcium supplementation is of any value. Since iron is stored by the fetus only during the last trimester of pregnancy, preterm infants have minimal iron stores. Iron supplementation usually begins before the baby leaves the hospital, either in the form of an iron fortified formula or iron drops. Iron is not given to babies with excessive red blood cell hemolysis (such as babies with Rh and ABO incompatibility; page 588) because the iron stores from red blood cell breakdown are not excreted.

Vitamin supplements are also frequently given to preterm babies, including vitamin E when the baby is believed to have a vitamin E dependent anemia.

Preterm infants have a number of conditions that may contribute to a high renal solute load, including low fluid intake, high extrarenal water loss, and a decreased ability of the kidney to concentrate urine.

In view of the differences between the digestive capabilities of preterm and term infants, we may well wonder what the ideal feeding for preterm infants might be. In spite of a great deal of research, the answer to this question remains unclear. The use of human milk is again coming into favor in some preterm nurseries (below); the advan age of giving the mother an opportunity to participate in her baby's care by pumping her breasts if she so chooses is obvious. Formulas with added oil, along with added vitamins and iron, are also used. Researchers continue to search for an "ideal" preterm feeding.

Human Milk and the Preterm Infant

Historically human milk has been considered the most appropriate food for preterm infants; in recent decades, however, the inadequacy of its protein for the rapid growth needs of the preterm baby has placed human milk in disfavor. Both the advantages and disadvantages of human milk for preterm infants are now under review.

Psychologic Advantages. A major rationale for human milk, quite apart from the nutritional significance, is the opportunity that providing the milk gives the mother to participate in the care of her baby. As noted in Chapter 22, producing a less than perfect baby (e.g., a baby born prior to term) is a blow to a mother's self-esteem and her image of herself. If she had also planned to breast-feed and is now told she cannot (or believes she cannot), this is a second disappointment.

However, if she can provide milk for her baby, this positive step can promote both feelings of self-worth and feelings of attachment for her baby.

What if the baby is at high risk of dying? As we emphasize in Chapter 22, attachment is important to normal grieving. Mothers who have provided milk for their high risk infant have said after the baby's death, "I would do it again; giving my baby my milk made me feel that I did everything possible for him."

Immunologic Advantages and Disadvantages. The immunologic factors in human milk include secretory IgA,

complement, macrophages, lymphocytes, neutrophils, and several others. Freezing and pasteurizing human milk may eliminate many of these constituents, but when the mother can provide fresh milk for her baby, she is also providing some protection against infection.

The immunologic disadvantages are rare when the mother is providing milk for her baby. If the mother is allergic to a medication that the baby is receiving, there is a possibility that the baby may have a reaction to that medicine. If the mother has a viral infection, the virus may be passed to her baby through breast milk. She can, however, continue to express her milk to maintain her milk supply until the infection is resolved and then again give her milk to the baby.

When human milk from a donor other than the baby's mother is used, there is a *potential* problem of an immunologic graft versus host reaction, but there is little evidence that this really does occur.

Nutritional Advantages and Disadvantages

PROTEIN. The lower amount of protein in human milk in comparison to cow milk formulas has already been mentioned. The quality of the protein is different, however. The ratio of lactalbumin to casein, which is important in digestibility, is 60:40 in human milk and in certain commercial formulas; it is 18:82 in cow milk.

When large amounts of protein are given, the level of amino acids can be excessive, which can be a detrimental factor in brain development.

Considering total protein needs, it appears that human milk does need supplementation to provide adequate protein, but this does not contraindicate the use of human milk.

FAT. The fat content of human

milk is slightly higher than that of cow milk. Moreover, the fat in human milk is better absorbed by infants, including preterm infants.

CALCIUM. The preterm infant's requirement for calcium is not met by human milk, but human milk is better for the baby because it also contains much less phosphate. Calcium supplementation will be necessary.

RENAL SOLUTE LOAD. The decreased renal solute load of human milk is an advantage for the preterm baby.

Providing Human Milk for the Preterm Baby

Because of immature sucking and swallowing reflexes (below), preterm babies will rarely be able to nurse at the mother's breast following delivery. Often the baby may be transferred to a medical center, while the mother remains in a community hospital.

How can the nurse who cares for the mother help her succeed in providing milk for her baby?

Initial assessment begins as we ask the mother if she planned to breast-feed. So often the assumption is made, by parents, nurses, and physicians, that because she has had a preterm baby (or a baby with some other problem that necessitates care in a high risk nursery), breast-feeding is not possible for her. This isn't true. If she had planned to breast-feed, we can help her to accomplish her goal by expressing her milk until the baby is able to nurse at the breast.

Expression can begin immediately after birth. The colostrum can then be given to the baby. If the mother is uncertain at first, but later decides that she wishes to breast-feed, lactation may be induced at this later time. Methods of expression are described in Chapter 20.

Milk expressed by any method is labeled with the name of the mother an the date and time of expression. If it is t be brought to the hospital that day (or it is expressed at the hospital), the mil may be refrigerated and must then b used within 24 hours. Milk for futur use is frozen. Freezing destroys many c the protective functions (e.g., mac rophages) but does not appear to affec the nutritional components. If a mothe lives at a great distance from the hosp tal and can only visit once or twice week, freezing may enable her to pr vide breast milk for her baby and thu feel she is doing something for him even when she is not with him.

Relactation and Induced Lactation

The mother of a preterm infant ma not choose to breast-feed or express he milk initially, but may later change he mind. A mother who was ill following delivery but subsequently recovers ma also wish to breast-feed. If the baby wa formula-fed but is not doing well, th mother may want to try breast-feeding Or the mother who started breast feeding and stopped for some reason may wish to try again. Under these cir cumstances *relactation* is possible.

Using a similar technique, lacta tion may also be induced in some womer who have not been pregnant. Some adoptive mothers induce lactation ir order to breast-feed their adopted in fants. Although they may never totall meet their infant's nutritional needs b induced lactation, mother and baby are able to share the close relationship tha the mother desires.

A Plan for Relactation. The key to lactation is nipple stimulation, which leads to the production of prolactin which in turn stimulates milk produc tion. Sucking by the infant every hours, or 10 to 12 times in 24 hours fo several weeks, is necessary to achieve actation. Night feedings are essential. The mother must know this before she begins. Unless her motivation and her patience are high, her milk supply will not develop, and she is likely to become very discouraged.

In addition to assessment of the mother, her support systems must also be evaluated. How does the father feel about her desire to lactate? Are there other children? Will she have help in caring for them? Is there a public health nurse, a La Leche member, or a supportive neighbor available to give her counsel when she gets discouraged?

The mother's nutritional status should be good.

The personality of the baby can also be a factor in the success or failure of lactation. A very fussy baby may produce tension in the mother, which can interfere with milk production. On the other hand a very passive baby may not be sufficiently interested in frequent sucking to stimulate production.

During the lactating period the mother's milk must be supplemented by formula. After the first 48 hours, giving the supplement by dropper rather than by bottle will encourage the baby to suck from the breast, a more difficult task than sucking from the bottle. Another method of giving supplement is with a Lact-Aid (Fig. 18–12), which car-

ries the supplement to the baby while he is nursing at the mother's breast. Adoptive mothers may use the Lact-Aid continuously.

The mother keeps a daily record, which includes:

1. The ounces of supplement given.
2. The number of times and length of time the baby nurses.
3. The number of wet diapers. (There should be at least eight wet diapers a day as evidence of adequate fluid intake.)

How long will it take for the mother of a preterm baby to lactate? A general guide is 1 week for every month she has not nursed plus 1 additional week to build up a strong milk supply. For example, if it has been 2 months since her baby delivered, it should take approximately 3 weeks (2 weeks plus 1 week) for her milk supply to develop. When the baby is taking only 4 ounces of supplement in 24 hours, supplement can usually be reduced to 4 ounces in 48 to 72 hours and subsequently eliminated entirely.

Immature Sucking and Swallowing Reflexes

The sucking and swallowing reflexes of most preterm babies are insufficiently developed to enable sucking from either bottle or breast. Alternate routes of feeding include:

1. Intravenous feeding of glucose and electrolytes.
2. Intravenous feeding of protein solutions (hyperalimentation).
3. Formula fed by gavage.
4. Continuous intragastric drip and transpyloric feeding.

Intravenous Feeding of Glucose and Electrolytes. Because of the danger of hypoglycemia in the first hours of life, intravenous glucose solution is started early and continued until

Figure 18–12 The Lact-Aid enables this infant to nurse at his mother's breast and induce lactation while receiving supplementary feeding from the Lact-Aid bag.

the baby is able to take approximately 120 ml. per kg. per day orally (gavage or nipple). The amount of parenteral fluid is decreased as the oral intake is increased (Fig. 18–13).

The type of solution and the total amount to be given, as well as the amount of solution to be given each hour, should be a part of the physician's order. Once the fluids are started, their maintenance at the proper rate becomes a nursing responsibility that involves the monitoring of both baby and intravenous equipment at the minimum of once every hour. If too small an amount of fluid is given, the baby will become increasingly dehydrated, and circulating fluid volume will be decreased. If the proper fluid level is not restored, he will die in a relatively short period of time. On the other hand, too much fluid in too brief a period of time will lead to pulmonary edema and water intoxication, and again, if uncorrected, to death. The margin for error is narrow in a newborn baby.

A first requirement for assuring accurate intake is an intravenous set designed specifically for pediatric patients. A small amount of fluid can be transferred from the main fluid bottle to the burette—not more than the baby is to receive in a 3 hour period. In this way, even if by some accident the fluid should begin to run at a faster rate than ordered, the baby will be protected against an overwhelming fluid intake. From 5 to 10 cc. of fluid should remain in the burette at all times as a buffer, so that if an emergency does arise and fluid intake cannot be checked exactly on the hour, all of the fluid will not be gone, and the needle will not be clogged with blood.

The amount of fluid the baby receives should be checked and charted each hour. Readings are made at the fluid level at the bottom of the meniscus. The chart should be a type that can be kept at the baby's bedside and quickly checked to see the kind of fluid he is receiving, the amount he has received, and the rate of flow.

The fluid site is one area to be observed in the baby. A scalp vein, an umbilical artery, and veins in the hands and feet are frequent sites for the administration of intravenous fluids in newborns. If it is suspected that the baby will receive fluids for a number of days, a "cut-down" to deeper vessels may be done. The site needs to be checked for swelling at least every hour. Occasionally, in adults, the continued postion of a needle in a vein is ascertained by lowering the fluid bottle to see if blood returns in the tubing. This should not be done in newborns because of the small gauge of the needle; the back-up blood may easily clog the needle, and the fluids will have to be restarted at another site. Swelling at the

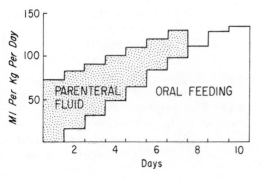

Figure 18–13 Schema of combined parenteral and oral feeding for a newborn infant weighing less than 1500 Gm. at birth and with poor ability to suck. As the quantity delivered orally is increased, the amount delivered parenterally may be decreased. Individualization of management is necessary. (From Babson: *J. of Pediatrics, 79*:694, 1971.)

uid site may indicate infiltration of
uids or merely that the tape holding
ae needle in place is too tight.

Umbilical artery catheterization,
hich allows frequent blood sampling
s well as the administration of fluids, is
procedure developed in the early
960's. It is usually reserved for very
nall premature babies who have tiny,
agile veins and respiratory distress
yndrome or another serious illness
aat will require fluid therapy for sev-
al days. An umbilical catheter can
inimize the number of times a sick
aby must be handled during the first
eek, which is decidedly to his advan-
age.

After the cord and surrounding
rea are washed with an antiseptic so-
ation, a catheter is inserted into one of
ae umbilical arteries and fixed in place
ith a silk thread. The tip of the cathe-
r should be in the abdominal aorta at
ae level of the diaphragm. The position
f the catheter is usually confirmed by
-ray.

Because there is always the possi-
ility of infection through the cord
tump, even in healthy newborns, an
ntibiotic ointment may be ordered for
ae area surrounding the stump.

Babies with umbilical catheters
nould be checked for leg blanching.
his is due to arterial thrombosis that
an occur shortly after the catheter is
aserted, during the time the catheter is
a place, or after the removal of the
atheter. The baby's leg may appear
ald and white with no pulse, or it may
e mottled, pale, and dusky.

After an umbilical catheter has
een removed, there may be bleeding
om the cord stump.

Even small babies have to be re-
trained while they are receiving fluids.
ike older people with restraints, they
eed to have their position changed fre-
uently and the restraints checked of-

ten, as well as having the skin under the
restraint checked, which is so very delicate and can easily be injured. If a baby
is to receive oral fluids while he is re-
strained, his head should be lifted for
feeding, and after feeding he should be
turned on his side or abdomen, depending upon the fluid site. Each time the
baby is turned or moved, the site and
flow must be rechecked.

If medications are added to the
fluids, this must also be included in the
record, just as any other medications
would be. Some medications, calcium
gluconate, for example, may have a
sclerotic effect on surrounding tissues
if the needle becomes dislodged from
the vein.

*Intravenous Feeding of Protein
Solutions (Hyperalimentation).* Hyperalimentation solutions provide
protein, vitamins, and electrolytes as
well as glucose. The intravenous solution is specifically prepared for each
baby under sterile conditions; hyperalimentation solutions must not be
interchanged. Laboratory studies of
each infant serve as a guide to determining his specific solution.

For short-term supplementation,
certain hyperalimentation solutions
are given in peripheral veins. More concentrated solutions for long-term
hyperalimentation are administered
through a catheter in the superior vena
cava (Fig. 18–14).

The intravenous system for central
hyperalimentation includes a millipore
filter, which serves to remove particles
or micro-organisms from the solution
before they can reach the baby, and an
infusion pump, to insure that the solution is delivered at a constant rate
throughout the 24 hour period. Both
filter and pump are changed at least
every 48 hours. The intravenous line
should be labeled with the date and time
of changing.

CONSTANT
INFUSION
PUMP

MILLIPORE FILTER

FINAL
POSITION OF CATHETER

Figure 18–14 Technique
catheter insertion and delivery
fluids for total intravenous alime:
tation. (From Moore: *The Newbo*
and the Nurse. Philadelphia, W.
Saunders Co., 1972.)

Because a number of serious complications are possible when hyperalimentation solution is administered, constant nursing attention is an absolute necessity. Septicemia is a major danger, because the glucose-protein solution is a nearly perfect medium for the growth of bacteria. The prevention of infection depends upon careful technique, not only at the time the catheter is inserted but throughout the period it is in place. The central hyperalimentation catheter should never be used for the administration of medications or for the withdrawal of blood; both procedures heighten the possibility of contamination. Babies must be observed carefully for any early signs of sepsis (page 577).

In order for the baby to utilize the protein of the hyperalimentation solution for growth, he must also receive sufficient glucose to stimulate insulin production. The insulin, in turn, stimulates both the transport of amino acids into the cells and the synthesis of protein. If relatively large amounts of glucose are not given, the amino acids will be utilized for energy rather than for growth.

However, the high level of glucose as we have already noted, can lead t rapid and severe dehydration. Urine are checked for glucose, and if glucos levels are 3+ or 4+ by Clinitest, either the rate of the infusion is decreased the glucose content of the solution decreased. Sometimes insulin is adde to the solution under these circum stances. Other regimens begin therap with a 10 per cent solution of glucos during the first 24 hours, a 15 per cer solution during the next 24 hours, and 20 per cent solution thereafter to pre vent this initial glycosuria.

Hypertonic sugar solutions in com bination with amino acids may, afte several days of administration, lead to hypoglycemic response within the body whether insulin has been added or no Therefore blood glucose levels ar carefully monitored.

The baby's growth in weigh length, and head circumference is a indication of the success hyperalimentation.

Feeding by Gavage. Gavage tubes come in sizes—size 5 for very tiny infants and size 8 or 10 for larger preterm babies.

The tube is measured from the bridge of the nose to the lobe of the ear to the xiphoid process. This distance is marked on the tube with tape. The catheter may be premarked, but since there are all sizes of even tiny infants, the tube should still be measured at each feeding.

A small quantity of sterile water run through the tube before it is inserted assures its patency. Nasal catheters may be lubricated with sterile water; oral catheters do not need to be lubricated. After the catheter is passed, the baby should be observed for a moment for signs of dyspnea, an indication that the tube may be in the trachea rather than in the esophagus. If the catheter is not already attached to a syringe, the syringe is attached and the formula poured into it and allowed to flow by gravity.

If the tube is not to be left in place, it is pinched and removed when every drop of formula has passed through it. A baby should be "burped" following gavage feeding, just as he is after a bottle- or breast-feeding. If he must remain in the incubator, he can be held in a sitting position and have his back gently stroked toward the neck. After feeding, the baby is placed on his abdomen or right side.

When a baby begins to suck on his gavage tube during feedings, he may be ready to begin the transition to bottle-feeding (Fig. 18–15). At first a few cc. of a feeding may be offered by nipple once or twice a day *after* gavage feeding. When the baby can take one feeding per day by bottle, he can graduate to two and then three feedings. If he appears tired during bottle-feeding, the next feeding should be by gavage. It is impor-

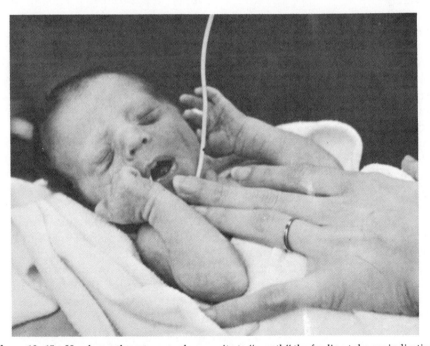

Figure 18–15 Hand-mouth gestures and a capacity to "mouth" the feeding tube are indications that this 3½ pound premature baby will soon take feedings from a nipple instead of a tube. (From O'Grady: *American J. Nursing*, 71:737, 1971.)

tant to carefully chart the way in which the baby takes each feeding in order to plan care for the next day. Patience is essential, both in increasing amounts of formula and in making the transition from gavage to bottle-feeding.

Continuous Intragastric Drip or Transpyloric Feeding. In some nurseries preterm babies are fed through a nasojejunal catheter inserted through the baby's nose and into his stomach. The baby is then turned on his right side to allow passage through the pyloric sphincter into the duodenum and ultimately into the jejunum. The position of the catheter is checked by abdominal X-ray when fluid aspirated from the catheter has reached a pH of 5.0 to 7.0.

First feedings through the catheter will be of water or dextrose, followed by half-strength and then full-strength formula. Approximately 10 to 15 ml. of formula is given by slow drip every 1½ to 2 hours.

Possible complications include occlusion of the catheter and infusion of an excess amount of formula, which may reflux into the stomach. Irrigating the tube with 1 ml. of sterile water following each feeding will help to prevent occlusion. A nasogastric tube placed in the stomach will prevent aspiration of any formula that regurgitates through the pylorus.

NECROTIZING ENTEROCOLITIS

Approximately 3 to 8 per cent of preterm infants acquire necrotizing enterocolitis (NEC), a life-threatening condition. The etiology is believed to be related to hypoxia, with a resultant shunting of blood from organs that tolerate ischemia comparatively well (such as the intestines) to those areas that must be continuously oxygenated

(such as the brain). Intestinal cells damaged by hypoxia, stop secreting mucus and become damaged; they are subsequently invaded by gas-forming bacteria that produce a characteristic picture of pneumatosis cystoides intestinalis (air in the intestinal wall) on X-ray. Intestinal perforation and death may follow if the baby's condition is not recognized. Other factors associated with NEC include sepsis, patent ductus arteriosus, exchange transfusion, umbilical vessel catheterization, low gestational age, and inappropriate oral feeding. Obviously, most babies in intensive care nurseries are potential candidates.

Nursing observations are invaluable in spotting early symptoms of NEC. A baby with abdominal distention is suspect, especially if rigidity is also present. The abdomen should be measured (Fig. 18–16) every 4 to 6 hours from the time distention is first noted; an increase of more than 1 cm. from the previous measurement should be immediately reported.

Failure to absorb feedings is another significant symptom. When a baby who has been taking feedings, either by nipple or gavage, begins to spit up formula, or when formula can be aspirated through the gavage tube at a subsequent feeding, he may have NEC. A shiny abdominal wall, absence of bowel sounds (listen with a stethoscope), and blood in the stools (check with Hemastix) are also symptoms nurses should assess.

Treatment includes the discontinuation of oral feedings for 7 to 10 days to rest the bowel and the administration of antibiotics. During this time the baby is carefully observed for signs of shock (inability to maintain temperature, decrease in blood pressure, bradycardia, and listlessness). He should be picked up as little as possible to avoid abdominal trauma, but his

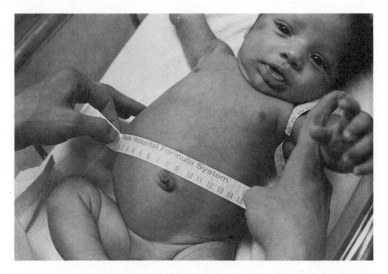

Figure 18–16 Select points on the right and the left, above or below the umbilicus, mark sites with indelible ink, and measure between them. (From Bliss: *MCN, 1*:37, 1976.)

hands and head should be stroked for emotional satisfaction. Surgery may be necessary to remove segments of inflamed bowel.

There is some evidence that the incidence of NEC is lower in babies fed breast milk, one major reason for the re-evaluation of the use of breast milk in preterm infants.

HYPERBILIRUBINEMIA IN PRETERM INFANTS

Hyperbilirubinemia is a common problem of preterm babies for several reasons. The preterm infant has a decreased ability to conjugate bilirubin in his liver, and thus the concentration of indirect, fat-soluble bilirubin increases more rapidly than in the term infant. Bruising, more frequent in preterm babies, leads to hemolysis and increased bilirubin levels. The delay in feeding that often occurs in the sick preterm infant is another contributing factor.

Moreover, kernicterus, the brain damage that results when bilirubin enters the brain cells, can occur at bilirubin levels lower than the 18 to 20 mg. per 100 ml. in the preterm infant with acidosis or with low circulating blood volume. This is because as long as bilirubin is bound to albumin it cannot enter the intracellular fluid compartment and is therefore nontoxic to cells. The excess of hydrogen ions present in acidosis; certain other ions; and drugs such as salicylates, sulfonamides, and others compete with bilirubin for albumin-binding sites. Thus more bilirubin is able to enter the cells, even though the total amount of bilirubin in the body may be lower.

In addition, any condition that leads to lower levels of albumin in the infant, such as decreased blood volume, has the same effect of decreasing the amount of bilirubin bound to albumin.

Two modalities are principally used in the treatment of hyperbilirubinemia. They are phototherapy and exchange transfusion.

Phototherapy

It was the careful observation of a nurse at the General Hospital in Rochford, Essex, England, that led to the use of phototherapy in the treatment of hyperbilirubinemia. The nurse, whose name unfortunately is not recorded in the published report, noted that jaundice faded after babies had been in direct sunlight for a short time. Cremer and his associates[9] then began to place naked babies in direct sunlight for 15 to 20 minutes, withdrawing them for similar periods before exposing them again. During exposure the babies' eyes were protected with a plastic shield. It was discovered that although jaundice quickly disappeared from the exposed areas, it remained in the shaded areas. Subsequently, Cremer devised a source of artificial light that was found to be effective in reducing serum bilirubin levels. Phototherapy has since become a common treatment in premature and intensive care nurseries.

Light causes bilirubin to break down into water-soluble products that are rapidly excreted in the bile, and to a lesser extent in the urine. Because of the mode of excretion, the stools of a baby who has been under the lights are brown or dark green; the urine may be a dark golden brown.

Blue light is more effective than white light in causing bilirubin breakdown. However, it is difficult to detect changes in the baby's color, particularly changes caused by cyanosis, under blue lights. They must be turned off frequently for observation of the baby. The baby will also appear "strange" to his parents under blue lights. Even white lights are frightening and should be carefully explained. Blue lights should be flicked off so the parents can see what their baby really looks like.

Nurses caring for babies receiving phototherapy must understand several aspects of care for these babies.

1. Because photodegradation of bilirubin takes place in the skin, the baby should be fully undressed while he is under the lights.

2. His temperature must be monitored; overheating with subsequent dehydration is a possibility. If a servomechanism is being used to monitor the baby's temperature, it should be covered with opaque tape.

3. Fluid intake should be increased because of increased insensible water loss, which may be increased by as much as 300 per cent in the preterm baby (and by approximately 40 per cent in the term baby). The baby should be weighed twice a day and fluid intake further increased if weight loss exceeds 2 per cent of body weight.

4. Both of the baby's eyes should be shielded completely. There is no data concerning human eye damage, but some retinal damage has been produced in experimental animals. When only one eye has been covered, permanent amblyopia (reduced vision) has been demonstrated in kittens.

5. Skin color is not an adequate guide to levels of serum bilirubin, because the skin will become less yellow during treatment. Bilirubin levels in the blood must therefore be measured.

6. Babies under the bilirubin light may have a rash from ultraviolet radiation. There should always be a Plexiglas shield between the baby and the light to filter out this radiation.

7. Light emission may decay over a period of time. Specific instructions for various types of lights are contained in instruction manuals and should be reviewed periodically.

Other than the findings of the animal research studies described above, no hazards of phototherapy have been identified in the 20 years since the inial discovery of the principle, although is recommended that lights be used nly when there is a specific reason (rising bilirubin levels) and never rophylactically.

How much radiant energy does a aby receive during phototherapy? ucey has calculated that a baby in an cubator near a window who is exposed 6 hours of summer sunlight receives 700 microwatts per square cm. in 24 ours.[39] A baby receiving 24 hours of hototherapy (daylight bulbs) receives 800 microwatts per square cm.

xchange Transfusion

A second method of treatment for yperbilirubinemia is exchange transsion. When bilirubin levels are rising apidly, exchange tranfusion is indiated rather than phototherapy. The lost common reason for exchange ransfusion is Rh incompatibility (below), although hyperbilirubinemia for ny reason may be treated by the exhange method.

Blood for exchange may be O negaive, which has been cross-matched gainst maternal serum. If it is uspected before delivery that an imnediate exchange will be necessary, his blood should be ready. If there is ime following delivery to type the aby's blood before exchange, negative lood of the baby's type that has been ross-matched against maternal serum s used. A sample of maternal serum hould be saved for future exchanges.)btaining additional maternal blood is lot a serious problem when the mother s in the same hospital as the baby. But is the transfer of very sick infants from maller community hospitals to the inensive care units of major medical ceners becomes increasingly more freJuent, the nurses at both hospitals must nake sure that maternal blood accom-

panies any baby with hemolytic anemia.

Why are Rh_D positive babies given negative blood? If Rh_D positive blood is used, the antibodies already present in the infant's circulatory system will destroy the new erythrocytes, just as they are destroying his own cells; nothing will have been accomplished by exchanging one set of positive cells for another.

In addition to proper type, blood for exchange must be the freshest available, never more than 3 to 4 days old. Older blood is more likely to hemolyze, exactly the process that exchange transfusion is attempting to prevent. Heparinized blood is always fresh, since it must be discarded if it is not used within a 24 hour period. Babies who receive heparinized blood must be watched for bleeding following transfusion; 10 mg. of protamine sulfate may be given intravenously following an exchange with heparinized blood. Blood that has had acid-citrate-dextrose (A.C.D.) added as an anticoagulant can lower blood calcium levels. Because of this, calcium gluconate is given through the exchange catheter after each 100 ml. of blood is exchanged.

The danger that the baby will be chilled during any procedure has already been discussed. In addition to the measures normally used to keep the infant warm, the blood for exchange should be warmed. An easy and safe way to do this is to place the blood in a basin of water warmed to, but not exceeding, 98.6°F. (37.0°C). Overheating the blood can damage erythrocytes and also increase the level of free serum potassium.

The amount of blood that will be used is figured at 85 ml. times the weight of the baby in kilograms times 2; 85 ml. per kg. being the assumed blood volume of the newborn infant. An amount equal to twice the blood volume is used because research indicates that this quantity will assure 85 to 90 per cent effective replacement of circulating erythrocytes.

During the exchange itself there must be one person—doctor or nurse—who can devote full attention to the baby by monitoring pulse and respiration, observing the infant's color and general condition, and suctioning him if necessary. The amount of blood injected and withdrawn and the baby's venous pressure must also be accurately recorded.

After the exchange is completed, the baby is observed closely both for evaluation of his general condition and for signs of hemorrhage from the exchange site.

PSYCHOLOGIC NEEDS OF PRETERM INFANTS

Our current knowledge of the psychologic needs of preterm infants, particularly those babies of very low gestational age, is limited. There are many questions we need to be asking. For example, in caring for the baby of 30 weeks' gestation, should we try to approximate his environment in utero? Should we try to treat him as nearly as possible like a full term infant? Or are his needs very specific and unlike either other group? The opportunities for nursing and interdisciplinary research are virtually unlimited.

To a certain extent approximating the environment of the uterus is impractical. The uterus is dark; light seems to be necessary for newborn care. The fetus lives in a fluid-filled world, but this does not seem feasible to simulate. One attempt to simulate the gentle rocking of the fluid environment has been to use a water-filled mattress be-

neath the baby. Other devices that roc the baby gently have also been used i isolettes to simulate the gentle rockin of the uterus.

Touch, so important to the de velopment of term infants, would als appear to be significant for preter babies. Both animal research and ol servations of human infants who hav not been touched have shown that ther are differences in the behavior of thes babies when they are compared wit babies who receive normal motherin The significance of touch for both par ents and babies is discussed in Chapte 22.

Young preterm babies have yet t develop sucking reflexes, so it would aj pear that sucking is not a need at thi time. Obviously, sucking needs ar going to become important as the bab grows older.

Our care of preterm babies (an other high risk infants) involves pai for the babies—the starting of in travenous fluids, the use of restraints blood tests, intramuscular injections and the like. It is hard to know hov much this pain during early week means in terms of long-term emotiona development, but it would seem impor tant to keep painful experiences to a minimum and to attempt to comfort th baby after painful treatment, just as w would comfort an older child.

Another area about which we hav more questions than answers is the im portance of auditory and visual stimu lation to preterm babies. Studies of th value of auditory stimuli (records o maternal heartbeat, music, and so on in accelerating weight gain have pro duced varying results. Are there long range advantages, or possibly disad vantages, to such stimuli? Are the ef fects different with babies of varyin gestational age? What about the leve of noise in an incubator from the con tantly running motor? What about the level of noise in the nursery?

What does the preterm baby see? Should we provide mobiles and toys for him to watch, as we do for the term baby?

The answers to all of these questions are important if we are to provide care for preterm babies that will enable them to develop their optimum potential.

PLANNING THE PRETERM INFANT'S DISCHARGE

As with every patient who enters the hospital, discharge planning begins at the time of admission. In the case of the preterm infant, or any high risk baby who has been separated from his parents, this is particularly important because the extent to which we are able to facilitate attachment in the days immediately following birth will be a significant factor in assuring that the baby is welcomed at home at the time of discharge, which may be weeks or even months later. Moreover, even when initial attachment is achieved successfully, the long period of hospitalization, which may be at a medical center many miles from the parents' home, may strain the bonds. We need to keep good records of the frequency of parental visits and telephone calls, to check out the reasons when they do not occur, and to work actively to maintain bonds between parents and their babies (Chapter 22). Otherwise, the time for going home may arrive with very little attachment between parent and baby.

A home visit by a public health nurse, working in close communication with the hospital, is very important before the baby is discharged. The community nurse's report to the hospital about the physical environment of the home, the preparations that have been made for the baby, and the feelings of the family is significant. If the home is found inadequate in one or more aspects, discharge may be delayed until either community or hospital nurses can help the family to better prepare for the baby. On the other hand, a baby may be discharged somewhat earlier into a home that is well prepared to care for him.

It is desirable for parents to take an increasingly greater role in the care of their baby throughout his hospitalization. In this way they will be more comfortable and confident in caring for him at home. If this is not possible throughout the period of hospitalization, perhaps because of the distance the parents live from the hospital or because of other small children in the home who cannot be left alone each day, there must be ample opportunity in the days preceding discharge for the parents to become acquainted with their baby—to feed, hold, bathe, and dress him and to understand his communication with them.

The ability of the baby to maintain his body temperature at 97.8°F. (36.5°C.) in an open bed is necessary before he can be discharged. He needs to be moved to an open bed several days before the discharge is anticipated. In addition, he must be able to gain weight while he is in the open bed. If he maintains temperature but is unable to gain weight, he is probably using too many calories for temperature control and needs to be returned to the warmer environment of the isolette for somewhat longer. Usually a baby is able to maintain his temperature at about 36 to 38 weeks of gestational age and about 1800 to 2000 grams of weight.

Many parents find this waiting period difficult. Once their baby is no longer critically ill and is beginning to gain weight, they want to take him home with them right away. Sometimes it helps them to gain perspective if we ask them what their expected date of delivery was. That date may be a relatively realistic one on which they can expect to take their baby home.

INFANTS WHO ARE SMALL FOR GESTATIONAL AGE

About one-third of all low birth weight babies are preterm, term, or post-term and small for gestational age (SGA) rather than preterm and appropriate for gestational age (AGA). Criteria for determining into which category a particular baby falls are discussed in Chapter 15.

Several factors appear to be related to the low birth weight of these babies, including intrauterine malnutrition, maternal smoking, infection, and congenital anomalies.

The importance of diet to a pregnant mother has already been discussed in the section on prenatal care. Nutritional deprivation seems to influence the growth of the placenta, which in turn affects the development of the fetus. There is some evidence that brain growth is also impaired in SGA infants. Studies of infants born in Holland during the last months of World War II, a time of severe food shortages, and also in Japan, suggest that food deprivation during the last weeks of pregnancy affected the newborn's weight more significantly than did deprivation earlier in pregnancy.

Smoking appears to be the single maternal factor that can be statistically correlated with SGA births. In experiments with rabbits it seemed that a constituent of tobacco was at fault, as smoke produced by other sources failed to cause the same effect as the tobacco smoke. Moderate smokers have twice the incidence of SGA infants as nonsmokers; infants of mothers who smoke heavily are three times as likely to be small for gestational age. Moreover, one British report indicates that the effects of smoking extend beyond infancy. In a study of 17,000 children, the children of women who smoked 10 or more cigarettes a day after the fourth month of pregnancy were found to have poorer physical and social development than the children of light smokers or nonsmokers. Although still other studies confirm the correlation between smoking and low birth weight (remember that correlation does not mean the same as causation), one report finds a correlation between low birth weight and mothers who first smoked after pregnancy, suggesting another factor may be involved.

Genetic factors undoubtedly account for some babies who are small for gestational age. A woman who has delivered one SGA infant is likely to do so in a subsequent pregnancy. Therefore, the relationship between birth weight and gestational age is an important aspect of maternal history in every pregnancy.

Infections that have been demonstrated to cause SGA infants are cytomegalic inclusion disease and rubella.

Mothers who are hypertensive (whether or not they have toxemia) and mothers addicted to heroin tend to produce small babies. Still other variables include certain anomalies of the sex chromosomes, high attitudes, and exposure to X-rays and some drugs.

The smaller a baby is in relation to his age, the more likely the occurrence of congenital malformations. Particularly close inspection and observation of such newborns are therefore necessary.

Hypoglycemia is a frequent problem of SGA babies. Other common conditions were noted in Table 18–3 and are outlined in Table 18–7.

INFANTS WHO ARE LARGE FOR GESTATIONAL AGE

Preterm, term, or post-term infants may be large for gestational age (LGA). A major problem of the preterm baby

Table 18–7 NEEDS AND CHARACTERISTICS OF LOW BIRTH WEIGHT INFANTS WITH SIMILAR WEIGHTS BUT VARYING GESTATIONAL AGES

	Preterm Infant, AGA	SGA Infant
Length of gestation	Less than 37 weeks' gestation	28–44 weeks' gestation
Duration of intensive care	Varies in relation to gestational age	Requires major care first 3 to 4 days of life
Mortality rate	Higher mortality than for growth retarded baby of same weight	—
Incidence of anomalies	—	Incidence of major congenital anomalies higher; the greater the degree of growth retardation, the greater the chance of malformation
Initial feeding	—	Susceptible to hypoglycemia; cannot tolerate prolonged fasting
Respiratory distress	Apnea, respiratory distress syndrome principal problems	Asphyxia, aspiration syndrome, pneumothorax principal problems
Maintenance of body temperature	—	Usual tables for neutral thermal environment don't apply; attempt to maintain body temperature between 96.8–97.8°F. (36.0–36.5°C.)
General appearance	Moves and cries less	Alert appearance
Weight gain	Gain is slower than would have normally been expected if had remained in utero	Loses little, if any, weight in the first 24 hours; gains more rapidly than AGA infant of same weight
Liver function	Immature; likely to have hyperbilirubinemia	Appropriate to age; hyperbilirubinemia less likely
Potential mental retardation	—	Greater chance of mental retardation in later life than AGA infant with same birth weight
Feeding	Prior to 32–34 weeks cannot suck and swallow; gastric capacity limited; small amounts of formula at frequent intervals required	Susceptible to hypoglycemia; cannot tolerate prolonged fasting; many SGA infants can nipple-feed when AGA infant of same birth weight cannot, because of being greater than 34 weeks' gestational age
Other problems	—	Polycythemia, occasionally with symptoms

who is large for gestational age is that because of his size, his immaturity and the problems associated with it are not recognized readily. He may, for example, have respiratory distress syndrome or a level of hyperbilirubinemia that might be expected for an infant of his gestational age, but is not usually associated with a baby of his size. Because his sucking reflex is appropriate to his age rather than to his size, because his ability to maintain his temperature in an open bed may be poor, and because his muscle tone may be diminished (again appropriate to age but not size), he may be falsely labeled as ill.

For reasons that are unknown, infants with transposition of the great vessels (below) tend to be large for gestational age.

Infants of diabetic mothers (IDM), particularly diabetic mothers who have not been in good control during the last trimester of pregnancy, are typically large for gestational age. When delivered at 37 weeks, they may weigh 9 or 10 pounds. (About 10 per cent of the infants of Classes D through F diabetic mothers are small for gestational age and resemble infants with placental insufficiency.) The increased size of the large IDM is due to fat (and not to edema as once believed) produced by a process described below in the discussion of glucose metabolism. Characteristically, the large IDM is fat and red-faced, lying quietly, moving very little, and crying infrequently. Not only the baby but the cord and placenta are oversized.

With very careful control of the mother's diabetes, especially in the last weeks of pregnancy, some diabetic mothers are delivering babies who do not have this classic appearance and who have decreased neonatal mortality as well. Although fetal and neonatal deaths are still higher for the infants of all but Class A diabetic mothers than for infants of nondiabetic mothers, neonatal mortality has decreased from 40 per cent to 10 per cent.[24]

The newborn IDM needs very careful nursing observation in the first hours and days of life. Major potential problems are hypoglycemia, hypocalcemia, hyperbilirubinemia, and respiratory distress syndrome. The incidence of congenital anomalies is also higher in these babies.

About 50 per cent of the infants of diabetic mothers become *hypoglycemic* during the first 6 hours after birth, probably because of the following sequence: Diabetic mothers who are not well controlled are hyperglycemic. The excess sugar, like other nutrients in maternal blood, crosses the placental barrier, causing hyperglycemia in the infant as well. To metabolize this excess sugar, the islets of Langerhans in the fetal pancreas hypertrophy in order to secrete increased amounts of insulin. The sugar is converted to glycogen and stored as excess fat, hence the large size of the baby. When the baby is born, he is removed from the source of his sugar, but his pancreas continues to work overtime for several hours. Thus he becomes hypoglycemic. The more nearly the mother's blood glucose levels can be kept within normal limits during her pregnancy, the less likely her baby is to develop hypoglycemia following delivery. The higher the maternal blood glucose level, the greater the infant's problem may be.

Most of these infants will have a transient hypoglycemia, lasting from 1 to 4 hours, after which blood glucose levels will begin to rise. In a few infants the hypoglycemia will be prolonged and severe.

Monitoring blood glucose levels was discussed earlier in this chapter.

Waiting for clinical signs of hypoglycemia to appear (tremors, apnea, cyanosis, limpness, failure to feed well, convulsions) would seem to violate standards of good care. Treatment for hypoglycemia is a constant, slow infusion of 10 to 15 per cent glucose. Rapid infusion of 25 to 50 per cent glucose is contraindicated because insulin production is increased as a response, with a subsequent drop in blood glucose levels.

An increased incidence of *hypocalcemia* has been reported in infants of diabetic mothers. Tremors are the most obvious clinical sign. *Hyperbilirubinemia* at 48 to 72 hours occurs more frequently than in other infants of comparable weight or gestational age.

Respiratory distress syndrome is also increased in babies of Class A through Class C diabetic mothers. Apparently, high levels of insulin produced by the baby interfere with the synthesis of lecithin, which is necessary for lung maturation. In babies of Class D through Class F diabetic mothers, for whom the intrauterine environment is even less favorable, the stress resulting from poor blood supply to the uterus may lead to increased production of steroids and thus to acceleration of lung maturation.

Because infants of diabetic mothers have more fatty tissue than most babies in the nursery, their temperature must be monitored closely if they are in an incubator without a servomechanism, or they will become overheated.

INFECTIOUS DISEASE AND THE NEWBORN INFANT

Infections affect newborn infants in two ways. Neonatal sepsis is an acute infection in which the baby appears ill and has a blood culture that demonstrates the causative organism. About one baby in every 1000 live term births and one in every 250 live preterm births has neonatal sepsis.

Our care of the preterm baby—the use of umbilical catheters and respiratory equipment and attending to breaks in his skin caused by intravenous needles and even by the electrodes of heart and respiratory monitors—combined with his less mature defense mechanisms, adds to his risk of developing sepsis. For many babies congenital anomalies are in themselves a potential source of infection (gastroschisis, for example, or a myelomeningocele). Surgical procedures further add to the risk.

Other acute infections in newborns are gonorrheal conjunctivitis (Chapter 16), urinary tract infections (which may lead to sepsis), meningitis, and infectious diarrhea.

A number of infections, several of which are acquired transplacentally, may affect the baby's long-range development but are not always obvious in the immediate newborn period. The most frequent causes of chronic infection are the organisms that are collectively known as the TORCH group (Chapter 6).

NEONATAL SEPSIS

Signs of Sepsis

Signs of sepsis in newborn infants, like the signs of many other problems, are more general than specific. Traditionally clinical signs such as vomiting, failure to feed well, the baby's inability to maintain his body temperature, and gray or mottled skin color have been recognized as the first evidence of sepsis. However, by the time these signs appear, the infection may be generalized. And in spite of all the antibiotics developed in recent years, there has been little change in infant mortality due to generalized sepsis.

Although we need to carefully observe and report the symptoms listed above, the current emphasis is on detecting earlier signs of infection. These signs may be:

1. Changes in blood count, particularly in white blood cells and platelets.
2. Hypoglycemia or hyperglycemia (glucose intolerance).
3. Metabolic acidosis.
4. Decrease in blood pressure.
5. Hyperbilirubinemia.

None of these signs are routinely monitored in the apparently healthy term newborn, although these babies may become septic. However, for infants in premature and intensive care nurseries, where the risk of sepsis is even greater, these parameters are followed.

Normal white blood cell (WBC) count in newborns varies from 6000 to 25,000 WBC's and also changes from day to day, so a single value is of little help in recognizing sepsis. Any marked and sudden change, either increase or decrease, suggests sepsis. Bands, a form of white blood cell, increase in the presence of sepsis. Platelets decrease.

Either hypoglycemia or hyperglycemia may indicate sepsis. Metabolic acidosis (bicarbonate levels below 21 mEq./L) also suggests the possibility of an infection. Here again, a sequence of values is far more helpful than a single value in giving a clue as to what is happening to a particular baby.

Pustules or furuncles on the skin, often in the umbilical or diaper area, are a sign of staphylococcal infection. In scalded skin syndrome, an exotoxin of staphylococci causes reddening, swelling, and tenderness of the skin, and frequently desquamation as well.

Organisms Involved in Neonatal Sepsis

The types of organisms most responsible for neonatal sepsis change from time to time. Currently Group B beta hemolytic streptococci are the chief source of infection in most nurseries in the United States. Since this organism is a part of the normal vaginal flora of many women, it is difficult to prevent. Not all babies whose mothers have Group B streptococci in their vaginal tract will become infected, however; only a small percentage will.

Escherichia coli, once the leading cause of neonatal sepsis, remains a major source of infection in nurseries. Other significant organisms are Klebsiella, *Staphylococcus aureus,* and Pseudomonas. Table 18–8 summarizes important information about common infections in newborns.

Diagnosis of Sepsis

When sepsis is suspected, a number of studies are immediately indicated. Blood cultures are drawn from a peripheral vein after disinfection of the skin with iodine. Urine for culture is obtained by suprapubic aspiration, considered less dangerous than catheterization and more reliable than a clean catch specimen. Cerebrospinal fluid is aspirated via lumbar pucture. Any skin lesion should also be cultured.

Treatment

Good nursing care, with emphasis on careful handwashing, should effectively isolate every infant from every other infant in the nursery. Babies with sepsis may be isolated in separate rooms as well, but never where they cannot be

Table 18–8   ORGANISMS IMPORTANT IN NEONATAL SEPSIS

Organism	Source	Form of Sepsis	Notes
Group B beta hemo- lytic streptococcus	Mother: vaginal flora	Septicemia within first 12 hours of life with 50% mortality	Leading cause of neonatal sepsis
	Environment: nursery personnel and infected infants	Meningitis at 2–12 weeks of life with 20–40% mor- tality	
E. coli (gram- negative)	Mother (initial case in nursery); hands of nursery personnel for subsequent cases	Diarrhea Sepsis Meningitis	Until recently the leading cause of neonatal sepsis
Aerobacter (gram- negative)	Intubation Surgery	Pneumonia Sepsis	
Klebsiella (gram- negative)		Meningitis	
Staphylococcus	Nursery personnel, particularly hands of personnel; other infants	Septicemia (Phage I group) Skin infection- scalded skin syn- drome (Phage II group)	
Pseudomonas (gram-negative)	Respiratory equip- ment; bottles of distilled water and so on; sink traps	Bacteremia Pneumonia Meningitis	Difficult to treat

closely observed, for they are usually very sick. A septic baby in a normal term nursery should be transferred to a high risk nursery to protect other healthy infants as well as to assure him the special care he needs.

In addition to the supportive treatment that all sick newborns need, babies with sepsis receive parenteral antibiotics. Because drugs are excreted more slowly by the immature kidneys of newborns, blood levels of antibiotics remain high for a longer period of time than in older children and adults. Therefore, a 12 hour schedule is usually

satisfactory. Dosage is calculated on the basis of body weight. Antibiotics commonly used in the care of new-borns are listed in Table 18–9.

Four antibiotics have been found to be highly toxic to newborn infants: the sulfa drugs, tetracycline, chloram-phenicol, and potassium penicillin. The sulfas compete with bilirubin for albumin-binding sites and can thus cause kernicterus and death at levels of serum bilirubin that would generally be considered safe. Tetracycline inhibits the linear growth of infants because it is deposited in the growing epiphyses and

Table 18–9   ANTIBIOTICS FREQUENTLY GIVEN TO NEONATES WITH SEPSIS

Drug	Dosage	Route	Expiration after Mixing	Comment
Ampicillin	200 mg./kg./day (every 6 hours)	IV or IM	1 hour	Against certain gram-negative organisms, along with kanamycir
Carbenicillin	200–400 mg./kg./day (every 2–4 hours)	IV only	72 hours	Used only for Pseudomonas in newborn
Gentamicin	3–7.5 mg./kg./day (every 12 hours preterm; every 8 hours term)	IM	Indefinite	Against staphylococci and resistant gram-negative organisms
Kanamycin	15 mg./kg./day (every 12 hours)	IM	Indefinite	Against gram-negative organisms, except Pseudomonas, not used more than 12 days
Nafcillin	100–200 mg./kg./day (every 6 hours)	IV or IM	48 hours	Nephrotoxic; watch for hematuria
Penicillin G	100,000–200,000 units/kg./day (every 12 hours)	IV or IM	72 hours	Against gram-positive organisms
Polymyxin	2–2.5 mg./kg./day (every 6 hours)	Deep IM		Most effective agent against Pseudomonas; nephrotoxic

also causes permanent yellow-green staining of the enamel of the baby teeth (as does the ingestion of tetracycline by the mother during late pregnancy). Chloramphenicol, because it is poorly excreted by newborns, can lead to sudden collapse and death. This is known as the "gray baby" syndrome. Potassium penicillin can cause heart block in infants.

Parents must receive careful explanations when sepsis is suspected or proved. They need to understand why their baby has been moved from the regular nursery, if this is the case, and what special care is being given to him.

They will need all of the kinds of support described in more detail in Chapter 22

INFANTS WITH CONGENITAL HEART DISEASE

About 7.5 babies out of every 1000 will have congenital heart disease Slightly more than 2 infants of every 1000 will have defects serious enough to require attention during the newborn period. Congenital heart disease is a major cause of death in term infants and contributes to death in preterm infants

By careful nursing assessment, in

many instances we may detect early clues that a baby has a heart defect. In this section we will discuss only those aspects of congenital heart disease significant during the first days of life. For a more detailed discussion of heart defects, see pediatric nursing texts and the texts of Avery[2] and Klaus.[31]

Recognizing the Baby with a Cardiac Defect

Cyanosis is a sign of certain heart defects. The most common cyanotic heart conditions are *transposition of the great vessels* (Fig. 18–17) and *tetralogy of Fallot* (Fig. 18–18).

Transposition needs attention during the first hours of life because the blood perfusing the baby's body is not reaching his lungs and therefore carries no oxygen. Some oxygenated blood may be carried throughout the system because of other congenital conditions, such as a patent ductus arteriosus (below). Babies with transposition have marked cyanosis from the time of birth.

Initial treatment of transposition is a palliative procedure, a balloon septostomy, in which a deflated balloon, introduced during cardiac catheterization, is pulled back through the atrial septum at the site of the foramen ovale, creating an opening that will allow mixing of arterial and venous blood (Fig. 18–19). Corrective surgery is deferred until the baby is older and larger.

Tetralogy of Fallot involves four major defects:

1. Pulmonary stenosis.
2. Ventricular septal defect.
3. Overriding aorta.
4. Hypertrophy of the right ventricle.

Babies with tetralogy of Fallot may have varying levels of cyanosis and mild tachypnea soon after delivery, or they may be asymptomatic for 1 or 2 months. If they are severely hypoxic, they may be hypotonic and have low blood pressure and bradycardia. Surgery is performed in the neonatal period only when symptoms are severe.

Dyspnea is an important symptom of infant cardiac disease, as well as of respiratory problems in newborns.

Tachycardia, with rates consistently above 60 beats per minute and as high as 200 beats per minute, may precede the appearance of other symptoms.

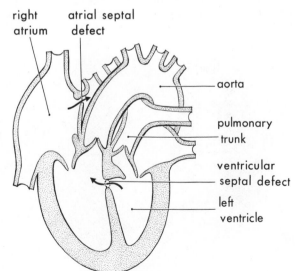

Figure 18–17 Diagram of a heart illustrating complete transposition of the great arteries. The ventricular and atrial septal defects allow mixing of the blood. (From Moore: *The Developing Human: Clinically Oriented Embryology.* 2nd Ed. Philadelphia, W. B. Saunders Co., 1977.)

right atrium

atrial septal defect

aorta

pulmonary trunk

ventricular septal defect

left ventricle

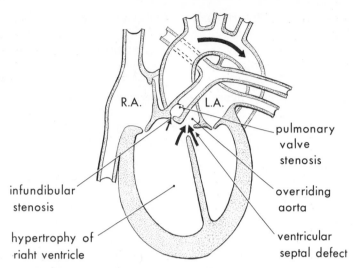

R.A.

L.A.

pulmonary
valve
stenosis

infundibular
stenosis

overriding
aorta

hypertrophy of
riaht ventricle

ventricular
septal defect

Figure 18–18 Frontal section of a heart illustrating the tetralogy of Fallot. (From Moore: *The Developing Human: Clinically Oriented Embryology*. 2nd Ed. Philadelphia, W. B. Saunders Co., 1977.)

Murmurs may be heard during the first days following birth. However, some murmurs heard during this period are "functional," i.e., they do not indicate pathology. On the other hand, pathology may exist during the first days without causing a murmur, which will appear later. Recognition of varying types of murmurs comes only with practice, but it is a skill well worth developing. Significant murmurs often do not appear until the third day of life, as the change from fetal to neonatal circulation stabilizes. If babies are discharged from the hospital before the third day, as a great many are, a follow-up physical examination should be done much earlier than the traditional 4 to 6 weeks, in order to detect possible heart conditions unrecognized in the nursery.

Failure to feed well and other signs that the baby is not behaving as he should may be the earliest symptoms of a cardiac defect, again usually recognized initially by the nurse.

Figure 18–19 Medical creation of an atrial septal defect in transposition of the great arteries. The method of Rashkind and Miller. The anteroposterior projection of the particular cine frame shown was recorded as the balloon filled with 3 ml. contrast medium passed without deformity through the created defect. (From Rowe and Mehrizi: *The Neonate with Congenital Heart Disease*. Philadelphia, W. B. Saunders Co., 1968.)

A *widened pulse pressure* may be a symptom of patent ductus arteriosus (Fig. 18–20). In intensive care nurseries, where blood pressure is usually monitored routinely, it is not difficult to note a widened pulse pressure. Should blood pressure be monitored, perhaps once a day, in all newborns?

Nurses should check *femoral pulses* in all babies during their daily bath. Bounding femoral pulses are associated with patent ductus arteriosus. Because the ductus arteriosus often remains open if the Pao₂ is below 50, babies with respiratory distress syndrome often have a patent ductus. In addition to the bounding femoral pulse, they also have a bounding posterior pedis pulse. If the ductus is large and blood is shunted from the systemic circulation to the lung, the baby may have congestive heart failure (below). Treatment may at first be with digoxin (Lanoxin), furosemide (Lasix), and other medications. If symptoms of congestive failure persist after medical treatment, the ductus is surgically ligated.

The absence of femoral pulses is usually a sign of *coarctation of the aorta* (Fig. 18–21). Babies with coarctation have good carotid and radial pulses. They may have no other symptoms during the first days of life, but signs of congestive failure may occur when they are 10 to 15 days old. Babies with coarctations may also be hypoglycemic because of decreased blood supply to the liver.

The most frequently occurring of all congenital heart defects, the ventricular septal defect (VSD) (Fig. 18–22), is rarely symptomatic in the newborn period because the normally high pressure in the blood vessels of the lung prevents shunting from the left side of the heart to the right side through the defect. As pulmonary pressure drops, from the second week to the third month after birth, blood is shunted from the left to the right side of the heart through the VSD. The lungs are flooded, and signs of congestive heart failure develop. Banding of the pulmonary arteries is a palliative procedure to keep blood from flooding the lungs. When the baby is larger (over 20 pounds), the septal defect itself is repaired and the band removed.

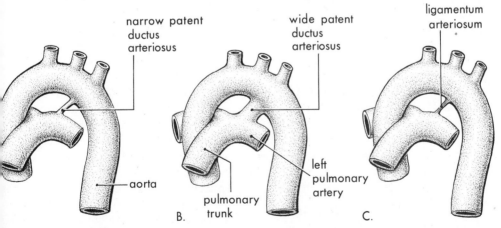

Figure 18–20 *A,* The ductus arteriosus of a newborn infant. The ductus is normally patent for about 2 weeks after birth. *B,* Abnormal patent ductus arteriosus in a six month old infant. The ductus is nearly the same size as the left pulmonary artery. *C,* The ligamentum arteriosum, normal remnant of the ductus arteriosus, in a six month old infant. (From Moore: *The Developing Human: Clinically Oriented Embryology.* 2nd Ed. Philadelphia, W. B. Saunders Co., 1977.)

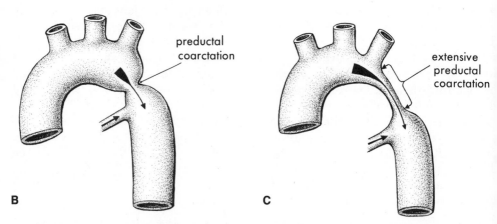

Figure 18-21 *A,* Postductal coarctation of the aorta, the commonest type. *B* and *C,* Preductal coarctation. The type illustrated in C is usually associated with major cardiac defects. (From Moore: *The Developing Human: Clinically Oriented Embryology.* 2nd Ed. Philadelphia, W. B. Saunders Co., 1977.)

It is important to understand why symptoms are delayed, because parents often feel that a diagnosis was missed or that their baby was not carefully examined at birth, when in fact it was not possible to recognize the defect at that time.

Diagnosis of Cardiac Defects

Once a heart defect is suspected, diagnosis is made on the basis of:

1. Clinical signs that have been observed and recorded.

2. X-ray.

3. Electrocardiogram (EKG).

4. Cardiac catheterization.

The clinical signs associated with individual defects have already been mentioned. The role of X-ray in evaluating heart size and some outstanding anatomic changes seems obvious. It is very important that the baby be comfortably at rest and not crying when chest films are taken, if they are to be detailed enough to be of any real value. Portable chest films can be taken through isolette walls. If the baby is to

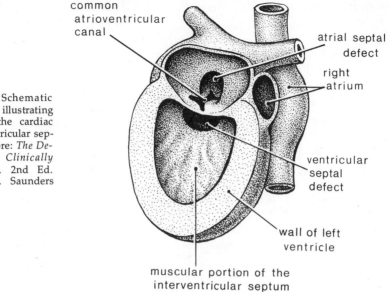

common
atrioventricular
canal

atrial septal
defect

right
atrium

ventricular
septal
defect

wall of left
ventricle

muscular portion of the
interventricular septum

Figure 18–22 Schematic drawing of a heart illustrating various defects of the cardiac septa, including ventricular septal defect. (From Moore: *The Developing Human: Clinically Oriented Embryology*. 2nd Ed. Philadelphia, W. B. Saunders Co., 1977.)

o to the X-ray department for films, he eeds to be transported in a heated bed nd to spend as little time as possible utside of it. A nurse should go with him nd remain with him throughout the ntire procedure, wearing a protective pron to shield her from radiation while he pictures are being taken. A bottle of ater or a pacifier will help to soothe the aby and keep him from crying. A bulb yringe for suctioning and a hand-perated bag resuscitator should go ith the baby; infants at times become pneic in X-ray departments and other reas of the hospital away from the nur-ery, and equipment for resuscitation is ot always immediately available. Iouth-to-mouth resuscitation can be sed in an acute emergency, of course, ut there is always a risk of introducing athogens into the respiratory tract of n already sick baby. How much easier is to be prepared.

Electrocardiograms of newborns iffer from those of children from age 2 ears through adulthood, and those of remature infants often vary from the

EKG's of term babies. The problems involved in the interpretation of newborn EKG's are beyond the scope of this book (see Rowe and Mehrizi,[53] Chapter 4). As with babies who are to be X-rayed, the infant should be warm and comfortable, with a full stomach, so that he will lie quietly during the procedure.

Cardiac catheterization presents a somewhat different problem in the newborn period than those problems encountered in other periods. Yet catheterization is highly essential; those conditions that can be treated must be distinguished from those that cannot. Although the mortality rate in newborns is in the neighborhood of 5 per cent, a large proportion of the babies who die have inoperable defects and would have died under any circumstances. Nevertheless, it is a hazardous procedure during the newborn period for several reasons:

1. The hazards of chilling the baby during the procedure are greatest in newborns.

2. The baby is often in very serious

condition before the catheterization—
he may be cyanotic or acidotic or in congestive failure.

3. Needle punctures and even traction on small vessels can cause thrombosis and impair circulation.

4. Catheterization in newborns is often combined with angiography so that an accurate anatomic diagnosis can be made, thereby necessarily increasing the risk.

5. Full exploration of the heart, rather than just right-heart catheterization, is felt to be necessary in a great many instances.

Measures that minimize the risk include:

1. Early detection of the possibility of a heart defect before the baby is critically ill.

2. Avoidance of premedication and anesthesia; local anesthesia and a cutdown are used. The umbilical artery is sometimes used during the first days of life.

3. Treatment of acidosis with bicarbonate.

4. Treatment of serious arrhythmias by electrical conversion.

5. The use of a minimum of contrast material.

Once the baby returns from catheterization, there must be careful monitoring of temperature, which often drops during the procedure; of apical pulse and respiration; and of acid-base balance and fluid intake. The cut-down site needs to be checked for bleeding, and the color and pulsation in the limb in which the cut-down was done should be observed. Thrombosis is a particular danger in tiny newborn vessels. If there is no pulse 4 hours after the study has been completed, arterial thrombosis has usually occurred. Fortunately, collateral blood supply usually prevents gangrene, but occasionally surgery will be necessary.

Recognizing Signs of Congestive Heart Failure

The signs of impending congestive heart failure may be very similar to the symptoms just described as evidence for the presence of heart disease. Cyanosis and dyspnea are almost always present. The liver, normally 1.5 cm. below the right costal margin with a sharp edge, is down to 3 cm. below the margin, with the edge feeling round and firm. Frequently a gallop rhythm can be recognized, in which three sounds are heard, as if a horse were galloping (in rhythm with the word "Tennessee").

Caring for the Baby with Congenital Heart Disease

Although care will vary with the type of heart lesion and the severity of symptoms, there are common principles. Care focuses on observation and support of the baby in the hospital and teaching his parents to care for him after discharge.

For the baby with a cardiac problem who is having respiratory distress, the semi-Fowler's position is often helpful. The mattress may be supported at an angle, or an infant seat can be used. Be sure that the baby maintains good position in the infant seat, and show his parents how they can do this at home. A diaper roll under the shoulders may be an additional help to breathing. Watch for abdominal distention, which can lead to respiratory embarrassment. Distention may be relieved by passing an oral gastric tube and gently aspirating the stomach.

Digoxin is given to babies with symptoms of heart failure. The digitalizing dose of digoxin is 0.04 to 0.0

mg./kg./day. Maintenance dosage is 0.01 mg./kg./day. The daily dose is usually given in separate doses at 12 hour intervals. Giving these very small doses requires great care in calculation and preparation. A second nurse should always be asked to check the dosage before it is given. If the baby is to receive 0.0025 mg., a dose of 0.025 mg., which seems very small, is actually ten times greater than that prescribed.

The dose is withheld if the heart rate is below 100 beats per minute, until we check with the physician. Often a rhythm strip (EKG) is run prior to giving the medication; lengthening of the P-R interval is a sign of digoxin toxicity. Other signs of toxicity are vomiting, diarrhea, and evidence of heart block on EKG.

A weight gain of more than 2 per cent indicates accumulation of fluid. Furosemide (Lasix) may be ordered as a diuretic. The intravenous dose is 0.5 to 1.0 mg./kg.; the oral dose is 1.0 mg./kg. A record of output may be kept by using an infant urine bag (be sure to give very good skin care) or by weighing diapers before and after use. Intake must also be monitored carefully. The baby who is acutely ill will probably be receiving intravenous fluids, which must be checked hourly to avoid overloading. We need to observe carefully for air bubbles in all intravenous lines, but particularly in those lines for babies who have intracardiac shunts.

Babies with heart disease often feed slowly, tiring easily. Parents need ample opportunity to feed their baby before taking him home so they can become accustomed to his ways. The baby will usually do best when he is held in an upright position and allowed to rest frequently. He may need to be burped after every 1/2 to 1 ounce. Because he is able to take less formula at a feeding, he is usually fed every 3 hours rather than every 4 hours. If we fail to help the mother understand his special feeding needs before his initial discharge, the baby may be back in the hospital at an early date because he has failed to gain weight. Because the baby is easily fatigued, all of his care should be planned to allow him uninterrupted periods of rest.

Before their baby is discharged, the parents need to know:

1. What type of problem their baby has.

2. Specific symptoms that need to be brought to the physician's immediate attention (e.g., heart rate below 100 beats per minute) and how to reach help should they not have an individual physician or should he be unavailable.

3. How to count pulse rate.

4. How to give any prescribed medications.

5. Signs of digoxin toxicity.

6. How to use a thermometer to check the baby's temperature.

7. How to feed their baby.

They should also be told that their baby has an increased susceptibility to infection in such a way as to provide protection, but not overprotection—no easy task. In spite of the best of care, their baby may still get an infection, such as pneumonia, and may have to be readmitted to the hospital, adding to the guilt they already feel for failing to bear a "normal" child (Chapter 22). Counseling concerning the way they treat this baby in relation to the treatment of the other children in the family is also essential.

These babies and their families will have a long-term relationship with hospitals and doctors; our care during the first days of life will have a great influence on their feelings about that relationship.

HYPERBILIRUBINEMIA DUE TO BLOOD GROUP INCOMPATIBILITY

"Physiologic" jaundice was discussed in Chapter 17, and the hyperbilirubinemia of premature infants was covered earlier in this chapter. Jaundice may also reflect neonatal sepsis, intrauterine infection, and a number of relatively rare conditions. Hyperbilirubinemia caused by blood group incompatibility may be due to the Rhesus factor (Rh factor), to ABO incompatibility, or to minor blood groups.

Rh$_D$ Incompatibility

The genetic basis for Rh$_D$ incompatibility was discussed in Chapter 2.

As soon as the baby is delivered, blood is Rh typed and a Coomb's test for the presence of antibodies is done. The Coombs' test is important, in addition to blood typing, because a baby with negative blood who has a great many antibodies may type positive. If the Coombs' test is negative, there are no antibodies present, and the baby should have no difficulty from Rh$_D$ incompatibility. If the Coombs' test is positive, indicating that the infant's red blood cells are coated with antibodies, further blood studies are done (hemoglobin and hematocrit determinations, indirect bilirubin level and reticulocyte count).

Some D positive babies are in obvious distress at the time of birth. They are not immediately jaundiced, because the bilirubin produced in utero has been cleared through the placenta, although the cord may be stained yellow. Commonly they are pale and edematous and have an enlarged liver and spleen. Blood studies show marked anemia, which can lead to heart failure and metabolic acidosis. Exchange transfu-

sion shortly after birth is usually necessary for these infants, whose condition is termed *hydrops fetalis*.

Erythroblastosis fetalis describes the condition of D positive babies who become significantly jaundiced, usually in the first 24 to 36 hours, from the high level of bilirubin that results from the destruction of their red blood cells by maternal antibodies at a rate so rapid that the liver cannot conjugate the bilirubin.

Not all babies with erythroblastosis require exchange transfusion. The decision is based on laboratory evaluation of hemoglobin levels (which indicate the destruction of the baby's red blood cells) and levels of bilirubin (which is the breakdown product of the destroyed red blood cell, as previously described); on the presence of signs of kernicterus (which always call for exchange transfusion at any level of bilirubin); and on other parameters that affect the binding of bilirubin to albumin (which were discussed earlier in this chapter in relation to the hyperbilirubinemia of prematurity). The blood for exchange transfusion is Rh negative, cross-matched with the infant's blood or type O. Phototherapy is usually used in conjunction with exchange transfusion.

ABO Incompatibility

ABO incompatibility exists in approximately 20 per cent of all pregnancies, but the incidence of severe hemolytic disease is very low. The mother is blood group O; the baby is blood group A or B. Antibodies to types A and B occur naturally in the plasma of type O individuals in response to A and B substances that are present in foods and in gram negative bacteria. Why some women develop high levels of antibody and others do not is unknown. It is the type A and B infants of those women with high antibody titers who may develop ABO disease. However, because there are a limited number of sites on the fetal red blood cells that will accept the antibody, the disease is usually not severe, and the Coombs' test may be only weakly positive.

There are no preventive measures against ABO incompatibility that can be taken during pregnancy. Unlike Rh_D incompatibility, ABO incompatibility may occur in first pregnancies. Occurrence in second and subsequent pregnancies does not produce more severe disease.

A Coombs' test on cord blood should be done at the time of delivery for the infants of all type O mothers. A positive Coombs' test will alert the nursery staff to the presence of antibodies.

Phototherapy, and occasionally exchange transfusion, is the treatment for ABO incompatibility if treatment is needed. Blood for exchange transfusion is always type O, with Rh factor the same as the baby's.

It is possible, of course, for a mother-infant pair to have both Rh and ABO incompatibility, as in the case of a type O D-negative mother with a type A or B D-positive baby.

Table 18–10 summarizes major factors in Rh and ABO incompatibility.

Minor Blood Groups

In less than 5 per cent of all infants with hemolytic anemia, a blood factor other than Rh_D, A, or B is involved. E, C, and the Kell (K) factors may be responsible for severe hemolytic disease and even for hydrops fetalis. The Coombs' test is positive. Very careful cross-matching with maternal serum is necessary, so that the blood used for transfusion will not contain the antigen responsible for maternal sensitization.

Table 18–10   COMPARISON OF Rh_D AND ABO INCOMPATIBILITY*

	Rh_D	ABO
BLOOD GROUP SET-UP		
Mother	Negative	O
Infant	Positive	A or B
CLINICAL ASPECTS		
Occurs in firstborn	5%	40–50%
More severe in subsequent pregnancy	Usually	No
Stillbirth and/or hydrops	Frequent	Rare
Severe anemia	Frequent	Rare
Degree of jaundice	—	—
Hepatosplenomegaly	—	—
LABORATORY FINDINGS		
Direct Coombs' test (infant)	Positive	Not always positive
Maternal antibodies	Always	Not clear-cut
TREATMENT		
Antenatal measures	Yes	No
Exchange transfusion		
Frequency	Approximately 66%	Approximately 10%
Donor blood type	Rh_D negative; group specific	Rh as infants; group O only
Late anemia	Common	Rare

*Adapted from Oski. *In* Avery: *Neonatology*. Philadelphia, J. B. Lippincott Co., 1975.

INFANTS WITH SPECIAL NUTRITIONAL NEEDS

The special feeding needs of preterm babies were mentioned earlier in this chapter. Other infants present feeding problems that may be mechanical (a cleft palate, for example, or the need for a gastrostomy tube) or physiologic (an inborn error in metabolism, for example).

The Infant with a Cleft Palate

Since the hard palate is essential to sucking, the baby with a cleft palate may have to be fed by some means other than breast or bottle. Some babies with cleft palates can be successfully bottle-fed; others seem to feed more easily with a Breck feeder. Only the tip of the nipple should be in the baby's mouth. Then, with a little practice, the baby will gently suck the tip. Nipple holes need to be small enough to keep the baby from being flooded with milk, which will then flow into his respiratory tract, depositing curds in the nasal passages and making the danger of infection of both the nasopharynx and the ears a very real possibility. Holding the baby upright to feed him also helps to prevent this regurgitation.

If the cleft is large, the baby may push the nipple up into the open area with his tongue. This can be avoided both by keeping most of the nipple outside of his mouth and by positioning it at an angle to the cleft.

Once the baby has begun to feed well, his mother should begin to feed him under nursing supervision. I am continually amazed at how well and how quickly many mothers are able to feed their babies with a Breck feeder. The baby is ready for discharge (barring other complications) when the mother feels comfortable about caring for him and feeding him.

The Infant with Gastrostomy Feeding

The most common reason for gastrostomy feedings in newborns is the repair of a tracheoesophageal fistula. The tube is inserted during surgery and sutured in place. Initial feedings of glucose and water (5 to 10 cc.) begin on the second to third day after surgery. If such feedings are well tolerated, they are followed by feedings of small amounts of milk, which are gradually increased as the baby shows his ability to handle these. Either vomiting or abdominal distention is a sign that feedings need to be decreased for a period.

The gastrostomy tube is connected through the hole in the top of the isolette to an Asepto-syringe without the bulb. It is never clamped until the baby is taking oral feedings and then only during the feedings themselves. This allows any gas and the contents of the baby's stomach to reflux up the tube and into the syringe when the baby cries or strains. Because of this reflux, there is no advantage to rinsing the tube with water after each feeding. If the baby is able to tolerate the extra amount of fluid that would be used to rinse the tube, his milk intake should be increased, giving him needed calories and nutrients as well as liquid.

The Infant with Phenylketonuria

Phenylketonuria (PKU) is an autosomal recessive disease (Chapter 2) that, when undetected, leads to irreversible mental retardation in affected infants. Mass screening for the presence of phenylalanine in urine or blood is now required by law in a number of states. This is only the preliminary step in the recognition of PKU, for there are other conditions in which phenylalanine is found in urine and blood. Children with conditions other than PKU will be harmed by a low phenyl alanine diet and by the use of Lofenalac, which is essential for children with PKU.

The dietary treatment of PKU must be constantly monitored by regular blood testing (daily during the first week, then weekly until the baby is 2 months old, twice a month from 2 months to a year, and monthly after that) and urine testing (daily during the first month, twice weekly until the baby is 6 months old, weekly until his first birthday, and twice a month from that time on). The reason for this constant monitoring—one that parents must understand—is that although a normal dietary level of phenylalanine will cause mental retardation, a diet too low in this essential amino acid will not meet the baby's growth requirements. In the newborn period the restriction of phenylalanine is met by the use of Lofenalac, with a small amount of cow milk added to the diet to provide the phenylalanine needed for growth. Later, strained foods low in protein are added to the diet.[25] Special dietary requirements are not necessary throughout life. Usually by the time a child is old enough to begin school, he can eat the same foods as his family and friends.

The Infant with Galactosemia

Like PKU, galactosemia is also inherited as an autosomal recessive trait. An infant with galactosemia lacks a specific enzyme, i.e., galactose-1-phosphate uridyl transferase. Because of this he is unable to metabolize lactose and galactose, so that galactose-1-phosphate accumulates in the red cells (hence galactosemia), and reducing sugars, for which specific tests are available, are found in the urine. Glucose, however, is not present in the urine.

The symptoms of galactosemia are not always easy to detect. Common findings are failure to gain weight and jaundice, which, unlike physiologic jaundice, persists beyond the first week. There may also be subcutaneous bleeding, vomiting, diarrhea, and subsequent dehydration. If the disease is not detected, the baby usually deteriorates progressively, developing physical and mental retardation, signs of malnutrition, cirrhosis of the liver, and cataracts.

The treatment is simple in theory. Since lactose occurs naturally only in milk, the newborn infant who shows signs of galactosemia is fed a formula, such as Nutramigen, that does not contain milk. Soybean formulas have also been found to be satisfactory if the baby does not have diarrhea. Problems in feeding arise as the baby grows older and needs a more varied diet, since milk and milk components such as lactose, casein, and whey are incorporated into so many commercial foods. Lactose, for example, is added to many canned and frozen fruits and vegetables during processing.

The removal of lactose from the diet changes the course of galactosemia markedly, even when the condition has gone unrecognized for several months. Appetite improves; vomiting, diarrhea, and jaundice subside; and liver function improves. In some instances, cataracts disappear.[8]

The Infant with Cystic Fibrosis

In the newborn nursery the recognition that a baby has an obstruction due to meconium ileus (thick, putty-like meconium) leads to the diagnosis of cystic fibrosis. Only about 10 per cent of cystic fibrosis babies are diagnosed this early; the remaining 90 per cent are recognized in later infancy or early childhood. Obstruction in the bronchi may not appear for weeks or even years after birth. The characteristic bulky, foul stools may or may not be evident in the newborn period.

Several dietary changes are necessary for babies with cystic fibrosis. Total caloric intake has to be increased because of the abnormally high loss of calories in stools. Fecal losses are reduced, but not entirely eliminated, by giving the baby pancreatic enzymes before each feeding. A formula is chosen that is high in protein and carbohydrate but has a low-to-moderate fat content, the fat being one that is readily absorbed. Fomon[25] suggests Olac as the best choice because corn oil is the source of fat; Nutramigen (which also utilizes corn oil) and Probana are also used. Banana flakes may be added to the diet to supplement caloric intake.

Water-miscible preparations of the fat-soluble vitamins A, D, E, and K are given to the baby. The dosage of vitamin D is adjusted according to blood levels of calcium, phosphorus, and alkaline phosphatase and to wrist X-rays, while the dosage of vitamin E is correlated with levels of blood alpha-tocopherol. The adequacy of vitamin K intake is determined by checking prothrombin times at intervals of 1 to 2 months.

The Infant of a Mother Addicted to Narcotics

As drug use among young women increases, as it has during recent years, the incidence of infants being born to mothers addicted to narcotics has increased. In some urban medical centers relatively large numbers of newborns addicted to morphine, heroin, and methadone are currently being seen. The problem for the nurse is to recognize these babies.

The most prominent sign is central nervous system irritability. The baby is frantic and inconsolable, he may have tremors, and the Moro response may be incomplete. His shrill cry is not unlike that of babies with central nervous system damage. In addition, there may be a large amount of mucus or such generalized symptoms as diarrhea and vomiting. Either excessive weight loss, because of fluid loss from vomiting or diarrhea, or failure to gain weight, because of a very high expenditure of energy, prevents these babies from growing normally in the nursery.

Since all these symptoms are common to many other kinds of newborn problems, it is important that the nurse be alert to signs of addiction in mothers, such as scarred veins and withdrawal symptoms, in order to evaluate the symptoms in babies. Addiction should be suspected and the possibility should be evaluated in mothers with venereal disease, hepatitis, cellulitis, and thrombophlebitis.

The diagnosis in the baby is confirmed by the discovery of narcotic breakdown products in the blood and urine. Specimens need to be collected shortly after birth, because these narcotic metabolites disappear quickly.

The care of addicted babies includes minimal handling, because of their hyperirritability; adequate hydration; and correction of any electrolyte imbalance. Phenobarbital and chlorpromazine (Thorazine) are the medications most commonly used for treatment; paregoric may be given for diarrhea. Methadone has been used experimentally for newborn withdrawal symptoms but is not, at the present time, commonly employed in treatment.

TRANSPORT OF THE HIGH RISK NEWBORN

When an infant with a condition that puts him at risk of serious illness or death is born in a community hospital, he may require transport to a large medical center in order to receive the specialized care he needs. The ideal form of transport is probably within his mother's uterus, with the delivery of the baby taking place in the medical center. This is occurring with increasing frequency, but it will never be possible for all high risk babies for two basic reasons.

First, not all high risk deliveries can be anticipated. Although some mothers can be identified as likely to produce a baby needing special care even before they become pregnant (for example, the mother with diabetes or the mother who has previously delivered a child with erythroblastosis; see Chapter 10), other mothers have sudden, premature labor, or have unanticipated difficulty during labor or delivery, or have a child with a major congenital anomaly without any prior indication. Under these circumstances baby transport will always be essential.

Second, even when a high risk baby is expected, it will not always be possible for the mother to leave her own community to be cared for in a hospital many miles away for a period of time that may involve 1 to 2 weeks or longer. Not only the economic cost but the social cost in terms of separation from husband and family may be too high. Planning for hospitalization of such a mother will have to include planning for all the needs of the family, not just for the mother's (and later the baby's) medical problems.

Systems of Transport

There are three basic ways in which newborn transport is accomplished, regardless of the mode of transport (ambulance, helicopter, fixed wing aircraft). A team (nurse and/or physician and/or respiratory therapist) may go from a med-

ical center to the referring hospital to begin intensive care from the moment they receive the baby, often in a specially equipped vehicle that is an intensive care unit in itself. Obviously such a vehicle is very expensive and by no means universally available. A team may also go from a medical center to receive the baby with far less in terms of equipment but with special experience in caring for the baby during transport.

The referring hospital may also have specially trained nurses or teams to send with the baby and have access to a modern transport incubator in which most babies can be cared for quite well. One problem with this system is if the community hospital sends its best trained person (who may be the only registered nurse in the neonatal area, or even in the entire obstetric area), their own coverage becomes inadequate.

A third possibility is to use emergency medical personnel to care for the baby during transport. It is essential that these men and women be given adequate initial training and continuing education in the care of high risk babies.

Before Leaving the Community Hospital

It is very important for the mother to *see and touch* her baby before the baby is moved to another hospital. Fathers often come with the baby or are able to see him soon after at the medical center. Mothers must remain in the community hospital for several days until the time of their own discharge. Over and over fathers tell us, "She (i.e., the mother) doesn't even feel like she has had a baby . . . it is totally unreal to her." Mothers share the same kinds of comments with us when they are able to come to the nursery several days later for the first time. (See also Chapter 22).

An explanation of why the baby must be transported is also essential. Parents will not understand a great deal of what we tell them at this time. They may hear nothing more than "we feel your baby should be transferred to the intensive care unit at the Medical Center." Later we will need to go back over what we have told them. But it is nevertheless important to give honest, realistic information prior to the transport of their baby. (Again, see Chapter 22 for further discussion.)

Physical preparation includes maintaining the baby's warmth; providing oxygen if it is needed; and starting intravenous glucose via umbilical artery catheter, if possible, or via a peripheral vein line. If an umbilical line cannot be inserted in the community hospital, leaving approximately 1 inch of stump when the cord is cut at delivery will make it easier to insert a catheter in the receiving hospital. Umbilical artery catheters can usually be inserted up to 24 hours after delivery; it is possible to insert an umbilical vein catheter for 5 days following birth.

Prophylactic vitamin K and silver nitrate should be given and charted, so that the dose will not be repeated at the receiving hospital. A gavage tube is passed into the stomach, and the contents are gently aspirated to prevent aspiration during transport. The baby must also be properly identified.

In addition to preparing the baby, records must be available to send to the receiving hospital. These include copies of:

1. The baby's record.
2. The mother's prenatal history and labor and delivery record.
3. The mother's admission sheet, which contains valuable information such as telephone numbers and places of employment that can facilitate communication.

Two tubes of the mother's blood, one clotted and one unclotted, and of the baby's cord blood, if available, should be sent.

Finally, it seems a simple thing to be sure that the gas tank of the ambulance is full, but our experience indicates that this phase of the transport plan is easily overlooked.

Care en Route

Throughout transport, warmth, oxygen, glucose, and suction continue to be essential.

The tremendous importance of *warmth* for all babies, and particularly for the high risk baby, has already been discussed in detail. A transport incubator that provides warmth as well as visibility is ideal. The battery should be fully charged at all times so that warmth is continuous. Alternatives include the careful use of hot water bottles filled at 105°F. (40°C.) (not really satisfactory but better than nothing at all) wrapping aluminum foil around the baby's blanket (good insulation but visibility, which is very important, is compromised), and wrapping the baby's arms and legs in cotton batting. This last measure, frequently used in baby surgery, is a useful adjunct to other methods and will reduce heat loss without compromising visibility.

The baby's temperature should be checked prior to transport and en route if the trip lasts more than an hour, and recorded in the nurse's notes.

Oxygen can be given by bag and mask during transport when it is needed. An extra full cylinder of oxygen should be taken along, for any lapse in oxygenation, even of short duration, can lead to possible brain damage. Plan for twice the amount of oxygen that you would appear to need (based on flow rate and amount of time in transport). The trip may be prolonged beyond the anticipated time. During a trip of more than 30 minutes, it is ideal to monitor oxygen concentration.

Hypoglycemia during transport is a major concern. How often a baby arrives at a medical center with an initial Dextrostix of 0, with no indication of how long his blood glucose has been that low. As noted above, glucose may be given through an umbilical artery catheter or through a peripheral line. Ten or 15 per cent is the common solution, given at approximately 10 cc. per hour for term infants and 3 to 4 cc. per hour for preterm babies. A battery-run infusion pump will assure a constant rate. Spare sterile supplies, both fluids and peripheral intravenous equipment, should be taken on the trip.

If it is not possible to get an intravenous started, some physicians suggest that a small amount of glucose may be gavaged into the stomach. If this is done, the baby must be transported on his abdomen with his head up to minimize the danger of aspiration.

A number of special points of care for specific conditions are summarized in Table 18–11.

A record of nursing care during transport is just as important as records kept in a hospital or health agency. The record should include:

Table 18–11 NURSING CARE DURING NEONATAL TRANSPORT

Condition	Special Points in Care
Tracheoesophageal fistula	Head must be elevated at a 45° angle Suction bubbly secretions in mouth and oral pharnyx
Pneumothorax	Normal side uppermost May have chest tube or needle to aspirate air Watch for sudden worsening of respiration and/or shift in position of apical heart sounds
Diaphragmatic hernia	Side with better lung function uppermost (usually is the right side) Head elevated so abdominal organs do not compromise limited lung function
Abdominal distention (e.g., intestinal block)	Nasogastric tube; aspirate gently with syringe and record amount aspirated
Exposed internal organs (e.g., gastroschisis, ectopic bladder)	Cover exposed internal organs with warm sterile saline dressings, then with Vaseline gauze. At high risk of heat loss because of exposed organs
Meningocele	Transport prone Use do-nut support around meningocele Cover with sterile saline dressing or dry sterile dressing
Hypognathia, Pierre Robin syndrome	Transport face down so that tongue will fall forward; tongue falling back will lead to respiratory obstruction
Choanal atresia or stuffy nose for some reason	Baby is obligate nose breather; to assist him to breathe through mouth, cut a large hole in a nipple and tape it to mouth
Eyelids open (as in severe facial palsy, occasionally in hydrocephalus)	Eye drops and ophthalmic ointment

1. Vital signs.

2. The type of fluids given, the rate, and the amount absorbed each hour.

3. The amount of oxygen given.

4. Observations of the baby's condition, including color, respirations, seizure activity, and so on.

SUMMARY

The concepts presented in this chapter serve only as an introduction to the care of newborn infants with special problems. Perinatal Nursing Standards (Appendix F) further indicate the scope of this special area of nursing practice. As in every type of practice, each day is a learning experience.

REFERENCES

1. Alfonso, D., and Harris, T.: Continuous Positive Airway Pressure. *American Journal of Nursing, 76:*570, 1976.
2. Avery, G. B.: *Neonatology.* Philadelphia, J. B. Lippincott Co., 1975.
3. Bliss, V. J.: Nursing Care for Infants with Neonatal Necrotizing Enterocolitis. *MCN,* January/February, 1976, p. 37.
4. Brown, J., and Helper, R.: Stimulation—A Corollary to Physical Care. *American Journal of Nursing, 76:*578, 1976.
5. Brown, J., Purvis, R., Forfar, J., et al.: Neurological Aspects of Perinatal Asphyxia. *Developmental Medicine and Child Neurology, 16:*567, 1974.
6. Chernick, V.: Continuous Negative Chest Wall Pressure Therapy for Hyaline Membrane Disease. *Pediatric Clinics of North America, 20:*407, 1973.
7. Chernick, V.: Continuous Distending Pressure in Hyaline Membrane Disease. *Pediatrics, 52:*114, 1973.
8. Cornblath, M., and Schwartz, R.: *Disorders of Carbohydrate Metabolism in Infancy.* 2nd Edition. Philadelphia, W. B. Saunders Co., 1976.
9. Cremer, R., Perryman, P., and Richards, D.: Influence of Light on Hyperbilirubinemia of Infants. *The Lancet, 1:*1094, 1958.
10. Dahl, N., and Frazier, S.: Neonatal Thermoregulation. Module 1 in the series:

The First Six Hours of Life. National Foundation/March of Dimes, 1976.
11. Dar, H., Winter, S., and Tal, Y.: Families of Children with Cleft Lips and Palates: Concerns and Counseling. *Developmental Medicine and Child Neurology, 16:*513, 1974.
12. Davis, J. A., and Dobbing, J. (eds.): *Scientific Foundations of Paediatrics.* Philadelphis, W. B. Saunders Co., 1974.
13. Drillien, C.: Abnormal Neurologic Signs in the First Year of Life in Low-Birthweight Infants. *Developmental Medicine and Child Neurology, 14:*575, 1973.
14. Dulock, H., and Swendsen, L.: Hypoglycemia in the Newborn. Module 2 in the series: *The First Six Hours of Life.* National Foundation/March of Dimes, 1977.
15. Dunn, D., and Lewis, A. T.: Some Important Aspects of Neonatal Nursing Related to Pulmonary Disease and Family Involvement. *Pediatric Clinics of North America, 20:*481, 1973.
15a. Dweck, H. S., Saxon, S. A., Benton, J., et al.: Early development of the tiny premature infant. *American Journal of Diseases of Children, 126:*28, 1973.
16. Fantz, R. L., and Fagan, J. F.: Visual Attention to Size and Number of Pattern Details by Term and Preterm Infants during the First Six Months. *Child Development, 46:*3, 1975.
17. Feigun, R.: The Perinatal Group B Streptococcal Problem: More Questions than Answers. *New England Journal of Medicine, 294:*1063, 1976.
18. Fisch, R., Gravem, H., and Engel, R.: Neurological Status of Survivors of Neonatal Respiratory Distress Syndrome. *Journal of Pediatrics, 73:*395, 1968.
19. Fisher, D., and Behrman, R.: Resuscitation of the Newborn Infant. *In* Klaus, M., and Fanaroff, Al (eds.): *Care of the High-Risk Neonate.* Philadelphia, W. B. Saunders Co., 1973.
20. Fitzhardinge, P.: Early Growth and Development in Low-Birth-Weight Infants Following Treatment in an Intensive Care Nursery. *Pediatrics, 56:*162, 1975.
21. Fitzhardinge, P., Pape, P., Arstikaitis, M., et al. Mechanical Ventilation of Infants of less than 1501 Gm. Birth Weight: Health, Growth and Neurologic Sequelae. *Journal of Pediatrics, 88:*531, 1976.
22. Fitzhardinge, P., and Ramsay, M.: The Improving Outlook for the Small Prematurely Born Infant. *Developmental Medicine and Childhood Neurology, 15:*447, 1973.
23. Fitzhardinge, P. M., and Stevens, E. M.: The Small-for-Date Infant: 1. Later Growth Patterns. *Pediatrics, 49:*671, 1972a.

24. Fletcher, A. B.: The Infant of the Diabetic Mother. *In* Avery, G. B. (ed.): *Neonatology.* Philadelphia, J. B. Lippincott Co., 1975.

25. Fomon, S. J.: *Infant Nutrition.* 2nd edition. Philadelphia, W. B. Saunders Co., 1974.

26. Gluck, L., and Kulovich, M. V.: Fetal Lung Development: Current Concepts. *Pediatric Clinics of North America, 20:*367, 1973.

27. Gregory, G. A.: Respiratory Care of Newborn Infants. *Pediatric Clinics of North America, 19:*311, 1971.

28. Gregory, G., Kitterman, J., Phibbs, R., et al.: Treatment of Idiopathic Respiratory Distress Syndrome with Continuous Positive Airway Pressure. *New England Journal of Medicine, 284:*1333, 1971.

29. Hubel, D. H., and Wiesel, T. N.: The Period of Susceptibility to the Physiological Effects of Unilateral Eye Closure i.a Kittens. *Journal of Physiology, 206:*419, 1970.

30. Jacobson, S.: Long Term Parenteral Nutrition Following Massive Intestinal Resection. *Nutrition and Metabolism, 14*(Suppl.):150, 1972.

31. Klaus, M., and Fanaroff, A. (eds.): *Care of the High-Risk Neonate.* Philadelphia, W. B. Saunders Co, 1973.

32. Korner, A., Kraemer, H., Hoffner, E., et al.: Effects of Waterbed Flotation on Premature Infants: A Pilot Study. *Pediatrics, 56:*361, 1975.

33. Krugman, S., and Gershon, A. A. (eds.): Infections of the Fetus and the Newborn Infant. *Progress in Clinical and Biological Research.* Vol. III. New York, Alan R. Liss, Inc., 1975.

34. Kuhns, L. R., Bednarek, F. J., Wyman, M. L., et al.: Diagnosis of Pneumothorax or Pneumomediastinum in the Neonate by Transillumination. *Pediatrics, 56:*355, 1975.

35. Lubchenco, L.: The Relationship of Fetal Size to Later Physical Growth of Prematurely Born Children. *American Pediatric Society Abstracts,* 1962, p. 45.

36. Lubchenco, L.: *The High Risk Infant.* Philadelphia, W. B. Saunders Co., 1976.

37. Lubchenco, L. O., Delevoria-Papadopoulos, M., Butterfield, L. J., et al.: Long-term Follow-up Studies of Prematurely Born Infants. I. Relationship of Handicaps to Nursery Routines. *Journal of Pediatrics, 80:*501, 1972.

38. Lubchenco, L. O., Delevoria-Papadopoulos, M., and Searls, D.: Long-term Follow-up Studies of Prematurely Born Infants. II. Influence of Birth Weight and Gestational Age on Sequelae. *Journal of Pediatrics, 80:*509, 1972.

39. Lucey, J. F., Wolk, T., Bottogi, J., et al.: A Flux Day—Observations on Factors Influencing the Light Environment of Infants. *Pediatric Research, 7:*169, 1973.

40. Mims, L. C., Estrada, M., Gooden, D. S., et al.: Phototherapy for Neonatal Hyperbilirubinemia—a Dose: Response Relationship. *Journal of Pediatrics, 83:*658, 1973.

41. Monif, G., Egan, E., Held, B., et al.: The Correlation of Maternal Cytomegalovirus Infection during Varying Stages in Gestation with Neonatal Involvement. *Journal of Pediatrics, 80:*17, 1972.

42. *National Study of Maternity Care.* Committee on Maternal Health, The American College of Obstetricians and Gynecologists. Chicago, 1970.

42a. Northway, W., Rosan, R., and Porter, D.: Pulmonary disease following respirator therapy. *New England Journal of Medicine, 276:*357, 1967.

43. O'Donnell, M., Ziegler, E., and Fomon, S. J.: Ingestas Recommendadas de Nutrientes para Prematuros en Crecumiento. *Archivio Argentinos de Dedeatr., 72:*126, 1974.

44. Oski, F.: Hematological Problems *In* Avery, G. B.(ed.): *Neonatology.* Philadelphia, J. B. Lippincott Co., 1975.

45. Palmquist, H.: The Effect of Heartbeat Sound Stimulation on the Weight Development of Newborn Infants. *Child Development, 46:*292, 1975.

46. Powell, L. F.: The Effect of Extra Stimulation and Maternal Involvement on the Development of Low Birth Weight Infants and on Maternal Behavior. *Child Development, 45:*106, 1974.

47. Raiha, N.: Biochemical Basis for Nutritional Management of Preterm Infants. *Pediatrics, 53:*147, 1974.

48. Rawlings, G., Reynolds, E., Stewart, A., et al.: Changing Prognosis for Infants of Very Low Birth Weight. *Lancet, 1:*516, 1971.

49. Reynolds, E., and Taghizadeh, A.: Improved Prognosis of Infants Mechanically Ventilated for Hyaline Membrane Disease. *Archives of Diseases of Children, 49:*505, 1974.

50. Rickard, K., and Gresham, E.: Nutritional Considerations for the Newborn Requiring Intensive Care. *Journal of the American Dietetic Association, 66:*592, 1975.

51. Robert M. F., Neff, R. K., Hubbell, J. P., et al.: The Association between Maternal Diabetes and the Respiratory Distress Syndrome. *Pediatric Research, 9:*370, 1975.

52. Robert, M. F., Raymond, K. N., Hubbell, J., et al.: Maternal Diabetes and the Respiratory Distress Syndrome. *New England Journal of Medicine, 294:*357, 1976.

53. Rowe, R. D., and Mehrizi, A.: *The Neonate with Congenital Heart Disease.* Philadelphia, W. B. Saunders Co., 1968.

54. Sausville, J., Sisson, T., and Berger, D.: Blue Lamps in Phototherapy of Hyperbilirubinemia. *Journal of IES,* January, 1972, p. 112.

55. Scopes, J. W.: Thermoregulation in the New-

born. *In* Avery, G. B. (ed.): *Neonatology.* Philadelphia, J. B. Lippincott Co., 1975.

56. Segal, S. (ed.): *Manual for the Transport of High Risk Newborn Infants: Principles, Policies, Equipment, Techniques.* Vancouver, Canadian Pediatric Society, 1972.

57. Smith, B. T., Giround, C., Robert, M., et al.: Insulin Antagonism of Cortisol Action on Lecithin Synthesis by Cultured Fetal Living Cells. *Journal of Pediatrics, 87*:953, 1975.

58. Snodgrass, G.: Seizures in Newborn Infants. *Developmental Medicine and Child Neurology, 16*:92, 1974.

59. Stahlman, M., Hedvall, G., Dolanski, E., et al.: A Six-Year Follow-Up of Clinical Hyaline Membrane Disease. *Pediatric Clinics of North America, 20*:433, 1973.

60. Tabb, P. A., Inglis, J., Savage, D. C. L., et al.: Controlled Trial of Phototherapy of Limited Duration in the Treatment of Physi-ological Hyperbilirubinemia in Low-Birth-Weight Infants. *Lancet, 2*:1211, 1972.

61. Warrner, R. A., and Cornblath, M.: Infants of Gestational Diabetic Mothers. *American Journal of Diseases of Children, 117*:678, 1969.

62. Wennberg, R. P., Schwartz, R., and Sweet, A. X.: Early Versus Delayed Feeding of Low Birth Weight Infants: Effect on Physiologic Jaundice. *Journal of Pediatrics, 68*:860, 1966.

63. Wiener, G.: The Relationship of Birth Weight and Length of Gestation to Intellectual Development at Ages 8 to 10 Years. *Journal of Pediatrics, 76*:694, 1970.

64. Zelson, C., Sook, J., and Casalino, M.: Neonatal Narcotic Addiction: Comparative Effects of Maternal Intake of Heroin and Methadone. *New England Journal of Medicine, 289*:1220, 1973.

Chapter 19

NORMAL PHYSIOLOGIC AND PSYCHOLOGIC VARIATIONS DURING THE PUERPERIUM: THE BASIS OF NURSING CARE

BY ORA STRICKLAND DAVIS, R.N., PH.D.

When labor is completed and the infant, placenta, and membrane have been delivered, the *puerperium*, also called the *puerperal period* or the *postpartum period*, has begun. The term puerperium usually refers to the 6 weeks of physical restoration that occur after parturition, wherein the reproductive organs are restored to their normal nonpregnant state. Rubin has extended the definition of puerperium to include the psychologic processes that occur after delivery.[14] She defines the puerperium as "a complex state of the childbearing experience, during which the physical and psychological work of gestation and delivery becomes final." The mother who has recently delivered an infant is often referred to as the *puerpera* or *parturient*.

The puerperal period is marked by rapid retrogressive and progressive changes in the mother's body. Retrogressive changes occur in the uterus, vagina, and genitalia, as these organs return to their nonpregnant state. Progressive changes occur in the breasts, as they are prepared for lactation. Psychologic and behavioral changes occur, as the mother adapts to the rapid physical changes common to the puerperal period and as she takes on her new role as mother. The puerperal period is an interval of physical and psychologic transition, and nursing care is based on the variations that occur during the puerperium.

ANATOMIC AND PHYSIOLOGIC CHANGES

THE PROCESS OF INVOLUTION

The term *involution* refers to the process by which the reproductive organs return to their normal size and functioning during the 6 week puerperium. However, not all of the changes of pregnancy are completely reversible. During pregnancy, physical modifications occurred gradually, but the process of involution is more rapid, with the most profound and distinctive changes occurring in the first 3 or 4 days of the postpartum period. As profound and rapid as these changes are, the process of involution is a normal physiologic process, and the normal postpartum period is not a period of illness. Because the physiologic changes associated with involution closely resemble pathologic problems, it is vital that the nurse understand the normal physiologic changes that occur during the puerperium and be able to quickly distinguish variations from the norm. Furthermore, these physiologic changes dictate and serve as the basis for a great deal of the nursing care provided to the postpartum woman.

Involution of the Uterus

Immediately after labor and delivery, the uterus is a large, flattened organ that weighs about 2 pounds and is about the size of a grapefruit. Its mucous surface is denuded, and the placental site is one large wound with exposed veins containing superficial thrombi. During the puerperium, remarkable retrogressive and restorative changes take place in the uterus, and by the end of the puerperal period the uterus is a much smaller organ that weighs approximately 60 to 80 grams. Its endometrial surface is epithelialized and ready for normal reproductive functioning again. These involutional changes in the uterus are caused by three main processes: (1) contraction of the uterus (2) autolysis of some of the protein substances of the cells of the uterine wall and (3) regeneration of the endometrium.

During pregnancy the walls of the uterus are thinned and stretched in order to accommodate the growing fetus and other products of conception. Immediately after placental expulsion, the uterine musculature contracts so that the walls of the uterus are thick and the anterior and posterior walls lie in close opposition. The fundus or corpus of the contracted uterus can be easily palpated through the abdominal wall as a solid mass of tissue between the umbilicus and the symphysis pubis. The contracted state of the uterus is one of nature's ways of preventing postpartum hemorrhage and reducing the bulk of the enlarged organ. Uterine contraction controls bleeding by compressing and sealing off the blood vessels that enter the area left denuded by the placenta. Therefore, as long as the uterus remains sufficiently contracted, the danger of excessive bleeding from the uterine cavity is reduced. The size and bulk of the uterus are also reduced as the uterus contracts because the muscle fibers become shorter.

Although the main mechanism that is responsible for the diminution in the size of the uterus is contraction, its reduction in size is also aided by the process of autolysis. In this process some of the protein materials in the cells of the uterus are reduced into simpler elements that are then absorbed by the bloodstream and are cast off, mainly in the urine. Thus, the nitrogen content of the urine greatly increases for several days because of the excretion of the components of broken-down protein. During the process of autolysis the uterine muscle cells become much smaller; however, the total number of muscle cells does not decrease greatly.

The approximate rate of the decrease in size of the uterus is estimated by noting the height of the uterine fundus in relation to the umbilicus. The

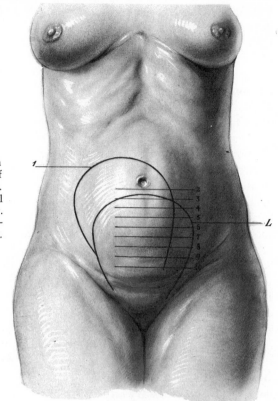

Figure 19–1 Frontal view of the abdomen indicating progressive changes in the height of the uterus postpartum with the bladder empty. *L*, Immediately after labor; *1* to *10*, fundal height on each successively numbered day. (From Greenhill and Friedman: *Biological Principles and Modern Practice of Obstetrics*. Philadelphia, W. B. Saunders Co., 1974.)

fundus is usually located below the level of the umbilicus immediately after delivery. It soon rises to the umbilical level, and about 12 hours after delivery the fundus is likely to be palpated a little above the umbilicus. The uterus then begins to decrease steadily in size and gradually descends into the pelvis as involution progresses. The diminution in the size of the uterus is reflected by the descent of the height of the fundus at a rate of about 1 fingerbreadth (1 cm.) each succeeding day (Fig. 19–1). Therefore, on the first day after the delivery the fundus of the uterus is palpable at 1 fingerbreadth below the umbilicus, on the second day postpartum at 2 fingerbreadths below the umbilical level, and so on. By the tenth to twelfth day it can no longer be felt through the abdominal wall.

Involution of the uterus tends to occur more rapidly in primiparas and in women who breast-feed their babies. In primiparas the rapidity of uterine involution is probably due to greater contractility of the uterine muscle because the woman's uterine muscle fibers are likely to be more elastic when only one full-term pregnancy has been experienced.

Secretion of oxytocin during breast-feedings, producing uterine contractions, is one explanation for the more rapid involution of the uterus during lactation. The diminished estrogen secretion during lactation may also be responsible for the more rapid uterine involution during lactation, since estrogens tend to enlarge the uterus.[7]

Methylergonovine maleate (Methergine) may be prescribed for some women for the first 3 to 5 days postpartum to encourage uterine contraction in an attempt to promote uterine involution. Adams and Flowers[1] found that methylergonovine administration had no appreciable effect on the amount of lochia flow nor on the fundal heights of women who had received the medication in comparison to those who did not receive it. Therefore, the administration of the drug seems to have minimal effect on the progress of involution. In addition, those who received methylergonovine complained of much more discomfort resulting from uterine cramping.

Nursing Care. Observation of the consistency and height of the fundus is an important aspect in the nursing care of the postpartum mother. These observations should be made at least every 15 minutes during the first hour after delivery and then at least every 4 hours for the next 23 hours. Daily observations are necessary on subsequent days. The uterus should feel firm upon palpation. A mother with a "flabby" uterus is likely to bleed heavily or hemorrhage. A well-contracted uterus seals off the open blood vessels at the former placental site and decreases blood loss.

As noted in Chapter 13, when palpating for the fundus, the nurse should first support the lower portion of the uterus with one hand, which is placed just above the symphysis pubis. The other hand is then used to palpate for the fundus. (See Chapter 13, Figs. 13–16 and 13–17.) The consistency and height of the fundus are then noted. If the uterus is not firmly contracted and the fundus feels soft or "flabby," the nurse should gently massage the uterine fundus with one hand until it is firm, while keeping her other hand in the position as described above to support the uterus. Care should be taken

not to overmassage the fundus because overstimulation can cause overcontraction of the fundus and subsequent muscle fatigue. If blood and clots have been retained in the uterine cavity, they should be gently expressed from the uterus with one hand while the other hand supports the lower portion of the uterus. Force should not be used while expressing clots from the uterus. Gentle pressure is all that is required.

Usually the fundus will be palpated at the midline of the abdomen rather than at either side. However, the ligaments that support the uterus are stretched and loose after delivery, and the uterus easily becomes displaced within the abdomen until these ligaments recover their tone. Therefore, observations of the fundal height should be made after the bladder is emptied, since a full bladder will displace the uterus and invalidate the measurement. A full bladder may push the uterus upward several centimeters, usually to the right side of the abdomen (Fig. 19–2). A distended colon can also cause a similar effect.

Observation of the rate of uterine involution by measurement of fundal height is important, and any marked

Figure 19–2   The uterus pushed up by a full bladder. (From Davis and Rubin: *De Lee's Obstetrics for Nurses.* 18th Ed. Philadelphia, W. B. Saunders Co., 1966.)

delay should be reported to the physician. Failure of the uterus to decrease progressively in size is an indication that involution is not proceeding satisfactorily. Failure of the uterus to return progressively to its normal size and condition within 6 weeks after delivery is called *subinvolution*. Retained placental fragments and infection are conditions that slow down the progress of involution and are among the most common causes of subinvolution.

Regeneration of the Endometrium

Just as the endometrium must undergo certain specific changes to prepare for pregnancy (Chapter 6), after delivery it must prepare to resume nonpregnant functioning. At the time of delivery both the placenta and membranes separate from the spongy layer of the decidua, leaving a portion of the decidua in the uterus. The denuded placental site is a raw, open surface that is infiltrated with blood. If we can imagine this jagged, bloody wound surface, it is not difficult to understand why so many new mothers died from infection in generations past and why protection from infection is still a vital part of care in the puerperium.

Within 2 or 3 days, the portion of the decidua that remained in the uterus after delivery becomes differentiated into two layers as healing begins. Leukocytes invade the remaining decidua, and a layer of granulation tissue is formed, which separates the necrosing, sloughing decidua on the surface from the deeper, healthier layer. This granulation tissue serves as somewhat of a protective barrier against infection. The superficial layer of the decidua then is cast off in the discharge from the uterus, referred to as the lochia (see below), leaving an inner layer adjacent to the uterine musculature. This remaining inner layer contains connective tissue and the bases of uterine glands. This is the source from which a new endometrium will regenerate. The regeneration of the endometrium is rapid except at the former placental site, which requires up to 7 weeks to heal completely. Elsewhere the endometrium is restored in about 3 weeks. The large blood vessels of the placental area that were present during pregnancy become invaded by fibroblasts, and there is recanalization of some of the vessels with smaller lumens.

The Lochia

After delivery, there is a vaginal discharge that usually persists throughout much of the puerperium, termed *lochia*. The amount and quality of lochia vary from day to day as involution progresses and provide an index of the healing process by which the endometrium of the uterus regenerates. Initially, the lochia consists of blood, along with small amounts of decidua and mucus, and occasionally contains vernix caseosa, lanugo, and meconium. Because the appearance of the lochia varies in the days following parturition, it has been classified into three groups according to its characteristics: lochia rubra, lochia serosa, and lochia alba (Table 19–1).

The early discharge is called *lochia rubra* because of its dark red color and persists for 3 or 4 days. Since the bleeding from the placental site is more copious during the early puerperium, lochia rubra consists mainly of blood. As the blood vessels of the placental site become thrombosed, the oozing of blood from the healing surface diminishes. Then the lochia appears as a sanguineserous discharge called *lochia serosa,* which is pink or a serous brown-red. Between the tenth to fourteenth day of the puerperium the lochia becomes

Table 19-1 LOCHIA

Type	Characteristics	Components	Duration
Lochia rubra	Consists mainly of blood	Blood Shreds of decidua Vernix (occasionally) Lanugo (occasionally) Meconium (occasionally)	3 or 4 days following delivery
Lochia serosa	Pink to red-brown Creamy consistency	Serous exudate Leukocytes Erythrocytes Shreds of degenerating decidua Cervical mucus Micro-organisms	From third or fourth day to 14 days postpartum
Lochia alba	Resembles cream	Decidual cells Leukocytes Epithelium Cells from uterus Mucus Bacteria	From tenth to fourteenth day until 6 weeks postpartum (may stop earlier)

thinner and greatly decreased in amount and assumes a yellowish or whitish color. These are the characteristics of *lochia alba,* which may last up to 6 weeks' postpartum.

At first the lochial discharge is somewhat heavy, but it gradually diminishes over time. The presence of frank, fresh bleeding from the vagina, however, is not normal at any time. Neither should there be large clots or a persistence of bright red blood in the lochia. In the first hour after parturition the woman can be expected to saturate no more than two perineal pads. During the next 8 hours a perineal pad may be saturated within 2 to 4 hours. After the first 8 hours, the vaginal discharge is not much heavier than a regular menstrual flow. Excessive lochia may indicate a relaxed uterus. If this is the case, corrective massage of the fundus should be done immediately. Excessive loss of blood should be reported immediately.

There is great variation in the amount of lochial flow in an individual mother and among mothers. The total discharge ranges from 150 cc. to 400 cc., but the average is about 225 cc. Multiparas tend to have more profuse lochia than primiparas. Mothers who breast-feed generally have a lesser amount of discharge, though there may be a temporary increase while the infant is nursing. During the night, when the mother is in a recumbent position, the lochial flow is less than during the day. Mothers who have had cesarean sections tend to have scanter lochia. The amount of discharge is increased when the mother is more active and when she is out of bed, particularly for the first time. If the woman has not been told that this is common, she may be frightened by the increase in lochial flow when she is more active.

Because the characteristics of the lochia are indicators of the progress of involution and the restorative changes of the uterine lining during the puerperium, it is vital to judge whether the discharge is or is not normal.

First, the *lochia should not be excessive in amount.*

Second, although the odor of lochia

varies, *lochia should never have an offensive odor*. The odor of the lochial discharge is determined by the kind of bacteria present in the vagina of an individual patient. A highly unpleasant odor of the lochia suggests infection, decomposing clots, or perhaps a retained sponge or packing. Investigation is imperative.

Third, *there should not be large pieces of tissue in* the lochia. The passage of distinguishable tissue in the lochia, particularly when accompanied by complaints of severe discomfort, may be indicative of retained placental fragments or membranes. If involution is to progress satisfactorily, tissues that are retained after delivery must be removed, since this predisposes the mother to hemorrhage and subinvolution. Passage of tissue in the lochia should be reported promptly.

Fourth, *lochia should not be absent* during the first 3 weeks of the puerperium. Normally, the flow of lochia does not cease until the endometrium is healed and the uterus has returned to its normal size and position in the pelvis. Supression of lochia may indicate postpartum uterine infection.

Finally, *the characteristics of the lochia should proceed from rubra to serosa to alba*. Once a mother's lochial flow has progressed to serosa or alba, there should not be a red flow of lochia again. An exception to this is when a mother has received a prolonged course of estrogen therapy for the suppression of lactation. The lochial discharge contains more red blood and increases somewhat in amount after such therapy.

The Cervix

The cervix, which became stretched and edematous during the birth process, is a soft, flabby, collapsed structure immediately after delivery. It is very succulent and may be bruised and infiltrated with blood and fluid. However, during the puerperium the cervix rapidly regains its tone, and small lacerations sustained during labor heal.

Within 18 hours after delivery the soft, spongy cervix becomes firmer and shorter. The cervical canal becomes progressively smaller, so that although two fingers can be passed through the internal os into the uterus on the second postpartum day, by the twelfth day only one finger can reach the internal os, but the finger cannot be passed through it into the uterus. By the fourth week the external os is a small, transverse slit in contrast to the oval pregravid external os. Once a woman has experience vaginal delivery, the external os of the cervix never regains its pregravid state. Although the internal os is closed as before, the external os remains somewhat open and has lateral indentations at the site of lacerations. These permanent changes in the external os distinguish the multiparous woman from the nulliparous woman.

The Vagina

Restorative changes in the vagina progress slowly following a vaginal delivery. The vagina is a soft, enlarged, and smooth-walled passage during the first part of the puerperium. As in the uterus, the muscles of the vagina slowly contract to diminish its diameter. About the third week of the puerperium, the vaginal rugae begin to reappear. Lacerations sustained during the delivery usually heal readily. The vagina does not completely return to its nulliparous condition, however. Residual tags of the torn hymen, called *carunculae myrtiformes,* remain and are characteristic of parous women. The vaginal introitus will remain slightly more distended than before.

Because of the amount of stretching that the vagina endures during a vaginal delivery, some parents may be concerned about the possible effects that this will have later on coitus and sexual gratification. Usually, changes in the vagina as a result of a vaginal delivery do not interfere with sexual functioning after involution is completed. Perineal or Kegal exercises, previously described, can promote the restoration of muscle tone in the vagina and perineal area. In addition, perineal exercises can help in the immediate postpartum period by helping to reduce edema and improve circulation. The exercise is performed by contracting and relaxing the perineal muscles, as if trying to stop a voiding. This exercise is more effective if it is done five times in succession three or four times each day.

The External Genitalia or Perineal Region

The appearance of the external genitalia reflects the stress that was placed on the perineal region during the vaginal delivery. The mucous surface of the vulva has a deep red, velvety appearance for several weeks following delivery. The muscles of the pelvic floor may be torn and overstretched, and the perineal tissues may be infiltrated with bloody serum. For several weeks after the delivery, the blood vessels of the perineum are fragile, and capillary oozing may complicate any perineal surgery that may be performed. Lacerations and bruises are often evident around the clitoris, vaginal introitus, and labia minora, particularly in primiparas. An episiotomy, which is an incision of the perineum frequently made during the second stage of labor to prevent perineal lacerations, may also have been performed. Edema often becomes more pronounced within 24 hours after delivery, giving a puffy appearance to the perineum.

In the absence of infection, the episiotomy and the lacerations of the perineal region heal with little inflammatory reaction. Restoration of the tonicity of the perineum is surprisingly rapid and takes about 6 weeks. Both the labia minora and the labia majora ordinarily remain flaccid in the parous woman.

Perineal Care

Special attention should be given to cleaning the perineal region and to promoting perineal comfort for each postpartum mother. Although the perineum is anatomically the area between the vagina and rectum, perineal care is more inclusive and involves cleansing of the perineum along with the vulva and rectal area. This procedure is done to prevent infection because perineal wounds and the build-up of dried lochia in the perineal region are conducive to bacterial growth. At the same time, cleansing of the perineum promotes maternal comfort because the procedure is refreshing to the perineal region. Hence, frequent perineal care is necessary to prevent infection and to promote healing and maternal comfort.

Perineal care is usually administered by the nurse in the early postpartum period and offers an opportunity for the nurse simultaneously to inspect the perineum for edema, and to check for capillary effusion of blood into the tissues of the perineum and the presence of hemorrhoids. After the mother becomes ambulatory, this aspect of care is usually attended to by the mother herself but the nurse will still want to inspect the perineum at least once daily to assess the progress of healing and to observe any evidence of infection Perineal care is done as part of the daily bath and after each time that the mother voids or evacuates her bowels.

Even though hospitals differ as to the type of cleansing solutions and articles used to carry out perineal care, the basic principles of the procedure are the same. At one time perineal care was done as a sterile procedure in some hospitals, but now most nurses agree that it should be conducted as *clean* procedure requiring clean technique. Thus sterile water, sterile gloves, and sterile utensils are not necessary. Hand washing prior to initiation of the perineal care is required.

Some hospitals use soap or detergent solutions for cleansing of the perineum, and others use plain tap water. A pitcher or spray can, washcloths, cotton balls, or gauze sponges may be used in the procedure. As just mentioned, the hands should be washed thoroughly prior to beginning perineal care. A hip pad should be placed under the mother's buttocks to prevent soiling of the bed. The nurse should note the color, amount, and odor of the lochia as she removes the perineal pad. The perineal pad should be removed from front to back, and the cleansing of the perineal region should proceed from the pubis toward the anal area. This approach is taken to prevent the contamination of the vaginal vestibule by bacteria from the anus. It is most effective to clean the anal area first, except when disposable washcloths are used. With the mother on her side, the buttocks are gently separated, and the anal area is washed with cleaning solution, rinsed, and dried. The sponges used to clean the anal area are discarded immediately after use.

In hospitals in which a pitcher or spray can is employed to cleanse the perineum, the cleaning solution is poured over the perineum as the mother lies in a dorsal recumbent position. The perineum is then rinsed with plain tap water in the same manner. The labia should not be separated during the procedure, since neither cleaning solution nor water should be allowed to seep into the vagina. Gauze sponges or cotton balls are then used to dry the area. The labia are dried, starting from the pubis, using a single downward stroke, and each gauze sponge or cotton ball should be discarded after each stroke. This is repeated with as many cotton balls or sponges as are necessary to dry the area.

When gauze sponges or cotton balls are used to cleanse the perineum, a sponge is moistened with cleaning solution, and the labia are cleaned first, proceeding from the pubis downward to the perineum. A single downward stroke is made with the sponge, and this is repeated with as many moistened sponges as are necessary to clean the area. Each sponge is discarded after use. Drying is done by using the same procedure described with dry sponges.

If disposable washcloths are used instead of gauze sponges, a similar technique is also used. The washcloth is first moistened with cleaning solution, and the labia are cleaned on one side down to the perineum. The other side is cleaned in the same manner. Then the anal area is washed last, and the washcloth is disposed of. The same technique is used to rinse and dry the perineal region; however, a second washcloth is used for rinsing the area and a third one for drying.

The perineal region is likely to be sore and tender from the trauma of delivery. Hence, perineal care should be done gently.

Once perineal care has been administered, the mother will want to put on a clean perineal pad. Contamination of the surface of the perineal pad, which will be next to the vulva, should be avoided. Therefore, the pad should be grasped on the outside when it is applied. Application of the pad should be from front to back. The sanitary belt is fastened in the front first; then the back of the pad is secured.

Perineal Care by the Mother. When the mother is ambulatory or is allowed to get up to go to the bathroom, she should be shown how to administer her own perineal care. The equipment that is to be used should be explained to her, and she should be shown where it is kept. Often it is best to give the mother simple instruction in perineal care as the nurse carries out the procedure. This can be done prior to the time the woman becomes ambulatory. When the mother ambulates for the first time, the nurse will want to review the procedure with her again. This instruction should also include the principles of perineal hygiene. Handwashing prior to initiating the procedure and cleaning the vulva from front to back should be particularly emphasized.

Measures to Promote Perineal Comfort. Complaints of perineal tenderness and pain are common among mothers who have had a vaginal delivery. Perineal discomfort is most often experienced by primiparas, who generally are more likely to have an episiotomy at delivery, and by women who have had difficult vaginal delivery.

Having the mother use a pillow or rubber ring to sit on will help relieve pressure on the perineum and decrease discomfort. A mild analgesic such as aspirin, Tylenol, or Darvon, which has been prescribed by the physician, is also helpful. However, local methods of treatment are immediately soothing and are effective in promoting perineal comfort. Local anesthetic sprays and ice packs are helpful when the mother complains of "pulling" or "tight"

perineal stitches. Perineal care should be done just prior to the application of local anesthetic sprays. A few women may be allergic to such sprays. Therefore, mothers should be watched for signs of an allergic response, such as a rash or itching. If a perineal ice pack is used, it should be placed on the perineum for about 15 minutes. When a perineal ice pack is not readily available, one can be devised by placing crushed ice in a rubber glove and sealing it securely. The ice pack should then be wrapped with gauze before applying it to the perineal area.

Heat lamps and warm sitz baths are also used during the early puerperium to promote perineal comfort. In addition to being soothing to the mother, both of these treatments stimulate circulation in the perineal area and thus promote healing of the episiotomy. Warm sitz baths are usually administered two or three times a day for 15 to 20 minutes. Generally, plain warm tap water is used for sitz baths. Care should be taken to make sure that the water is not too hot. Most sitz bath units fit easily over the bathroom commode. At many hospitals, disposable sitz bath equipment is available, which the mother may take home with her at the end of her hospital stay. If disposable equipment is not available, the sitz bath unit should be sterilized between users.

When a heat lamp is used, the perineum is exposed to heat from a 25 watt bulb two or three times a day for 20 to 25 minute period. Perineal cleansing should be done just prior to starting the treatment. The mother is instructed to lie in the dorsal recumbent position. The heat lamp is placed between the woman's legs about 10 to 12 inches away from the perineum, making sure that it is not so close that the heat from the bulb will be too hot. The light is adjusted so that it shines directly on the perineal area. The mother can be easily draped with the bed linen when the treatment is in progress.

CLINICAL CHANGES IN OTHER BODY ORGANS AND SYSTEMS

Since pregnancy brings about both local and general physiologic alterations, it can be expected that puerperal changes will also involve local and general readjustments. As the new mother's reproductive system is adapted and restored to a nonpregnant state, so too are other body systems that have been changed or affected by the pregnancy or delivery. The puerperal alterations in other body systems occur in varying degrees, and in the physically healthy woman there should be no significant effects of pregnancy once the puerperium is complete.

The Urinary Tract

During pregnancy the ureters become markedly dilated and lose much of their tone. This is due in part to softening of walls of the ureters as a result of endocrine influences. During the postpartum period the ureters regain their tone and return to normal within 4 to 6 weeks.

Proteinuria is typical in the first few days following delivery. This increased nitrogen content of the urine is caused by autolysis or protein catabolism in the walls of the uterus, whereby muscle cells become smaller as protein is broken down into its components. Some of the products of protein catabolism are absorbed while others are eliminated in the urine. Proteinuria usually disappears about the third day postpartum.

Substantial amounts of sugar may also be present in the urine during the early weeks of the puerperium because of lactose absorption from the mammary glands into the bloodstream. This lactose sugar is subsequently excreted in the urine.

One of the most significant aspects of the puerperium is the large volume of urine excreted by the kidneys between the second and fifth postpartum days. This puerperal diuresis represents a reversal of the hydremia that was necessary for the nurture and support of the growing fetus during pregnancy. Since the increased extracellular fluid is unnecessary, its volume is reduced by copious urination. Sometimes the daily urine output of a postpartum mother may be as high as 3000 ml., and as much as 500 to 1000 ml. may be excreted at one voiding.

Spontaneous voiding during the first 8 hours of the puerperium may be very difficult or impossible for some puerpera. There are several reasons for this problem. The fetal head exerts a great deal of pressure on the urethra and trigone during the second stage of labor. As a result of the trauma of labor and delivery, some edema and loss of bladder tone are present for a short time after parturition. Pain from a sutured episiotomy or laceration may cause reflex spasm of the urethral muscle, making voiding very difficult. General swelling of the vulva may also inhibit voiding.

Another result of the trauma sustained during labor and delivery is a transient loss of some bladder sensation. Therefore, the puerpera is not as sensitive to a full bladder. The condition is found most often in women who have had long labors or an instrumentally assisted delivery. The mother may not void because she does not feel that her bladder is full, since there is a lack of a sensation to void. Anesthetics can have a similar effect on bladder sensitivity. A spinal anesthetic or general anesthesia given during childbirth may also interfere with bladder sensation, and, until their effects diminish, may predispose the woman to bladder distention.

Related Nursing Care. Since the newly delivered mother may not sense a full bladder, she should be encouraged to void, even though she may not feel a desire to do so. The puerpera should be offered the bedpan within the first 4 hours following childbirth. However, the nurse must not stick strictly by a timetable to determine when the patient needs to void. It is well to keep in mind that women who have received or who are receiving intravenous fluids are more likely to develop a full bladder. Assessment skills should be used to help determine when the mother has a full bladder.

The bladder may fill to such an extent that it rises and protrudes above the symphysis pubis. If markedly distended, it can easily be observed bulging between the uterus and the symphysis pubis. The uterus may be pushed upward and to the side of the abdomen. Palpation and percussion of the lower abdomen can also determine a full bladder. When palpated by the examiner's palm, the distended bladder feels like a soft fluid-filled sac, while the fundus feels solid and has a firmer tone. On percussion the uterus emits a dull sound, while a full bladder sounds more resonant. A full or distended bladder requires immediate attention. A full bladder can interfere with the contraction of the postpartum uterus and can render the mother susceptible to postnatal hemorrhage. A distended bladder further diminishes bladder tone and is a cause of urinary retention, which can lead to cystitis resulting from urinary stasis.

Voiding for the first time after delivery will be difficult for some mothers.

However, when a mother has difficulty voiding spontaneously, several steps should be taken to encourage bladder activity. Voiding can be stimulated by exposing the mother to the sound of running water in the sink or shower, having her dabble her fingers in warm water, pouring warm water over her wrist or vulva, and having her drink a warm beverage.

Ambulation facilitates urination. Hence, the mother who is allowed to ambulate early is less likely to have difficulty voiding. If the mother is confined to bed, the nurse can facilitate urination by helping her to be more comfortable when she needs to void. Interventions that can encourage urination when the puerpera must use the bedpan include providing her with privacy, offering a warmed bedpan, and helping her to assume a comfortable upright position with body support. An upright sitting position facilitates urination because of the pressure on the urethra.

Since the mother may not have a spontaneous awareness of her need to void, it is advisable to offer the mother the bedpan at 2 to 3 hour intervals during the first 24 hours postpartum. The urine should be measured and recorded after each voiding for the first day of the puerperium until there is some certainty that the bladder is emptying completely.

Once the puerpera has voided spontaneously for the first time, she will usually not have difficulty with urination on subsequent attempts. The nurse will want to watch for signs of residual urine by noting the amount of urine voided at each attempt. At least 100 ml should be voided to be considered sufficient. Large voidings are expected during the first few days. If, after several frequent voidings, the mother tends to excrete only small amounts of urine, residual urine may be present. It is likely that these voidings result from an overflow of a distended bladder. At this point the nurse will want to determine whether the bladder is empty by judging fundal height and position and by palpating and percussing the lower abdomen for a full bladder. If the mother is not able to empty her bladder sufficiently, catheterization for residual urine is indicated.

Catheterization. When catheterization becomes necessary, every effort should be made to prevent the introduction of bacteria into the bladder. Therefore, strict asepsis is imperative. Perineal cleansing should be done prior to beginning the catheterization procedure in order to further reduce the possibility of introducing bacteria. The nurse should keep in mind that the perineum is sore and tender and that any manipulation to expose the meatus is painful. Hence, the procedure should be carried out gently to prevent further perineal pain and discomfort. Because of edema and distortion in the perineal area, the meatus may not be easily visualized, making catheterization of a postpartum mother difficult. To facilitate the procedure, good lighting should be available and should be directed on the vulva. The nurse must gently separate the labia to prevent pulling on the perineal sutures. The solution that is used to cleanse the urinary meatus and surrounding area should be at least room temperature so that it will not feel too cold for the mother. While cleaning the area, care is taken not to allow any of the solution to flow into the vagina, to prevent inadvertent contamination of the birth canal. Lochia may be prevented from spreading upward to contaminate the meatus by placing a dry sterile cotton ball at the vaginal introitus. The catheter tip is then inserted into the meatus.

An indwelling catheter, which remains in place for 2 or 3 days, is preferred by a few physicians. This eliminates the need for frequent catheterization and permits the bladder to rest until some bladder sensation returns. Other physicians prefer catheterization as necessary, rather than an indwelling catheter, with the hope that the bladder will regain its tone more readily if it is permitted to empty and fill with some regularity. Because an indwelling catheter is likely to result in an ascending infection, preventative precautions include encouraging an increased fluid intake, keeping the urine receptacle below the level of the bladder, and assuring good perineal cleansing.

The Gastrointestinal System

The enlarging pregnant uterus causes considerable displacement of the gastrointestinal organs, and the rise in the progesterone level during pregnancy causes the motility of the gastrointestinal tract to become more sluggish and less efficient. During the puerperium the normal motility of the gastrointestinal tract is restored, and gastrointestinal displacement is corrected. Pressure on the pelvic floor during delivery causes decreased tone of the anal sphincter. Therefore, the mother should be told that she may not have complete anal sphincter control for several days after childbirth, until sphincter tone returns.

Most mothers are able to eat and drink an hour after delivery if general anesthesia was not used and if there are no complications. However, a few mothers may feel nauseated and may vomit immediately after delivery. In general, the alert mother will usually have a good appetite after giving birth and may be ready to eat immediately.

Intestinal Elimination. The puerpera may experience some difficulty evacuating her bowels during the first week of the postpartum period, with constipation resulting. This sluggishness is mainly caused by a tendency of the bowels to remain somewhat relaxed during the early puerperium, along with the relaxed condition of the abdominal walls. Once the products of conception have been delivered, the abdominal walls, which have been stretched during pregnancy, do not exert enough pressure to readily cause a bowel movement. Hemorrhoids and perineal stitches may further contribute to constipation as the mother may be reluctant to try to defecate because of fear of pain.

Some women worry, probably more than is necessary, because they are having difficulty moving their bowels. If the woman had an enema during labor, there is probably little solid waste to be eliminated for the first several days.

Early ambulation after delivery will aid in preventing and correcting constipation. Some new mothers will need laxatives in order to produce spontaneous bowel evacuations early in the puerperium. To prevent constipation, many physicians routinely order a stool softener to be given each night after delivery. A laxative, suppository, or cleansing enema may be ordered if the mother has not defecated by the third postpartum day. If a suppository or an enema is given, these should be administered gently, as the anal sphincter may be tender and sore.

The new mother should be requested to employ measures that will encourage natural evacuation of the bowels. Roughage in the diet; adequate intake of fluids, especially of fruit juices; and exercise are effective in preventing constipation. If a mother is breast-feeding, she should be advised to consult her physician and follow his prescription if laxatives are required. Certain laxatives that are excreted in breast milk will affect the nursing infant.

Flatus. Flatus is also a common complaint during the early postpartum period. Although the displacement and replacement of the gastrointestinal tract during the childbearing experience contribute to flatus, the retention of waste products in the bowel produces flatus and resultant distention. Mothers can suffer great discomfort because of "gas pains." Drinking an effervescent beverage such as ginger ale will help provide some relief. Ambulation and bowel eliminations usually help to reduce flatus. Insertion of a rectal tube may be indicated.

Hemorrhoids. Hemorrhoids are a common problem for some women during the puerperium, as during pregnancy. They result from the entrapment and stasis of blood in the rectal veins. Pressure exerted on the pelvic floor by the presenting part and straining during labor and delivery may have precipitated the development of hemorrhoids or caused aggravation of the condition if hemorrhoids were present previously. Usually, hemorrhoids are most painful during the first 2 or 3 days after delivery. They tend to reduce in size and become less painful as the puerperium progresses.

Hemorrhoids can cause much discomfort for the postpartum mother. Painful hemorrhoids are relieved by anesthetic sprays, sitz baths, and cool astringent compresses. Cold witch hazel compresses are ordered by some physicians, and they are very effective in abating discomfort and in reducing hemorrhoids.

Further irritation and pressure on hemorrhoids should be prevented. The perineal pad should be loosened or detached to relieve irritation of the rec tum. The assumption of the Sim's position by the mother while she is in bed relieves some of the pressure and congestion of the rectal veins.

Hemorrhoids that were not present prior to pregnancy will probably disappear during the latter half of the puerperium. Hemorrhoids that were present prior to pregnancy are likely to return to their prepregnancy condition.

The Circulatory System

During the early puerperium, the total blood volume remains high. However, as the excess fluid that was necessary during pregnancy is excreted after childbirth, the blood volume decreases and returns to normal. The total blood volume returns nearly to its prepregnant level by the end of the first week postpartum. A high fibrinogen level that was pregnancy-induced persists during the same period. Consequently, an elevated sedimentation rate is found during the immediate puerperium. The leukocytosis that occurs during the labor and delivery process is reflected in the puerpera's leukocyte count for the first few days after delivery.

The hemoglobin and hematocrit levels and red blood cell count tend to be variable from woman to woman. If the mother is not well hydrated after a long labor, these values may be somewhat elevated for about 3 days postpartum because of hemoconcentration. On the other hand, if the woman has lost a considerable amount of blood, hemoglobin and hematocrit levels and red blood cell count may be low, with subsequent fluid redistribution. If a mother tended to be anemic during pregnancy, then anemia will likely persist in the puerperium. It is imperative to note hemoglobin and hematocrit levels, since women with low levels need rest and are liable to experience weakness and faintness.

Iron preparations, and possibly transfusions, may be ordered by the physician to help correct low hemoglobin and hematocrit levels. Dietary counseling with a focus on iron-rich foods is also indicated.

As during pregnancy, women with superficial varicosities will continue to require special attention. Usually, there is some improvement in varicose veins as the blood volume decreases after childbirth. Constricting garters or other clothing that causes pressure and interference with the flow of blood, particularly from the lower extremities, should not be worn. Although elevation of the legs may help varicosities of the lower extremities, the patient should not elevate her legs above the level of the buttocks while her head is also elevated, since this causes pooling of the blood in the pelvic region and engorgement of pelvic veins. Elastic stockings should be worn to give support to the weak walls of the veins.

Vital Signs

Pulse. The pulse rate is slower during the early puerperium than at other times. Puerperal bradycardia is a good prognostic sign and is a transient phenomenon. The pulse rate averages between 60 and 70 beats per minute, but sometimes is as low as 40 or 50 beats per minute on the first or second day postpartum. The heart rate returns to normal by the seventh to tenth day after delivery. Although the cause of the phenomenon is not known, it has been suggested that it results from a reduction in cardiac output without a reduction in stroke volume. A decrease in the pulse rate is a compensatory mechanism that results in a decrease in cardiac output, which may be related to the markedly lower flow of blood through the placental site.[8]

A rapid pulse rate in the early puerperium may be an indication of marked blood loss, cardiac disease, or nervousness.

Temperature.   The mother's temperature may increase slightly after delivery without an apparent cause. In the normal puerpera, temperature elevations should not exceed 100.4°F. (38°C.) in any two consecutive 24 hour periods, excluding the first 24 hours postpartum. A woman who has endured a long and difficult labor is likely to have a temperature that is slightly elevated in the first 24 hours after giving birth, but it rarely exceeds 100.4°F.

Any mother with a temperature exceeding 100.4°F. should have her temperature and pulse taken every 4 hours throughout the day and evening. The pulse rate is a helpful guide in judging the significance of an elevated temperature during the puerperium. A mother with a slightly elevated temperature along with a slow pulse rate is not likely to have a complication. However, an elevated temperature during the puerperium suggests the possibility of an infection of the genitourinary tract. The mother with an elevated temperature should be assessed for other signs of infection, such as general discomfort, chills, and local pain and tenderness.

The establishment of lactation on the third or fourth postpartum day was formerly believed to cause a natural elevation of temperature. This so-called milk-fever was regarded as a normal accompaniment of the early phase of lactation. However, today, milk-fever is not a recognized process and is considered a fallacy. Although extreme lymphatic and vascular engorgement of the breasts can on rare occasions cause a sharp elevation in temperature; this rise lasts longer than 12 hours.

The Skin

Most of the pigmentary changes that developed during pregnancy either disappear or regress during the postpartum period. Facial deposits of pigment (chloasma) usually disappear completely. The increased pigmentation of the breasts and abdomen becomes less pronounced. Spider nevi that developed during pregnancy disappear, and striae gravidarum become lighter in color.

In addition to the regression of skin changes, there is an increase in the activity of the sweat glands in the immediate puerperium. Diaphoresis occurs during the first few days of the postpartum period, as the body rids itself of the excess water retained during pregnancy. Perspiration is usually most profuse at night and may be accompanied by desquamation of the skin. By the end of the first week postpartum diaphoresis gradually subsides.

The postpartum mother should be reassured that profuse sweating during the puerperium is normal and is a process that aids the body in returning to its prepregnant state. Wearing of hospital gowns may be preferable at night, when perspiration is most profuse. Protection of the mother from chilling is important during periods of diaphoresis.

Bathing.   A bath or shower is refreshing and stimulating for the postpartum mother, particularly during periods of diaphoresis. Most mothers find a bed bath administered by the nurse in the recovery room a source of comfort. This is best done after the woman has rested and settled down somewhat from the labor and delivery experience. Mothers usually enjoy having the nurse give the first bath after delivery, and it provides an opportunity for the woman to talk to the nurse about the childbirth experience. It also is an excellent time for the nurse to introduce the mother to basic postpartum care, such as perineal care, breast care, elimination, and hospital routines. However, the discussion and teaching activities should be guided by the mother's readiness to learn. The new mother can only retain so much information during this early phase of the puerperium, and much of the information may need to be reviewed at another time. In the first few hours after delivery, most women are excited and caught up in their labor and delivery experience and have a need to talk with someone about it and about the new baby. Therefore, teaching and demonstration of basic postpartum care may need to be postponed until later.

Showers are usually permitted when the mother becomes ambulatory. The first few times that the mother takes a shower, it is particularly important that she be accompanied by a nurse or attendant, who should remain close by for safety. Some women become faint and light-headed while in the shower and need assistance. The patient who has had a cesarean section will need to keep her incision dry until healing is well underway. Thus she may not be allowed to take a shower although she is ambulatory.

Tub baths are not allowed by some physicians following delivery. The danger of introducing infection through the vagina from the bath water is the major rationale for prohibiting tub baths in the early puerperium.

The Abdominal Wall

The return of the prepregnancy "figure" is one of the concerns of many postpartum mothers. A minimum of 6 weeks is required for the abdominal wall to regain its muscle tone. Immediately after delivery, the abdomen is flat, soft, and flabby. The abdominal wall never regains its tone in some women, remaining soft and covered by loose, wrinkled skin. The return of abdominal tone is influenced by the degree of distention of the abdominal muscles and by the mother's individual constitution. Women who have generally poor muscle tone, who have pregnancies that follow each other in close succession, or who have had excessively distended abdomens because of multiple pregnancy or hydramnios are more likely to have difficulty regaining their original abdominal muscle tone.

If the abdominal wall is so weakened that the rectus muscles separate at the midline (diastasis recti), this will be recognizable as a dark groove down the middle of the abdomen. The width of the diastasis recti should be noted and recorded. With active exercise, the width of the separation will narrow. A good diet, proper posture, and rest will further aid in the restoration of abdominal muscle tone.

At one time tight abdominal binders or girdles were used by postpartum mothers in the hope that this would restore the mother's figure and aid involution. Today, the general consensus is that abdominal binding is not necessary for the postpartum mother. However, an abdominal binder or an ordinary girdle may help the puerpera feel more comfortable if her abdomen is flabby and pendulous.

Weight Loss

Weight loss after delivery is a special concern for most mothers who desire to return to their prepregnancy weight as soon as possible. One of the first acts of some new mothers after they become ambulatory is to weigh themselves. These mothers may anxiously anticipate the day that they can again wear the clothes that they wore prior to pregnancy, and may be disappointed after delivery because they do not quickly return to their prepregnancy weight and size.

The average weight loss at delivery is approximately 12 pounds. This initial weight loss is mainly due to the delivery of the products of conception, which include the fetus, placenta, membranes, and amniotic fluid. An additional 5 pounds is lost during the first 2 weeks after delivery. This loss in weight is largely due to the elimination of excess fluid in the tissues through urination and perspiration.

In his study of 200 mothers during the first 8 days following normal delivery, Sheikh found that weight loss occurred in some mothers and weight gain in others during the first 3 postpartum days.[16] Of the mothers included in his study, 28 per cent showed a weight gain during the first 3 days postpartum, 40 per cent showed a weight loss, and the other mothers' weight remained stable. However, from the fourth day onward most of the mothers began to lose weight. Primiparas and breast-feeding mothers were more likely to lose weight in the early puerperium. Mothers given lactosuppressants tended to have stable weights with little weight loss or gain. This was probably a result of the water and salt retention effect of estrogens given to suppress lactation.

The nurse should discuss weight loss with the mother after delivery and should point out that it usually takes the 6 weeks of the postpartum period for her to return to her prepregnancy weight. Except for the additional weight of the lactating breasts in the mother who is breast-feeding, excess weight at the end of the postpartum period represents additional fat. If the woman has had previous problems controlling her weight, the nutritionist should talk with her about her diet habits prior to pregnancy and should provide some suggestions that may be of help to her. If a nutritionist is not available prior to the mother's return home, the nurse should review her diet history and offer assistance to her.

Afterpains

As pointed out previously, contraction of the uterus is a major process by which the uterus returns to its nonpregnant size during the puerperium. Uterine contractions after childbirth cause cramping sensations in some women similar to those accompanying a menstrual period. These are called "afterpains." Multiparas experience afterpains more frequently than primiparas. The uterus tends to remain tonically contracted in primiparas, while it often contracts and relaxes at intervals in multiparas. Painful sensations may occur with contractions, which sometimes are severe enough to require an analgesic.

Afterpains are also more likely to be a complaint when the uterus has been greatly distended during pregnancy, such as following multiple births, a large baby, or hydramnios. Women who are breast-feeding will notice that afterpains tend to occur when the infant is put to breast. The release of oxytocin from the posterior pituitary during the infant's suckling increases contractions of the uterus and gives rise to afterpains. As the puerperium progresses, afterpains decrease in intensity and frequency. By 48 hour following the delivery, they are usually mild. Usually the administration of a mild analgesic will abate or alleviate afterpains and help the woman feel more comfortable.

The Breasts

Breast development begins at puberty and is stimulated by the estrogens of the monthly sexual cycles. These estrogens stimulate growth of the ductile system and stroma. With pregnancy, additional growth of the breasts occurs, as the glandular tissue of the breast becomes completely developed for the final goal of milk production after parturition. Estrogen, progesterone, and chorionic somatomammotropin (human placental lactogen), which are secreted by the placenta, are responsible for accelerated breast development during pregnancy. There is growth and branching of the ductile system, further fat deposition, growth of lobules, and budding of the alveoli of the breasts. Development of the secretory characteristics of the *acini cells,* or the milk-producing cells of the alveoli, also occurs. Thus by the end of pregnancy, the mother's breasts have become fully developed for actual milk production, and colostrum, a thin, yellowish milk precursor, is secreted in small amounts. The actual production of milk does not occur until after the baby is born.

After parturition, no change in the condition of the breasts will be noted until about 2 days postpartum. Colostrum continues to be secreted in small amounts until lactation begins. Milk secretion begins by the third or fourth day postpartum. The onset of lacteal secretion is accompanied by larger, firmer, and more tender breasts. The veins become more prominent, and the breasts feel heavier to the mother. Some women may complain of a burning or prickling sensation in the breasts. This early breast tenderness and congestion are referred to as *primary engorgement.* At about the same time, the secretion from the nipples changes from yellow, the color that is characteristic of colostrum, to bluish-white, the color of normal breast milk.

Secretion of Milk. After childbirth, milk is produced in response to the hormone prolactin (also called luteotropin, LTH, or the lactogenic or mammogenic hormone), which is secreted by the anterior pituitary. High levels of prolactin secreted after delivery of the placenta are responsible for the initiation of lactation. The high blood levels of progesterone and estrogens during pregnancy are believed to have an inhibitory effect on the secretion of prolactins by the pituitary gland, and thus on milk secretion by the breasts. The sudden loss of estrogen and progesterone secretion after the placenta is delivered allows production of prolactin by the anterior pituitary because of the removal of the inhibitory effects of these two hormones (Fig. 19–3). Prolactin secretion stimulates the synthesis of fat, lactose, and casein

Figure 19–3 Changes in rates of secretion of estrogens, progesterone, and prolactin at parturition and during the succeeding weeks after parturition, showing especially the rapid increase in prolactin secretion immediately after parturition. (From Guyton: *Textbook of Medical Physiology.* 4th Ed. Philadelphia, W. B. Saunders Co., 1971.)

by the acini cells in large quantities, and milk is produced.

The quantity of milk produced varies from woman to woman and from day to day in the same woman. Frequent and complete emptying of the breasts is necessary for the secretion of milk to continue. Milk production is inhibited by full breasts, and the amount of milk produced is generally dependent on the quantity of milk removed. Thus the infant's requirements for milk directly affect the quantity of milk produced. This is nature's way of insuring an adequate amount of milk for the infant. As more and more milk is suckled from the breasts, the production of larger quantities of milk occurs. Usually less than an ounce is withdrawn from the breasts at each feeding on the first day after delivery. Thereafter the baby's consumption increases steadily, and by the end of the first postpartal week he removes about 2 to 3 ounces of milk from the breasts at each feeding. At the height of lacteal secretion 1.5 liters of milk may be produced each day.

If the breasts are not emptied regularly, secretion of prolactin is not stimulated, and milk production decreases and eventually ceases. When milk is not continually withdrawn, lactation will cease with 1 to 2 weeks. Milk secretion continues for as long as the breasts are emptied frequently and sufficiently. Secretion of milk normally decreases by 7 to 9 months, but this mainly depends on the amount that is withdrawn continually. The suckling of the breasts seems to be the stimulus that fosters continued prolactin secretion and milk production. Lactation can continue for several years if the mother's breasts are suckled frequently.

Other factors that influence the amount and quality of milk produced are the mother's diet and fluid intake, her activity level, and the amount of rest that she gets. An increased caloric intake is vital for the nursing mother, along with increased amounts of protein, iron, calcium, vitamins, and fluids. The mother who is breast-feeding needs to stay well rested and prevent fatigue. A midday rest period may be necessary in addition to a good night's sleep of at least 8 hours. Although moderate exercise is beneficial, the woman should not overexert herself, because fatigue has an adverse effect on lacteal secretion.

Some mothers may be concerned that their breasts are not large enough for sufficient milk production. These mothers' concerns can be alleviated by the understanding that the quality and quantity of milk produced are not related to the size of the breasts but to the amount of glandular tissue in the breasts. Breast size is related to the amount of fatty tissue in the breasts and not to the amount of glandular tissue. Since the milk is produced from the secretory mammary glands of the breasts, the amount of fat in the breasts has no influence on lactation.

Nursing care of the breast-feeding mother is discussed in detail in Chapter 20.

Engorgement. Several days after delivery the mother may experience breast discomfort due to engorgement. Engorgement is local congestion and distention of the breasts and is related to the initiation of lactation. This condition has been attributed to an increase in the venous and lymphatic circulation in the breasts and to the filling of the lobules of the breasts with milk. *Primary or initial breast engorgement* occurs about the third or fourth day post partum and is caused mainly by lymphatic and venous distention as lactation is being established. Engorgement that occurs after lactation has been established is referred to as *secondary or* *ate engorgement* and is primarily due to he filling and distention of the lobules with milk.

When lactation is initiated, the breasts become heavier, larger, firmer, and more sensitive. The skin covering he breasts becomes tight and shiny. On palpation the breasts feel warm and ense. The individual lobules that are distended can be felt as hard lumps, and milk ducts can be felt as hard strings. There may be a darker or bluish coloration to the surface of the breasts, but rarely do they become reddened.

The degree of engorgement varies in severity. Varying degrees of discomfort are felt by the mother; however, engorgement is frequently quite painful. Primiparas usually suffer more discomfort from breast engorgement than multiparas. In addition to breast discomfort, the mother may complain of lassitude and headache. At one time, engorgement was believed to cause the mother to become febrile. Today engorgement is not accepted as a cause of fever in the postpartum mother. A mother's temperature may rise slightly (less than 1°F.) with engorgement, but if the mother's temperature exceeds 100.4°F. or 38°C., some other cause should be suspected.

Engorgement is a transitory condition that is usually present for 24 to 48 hours; however, it requires prompt attention. If the puerpera is nursing her infant, engorgement can interfere with the ease of nursing. If the condition is not corrected early in the nursing mother, emptying of the breasts becomes very difficult. Lactation will be terminated if the milk is not removed.

In the nursing mother, engorgement can be prevented, or at least decreased, by rooming-in. When rooming-in is practiced, the mother and infant are together constantly, and the mother can nurse according to the in-fant's demand and when her breasts feel full. Nursing can thus be initiated as necessary to maintain maternal and infant comfort. If the breast-feeding mother is not rooming-in, nursing staff need to make the infant available to her as often as is necessary to meet the infant's needs and to empty her full breasts.

Relief of the discomforts of engorged breasts is promoted by breast support, analgesics for pain relief, and application of heat or ice bags to the breasts. In the nursing mother removal of milk from the breasts can provide relief. A firm bra or breast binder can uplift and support heavy, engorged breasts. Bra straps should be wide enough to prevent cutting into the shoulders. Breast binders have an advantage over bras because they can be more easily adjusted and thus provide more rapid relief (Figs. 19–4 and 19–5).

Figure 19–4 A simple binder will provide moderate support to the breasts and decrease the discomfort of engorgement. (From Davis and Rubin: *De Lee's Obstetrics for Nurses.* 18th Ed. Philadelphia, W. B. Saunders Co., 1966.)

Figure 19–5 A straight binder fitted snugly to the breasts by means of darts and shoulder straps will reduce the discomfort incidental to drying up the breasts when lactation is to be discontinued. (From Davis and Rubin: *De Lee's Obstetrics for Nurses.* 18th Ed. Philadelphia, W. B. Saunders Co., 1966.)

Fifteen to 20 minute application of hot packs or ice bags to the breasts can be comforting to mothers with engorgement. Relief can also be provided by applying hot or cold wet compresses or by using a towel that has been wrung in hot or cold water. Some women find that warm water from a shower that falls on the breasts is soothing.

Analgesics need to be administered as necessary for headache and local pain that may result from engorgement. If the mother is nursing, analgesics should be administered early enough prior to nursing so that the effects can provide relative comfort during the nursing period.

Removal of milk from the breasts of nursing mothers can provide some relief. This may be accomplished by manual expression of the milk or by use of a breast pump. A nipple shield may be indicated when engorgement interferes with the infant's ability to grasp the nipple. If a mother is not breast-feeding, removal of milk from the breasts is no an appropriate treatment, since this en courages further milk production.

Suppression of Lactation.   When a mother chooses not to breast-feed, mill will still be produced by her breasts un less lactation is suppressed. The non nursing mother should wear a well fitting bra or breast binder to suppor and prevent manipulation of the breasts. The woman should be told no to remove any breast milk, as this en courages further milk secretion. If en gorgement is present, it generally sub sides in several days, since accumula tion of milk in the breasts prevents mill production. At one time it was believe that restriction of fluids and the admin istration of diuretics would aid in th suppression of lactation; however, suc treatment has not been found to be e fective.[17]

When women choose not to breast feed, the physician will usually pre scribe hormones to suppress lactation An estrogen-androgen combination c oral progestins, estrogens, or androgen alone have also been used.[18] These hor mones are believed to interfere with c suppress the release of prolactin in th nonnursing mother. Diethylstilbestro quinestrol, and chlorotrianisen (TACE) are hormone medications tha are usually prescribed for oral adminis tration over 2 or 3 days during the earl puerperium to suppress the secretion milk. Deladumone, a long-actin estrogen-androgen combination, is ad ministered intramuscularly. It is give in a single injection during the secon stage of labor or immediately after de livery.

Estrogen-androgen combination have been found to be most effective i preventing lactation.[18] Administratic of hormones does not always effective suppress lactation, however. Som women who have received lactosu pressants may experience filling of the breasts a few days postpartally, or as late as several weeks after delivery. Women who receive hormones for the purpose of lactosuppression should be told that filling of the breasts may occur, but this usually disappears spontaneously if milk is not removed from the breasts.

Side effects sometimes occur with the administration of lactosuppressant hormones. The administration of estrogenic hormones has been associated with heavier lochial discharge and with a greater proportion of bright red blood in the lochia, particularly after the treatment is discontinued. Thromboembolic diseases have been found to occur rarely after the use of estrogen for postpartum milk suppression. A delay in the onset of menstruation and the development of virilizing effects may be observed following the administration of androgens.

Breast Care. The importance of proper breast care for the postpartum mother cannot be overemphasized. Care of the breasts during the puerperium is aimed at providing good breast support and maintaining hygienic care. A supportive bra with wide straps is necessary. The bra should provide upward support for the breasts, but at the same time it should not be too tight. A bra or breast binder should be worn during the night as well as during the day. Some women, particularly breast-feeding mothers, may be concerned that their breasts will begin to sag after childbirth. If adequate support is given, pendulous, sagging breasts are not likely to result.

The mother should be instructed to wash the breasts daily with soap and water as she showers. In nursing mothers, soap and other drying agents should not be used to cleanse the nipples because such preparations may remove the natural protective oils and leave the nipples more prone to damage during suckling. In the breast-feeding mother, nipples should be cleaned with plain water before and after suckling. Dry nipples are less likely to become macerated than nipples that stay wet and damp. Therefore, nursing mothers should leave the bra flaps that cover the nipples down for a few minutes after nursing, so that the nipples will air and dry.

Massage of the breasts between breast-feedings in nursing mothers can be helpful, by keeping the lacteal ducts open.[17] Breast massage can also aid in preventing engorgement once lactation is established.

Fissures of the nipples are portals through which infection may be introduced into the breasts. When cracks and fissures of the breasts are present, the nurse should be alert for signs of mastitis or breast infection, which include local redness, swelling, pain and tenderness, general malaise, and a high fever. If breast infection occurs in a nursing mother, termination of breast-feeding may be recommended by the physician.

Menstruation and Ovulation

Prior to returning home, mothers will want to know when they can expect their menstrual flow to appear again and when ovulation is likely to occur. The menstrual flow usually returns within 6 to 8 weeks after delivery if the woman does not breast-feed her infant. Variations are observed in the recurrence of menstruation and in the return of ovulation.

Generally, menstruation does not occur while the woman is breast-feeding. This phenomenon is called *lactation amenorrhea*. Although the most common time for the reappearance of menstruation in the lactating mother is during the third to fourth month post-delivery,[8] El-Minawi and Foda[4] noted that the duration of postpartum lactation amenorrhea ranged between 6 weeks and 26 months. They also found that lactation amenorrhea persists for a longer period of time if breast-feeding is not supplemented.

A substantial degree of infertility occurs jointly with lactation, as long as lactation amenorrhea persists. However, the mother may ovulate while she is breast-feeding, even though the menstrual flow has not reappeared. Therefore, all breast-feeding mothers should be informed of the potential occurrence of a pregnancy. Some type of birth control method should still be used while breast-feeding if the woman wants to prevent a pregnancy at that time.

PSYCHOLOGIC AND BEHAVIORAL REACTIONS OF THE PUERPERIUM

After delivery there is a period of psychologic adjustment for the postpartum mother. This psychologic or emotional adjustment is directly related to the physical or bodily changes she is experiencing and to her role and relationship to her new baby.

Just as the woman had to adjust to a new body image during her pregnancy, a similar adjustment is required after delivery. Once again the mother's body image changes, and she may feel a void and emptiness where the baby once was. The change in her body shape tells her that her infant is an individual, separate and real. The mother must begin to feel whole and not empty before she can reconcile herself completely to the actual birth of her baby. Initially there may be a feeling of bewilderment in the

mother as she has difficulty feeling that the baby is really hers and because the sight of the newborn does not evoke an overwhelming feeling of maternal love.[11] However, as time passes she will become relieved as she begins to identify her infant as a separate individual to whom she has a binding emotional tie.

If the mother has experienced discomforts or difficulties related to the pregnancy or to the labor and delivery process, she may be anxious and fear that her body's level of functioning will never be quite the same again. When the mother has anticipated the return of her figure to the prepregnant state, she will be disappointed and frustrated during the early puerperium to see that she is still larger than she was prior to her pregnancy. It is imperative that the mother understands that these physical changes are normal, so that her anxieties and fears will be alleviated. Thus, the nurse should tell the mother about these normal alterations and should give her simple explanations about the cause of her discomforts and about their usual course before their end.

Phases of the Process of Regeneration and Restoration

Predictable psychologic and behavioral reactions occur during the course of the puerperium as physical healing and restoration process. Rubin has described the common reactions that occur in the hospitalized mother and has distinguished two phases of puerperal adjustment—the "taking-in" phase and the "taking-hold" phase.[14] How well these phases apply to the mother who delivers at home is not known, since these maternal reactions may be influenced by the mother's hospital confinement. However, we can safely ssume that the common physical changes that occur in the postpartum mother will affect her behavioral and psychologic processes similarly, whether she delivers her infant in the hospital or at home.

The Taking-in Phase. The first 2 or 3 days after the delivery the mother is in the taking-in phase of the puerperium. Characteristic of this phase is the importance of sleep and food to the mother. She tends to be passive and dependent during this period, and her psychic and physical energies are usually centered more around herself and the events of the immediate past.

Sleep and rest are necessary during the taking-in phase of the puerperium. Uninterrupted sleep is vital for the mother as she recovers from the labor and delivery experience. In the first hours after delivery the mother feels exhausted and will fall into a deep sleep. If she is not allowed to get the sleep that she requires, a "sleep hunger" may result, and the restorative processes of the puerperium may be prolonged. As a consequence the mother may become irritable and feel fatigued for several days. Therefore, the nurse will want to insure that the mother is allowed adequate periods of rest and sleep.

The mother's desire to ingest food is apparent during the taking-in phase. When she is not eating, she may talk about food until she eats and her hunger is satisfied. This reaction is probably partly physical and partly psychologic. Labor and delivery require hard work of the mother and a lot of energy. In addition, most mothers have gone for a long period of time without food during the labor and delivery process. Thus, the body requires food to aid in the restorative process. Food also has a great psychologic benefit for the mother, since the taking in of food may be emotionally satisfying and may signify an early step

in the recovery process. Recognizing the mother's need for nourishment, the nurse should foster the woman's intake of nutritious food in the early puerperium.

Since dependence and passivity are characteristic of the mother during the taking-in phase, she does not actively initiate self-care activities. As the receiver of care, she accepts the care given to her without much input, and she does what she is told without much autonomy. The nurse will want to respect this seemingly natural response during the early puerperium by meeting the woman's dependency needs. The mother should not be forced to carry out physical activities that she is not ready to do and that seem to fatigue her. The nurse will need to have a major role in providing physical care for the mother during the first 24 hours after childbirth and should be available to assist and guide her in any self-care activities that she may initiate. The nurse will also notice that the woman's expressed needs tend to center on herself more than on her infant. The mother requires help from the nurse while she is learning to meet her own puerperal needs before she can sufficiently reach out beyond herself to meet the needs of her infant.

During the taking-in phase the mother responds psychologically to the childbirth experience by reviewing the details of labor and delivery. The woman has a need to talk about the birth events repeatedly, so that she can comprehend and grasp the reality of the whole event and of her motherhood. She needs to pull the whole event together by discussing every detail. The mother may discuss her labor and delivery over and over with several different people, so that she can better realize the completeness of birth experience. The nurse should lend a receptive ear to the mother and expedite this assimilative work, so that the mother can move on to the realities of the immediate present.

The Taking-hold Phase.   In the taking-hold phase the mother reaches out more beyond herself and begins to focus on the order of things in the immediate present. This phase is marked by increasing independence and autonomy, as the mother becomes the initiator and producer of self-care and infant-care activities. The mother generally arrives at the taking-hold phase about the third postpartal day.

The mother seemingly was resting and recuperating after the events of labor and delivery in the taking-in phase. However, she now begins to move forward to deal with the events of the present in the taking-hold phase with an urgency, an immediacy that was not characteristic of her in the previous stage. Her focus is on the reality of "right now," and she presses forward to become involved and to get things organized. Her ability to carry out self-care activities becomes paramount initially, as she tries to take control of her own bodily functions. There is an element of anxiety about this, and she becomes less tolerant of delays and indications of her own inadequacies.

At this time she is concerned about her ability to evacuate her bowels and her bladder. If she is breast-feeding, she wants to know when the milk will "come in" or if she will be able to produce enough milk for her baby. As she becomes more confident of her own bodily functions, the woman begins to take hold of some of her mothering tasks with greater ease. It is as if the woman's involvement and concern with her bodily functioning are extended to her infant once she has successfully coped with the changes that occurred in her own body.

As her mothering tasks become paramount, the woman focuses on her ability to care for her infant. She ha high ideals about how she should per form as a mother and feels inadequat and frustrated when she has not per formed at the level that she expects. I she is having difficulty getting her bab to eat for her or if she feels awkward i providing his care, she may feel that sh is failing in her mothering tasks. He confidence is very delicate at this tim and she needs constant reassuranc that she is performing well.

The woman may be overwhelme by the dependence of the small, helples infant. She is curious about the infan care tasks and is concerned about h infant's bodily functions. Most ne mothers want to know the details of ir fant care—if the infant is gettin enough to eat or if he is evacuating h bowels satisfactorily. The mother's anx iety will increase if there appears to l any defect in the infant's functioning appearance (e.g., forcep marks, cap succedaneum, or jaundice), since sh may feel that these reflect on the ad quacy of her functioning during the ge tation period or during labor and deli ery. Thus, the nurse should discuss i fant behavior and any variations fro the expected with the mother. Whe explanations are given, they should l simple and easy for the mother to u derstand.

Because the woman is interest and curious during the taking-ho phase, it is a stage when receptivene and readiness for learning are heigh ened. The nurse will want to tal advantage of the mother's readiness f learning by providing instruction infant care, self-care, and person hygiene. She also can be of much a sistance by giving anticipatory guidan to the mother about what to expe in the coming weeks after her retui home and how to deal with the changes.

When the woman has begun to cope successfully with her mothering tasks in relation to her baby, her energies begin to extend beyond herself and her infant to encompass her role responsibilities as they affect other family members. Much of the taking-hold phase will take place at home, since this stage lasts about 10 days. Thus, prior to the mother's return home, the nurse will want to help her establish realistic expectations for herself. New mothers may involve themselves with too much activity during this phase and exhaust themselves in their drive for excellence.

Postpartum Blues

One of the emotional aftermaths of childbirth that some women experience is a depression or "blue" feeling for which the mother may not be able to determine an apparent cause. Postpartum blues, as it is called, usually appears between the third and tenth day postpartum, but may occur earlier or later. The incidence of this phenomenon has been shown to range from 50 to 80 per cent. Mild depression, anxiety, and a feeling of being a bit slow or "not quite with it" are most characteristic of the phenomenon.[12] The mother may also have periods of weepiness and irritability. All of these symptoms are transitory and usually last from 1 or 2 hours to several days.

Several psychologic and social factors interact to influence the mood of women during the puerperium. Even though this is the case, the transient depression of postpartum blues is believed to result from the impact of the additional responsibilities of motherhood on the woman. Another explanation that has been offered is that the reaction is precipitated by a drop in hormonal levels after childbirth. Fatigue and anxiety about the baby and

about her adequacy in carrying out the maternal role may also contribute to the condition.

The nurse can be of assistance to the mother by recognizing postpartum blues from the mother's behavior and by discussing the phenomenon with her. The mother will be relieved to know that her feelings are not unusual and that her crying is acceptable to the health care team. Since a large number of mothers are likely to experience postpartum blues after they return home, women and their mates should be warned of the possible occurrence of this condition after they leave the hospital. If the condition persists for several days or if the mother becomes deeply depressed, her physician should be contacted. Infrequently, a postpartum mother may develop a more serious depressive reaction for which she will need close psychiatric supervision.

SUMMARY

In general, the emotional state of the postpartum mother during the early puerperium tends to be somewhat labile and is affected by the mother's physical state and well-being. She is required to make adjustments to the rapid changes that have occurred and that continue to occur in her body. She is in a transitory period and is faced with stress and strain as she adapts to the new responsibilities of her maternal role. Although commonalities have been emphasized in this review of the mother's physical, psychologic, and behavioral reactions during the puerperium, the nurse must be aware of the great range of variability among postpartum mothers. Therefore, nursing care during the postpartum period must not be considered to be "routine," but each mother's individual situation and condition must be considered in planning and providing care.

REFERENCES

1. Adams, H., and Flowers, C. E.: Oral oxytocic drugs in the puerperium. *Obstetrics and Gynecology, 15*:280, 1960.
2. Barnes, J.: The aftermath of childbirth: Physical aspects. *Proceedings of the Royal Society of Medicine, 68*:223, 1975.
3. Dessouky, D. A.: Myometrial changes in postpartum uterine involution. *American Journal of Obstetrics and Gynecology, 110*:318, 1971.
4. El-Minawi, M. G., and Foda, M. S.: Postpartum lactation amenorrhea: Endometrial pattern and reproductive ability. *American Journal of Obstetrics and Gynecology, 111*:17, 1971.
5. Eppink, H.: Catheterizing the maternity patient. *American Journal of Nursing, 75*:829, 1975.
6. Greenhill, J. P., and Friedman, E. A.: *Biological Principles and Modern Practice of Obstetrics*. Philadelphia, W. B. Saunders Co., 1974.
7. Guyton, A. C.: *Textbook of Medical Physiology*. 5th Edition. Philadelphia, W. B. Saunders Co., 1976.
8. Hellman, L. M., and Pritchard, J. A.: *Williams Obstetrics*. 14th Edition. New York, Appleton-Century-Crofts, Meredith Corporation, 1971.
9. MacDonald, H. N., Good, W., and Stone, J.: Changes in common plasma solute levels during labor and the puerperium. *Journal of Obstetrics and Gynecology of the British Commonwealth, 81*:888, 1974.
10. Nott, P. N., Franklin, M., Armitage, C., et al: Hormonal changes and mood in the puerperium. *British Journal of Psychiatry, 128*:379, 1976.
11. Pines, D.: Pregnancy and motherhood: Interaction between fantasy and reality. *British Journal of Medical Psychology, 45*:333, 1972.
12. Pitt, B.: Aftermath of childbirth: Psychological reactions to childbirth. *Proceedings of the Royal Society of Medicine, 68*:22, 1975.
13. Rubin, R.: Basic maternal behavior. *Nursing Outlook, 9*:683, 1961.
14. Rubin, R.: Puerperal change. *Nursing Outlook, 9*:753, 1961.
15. Salazar, H., Tabon, H., and Josimovich, J. P.: Developmental, gestational and postgestational modifications of the human breast. *Clinical Obstetrics and Gynecology, 18*:113, 1975.
16. Sheikh, G. H.: Observations of maternal weight behavior during the puerperium. *American Journal of Obstetrics and Gynecology, 111*:244, 1971.
17. Stone, S. C., and Dickey, R. P.: Management of nursing and nonnursing mothers. *Clinical Obstetrics and Gynecology, 18*:139, 1975.
18. Vorherr, H.: Suppression of postpartum lactation. *Postgraduate Medicine, 52*:14, 1972.

Chapter 20

NURSING APPROACH TO THE POSTPARTUM FAMILY

BY ORA STRICKLAND DAVIS, R.N., PH.D.

The postpartum mother and her newborn are the major focus of nursing care on the postpartum unit. The parturient mother receives special attention because she is experiencing major physical changes with resultant emotional adjustments after giving birth. Special consideration is given to the newborn because he is making a delicate transition from intrauterine to extrauterine life.

In providing nursing care during the puerperium, we must remember that childbirth has implications for others beyond the mother-infant dyad. Reproduction and childbearing are a family experience that touches the lives of all family members. The mother's most intimate contacts, such as with her husband, her other children, and her own parents and siblings, will be most profoundly affected by the birth. The arrival of the newborn will require adjustments and adaptations to be made by all members of the immediate family. Family relationships will have to be modified to incorporate the new baby.

The quality of care that the family receives during the postpartum period can influence the family as it reorganizes and adjusts after the birth and can be viewed as an important basis of future family health.

We must recognize the importance of the birth to all family members and must realize that each mother, baby and family is unique and has different needs. Every effort should be made to make sure that those family members who are most important to the mother and who will be influential in the life of the newborn are incorporated into nursing care whenever possible.

In providing postpartum care, our nursing approach is based on two basic principles:

1. The mother's body is readjusting and is being restored to the nonpregnant state.

2. With each birth a "new" family begins, as new relationships are established with the newborn and former relationships are modified.

In assessing the needs of the post-

627

partum mother and her family, factors
to be considered are:

1. Maternal physical aspects of the
puerperium.

2. Parent-infant interaction.

3. Teaching needs.

The specific nursing needs of the
postpartum family must be determined
to insure that comprehensive nursing
care is provided.

THE POSTPARTUM MOTHER

The postpartum period is not an entity in itself, not does the mother start
the puerperium with a blank slate. She
brings with her a history that affects
her needs, expectations, and responses
during the postpartum period. Information regarding the mother's family, previous childbearing experiences,
sociocultural background, and other
maternal characteristics can be vital in
assessment and in planning nursing
care. The uniqueness of each mother's
history, along with her current physical
condition and behavioral responses,
will influence the care provided to her.

CARE IN THE IMMEDIATE POSTPARTUM PERIOD

During the first hours after birth,
much of the nursing care will be related
to the physical aspects of the puerperium to insure that the mother's
physical condition is good. The major
threat to the mother during the first 24
hours after delivery is the possibility of
excessive bleeding. The fundus should
be checked at least every 15 minutes
during the first hour postpartum to determine if it is firm and contracted. The
mother's lochia flow should be checked
at the same time intervals to assess the
amount of bleeding. After the first hour,

the fundus and lochia flow should b
checked at least every 4 hours for th
next 8 hours.

The patient's history should be con
sidered when making a judgment as t
whether she should be assessed for ex
cessive bleeding more frequently. If th
mother had an operative delivery o
lacerations of the perineum, vagina, o
cervix, she will need to be observe
more closely for bleeding. The olde
multipara who has delivered severa
children and the mother whose uteru
has been extensively distended (e.g., be
cause of a large infant, multiple preg
nancy, or hydramnios) are more pron
to uterine atony and hemorrhage an
also require closer observation.

If the uterus is atonic, it should b
gently massaged until firm again. Th
uterus must be supported at the su
prapubic area with one hand when it
being massaged and when blood tha
has pooled in the uterine cavity is bein
expressed. To prevent inversion of th
uterus with resultant hemorrhage an
shock, expression of blood from th
uterus should be done only when th
uterus is firm and well contracted.

A distended bladder can result in
less firmly contracted uterus. Som
mothers will need to void within th
first hour or two after delivery. Bladde
distention should be checked and th
mother should be offered the bedpa
within 2 to 4 hours after parturition.

The mother's pulse, respiration
and blood pressure are taken im
mediately after delivery and every 1
minutes during the first hour or unt
stable. It is usually best to take the vita
signs at the time when the fundus an
the amount of lochia flow are evaluate
during the first few hours after deliver
This is done in such a manner that th
mother will not be frequently disturbe
so that she can get more rest.

Some time in the first hours afte

childbirth, the mother is allowed a visit from her mate or another significant family member of her choice, if she feels like receiving company. In some hospitals the father is allowed to stay with the mother in the recovery room. This practice should be encouraged, since the father is important in the childbearing experience.

Parents often want to be together in the immediate puerperium. This provides the couple with an opportunity to talk about the birth and about their baby. If the infant is not having any problems, he can also remain with the parents in the recovery room, at least for a short while, so that the parents can cuddle and explore their newborn. Affectional bonding of parents to the infant is facilitated by this early parent-infant interaction. The few minutes that parents spend with each other and with their infant immediately after delivery can become a precious memory that is recalled with warmth and joy.

The mother should have a bed bath prior to the time that she is transferred from the recovery area to her room. Many newly delivered puerpera find the bath refreshing. Mothers who have not been able to relax previously may then settle down and get some sleep after the excitement of the delivery.

POSTPARTUM PHYSICAL ASSESSMENT AND RELATED PATIENT TEACHING

The mother's physical condition and the progress of involution are assessed daily while she is in the hospital. At the same time that the nurse is doing the postpartum physical assessment, she can teach the patient about involution and physical care. In addition, the nurse can help the mother feel that she is being included in the assessment by sharing her findings and discussing variations that are expected as the puerperium progresses. The approach to the postpartum physical assessment should follow a logical order, proceeding from the breasts downward. If the mother's bladder is full, it should be emptied prior to the initiation of the assessment. If the mother needs to void, her perineal pad should be checked before she uses the bathroom in order to observe her lochia flow.

The assessment is begun by taking the mother's vital signs. Temperature, pulse, respirations, and blood pressure are taken and recorded. If the temperature is elevated, along with a rapid pulse rate, the nurse should be particularly alert for signs of infection.

Breasts

The mother removes her bra so that the breasts can be easily inspected and palpated. The breasts are observed for contour, symmetry, color, fullness, firmness, venous distention, nodules, warmth, and secretion from the nipples. As the breasts are palpated, the mother is asked if there is breast tenderness or tingling. The firmness or fullness of the areola of the nursing mother is particularly noted, along with characteristics of the nipples. Nipple prominence is observed, and reddened, cracked, sore, or fissured nipples are noted. Full or firm breasts and the secretion of yellowish colostrum or bluish-white milk are characteristic in the lactating mother. Breasts that are bluish or darker in color (because of venous distention) and that are hard, tender, lumpy, and tingling are engorged. Proper treatment should be instituted immediately. Breasts that are red and hot may be indicative of breast infection, particularly if the mother's temperature is also elevated. In the nursing mother, fissured, sore, or cracked nipples must be treated promptly, and breast shields may need to be worn at feeding time.

Several teaching opportunities are provided during the breast examination. These include discussing the process of milk production, the characteristics of colostrum and human milk, manual expression of milk, nipple care, breast self-examination, and the importance of adequate breast support. Of course all of these things won't be covered at one time but can be taught during the several days before the mother returns home.

Back

The mother's back is checked for acute pain or tenderness. The presence of flank pain or pain in the area of the kidneys is also checked. Flank pain and deep tenderness are a sign of kidney infection. Mothers should be told about the importance of drinking adequate fluids daily.

Abdomen

The abdomen is observed for distention and diastasis. A large abdomen, with or without diastasis, indicates poor muscle tone. If diastasis is present, its width should be measured. Abdominal tightening exercises should be explained to the mother with poor abdominal muscle tone, and she should be encouraged to carry them out throughout the 6 weeks of the puerperium. One effective exercise is that of lying flat in bed and lifting the head to touch the chin to the chest for five times at least twice daily. If the mother places her hand on her abdomen while she does the exercise, she will be able to feel her abdominal muscles become more tense as she raises her head.

During the examination of the ab-domen, the fundus of the uterus is checked for firmness, tenderness, and height in relation to the umbilicus. The presence of bowel sounds and of abdominal tenderness is also checked. If a cesarean section was performed, the dressing is checked for drainage. The inguinal lymph nodes are also checked for enlargement.

Descent of the uterus is an indication of involution. The presence of bowel sounds is a sign of bowel functioning. Some mothers will have fundal tenderness, which is related to the intermittent contractions of the fundus during labor. However, this usually subsides in a few days. General abdominal tenderness is a sign of infection, particularly when accompanied by enlarged inguinal lymph nodes and an elevated temperature.

As the abdominal examination is performed, the patient can be taught what the fundus feels like and how to massage the fundus properly, without overstimulating it when it is not firm. Teaching should also include a discussion of the process of involution.

Suprapubic Area

The suprapubic area is examined for bladder fullness. The bladder should be empty if the mother voided prior to the initiation of the physical assessment. If the bladder is full, the mother should be encouraged to void. If the mother has difficulty voiding, special measures should be taken to stimulate urination (Chapter 19). Inability to empty the bladder spontaneously indicates that catheterization may be necessary. Since a full bladder interferes with accurate assessment of fundal height, the fundal height may need to be re-evaluated.

The amount and frequency of voidings, the odor of the urine, and whether pain, urgency, and burning occur on urination are also ascertained. Malodorous urine, urinary urgency and frequency, and pain and burning on micturition often occur with cystitis. However, the mother will normally excrete large volumes of urine during the first week of the puerperium. The mother should be taught about the normal diuresis that occurs in postpartum women and should also be told to void frequently, since she may have less of a sensation to void.

Vaginal and Perineal Area

With the mother lying on her back, the nurse inspects the vaginal area and lochial flow. She also checks the perineal pad to assess the type of lochial flow (rubra, serosa, or alba) and the odor of the lochia. The amount of flow can be estimated from the number of pads soaked in 1 hour. Asking the mother if her flow is heavier than, the same as, or less than a normal menstrual flow assists in estimating the amount of lochia. The presence of clots in the lochia should also be noted. Observation of the lochial flow can help determine if involution is progressing normally or if complications such as infection, hemorrhage, or retained placental fragments are present.

The mother can be told about changes in the appearance of the lochia, the proper application of perineal pads, and when she can expect the discharge to cease. She should be told not to use tampons while the lochia is flowing. The nurse should make sure that the mother has a clear understanding of the nature of the lochia flow. Some women may think that the lochia is a menstrual period if they do not understand its basis.

The perineal area is more easily in-spected if the mother turns on her side with her top leg flexed forward. Use of a pocket flashlight makes visualization of the perineum and anal area easier. The perineum is observed for bruising, hematoma, swelling, and tenderness. If an episiotomy or laceration repair was done, the site should be inspected for healing. The anal area is inspected for hemorrhoids. Information regarding the amount of sphincter control can be provided by the mother. While examining the perineum, the nurse can discuss perineal care with the mother. Exercise for perineal tightening (repeatedly tightening the perineal muscles as if stopping the flow of urine) should be encouraged.

Lower Extremities

The lower extremities are examined for edema, varicosities, symmetry, size, shape, temperature, and color. Range of motion is observed. Check to see if the mother experiences pain in her calf when her foot is flexed while her leg is extended flat on the bed (Homans' sign). If pain is experienced, this is a sign of possible thrombophlebitis.

The pulses of the lower extremities (femoral, popliteal, posterior tibial, and dorsalis pedis) are checked to determine if they are palpable. Fever, swelling, and absence of one or more of the pulses in an extremity are also signs of thrombophlebitis. The mother should be taught the signs of thrombophlebitis, since the condition usually occurs after she returns home rather than in the early days of the postpartum period. Advise the mother against leg massage and the use of constricting garters and other clothing that interferes with circulation.

Physiologic Changes

The nursing care related to the specific normal physiologic changes of the puerperium was discussed in Chapter 19.

OTHER CONSIDERATIONS

Rest and Sleep during the Puerperium

The postpartum mother needs adequate rest during the puerperium. While she is in the hospital, the mother's environment should be as conducive to rest as possible, and she should get adequate periods of uninterrupted sleep. The new mother is usually tired after labor and delivery and needs several hours of sleep. If not, the mother may feel tired and fatigued for several days and feel that she just cannot get enough sleep. The nurse may have to vary hospital routines in order for the mother to get adequate periods of sleep.

The mother needs to be comfortable and relaxed after delivery. Anxiety, tension, and worry can interfere with her ability to rest. Her mate and other significant family members need to be made aware of her need for relaxation and rest. If the mother becomes overly exhausted from frequent visitors both they and the length of their stay may have to be limited.

The mother should be told about her continued need for rest after she returns home. Some mothers may try to take care of a new infant along with carrying out all of their former household tasks. This will be too much for them to do. The mother should not expect to keep a thoroughly cleaned house when she has the responsibility of caring for a newborn. We must help the mother accept the idea that she will have to limit her activity at home dur-

ing the puerperium. Having someone assist her during the first week or two after she returns home is beneficial. Some husbands may be willing to stay home and help their wives for a few days after they return home. It is especially important that breast-feeding mothers get adequate rest and sleep, since fatigue can adversely affect the secretion of breast milk and interfere with the let-down reflex (page 638).

Ambulation

At one time the newly delivered mother was confined to bed from 1 to 2 weeks after delivery. However, early ambulation (within the first 4 to 8 hours after childbirth) has been found to be the most advantageous practice. When the mother is allowed to ambulate early, her circulation is increased and her bowel and bladder function is stimulated. Hence, early ambulation should be encouraged to prevent thrombophlebitis, constipation, and urinary retention.

Most mothers will be able to ambulate within 4 to 8 hours after parturition. Women who have had spinal anesthesia, however, should be kept in a recumbent position for 8 to 12 hours post delivery. Most physicians believe that spinal headaches occur because spinal fluid leakage through the puncture site in the dura causes a decrease in cerebrospinal fluid and pressure. Cerebrospinal fluid leakage is precipitated and spinal headache is more likely to occur when the head is elevated prior to the time that the puncture site seals.

A new mother may be weak and may easily become faint during the first few hours after giving birth. For this reason, the mother should begin to ambulate slowly. Rapid elevation of the head with rapid ambulation should be avoided to discourage fainting. The paient should first sit upright and "dangle" for a few minutes before she attempts to walk. Then she can be allowed to stand and walk for a short distance near the bed. If she feels faint, she can quickly be returned to bed.

After the mother has successfully ambulated for short distances, gradually longer excursions can be taken. The nurse should remain close by when the mother initially ambulates until she safely returns to bed. Standing for long periods of time should be discouraged at first, until the patient is strong enough to ambulate safely. The nurse should remain close by when the mother goes to the bathroom or showers during the first day after delivery, in case she becomes dizzy or faint.

Prior to ambulating for the first time, the mother should be told to call someone before getting up. Some mothers will try not to "burden" the nurse by attempting to get up for the first time alone. Others may feel that they are strong enough not to require assistance. We should explain to these women why it is necessary to have assistance when ambulating initially. On the other hand, some mothers may want to stay in bed rather than ambulate. The advantages of early ambulation should be discussed with these women, and they should be encouraged to get out of bed. When a mother ambulates for the first time, her reactions (whether she becomes dizzy or faint or whether she ambulates successfully) should be recorded.

Diet

The mother may begin to eat almost immediately after delivery unless she is nauseated or has received general anesthesia. Most mothers are hungry and ready to eat at this time.

The diet for the mother who is bottle-feeding her infant should be the same as that recommended for the average nonpregnant woman of her size and body build. The diet should be well-rounded, with adequate amounts of protein, iron, calcium, calories, and vitamins. Foods from the four basic food groups should be included in sufficient amounts.

The lactating mother has additional nutritional requirements. (See also Chapter 9.) Approximately 700 additional calories are needed to provide for milk production and for the calories contained in the milk. The amounts of some other nutrients required, such as calcium. iron, thiamine, ascorbic acid, and vitamin D, are similar to those needed during pregnancy. The lactating mother will need about 10 less grams of protein than she required during pregnancy. She will need about 1000 international units of additional vitamin A above the amount that she needed during pregnancy. More riboflavin and niacin are also necessary.

Since the average daily output of milk is 850 ml., a large volume of fluid intake is necessary to insure adequate milk production. The recommended fluid intake for the lactating mother is between 2500 ml. and 3000 ml. per day under usual circumstances. With increased physical activity and increased activity of the sweat glands, even more fluids may be necessary.

We must be sure that the breast-feeding mother is aware of how her present diet differs from her diet during pregnancy. Nursing mothers should also know that certain foods that they may eat can have adverse effects on their infant. Excessive amounts of chocolate or any food to which the infant is allergic can cause skin rash in the newborn. Foods that cause discomfort in the infant should be decreased or deleted from the mother's diet.

Postpartum Exercises

As with early ambulation, postpartum exercises can do much to prevent complications and speed the recovery of the muscles that were overstretched during pregnancy. In addition to promoting involution and a speedy convalescence, postpartum exercises aid in the restoration of the mother's figure by retoning the muscles.

10 Exercises after Pregnancy

Worried about your appearance? Your problem is largely temporary—if you avoid excessive weight-gain, wear an expertly fitted bra, even during sleep, and start these re-toning exercises before you leave the hospital. Add a new exercise each day. Do each one 4 times, twice each day, morning and evening, for a month or more.

3rd Day: Lying with your arms at your sides, draw your knees up slightly, arch your back.

1st Day: Breathe deeply, expanding your abdomen. Hiss as you slowly exhale, then forcibly draw in your abdominal muscles.

4th Day: Lying with your knees and hips flexed, tilt your pelvis inward and tightly contract your buttocks as you lift your head.

2nd Day: Lying on your back with your legs slightly parted, place your arms at right angles to your body and slowly raise them, keeping your elbows stiff. When your hands touch, lower your arms gradually.

5th Day: Lying with your legs straight, raise your head and left knee slightly, then reach for (but do not touch) your left knee with your right hand. Repeat, using your right knee and left hand.

Figure 20–1 Postpartum exercises. (From Benson, R.: *Handbook of Obstetrics and Gynecology*. 5th Edition. Los Altos, CA, Lange Medical Publishers, 1974.)

These exercises can be initiated on the first postpartum day. The mother should not overexercise initially. Exercises should be introduced gradually, as the puerperium progresses. As illustrated in Figure 20–1, a new exercise should be added during each succeeding day of the puerperium. Each exercise should be done four times in the morning and evening for at least the 6 weeks of the postpartum period.

8th Day: Leaning on your elbows and knees, keep forearms and lower legs together. Hump your back upwards, strongly contracting your buttocks and drawing in your abdomen. Then relax and breathe deeply.

6th Day: Lying on your back, slowly flex one knee and one thigh towards the abdomen; lower your foot towards your buttock, then straighten and lower your leg.

9th Day: Same as 7th day, but lift both legs at once.

7th Day: Lying on your back, toes pointed and knees straight, raise one leg and then the other as high as possible, using your abdominal muscles but not your hands to lower your legs slowly.

10th Day: Lying on your back with your arms clasped behind your head, sit up and lie back slowly. At first, you may have to hook your feet under furniture.

Figure 20–1 *Continued*

CARE OF THE NURSING MOTHER

The parents' decision to breast-feed or not to breast-feed their infant is affected by a wide variety of interrelated psychologic, social, and physical factors. With proper support and guidance during the antepartum period, the couple should have arrived at a decision regarding the method of infant feeding prior to delivery.

Because of modern technology and scientific knowledge, breast-feeding is not necessary for infant welfare. Thus, adequate nutrition for infant growth can be provided by artificial means as well as by breast-feeding. Therefore, the decision whether to breast-feed or not can more readily be made by the parents based on their own attitudes and personal situation, without fear of "short changing" the infant.

Health care personnel, particularly nurses who work with parents, have a definite bearing on breast-feeding behavior. The nurse can influence parents in their decision to breast-feed by her actions, which imply negative or positive attitudes. She must remember that whatever decision is made by the parents regarding the method of infant feeding must be accepted and respected. Thus, the nurse should not pressure parents to make a decision for or against breast-feeding. However, she should be able to provide parents with information that they may need in order to make their own decision about which method is best for them.

Once the parents decide to breast-feed, their success will be greatly influenced by the quality of guidance and care provided by the nurse who works with them. Breast-feeding is not a totally instinctive behavior in humans. Therefore, the parents will need much assistance from the nurse. The successful establishment of lactation is largely determined by the care and assistance that the mother receives during the first few postpartum days.

An environment conducive to breast-feeding must be established. In a favorable environment, the mother who is insecure or ambivalent about her ability to nurse her baby may be helped to have a highly successful breast-feeding experience (Fig. 20–2). Under adverse circumstances, even the mother who is confident and enthusiastic about breast-feeding may become discouraged. Therefore, comfortable physical surroundings and a positive emotional climate are necessary.

All too frequently, hospital routines interfere with the mother's attempt to breast-feed her infant. Often these routines have been established for the convenience of health care personnel rather than for the benefit of the parents. To provide the best opportunity possible for the nursing mother, we should consider whether established routines interfere with optimum care and whether these routines can be altered.

The Initiation of Breast-feeding

Breast-feeding should start as soon after delivery as possible, even though milk may not "come in" until about the third day postpartum. The infant will receive adequate nutrients from colostrum until milk is produced, as colostrum contains more protein and minerals, but less fat and sugar, than mature breast milk and is a substantial nutritional source for the infant initially.

The recommended time interval between delivery and the initiation of breast-feeding will vary according to the condition and readiness of the infant and mother and the recommendations of the pediatrician and obstetrician. Breast-feeding may begin within a few

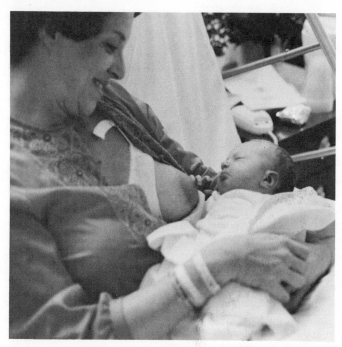

Figure 20–2 In a favorable environment, mothers are able to have highly successful breast-feeding experiences. Both Susan and daughter Alice seem content.

minutes after the baby's birth or as late as 12 hours following delivery.[54]

There are conflicting views about whether breast-feeding should begin immediately or several hours after birth. From the information available, there is not much support for delaying breast-feeding when the condition of the mother and infant is favorable. Initiating nursing immediately after birth has the advantage of stimulating uterine contractions and lactation in the mother. It also will fulfill the infant's need for sucking and orients the infant to the breast early. It has been conjectured that the length of the interval between the baby's birth and the first breast-feeding influences his acceptance of the breast. Early initiation of breast-feeding can also affect the mother's success at nursing her infant. In a study reported by Johnson[25] women

who were allowed to breast-feed their infants within 1 hour after delivery were found to be more likely to continue to breast-feed than those who waited 16 hours or more.

Some pediatricians recommend one or two feedings of water before breast-feeding begins. The ingestion of water is believed to help the infant to regurgitate any mucus or secretions that may have been swallowed during delivery. One disadvantage of initial bottle-feedings instead of initial breast-feedings is that the infant may have difficulty accepting the breast, because it was easier for him to get water or milk from the bottle.

Close nursing assessment and supervision in the early hours following delivery can indicate both the mother's and infant's readiness for the initiation of breast-feeding. When the mother and infant are alert and ready, the infant may be encouraged to breast-feed. It is preferable that breast-feeding begin within an hour after delivery when possible.

The "Let-Down" or "Milk-Ejection" Reflex

An important physiologic aspect of breast-feeding is the "let-down" or "milk-ejection" reflex. During lactation milk is produced and secreted continuously into the alveoli of the breasts, but milk does not flow easily into the ductile system. However, the milk must flow into the ducts before the baby can obtain it. The ejection of milk from the alveoli into the mammary ducts is stimulated by oxytocin, a hormone secreted by the posterior pituitary. This process of the "letting down" of milk from the breasts is called the milk-ejection reflex, the let-down reflex, or the expulsion mechanism.

The reflex is initially precipitated by the suckling of the breasts by the infant. The sensation of the infant's sucking is transmitted to the hypothalamus, which stimulates the secretion of oxytocin by the posterior pituitary. Oxytocin is released into the bloodstream, and when it flows to the breasts, it causes the contractile tissues that surround the alveoli, the *myoepithelial cells,* to contract and express milk from the alveoli into the mammary ducts. After milk is impelled into the lactiferous ducts, it is easily removed from the breasts by compression of the areola and suction of the nipple resulting from the infant's nursing.

The milk-ejection of let-down reflex causes milk to flow within 30 seconds to a minute after the baby begins to nurse. Suckling on one breast also causes milk to flow in the opposite breast. Hence, milk may drip from the unsuckled breast while the infant is nursing at the other breast.

In the early puerperium, the breast-feeding mother may feel painful uterine contractions while nursing her infant, as oxytocin also causes the muscle fibers of the uterus to contract. Because of the role that oxytocin plays in the let-down reflex, this hormone is sometimes administered to a nursing mother for the first few days postpartally to expedite milk flow. Oxytocin may be administered parenterally or via nasal spray just prior to nursing time. The administration of oxytocin is also effective when the let-down reflex is inhibited, such as during periods of maternal stress.

Psychogenic factors and the emotions of the mother greatly influence the let-down reflex. Such influences may be either positive or negative. For example, stimuli that are associated with nursing (e.g., the infant's crying at feeding time or actions associated with nursing) may cause milk to drip from the mother's breasts. On the other hand, pain, fear, fatigue, and emotional stress can inhibit the let-down reflex and adversely affect the flow of milk. Thus the mother needs to avoid emotional stress and strain as much as possible. The nurse can help by fostering a quiet and relaxed hospital environment; by encouraging optimum comfort for the mother, particularly at feeding time; and by maintaining a supportive attitude.

The nursing mother and her mate should be given an explanation of the let-down reflex, so that they will understand how psychogenic factors may adversely affect breast-feeding. They should be aware that a pleasant and relaxed milieu is important during periods of nursing and that various disturbances and emotional stress may interfere with breast-feeding.

Preparation and Assistance of the Breast-feeding Mother

A nurse knowledgeable about breast-feeding needs to be present to assist the mother and infant, particularly during their first attempt to breast-feed. Even if a woman has breast-fed before, she may still need assistance and guidance. No two infants are the same; thus, a breast-feeding experience with a subsequent infant may be quite different from a previous one. Hence, the type of intervention that is necessary for each mother-infant team is assessed, based on their individual situation.

Prior to placing the infant at the breast, the mother needs to be prepared for nursing. She is given instructions about the necessity for handwashing prior to each breast-feeding. The nipples are also cleansed with plain water just prior to nursing. Ideally, the mother should wash her hands and clean her nipples immediately before she takes the infant for nursing.

Mothers need guidance about how to hold the infant while breast-feeding, how to position themselves, and how to help the infant suckle successfully. It will take some mothers a while to determine the position that is most comfortable for them. A sitting position or a sidelying position may be equally comfortable for some women, but not for others. If the sidelying position is used, the mother's arm should be raised on the side at which the infant is placed to nurse, and her head should be supported by a pillow. The infant must be supported at the breast. Some mothers need to be shown how to hold the infant at the breast, since some women feel awkward when holding a small baby. Generally, it takes about a week for the mother and infant to establish a good nursing technique.

When the infant is placed at the breast, he may not display immediate interest in feeding. Usually the infant will turn toward the nipple as he smells the milk and will begin to nurse. The rooting reflex can be used to orient the infant to the breast. If the mother gently brushes the infant's cheek on the side nearer to the breast, he will turn toward the breast and grasp the nipple. Gently directing the infant's head toward the breast will also encourage nursing.

Both the nipple and areola should be grasped by the infant while he is nursing. If the areola and nipple are not grasped, milk will not be withdrawn well. Furthermore, the mother's nipples are likely to become extremely sore and possibly damaged. Mothers should be told about the correct position of the infant's mouth on the nipple and areola. The nipple should be placed well into the infant's mouth, so that his lips are fitted well around the areola. Thus, when the infants sucks, the alternating pressure of the tongue and palate on the lactiferous ducts will encourage withdrawal of milk. The mother can make the nipple and areola more easily grasped by the newborn by compressing the tissues above the areola between two fingers while placing the nipple and areola into the infant's mouth.

Once the baby has accepted the breast, the mother should make sure that the breast does not occlude the infant's nostrils and interfere with his breathing. This can be done by holding the breast away from the infant's nose while indenting that part of the breast near the infant's nose with a finger.

Mothers consider several factors in their self-evaluation of the success of their maternal abilities. One is the reaction of the infant during feedings. If the baby does not take the nipple easily, the mother may feel rejected by the infant. Mothers want and need to feel accepted by the infants. New mothers need to be told that it may take a day or two for the infant to be easily oriented to the breast. Once the infant learns to associate the nipple with food, he will readily grasp the nipple when it is time to feed.

The vigorousness of sucking by the infant is often important to new mothers. If the baby does not suck as soon as he takes hold of the nipple, some women may become concerned. If the infant stops nursing at any time during the feeding, it is probably because he is not hungry or has stopped to rest for a while.

The mother needs to be made aware that individual differences do exist in infants' sucking behavior. Some infants will hold the nipple in their mouth for a while before they begin to suck. Other infants will first suck and then stop at intervals during the feeding to rest. Others will suck vigorously throughout the feeding until they are full. The infant should not be prodded into a sucking pace that is not natural for him. As the mother becomes more experienced in breast-feeding, she will become familiar with her infant's sucking pattern.

Alternate Massage

To expedite early breast-feeding, alternate massage should be taught to new mothers. This procedure encourages emptying of the breasts by the nursing infant.

The mother is first taught to observe the characteristics of her infant's nursing behavior as nursing proceeds. Long, slow, and rhythmic movement of the baby's mouth indicates that the infant is compressing the milk reservoirs behind the areola (lactiferous ducts) with his palate and tongue and is withdrawing milk satisfactorily.

During the course of the feeding, the infant will rest more frequently, and the character of nursing becomes rapid and shallow. This type of nursing behavior indicates that the milk is not flowing from the breasts as freely. When the baby's mouth movements become shallow and he seems to be sleeping, the mother begins alternating breast massage with infant nursing. The baby should not be removed from the breast, but the mother should slip her hand "to the back and middle portion of the breast near the armpit and gently massage the breast several times."[24] At the same time the baby usually stops nursing; then he begins to nurse again with long, slow strokes. Only two or three strokes may be taken, since the infant quickly withdraws the milk that has flowed from the alveoli to the milk reservoirs after the massage. The massage is then repeated and the baby permitted to nurse again.

Mothers often feel the breasts softening beneath their fingers during the massage. When one area has softened, the mother should move her fingers to a new position and resume alternate breast massage, along with the infant's nursing, until the entire breast softens.

The mother is taught not to use alternate massage "until the character of the baby's nursing has changed from long, slow mouth movements to sleeping for the most part or to rapid shallow nursing. If massage is used before this time, the milk flows too fast for the baby to manage."[24]

Occasionally some mothers will have flat or inverted nipples, which the infant has difficulty grasping. Flat or inverted nipples are tested for protractility by pinching or compressing the areola between the thumb and forefinger. If the nipple elongates, this is an indication that the nipples can be pulled out manually with the fingers or with the suction from a manual breast pump just prior to placing the infant at the breast. A breast shield can also be used for the first few minutes of nursing to draw the nipples out for the infant to grasp. Usually flat or inverted nipples become more erect when the infant sucks.

Time Interval for Nursing

During the first 2 or 3 days of the puerperium, the length of the nursing period is limited to 5 minutes on each breast. This includes actual nursing time and does not include the time spent getting the infant started. As the mother's nipples become tougher and are able to tolerate longer intervals of nursing, the time interval at each breast is gradually increased.

In the first days before milk production is established, the colostrum in the breasts can usually be withdrawn during 5 minutes of nursing time on each breast. Prolonged nursing after colostrum has been removed creates undue negative pressure, which causes sore nipples.[24] The nursing period is increased up to 20 minutes as lactation becomes well established. Of course the length of the nursing period will vary according to the individual infant's need. If the infant nurses for long intervals, the mother should not be greatly concerned, as long as he is sucking intermittently and her nipples can tolerate the length of the nursing period without becoming sore. However, long intervals of nursing may be an indication that the infant's hunger is not satisfied because there is not enough milk present. If the amount of milk is adequate, the infant's own pace of nursing should not be rushed.

The mother can nurse her infant on one or both breasts at each feeding once lactation is well established. What is most important is that the mother should alternate the side that is emptied at the next feeding and that at least one breast is emptied at each feeding. Remember that thorough emptying of the breast stimulates the natural production of larger volumes of milk. Less milk will be produced if the breast is not emptied well.

Removing the Infant from the Breast

The suction created by some infants while nursing is so strong that it is not an easy task for some inexperienced mothers to remove the infant from the breast. To break the suction, the mother needs to apply gentle downward pressure on the infant's chin. If the baby continues to hold on after the pressure is first applied, the pressure should be loosened and reapplied.

Burping

Infants who breast-feed do not usually swallow as much air as bottle-fed babies; however, this does not exclude breast-fed infants from the need to be bubbled or burped. Breast-fed babies are usually burped midway through the nursing period or before the mother changes the infant to the other breast, and again when the feeding period is completed. For most infants the most effective position for burping is one in which he is held in an upright position. This is done by having the mother place the infant with his head at her shoulder and his body against her chest. Some mothers find it easier to hold the infant in a sitting position in her lap, with the infant's torso supported by her forearm and with his head supported by positioning her thumb and index finger on each side of his mandible. The other arm is left free to rub the infant's back gently.

Supplementary Feedings

The use of supplementary, complementary, or prelacteal bottle-feedings for the breast-fed infant is a controversial issue. Some physicians and nurses point out that this practice reduces the success of breast-feeding by decreasing the sucking stimulation received by the breasts and thus causes less milk to be secreted. This is based on the belief that bottle-feeding causes the infant to develop a weaker sucking reflex resulting from the easy flow of milk from the bottle as opposed to removing milk from the breast. Hence, supplementary feedings are believed to cause the infant to suck less vigorously when he is placed at the breast.[36] When supplemental feedings are given, plain water, glucose water, or formula may be used.

The mother who is to use supplemental feedings at home must understand their proper function. The nurse should discuss the kind, amount, preparation, and indication for supplemental feedings with the parents before they return home. Supplemental feedings are needed when the infant remains hungry after he has nursed at the breast. When used for this reason, supplemental feedings should be given to the infant immediately following breast-feeding, when he has obtained as much breast milk as possible.

Care of the Nipples

In the early puerperium, sore nipples are a frequent complaint of breast-feeding mothers. Mothers should be encouraged to report any nipple discomfort, so that immediate intervention will be taken. When the mother's nipples are sensitive, applications of plain unmedicated hydrous lanolin after each feeding will help toughen the nipples. Commercially prepared compounds, such as vitamin A and D ointment, may also be used.

Sore nipples should be examined for cracks, blisters, or erosion, since cracked and raw nipples are potential portals of entry for bacteria that may cause infection of the breast. Nipple or breast shields can be used during nursing periods when nipples are sore to prevent further irritation until the soreness subsides. If the mother prefers not to use a breast shield and can still withstand suckling, more frequent feedings of a shorter duration can be instituted to prevent prolonged sucking. This approach will also prevent overfilling of the breasts and engorgement, which can make the nipple difficult for the infant to grasp.

Expression of Milk

There are some situations in which the infant cannot be put to the breast to nurse or in which milk needs to be removed from the breasts because they have not been emptied sufficiently by the infant. With either of these situations, artificial means are instituted to remove milk from the breasts. *Manual expression* or a *breast pump* may be used.

Manual expression of milk can be done by the nurse or by the mother. Preferably, the nursing mother will practice manual expression of milk in the hospital, with the nurse's supervision before she goes home so that she will know the proper procedure.

Prior to beginning manual expression, the woman should wash her hands and cleanse her nipples with plain water. The breast is gently massaged just prior to expression to stimulate the flow of milk. During breast massage one hand is placed beneath the breast while the other is placed on top. Gentle but firm pressure is exerted, with a gliding notion from the upper portion of the breast downward. Manual expression is then initiated (Fig. 20–3). One hand is used to hold the sterile receptacle for the breast milk. The fingers and palm of the other hand are placed underneath the breast for support, and the thumb of the same hand is placed above the upper edge of the areola. The thumb and forefinger are then used to gently and rhythmically compress and release the breast area just above the areola. Milk is then forced out of the breast into the receptacle.

The fingers and thumb should not touch the areola and nipple, but they should be gradually moved around the area above the areola during the "milking" procedure to empty the breast. Manual expression should not be carried out any longer than 15 minutes at each breast.

When the breast pump is used, intermittent suction is employed to withdraw milk from the breast. Because suction is necessary to remove milk, breast pumps can cause some trauma to the breast if used improperly. Therefore,

the mother is always supervised by the nurse when a breast pump is required in the hospital.

When expression of milk is implemented by an electric breast pump, low, gentle pressure can remove milk with little danger of irritation. If more suction is needed to withdraw the milk, suction must be gradually increased to prevent nipple trauma and pain.

The suction apparatus of the pump is attached to a funnel that collects the milk. This sterile glass or plastic funnel is placed over the areola so that it does not touch the nipple. As intermittent suction is applied by the pump, milk flows through the funnel to a larger sterile container. The woman is told to inform the nurse if she feels chest pain or back pain. These signs are indications that the breast has been emptied and that pumping should cease immediately. A breast pump should not be used for more than 10 minutes on one breast. If milk stops flowing during the procedure, the pumping should be promptly discontinued.

The electric pump must be cleaned well after use, since it will be used by more than one mother. The funnel, milk container, and rubber tubing should be washed thoroughly and autoclaved.

A hand pump may also be used to empty the breasts. This is a funnel-like receptacle that fits over the areola. A trap to catch the milk is located at the end of the receptacle, and a bulb syringe is attached to the container. The bulb is compressed and released intermittently to withdraw the milk. The principles that underlie the use of the electric breast pump also apply to the hand pump. The hand pump is also washed immediately after use. If more than one mother will be using the same apparatus, it should be autoclaved.

Whenever breast milk is expressed in the hospital, the amount obtained is

Figure 20–3 Hand expression of milk from the breast.

recorded. The record should also indicate the method used to express the milk and whether one or both breasts were emptied. When only one breast is emptied, it is important to note which one it was, so that the other breast will be emptied the next time. When the milk is obtained, it should be placed in a sterile container and labeled with the mother's name and/or infant's name, the date, and the time it was collected. If the milk is not fed to the infant immediately, it must be sterilized prior to feeding.

Excretion of Drugs in Breast Milk

The mother must understand that almost all products ingested by her are excreted in some form in her milk. Therefore, any medication that is taken by a nursing mother may be inadvertently administered to her infant.

Because a newborn has an immature enzyme system, along with incompletely developed kidney function, he is susceptible to accumulation of toxic levels of drugs. Though only small amounts of a particular drug may be in the breast milk, the cumulative amount in the milk ingested by a small infant during a 24 hour period could result in a full therapeutic dose.[37] Irritant-type laxatives taken by the nursing mother can cause abdominal pain, diarrhea, colic, and nausea in the nursing infant.

Breast-feeding mothers must not take any medication without the physician's knowledge. The mother should remind her physician that she is breast-feeding if medications are ordered for her while she is still nursing her infant.

Further Guidance and Instruction for the Nursing Mother

Although breast-feeding is a rewarding experience for most mothers, it can be frustrating when the woman has not received adequate guidance about concerns that she may have when she returns home. It is often after the mother leaves the hospital or is no longer under the direct care of the nurse that she has questions or concerns that she had not considered previously. We can help to moderate or eliminate factors that may interfere with the success of breast-feeding by anticipating these concerns.

Prior to returning home, the nursing mother needs to be given information about painful and fissured nipples. The treatment of painful nipples should be discussed. A demonstration of the use of a breast or nipple shield will also be helpful.

Leakage of milk from the breasts is often a problem for breast-feeding mothers, as lactation becomes well established and increasing amounts o. milk are produced. Some mothers become distressed and embarrassed because their blouse may become soiled by leakage of milk. The nursing mother needs to be told about this before she returns home. She should be advised that wearing bra pads will prevent soiling of clothes.

Nurses need to be supportive o' mothers who breast-feed their infants Positive feedback regarding thei ability in their maternal role and reas surance that their infant is nursing properly are needed. Even after the mother and baby return home, telephone calls or home visits are indicated for breast-feeding mothers until they are secure in their ability to success fully nurse their infant.[25]

As the infant grows older and the parents feel more comfortable abou leaving the baby with a babysitter some nursing mothers may feel tha they cannot be away from their infan for more than a few hours. Such mother should know that breast-feeding doe not have to tie the woman down to her infant or her home. Breast milk can be expressed by the mother and left for the babysitter to feed to the infant. The mother should be reminded that breast milk should be stored in a sterilized bottle and refrigerated until the time that it is used.

Weaning

The duration of breast-feeding and weaning is an issue that should be discussed with parents. The mother needs to know that there is no set length of time to breast-feed her infant. Some infants may stop nursing as early as 3 or 4 months after birth, while others may still be breast-feeding at over 12 months of age.

In the United States, weaning from the breast usually occurs between 4 and 9 months of age. Ideally, the baby's willingness to wean rather than the mother's decision to stop breast-feeding will be the major determinant of the time for weaning. Once begun, weaning should be a slow process for mother and baby. The mother should be aware that weaning may proceed from the breast to the cup, or from the breast to the bottle and then to the cup, depending upon the infant's sucking needs.

Problems that May Complicate Breast-feeding

Breast-feeding may be complicated by problems that occur in the infant or in the mother. Oral defects in the infant may make sucking difficult. Although a cleft palate can interfere with the ability of an infant to suck, occasionally such an infant can be fitted with a prosthesis by a dentist to enable him to breast-feed.[38] Infants with facial deformities, macroglossia, or trauma or fractures to the jaw may also have dysphagia with breast-feeding. The effect of these conditions on the infant's sucking ability should be evaluated in each individual case before a definite decision regarding permanent or temporary discontinuance of breast-feeding is made.

As noted in Chapter 18, prematurity and low birth weight are not contraindications if the mother wants to breast-feed her infant. If the premature baby is able to suck well, prematurity presents no special problem, except that more frequent nursing around the clock may be necessary for adequate infant intake. When small babies and premature infants have a weak sucking ability, the mother can express her breast milk into sterile containers for feeding by dropper or by a nasojejunal tube until the infant is able to nurse at the breast.

Deficient secretion of milk and illness of the mother are maternal conditions that may interfere with breast-feeding. Some bacteria and possibly some viruses can be passed to the infant through the breast milk. Active tuberculosis is one absolute contraindication to breast-feeding. In some instances mothers with an infectious disease may be allowed to breast-feed, depending on the nature of the infection.

When a mother has a fever of undetermined origin, febrile respiratory infection, gastroenteritis, or any communicable infection, she should not have contact with her infant until she is receiving appropriate treatment and is no longer contagious. During the interim when the mother is unable to breast-feed, the infant may receive donor human milk or a suitable proprietary formula. The mother's breast milk should be expressed at frequent intervals to maintain lactation until the infant can be put to breast again.

When the mother is not able to continue breast-feeding because of hypogalactia (insufficient milk secretion) or agalactia (failure of the secretion of milk), she may feel frustrated or guilty if she believes that she is not getting her infant off to the best start. This mother needs reassurance that artificial means of feeding can be just as nutritious for the infant as breast-feeding.

SEXUALITY IN THE PUERPERIUM

Sexual Relationships

Most couples usually have some concern about when it is safe to resume sexual intercourse after pregnancy. The recommendations of physicians regarding the time to resume sexual intercourse vary widely. Some may not restrict intercourse at all as long as there is no bleeding, while others may recommend abstinence for as long as 6 weeks or more postpartum.

Abstaining from intercourse should be suggested until lochia serosa ceases, because of the possibility of introducing infection to the placental site.[15] Physical discomfort that results from perineal wounds and the episiotomy is also a factor that the couple will want to consider when resuming coitus. If sexual intercourse is very painful for the woman, the couple will want to refrain from coitus for a while longer. Perineal wounds have usually healed sufficiently for the resumption of intercourse within 2 to 4 weeks postpartum.[34] Many women will suffer some discomfort from the episiotomy scar for 10 days to 2 weeks postpartum, while others may have slight discomfort for as long as 3 weeks. Clark and Hale[15] suggest that a change in position for intercourse, so that the penile shaft does not press directly on the posterior area, will reduce physical discomfort in the early puerperium.

Usually, continuing sexual intercourse is beneficial because it tends to soften the episiotomy scar and thus decreases problems.[15]

Many changes in the sexual relationship of couples are likely during the postpartum period. Falicov[18] reports that a great deal of anxiety surrounds the resumption of coitus after the birth of the baby. Additionally, the ability to relax during intercourse may be affected by tension and fatigue from caring for the infant. Falicov also found that a large portion of the women in her study reported that sexual intercourse at 7 months postpartum was considerably less frequent than before pregnancy. The husbands' manifestations of eagerness and affection seemed to play an important role in facilitating sexual adjustment in the puerperium. The level of prepregnancy sexual investment was associated with sexual adjustment during pregnancy and in the late postpartum period.

Landis and associates[30] reported that the general level of sexual desire of husbands and wives in their study was lower after the birth as compared with prepregnancy levels. However, several factors were related to postchildbirth sexual adjustment. When wives had confidence in the contraceptive being used, the couple experienced better sexual adjustment following childbirth. Good sexual adjustment after childbirth was hindered by fear of another pregnancy.

In their investigation of the transition to parenthood, Meyerowitz and Feldman[35] found that the area of sexual adjustment was the major cause of complaint between new parents. Wives were frequently confused about what they should do regarding sexual intercourse. Psychic trauma was created for the wives when intercourse was resumed against the recommendations of the obstetrician. The mother was also found to be less interested in sexual relations than her husband at 1 month postdelivery, when she was still defining and adjusting to the maternal role.

It has become increasingly clear that health care providers should not ignore the sexual life of the new parents following delivery. Individual needs, desires, and circumstances affect sexual adjustment in the puerperium and must be considered. The personalities of the husband and wife will play a major role in molding sexual behavior during the puerperium. The new baby can also affect the sexual relationship of new parents, particularly as adjustments are made to his presence and the additional demands that he may place on the parents. A sickly baby or an infant with deformities may place such an additional strain on the emotional lives of the parents that their coital relationship may be disrupted. Discussion of puerperal sexuality should therefore be included in the plan of care for the parents.

Sexuality and Breast-feeding

Some breast-feeding mothers find that sexual arousal occurs when their infant is nursing at the breast. This reaction may be guilt-provoking or distressing if the mother does not understand that this is a normal and frequent response. The possibility of sexual arousal during periods of breast-feeding should be discussed with the mother so

that she will be aware that this reaction may occur.

Another common reaction that breast-feeding mothers may experience is the flowing of milk from their breasts when they are sexually stimulated, just as it does when they are stimulated by their baby's cry or even by the thought of their baby. This may also be distressing to some women and is another important piece of information for nurses to share with mothers while they are still in the hospital.

Just as coitus and labor and delivery have many similarities, breast-feeding and sexual intercourse can also be compared (Table 20–1). The similar physiologic responses during breast-feeding and sexual excitement are due to the release of the pituitary hormone oxytocin. The breast is an erogenous zone for most women. Sexual arousal occurs with stimulation of the breasts, regardless of the type, because of the nerve pathways to the hypothalamus from the nipples.

THE NEW FAMILY: ACCOMMODATING A NEW MEMBER

THE FAMILY-CENTERED APPROACH TO POSTPARTUM CARE

Several decades ago, childbirth was a family affair that was almost totally controlled by the parents. Because the parturient woman was attended at

Table 20–1   COMPARISON OF BREAST-FEEDING AND SEXUAL INTERCOURSE

Breast-feeding	Sexual Excitement and Orgasm
1. Uterus contracts	1. Uterus contracts
2. Nipples become erect; breasts are stimulated	2. Nipples become erect; breasts are stimulated
3. Skin changes; body temperature raised in submammary and mammary areas	3. Skin changes; body temperature raised in submammary and mammary areas

home, she was surrounded by family members from the time she began labor throughout the puerperium. Since the mother was confined in her own home, the father and siblings had the freedom to spend an almost unlimited amount of time with the mother and new baby. Family contact with the newborn and newly delivered mother often began within a few moments after childbirth, and the father was often present at birth.

Today, the hospital has become the major setting for childbirth. The transition of childbirth from the home to the hospital has major implications for the family. Although childbirth occurred in the family's own territory during home deliveries, movement of the event into the hospital made the family members intruders on foreign grounds.[33] When moved out of the home setting, care connected with childbirth became primarily centered around the mother and newborn infant. Even the mother and infant were separated from each other with the mother in her own room and the infant in a separate nursery.

In many hospitals the father is allowed to visit for only short intervals, and young siblings are totally excluded from visitation. The father and siblings do not have much of a choice about what their level of participation will be because the mother and infant are confined on others' territory. The major reason given for such restrictions is that the mother and newborn must be protected from harmful infectious organisms that family members may harbor. Although there is no real justification for the practice, many hospitals still place barriers to mother-infant interaction and to the participation of fathers and siblings on postpartum units.

The family-centered approach to nursing care recognizes the need and right of fathers and other family members to be actively included in the childbearing experience. Childbirth is viewed as an experience that belongs to the family as a whole. The family on the maternity unit is viewed as a complete unit. The family-centered approach to nursing care recognizes that each family has "lines of attachment" to one another. Therefore the birth of a new family member requires readjustment by all members of the family unit. The quality of postpartum care that the family receives influences family relationships, as adjustments are made to the arrival of the newborn. Thus fathers and other family members are allowed to share in the postpartum experience to whatever extent is desirable.

In the postpartum hospital suite, the family is cared for as a unit. The father is not considered a visitor and is recognized as a vital and inseparable family member. He is considered in the nursing care plan and his needs are of paramount importance. Fathers are included in parenting classes and are allowed to come and go at will.

Rooming-in

Many more nurses and health care personnel have become aware of the importance of early and continuous contact between parents and their infant after birth. Through rooming-in, parents have increased levels of contact with the infant during the early puerperium and parent-infant bonding is facilitated. In the rooming-in arrangement, the newborn is kept in a cot at his mother's bedside and receives most of his care from the mother. However, each mother's individual situation must be considered. Mothers who have had complicated deliveries or who are inexperienced with babies cannot be expected to care for the infants by themselves for the first few days. All mothers will require assistance from the nurse when rooming-in is practiced during the first day or so.

Father are also afforded greater contact with the infant when rooming-in is practiced and are likely to be more actively involved in infant care. Mothers and fathers can be taught infant care skills more easily when the infant is kept at the mother's bedside.

In some hospitals, infants are returned to the nursery at night or whenever the mother needs rest. This keeps the mother from becoming overly tired and encourages her to get adequate rest and sleep. When the mother seems not to be getting the rest that she needs, the infant should be returned to the nursery for a while. When rooming-in is practiced on units where other mothers are not utilizing such services, rooming-in infants are placed in a separate nursery.

The nurse on a rooming-in unit is in a better position to assess parenting skills and to do much more teaching. The nature of parent-infant interaction can also be more easily ascertained.

The chances of cross-infection are minimal on a rooming-in unit. Parents should be reminded, however, that they should practice frequent handwashing. Parents should wash their hands prior to handling their infant, and visitors should wash their hands upon entering the unit. Special gowns are usually worn by the father and visitors to cover their street clothes while they are with the mother and infant.

Sibling Visitation

Sibling visitation is another dimension of the family-centered approach that is practiced at some hospitals. Other children in the family should not be excluded from the childbearing experience. Visitation by siblings is beneficial for the visiting child and for the mother.

Young children are often heartbroken and feel rejected for the 3 or 4 days that their mother is away from them in the hospital. Toddlers and other young children who cannot fully understand the mother's temporary absence suffer the most adverse effects from this separation. Often these children may exhibit detachment from the mother and regress after the separation. This lack of contact between the older child and the hospitalized mother can be a major contributor to sibling rivalry when the new baby is brought home. Mothers are often also heartbroken when they have left a young child at home, particularly if the separation is the first one.

When siblings are allowed to visit, they can see their mother and their new brother or sister prior to the time that he or she is brought home. This helps the older child feel that he is also part of the birth experience.

Of course children (and adults) who are sick or who have infectious diseases are not allowed to visit. Whenever this is the case, the nurse should encourage the mother to maintain contact with the child at home by daily telephone calls. The father and other family members who visit should be encouraged to share their visits with the child at home. Both parents should talk with the older child about the newborn, thus helping to prepare him for the infant and mother's return home.

PARENT-INFANT ATTACHMENT

When the newborn enters the world, he is in a totally dependent state. The infant is helpless and is incapable of surviving without the care of an adult. The caring adult(s), usually the mother and/or father, compensates for the newborn's incapabilities because of their attachment to him. The relationship of parents to their infant is one of the most important emotional ties that exists. This bond is vital because it promotes the survival of the infant and the species, by insuring that the helpless infant's needs will be met.

The literature concerning attachment of parents to their infant has great significance for nurses who care for infants and their families. Many of the "routine" practices of hospitals in the United States interfere with the kind of activities that seem to foster attachment. In many hospitals fathers are still excluded from delivery rooms and from direct contact with their babies. Even many mothers are only allowed to see their newborns for short periods of time during each 24 hour period, and this is usually for short periods at each feeding. Rarely are concepts such as attachment discussed with parents, either prenatally or postpartally. Even when practices such as rooming-in exist, they may be structured so they are more punitive than helpful to parents and infants.

The Nature of Attachment

Attachment involves affects and is an affectional bond between two persons or a dyad. Therefore, attachment is specific and discriminating, as it is a special tie that binds one individual to another. Because positive feelings usually predominate, attachment usually implies affection or love.[1] Attachment is a bond that is enduring over time. Once formed, this affectional tie is amazingly persistent; however, contact and interaction between two individuals are necessary for attachment to continue over time.

Behavior that promotes contact, proximity, and communication with a specific individual is characteristic of attachment. Among the common attachment behaviors are those that are signals to another (crying, talking, and vocalizing), those that include actual physical contact behavior (embracing, clinging, and touching), and those behaviors that orient the individual to the person to whom he is attached (looking, following, or approaching). Such behaviors are indicative of attachment when they are differentially directed toward an individual to maintain a long-term affectional tie or relationship.[1]

The nature of parent-infant attachment is a unique kind of bond because at least some degree of parental attachment has begun to evolve prior to the infant's birth. Many factors interact to influence the degree of parental attachment to the child. Among the factors that may influence the prenatal and postnatal attachment of parents to their infant are the quality of the relationship between the parents, experiences with previous pregnancies, the parents' attitude about the addition of a new member to the family, and specific events that may occur during the pregnancy or during the labor and delivery.

Parents who have a good relationship with each other are more likely to have positive feelings toward their unborn child. When a pregnancy is welcomed and anticipated, parents will usually have positive feelings toward the child who is the product of that pregnancy. If prior experiences with pregnancy and with labor and delivery were positive and the events that surround the course of the present pregnancy are positive, a positive affect toward the baby will most likely develop.

Any information regarding the parents' attitude toward the pregnancy should be evaluated, when it is available. Mothers and fathers who had negative feelings toward the pregnancy may have some difficulty attaching to their infant and moving into their parental roles during the puerperium. Nursing support of parents who are ambivalent toward their newborns can aid the progression of parent-infant attachment by providing appropriate guidance and by facilitating parent-infant contact.

The Attachment of Parents to Their Infant

Contact and interaction between parent and child are essential parts of parenting. Contact is vital for attachment to evolve. Mother-infant contact has generally been accepted as a requisite for the evolution of maternal attachment to the newborn. However, little emphasis has been placed on the need for early father-infant contact. Biller and Meredith[5] and Lynn[31] have pointed out that frequent contact with the infant encourages love, attachment, and nurturing behaviors in the father. Parents need frequent contact with their infant so that the evolution of a strong parent-infant bond will not be hindered.

There seems to be an innate potential for parents to become attached to their newborn, and this potential for attachment is released by early contact with the infant. Hess[22] states that Lorenz has postulated that the characteristic baby features of an infant stimulate a biologically based affection for the infant by the adult. Thus, contact by the adult with an infant encourages the adult to respond positively and to become attached to the infant.

The findings of several studies support Lorenz's contention. Hess[22] reported the results of a study by Cann that gauge the positive responsiveness of men and women to pictures of both infants and adults of several different animal species. Findings indicated that women preferred the "baby" pictures over adult pictures and that men's responses to the "baby" pictures increased as a function of marriage and parenthood. Hess[21] used enlargement in pupil size as an indication of positive response to drawings of faces progressively stylized toward greater babyishness. He found that greater babyishness of the faces elicited correspondingly greater pupil sizes. Hence, these studies not only lend support to Lorenz's thesis but also imply that positive affect and interest can even be aroused in adults by "baby" pictures.

Not only is parent-infant contact necessary for attachment to evolve but contact should occur early and frequently. Studies of parents who have been separated from their infants during the early puerperium suggest that the degree of contact and parent-infant interaction during the early days following childbirth affects later bonding to the infant and possibly affects infant development.

A study to determine whether limited maternal contact with the newborn would affect maternal behavior revealed that mothers who had extended contact with their infants in the immediate postpartum period were more attached to their infants at 1 month of age.[3] These mothers reported that they picked up their babies more in response to infant crying and that they were more likely to stay home with their babies than were those mothers who had limited contact with their infants. The mothers who had extended contact with their infants were observed to fondle their infants more, to have increased eye-to-eye contact while feeding the infants, and to comfort their babies more during doctor's office visits.

In a follow-up study a year later, there were still distinct differences in reported attachment and in observed attachment behaviors between the two groups.[27] After 2 years the mothers' patterns of speech revealed "that those who had been given extra contact with their infants during the neonatal period used significantly more questions, adjectives, words per proposition, and fewer commands and content words" than did the group of mothers who had limited contact.[42]

Fathers begin to develop a bond to their infant when they are allowed contact with their baby early in the puerperium (Fig. 20–4). Greenberg and Morris[19] found that fathers begin to develop an attachment to their infant by 3 days after birth or sooner when they have early contact with their newborn. The fathers in this study reported that they felt preoccupied, absorbed, and interested in their newborn. These fathers found that their newborn's face, activity, and eye movements held tremendous importance for them. The men often interpreted any infant activity that occurred in their presence as their infant's response to them. A new self-perception was recognized by these fathers, who described themselves as bigger, older, and more mature after seeing their newborn initially.

Parents should be helped to become acquainted with their infant by frequent and early contact. They should be encouraged to unswaddle and explore their infant. When parents can feel their infant's warm skin and cuddle the infant, bonding is further facilitated.

For the baby contact provides a source of essential security, warmth, and comfort. The infant's sense of kinesthesia is highly developed at birth and is a dominant mode of adjustment for him.[46] Therefore, touch is a major mode of stimulation and communication for the newborn. Parents should be aware of the infant's need for stimulation through touch, as well as his need for auditory stimulation from a warm and loving voice.

The attachment of parents to their infant is also affected by infant behav-

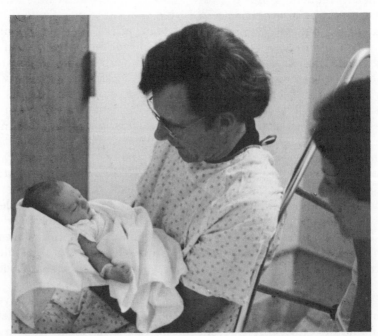

Figure 20–4 A father begins to develop a bond to his infant when they are allowed contact in the early puerperium. Bob's attachment to two day old Alice seems evident.

iors. A one-way relationship is often difficult to maintain. The parent-infant relationship is tenuous until the infant is able to actively participate and contribute to the relationship. Some mothers and fathers may have difficulty establishing a strong bond to the infant until he responds meaningfully. It is postulated that reciprocal and spontaneous infant attachment behaviors (such as crying, smiling, clinging, sucking, and rooting) are genetically determined biologic safeguards to sustain parental attachment and care of the infant.[1]

Assessing Parent-Infant Interaction and Attachment

A good parent-infant relationship is necessary to insure that the child's needs will be met and that his development will be optimally facilitated. It is therefore vital that the nurse assess the parent-infant relationship to evaluate the future relationship and its ability to withstand stress. The immediate neonatal period presents a unique opportunity for the nurse to evaluate this relationship. If there are indications that the relationship between the infant and his parents is not progressing satisfactorily, the nurse should refer the family to the public health nurse for follow-up visits.

The parents' attitude about themselves in the maternal or paternal role is important. A parent's self-concept can be a help or hindrance to his or her bonding ability.[14] The parent's ideal self-image interacts with the actual self-image to contribute to her or his attitude in regard to the mothering or fathering role. Those traits, characteristics, abilities, and attitudes that are deemed desirable for the parental role combine to form the ideal image. How the parent views himself or herself

currently constitutes the self-image. The comparison of one's self-image with the ideal image will have an impact on the developing parent-child relationship. Parents who have a positive self-image are likely to establish a positive relationship with their infant and vice versa.

Both parents' attitudes toward the newborn must also be assessed. Positive attitudes toward the infant facilitate bonding and movement of the mother and father into their parental roles. Negative attitudes will delay bonding. Assessing parental attitudes toward the infant includes consideration of whether the parents are happy about the infant's sex, whether they talk positively or negatively about the infant, and whether they move to immediately meet the newborn's needs.

The characteristics of the parents' touch can also provide information about the parents' progress in bonding to the infant. In the beginning parental relationship, there is a definite progression in the nature and amount of contact when parents touch their newborn. Movement is made from very small areas of contact to more extensive contact. Rubin[46] indicates that at first only the fingertips are used in touching, then the hands, and later the whole arms are brought in contact with the newborn. The direction of contact areas is from the periphery of the body during early stages of bonding. Then there is progression inward, centripetally, as bonding continues to evolve and the parent feels more confident in the maternal or paternal role (Fig. 20–5).

The characteristics of the parent's communication with the infant also give an indication of the ensuing parent-infant relationship. Whether the parent talks to the infant and whether the voice is warm and loving should be noted. The expression on the

Figure 20–5   Alice is incorporated into the family.

parent's face should be observed to determine if this is positive when interacting with the infant. Eye-to-eye contact with the infant by the parent is a positive sign of parental bonding. Whether parents call their infant by name should also be noted. Parents who do not name their infant or do not call their newborn by name may be experiencing difficulty recognizing or accepting him as a separate, whole individual, which will interfere with the parent-infant relationship.

Finally, how the parent stimulates the infant should be noted when evaluating the parent-infant relationship. Observe if the parent attempts to elicit responses from the infant or if the mother or father is passive, with little contact with the infant. Overstimulation of the infant by slapping, pinching, hitting, poking, and the like are negative signs for the ensuing parent-infant relationship.

INCORPORATION OF THE NEWBORN INTO THE FAMILY

At the time that the newborn is added to the family there are changes in family relationships and in the roles of the individual family members. The newborn is not quickly assimilated into the family without an internal change occurring in the family system. The newborn is an additional person with individual needs and demands that have to be considered in relation to the desires and needs of the other family members. Thus, the family must accommodate the new arrival.

Each family member's role within the context of the family changes with the new addition, and each obtains a new status. Rubin points out that "one becomes a mother or father, another a brother or sister, an aunt or uncle, a grandfather or a grandmother, simply by virtue of someone else's birth."[47] In any case, the arrival of the newborn introduces an additional person to whom the family members, particularly the immediate family members, must relate and adjust. In essence, with the newborn's arrival a new family is born.

The postpartum period is a phase accompanied by the incorporation of the infant into the family unit and by the incorporation of new roles and identities by family members. The taking on of a new role consequently brings about a new identity. The period during which the parents take on their new roles and identities is a critical time for mothers and fathers. Many parents need some assistance in order to feel comfortable about their new role. The infant is not completely incorporated into the family until each member is comfortable about his or her unique dyadic relationship with the newborn. Hence, parents must feel reasonably competent and comfortable about their parenting ability in relation to the newborn.

The postpartum nurse is in a unique position because she is an active participant in the care of families when the parents are in the early stages of their relationship with the newborn. She is accessible to the new parents as they begin to take on their parenting roles and can intervene to assist them when needed.

The Attainment of Parenting Roles

A first step in the attainment of the role of mother or father is the identification of the infant as a whole, separate individual. Part of this process involves obtaining relevant information about the newborn—sex, condition, and size.[47] Once the parents have received this information they each must weigh it in relation to their own fantasies and ideals regarding what the infant would be like. It is only after they have satis-

factorily accepted and dealt with this basic information that the identification process can continue onward in an easy, eager manner.

When parents have a less-than-perfect baby or are disappointed about the basic characteristics of the infant, the identification process is delayed while disappointments are coped with. This point is of particular significance to the postpartum nurse, since these parents are likely to have difficulty in carrying out their roles. The initial step in assisting such parents is to help them accept their infant by encouraging contact with the newborn and by discussing the realities of the infant's condition with them.

Once parents have realistically dealt with their disappointments and have accepted their infant, a realignment of their anticipated relationship with the newborn can be made and the identification process can continue. Until the parents are able to accept their infant, they grieve about their disappointment. Each of their specific disappointments must be reviewed and mourned, so that their attachment to the previously desired relationship can be loosened.[47]

The identification process is fostered by direct contact and interaction with the infant. Through such contact and interaction, parents begin to differentiate the identity of the newborn. Both the infant and their parenthood become more real to them. Once parents identify their infants as separate individuals, they can more effectively proceed to carry out their roles of mother or father.

Although much of the attainment of parental roles occurs after delivery, there is evidence that a great deal of role anticipation occurs during childhood and again during the prenatal period, as parents prepare to move into their roles.[48, 49] However, Rossi[44] points out that most individuals do not receive any realistic training for parenthood in our society.

In her study of the attainment of the maternal role, Rubin found several operations by which mothers incorporated their roles.[48] Although fathers were not considered in the investigation, it is likely that similar operations influence the attainment of the paternal role. Six operations were identified: mimicry, role play, fantasy, introjection-projection-rejection, identity, and grief work.

1. In mimicry the parent adopts simple behavioral manifestations that are recognizable symbols of parenthood, such as speech, affects, or gestures.

2. Role play involves the acting out of what a parent does in a specific situation.

3. In fantasy, the daydreams, wishes, and fears of the person proliferate to help her get an idea of what the parenting role that she fantasizes will actually be like.

4. In introjection-projection-rejection the parent finds a model to emulate whose own behavior seemed to work toward resolving a specific event that the parent is presently experiencing. If the "fit" is workable, then the behavior is reinforced; however, if it is unsatisfactory, the behavior is rejected.

5. Identity is the end process in the attainment of the parenting role. When the parent reaches a sense of confidence and comfort about the role, then parental identity is reached and role attainment is complete.

6. However, final grief work occurs as the parent lets go of the former identity in some previous roles that are incompatible with the assumption of the new parenting role. It involves the review and mourning of the attachments to a former role that had to be dropped during the attainment of the new parenting role. Thus the incorporation of the parenting role and of the infant into the family requires some degree of loss of former life patterns that must be mourned and resolved. Resolution may involve reduction of social roles or career pursuits.[20]

Rubin[49] also found that mothers most often selected their own mother or mother substitute as their role model, as they incorporated their maternal role. However, peers were also extensively used. It is also likely that fathers use peers as models to a great degree. In her study of expectant fathers, Marquart[33] found that expectant fathers reported that they sought out and spent more time with other expectant fathers or with actual fathers. These findings point to applicability of parent group discussions on the postpartum unit as a means of peer teaching.

The nurse is also used as a model by parents as they begin to carry out their parenting roles. Thus, as she interacts with the infant, parents observe her and may adopt certain aspects of her approach. This is why it is important for nurses to relate to the infant on an individual basis. She should cuddle, talk to, and smile at the infant during her contact with him, since these are behaviors will hopefully be modeled by the parents. The nurse can also serve as a role model by communicating her knowledge about parenting to new mothers and fathers.

Postpartum Teaching—Helping Parents to Incorporate Their Roles

Learning to be a good parent is difficult, and few people are truly prepared for parenthood. Now that the nuclear family has replaced the extended one, parents, grandparents, cousins, aunts, and uncles are often not available to young couples to offer advice and assistance. Teaching parenting skills to new mothers and fathers is of paramount importance and should be a part of postpartum nursing care. New parents need assistance and instruction in the areas of infant care, infant behavior and characteristics, and infant development. Parents must also be knowledgeable about other areas of family life, such as sexuality, contraception, and family dynamics, in order to function well in their parenting role. Hence, the postpartum teaching needs of parents may touch on many facets of family life.

Individual Parent Teaching. Not all parents have the same parenting capabilities. Individual instruction is a recognition of the differences in the background and experience of parents that result in specific capabilities and individual learning needs.

Certain factors must be considered when assessing the parents' individual learning needs. The most important factor is what the parents feel they need to know. People learn best what they are ready to learn and what they want to learn. The parent's own perceived need is important to her or him and is a strong motivator for learning. Most often it is best to give consideration to what the parents want to learn when they express this, so that they can then move on to accept other needed teaching.

Other factors that should be considered when assessing the learning needs of parents are the specific characteristics of the parents' individual situation, which determine the need for specific knowledge. For example, parents who have an infant with a cleft palate, hypospadias, or even a cephalhematoma require additional information regarding their infant. Indi-

vidual teaching allows the nurse to relate information to the parents' particular situation at a time when the situation presents an optimum opportunity for teaching. For example, it may be more effective to explain and demonstrate perineal care to a mother as it is being done by the nurse, rather than waiting to teach it in a formalized group session. Often individualized instruction, when a teachable situation presents itself, can be used to reinforce information that was given in a group session.

Information that should be shared with all postpartum parents, that is, information that all postpartum parents can generally benefit from, is usually given in group classes.

Group Postpartum Teaching. Group teaching is an effective method of postpartum instruction because many people can have their need for similar knowledge met at the same time. Group teaching can also insure that a large number of parents get certain information that all parents need but are not likely to know. Information that all parents generally need to know during the puerperium includes infant care skills, infant development, normal newborn behavior, and contraceptive methods. A well coordinated program of group classes can be very effective in teaching a broad range of parenting skills, particularly when a topic requires a longer interval of time to be covered well. More parents are likely to be reached and taught a topic that requires 45 minutes than if each individual is taught separately.

In selecting topics and planning group classes for parents, the nurse should ask herself several questions: "What common information do a number of parents need to know? Is this information best taught in a group situation or on an individual basis? If this information is not taught in a group session, are parents who need to be reached likely to be taught this individually, based on the number of qualified staff who could provide the information?"

Once the topics to be included in the program of group classes have been selected, the instructor must determine what resources and approaches to teaching will be most effective. Films and other audiovisual aids, demonstrations, discussion groups, or lecture-discussions are teaching approaches and methods that can be used for group classes. Mothers may also bring their infants with them to the group class, so that they can practice what they were taught while the instructor is available to guide them.

The instructors of the classes may be staff nurses only or may also include nutritionists, public health nurses, physicians, and social workers. No matter who is included in the classes as instructors, *nurses must remember that it it their responsibility to initiate, plan, and implement an organized postpartum group teaching program.*

An often unrecognized benefit of group teaching is the peer teaching that often occurs when parents begin to discuss topics in a group. Often multiparas and experienced fathers share valuable information with their peers based on their previous experience. As previously mentioned, parents often use their peers as models as they attain their parenting roles. Parents may informally share problems and teach each other as they gather around a table for tea or recreation. A parent who is returning home to older children can exchange notes with an inexperienced parent. This informal interaction can also be facilitated by insuring that parents have a place to gather informally.

All of the group class sessions may not be needed by all parents. Some maternity units establish special ses-

sions for smaller groups of parents with common special concerns. Examples are classes for breast-feeding mothers, for parents of infants requiring intensive care services, or for parents with premature infants. Of course the type of special group sessions offered will depend on the number of clients on the unit with common special concerns.

Outpatient Teaching. Once parents leave the hospital, they may be cut off from needed supportive and teaching services. Studies by Sumner and Fritsch[55] and by Gruis[20] show that parents still have teaching needs and parental concerns when they return home. Once faced with the care of the infant in their home without assistance, the parents find that questions and concerns arise that had not surfaced previously. In many communities postpartal parent groups have been established to assist those who need further instruction and support. Usually some of the purposes of these groups are to increase parents' knowledge of childrearing and child development and to provide a supportive atmosphere while parents incorporate their roles.

Parents may receive a similar type of assistance during the postpartum period from the public health nurse, a community liaison nurse from the hospital postpartum unit, or through the private sector. A telephone service whereby parents can share their concerns with nurses and have their questions answered can be beneficial, particularly for those parents who may not be able to attend group classes outside their home.

DISCHARGE FROM THE HOSPITAL

At the time that the mother and infant are discharged from the hospital, the nurse or the mother's obstetrician usually gives her special discharge instructions. One of the things discussed is a short review of self-care between the time of her release from the hospital and the time of the 6 week postpartum check-up. Usually the mother is advised to return to her usual activities gradually. She is advised against heavy work and lifting. Stair climbing is also limited until after the second week postpartum. The mother is told not to douche until after her 6 week check-up. She is encouraged to get adequate rest and sleep to prevent fatigue. The mother should be aware that she can take tub baths and showers and wash her hair when she returns home. The resumption of sexual activity by the couple is also included in the discharge discussion.

Special instructions regarding infant care may be given by the pediatrician. If the infant is bottle-feeding, the type of formula to be used is reviewed with the parents, and they may be given other special instructions about their infant's care.

Even though the major points above are reviewed at the time of discharge, the family was constantly being prepared for discharge while they were at the hospital. Therefore, a more in-depth discussion of this information should have been led by the nurse at some time prior to the discharge.

The family's need for support systems should have been assessed before they return home. Mothers or infants with special problems or conditions should be followed at home by a visiting nurse or a public health nurse. Appropriate referrals should be made to other health care providers when needed.

REFERENCES

1. Ainsworth, M. D. S.: The Development of Infant-Mother Attachment. *In* Caldwell, B. M., and Ricciuti, H. R. (eds.): *Review of Child Development Research.* Vol. 3. Chicago, The University of Chicago Press, 1973.
2. Atkinson, L. D.: Is Family-centered Care a Myth? *American Journal of Maternal Child Nursing, 1*:256, 1976.
3. Barnett, C. R., Leiderman, P. A., Grobstein, R., et al.: Neonatal Separation: The Maternal Side of Interactional Deprivation. *Pediatrics, 45*:197, 1970.
4. Benson, R. C.: *Handbook of Obstetrics and Gynecology.* 5th Edition. Los Altos, Ca., Lange Medical Publications, 1974.
5. Biller, H. G., and Meredith, D.: *Father Power.* New York, David McKay Co., Inc., 1975.
6. Bishop, B.: A Guide to Assessing Parenting Capabilities. *American Journal of Nursing, 76*:1784, 1976.
7. Bowlby, J.: *Attachment and Loss.* Vol. 1. New York, Basic Books, 1969.
8. Brazelton, T. B.: The Parent-Infant Attachment. *Clinical Obstetrics and Gynecology, 19*:373, 1976.
9. Cahill, A. S.: Dual-purpose Tool for Assessing Maternal Needs and Nursing Care. *JOGN Nursing,* Jan./Feb., 1975, p. 28.
10. Childbirth and Postnatal Care a Family Experience Shared by the Father. *Nations Hospitals, 2*:40, 1972.
11. Clark, A. L.: The Adaption Problems and Patterns of an Expanding Family: The Neonatal Period. *Nursing Forum, 5*:93, 1966.
12. Clark, A. L.: Introducing Mother and Baby. *American Journal of Nursing, 74*:1483, 1974.
13. Clark, A. L.: Recognizing Discord between Mother and Child and Changing it to Harmony. *American Journal of Maternal Child Nursing, 1*:100, 1976.
14. Clark, A. L., and Affonso, D. D.: Infant Behavior and Maternal Attachment: Two sides to the Coin. *American Journal of Maternal Child Nursing, 1*:95, 1976.
15. Clark, A. L., and Hale, R. W.: Sex during and after Pregnancy. *American Journal of Nursing, 74*:1430, 1974.
16. Cox, B. S.: Rooming-In. *Nursing Times,* Aug. 8, 1974, p. 1246.
17. Eckes, S.: The Significance of Increased Early Contact between Mother and Newborn Infant. *JOGN Nursing,* July/Aug., 1974, p. 42.
18. Falicov, C. J.: Sexual Adjustment during First Pregnancy and Post Partum. *American Journal of Obstetrics and Gynecology, 117*:991, 1973.
19. Greenberg, M., and Morris, N.: Engrossment: The Newborn's Impact upon the Father. *American Journal of Orthopsychiatry, 44*:520, 1974.
20. Gruis, M.: Beyond Maternity: Postpartum Concerns of Mothers. *American Journal of Maternal Child Nursing, 2*:182, 1977.

21. Hess, E. H.: Ethology. *In* Freedman, A. M., and Kaplan, H. I. (eds.): *Comprehensive Textbook of Psychiatry*. Baltimore, The Williams and Wilkins Co., 1967.

22. Hess, E. H.: Ethology and Developmental Psychology. *In* Mussen, P. H. (ed.): *Carmichael's Manual of Child Psychology*. 3rd Edition. New York, John Wiley and Sons, Inc. 1970.

23. Hogan, A. I.: The Role of the Nurse in Meeting the Needs of the New Mother. *Nursing Clinics of North America, 3*:337, 1968.

24. Iffrig, Sis. M. C.: Nursing Care and Success in Breast Feeding. *Nursing Clinics of North America, 3*:345, 1968.

25. Johnson, N. W.: Breast-feeding at One Hour of Age. *American Journal of Maternal Child Nursing, 1*:12, 1976.

26. Jones, W. L.: The Emotional Needs of the New Family. *Nursing Mirror*, Oct., 1975, p. 49.

27. Kennell, J. H., Jerauld, R., Wolfe, H., et al.: Maternal Behavior One Year after Early and Extended Post-partum Contact. *Developmental Medicine and Child Neurology, 16*:172, 1974.

28. Klaus, M. H., Jerauld, R., Kreger, N. C., et al.: Maternal Attachment. *New England Journal of Medicine, 286*:460, 1972.

29. Knafl, K.: Conflicting Perspectives on Breast Feeding. *American Journal of Nursing, 74*:1848, 1974.

30. Landis, J. T., Poffenberger, R., and Poffenberger, S.: The Effects of First Pregnancy upon the Sexual Adjustment of 212 Couples. *American Sociological Review, 15*:766, 1950.

31. Lynn, D. B.: The Father: His Role in Child Development. Monterey, Ca., Brooks/ Cole Publishing Co., 1974.

32. *The Mammary Glands and Breastfeeding*. Ross Laboratories, 1972.

33. Marquart, R. K.: Expectant Fathers: What are their Needs? *American Journal of Maternal Child Nursing, 1*:32, 1976.

34. Masters, W. H., and Johnson, V. E.: *Human Sexual Response*. Boston, Little, Brown and Co., 1966.

35. Meyerowitz, J. H., and Feldman, H.: Transition to Parenthood. *Psychiatric Research Report 20*, Washington, D. C. American Psychiatric Association, Feb. 1966, p. 78.

36. Newton, N., and Newton, M.: Lactation—Its Psychologic Components. *In* Howells, J. H. (ed.): *Modern Perspectives in PsychoObstetrics*. New York, Brunner/ Mazel Publishers, 1972.

37. O'Brien, T. E.: Excretion of Drugs in Human Milk. *American Journal of Hospital Pharmacy, 31*:844, 1974.

38. Oseid, B. J.: Breast-feeding and Infant Health. *Clinical Obstetrics and Gynecology, 18*:149, 1975.

39. Otte, M. J.: Correcting Inverted Nipples—An Aid to Breast Feeding. *American Journal of Nursing, 75*:454, 1975.

40. Penfold, K.: Supporting Mother Love. *American Journal of Nursing, 74*:464, 1974.

41. Rich, O. J.: Hospital Routines as Rites of Passage in Developing Maternal Identity. *Nursing Clinics of North America, 4*:101, 1969.

42. Ringler, N. M., Kennell, J. H., Jarvella, R., et al.: Mother-to-Child Speech at 2 Years—Effects of Early Postnatal Contact. *The Journal of Pediatrics, 86*:141 1975.

43. Rising, S. S.: The Fourth Stage of Labor: Family Integration. *American Journal of Nursing, 74*:870, 1974.

44. Rossi, A. S.: Transition to Parenthood. *Journal of Marriage and the Family, 30*:26, 1968.

45. Rubin, R.: Basic Maternal Behavior. *Nursing Outlook, 9*:683, 1961.

46. Rubin, R.: Maternal Touch. *Nursing Outlook, 11*:828, 1963.

47. Rubin, R.: The Family-Child Relationship and Nursing Care. *Nursing Outlook, 12*:36, 1964.

48. Rubin, R.: Attainment of the Maternal Role: Part I. Processes. *Nursing Research, 16*:237, 1967.

49. Rubin, R.: Attainment of the Maternal Role. Part II. Models and Referrants. *Nursing Research, 16*:342, 1967.

50. Rubin, R.: Maternity Nursing Stops too Soon. *American Journal of Nursing, 75*:1680, 1975.

51. Schroeder, M. A.: Is the Immediate Postpartum Period Crucial to the Mother-Child Relationship? *JOGN Nursing*, May/ June, 1977, p. 37.

52. Shaw, N. R.: Teaching Young Mothers Their Role. *Nursing Outlook, 22*:695, 1974.

53. Sonstegard, L. J., and Egan E.: Family-centered Nursing Makes a Difference. *American Journal of Maternal Child Nursing, 1*:249, 1976.

54. Stone, S. C., and Dickey, R. P.: Management of Nursing and Nonnursing Mothers. *Clinical Obstetrics and Gynecology, 18*:139, 1975.

55. Sumner, G., and Fritsch, J.: Postnatal Parental Concerns: The First Six Weeks of Life. *JOGN Nursing*, May/June, 1977, p. 27.

Chapter 21

PHYSIOLOGIC AND PSYCHOLOGIC VARIATIONS IN THE PUERPERIUM

In Chapters 19 and 20 we described the puerperium as a time of physiologic restitution and of individual and family integration. For some women and families, these goals are more difficult to achieve. Two major barriers are complications in the mother and illness in the infant. In this chapter we will examine maternal complications; in the chapter that follows we will look at the effect of a sick infant or an infant with a congenital defect on the family.

THE MOTHER WHO IS ILL DURING THE PUERPERIUM

The immediate postpartum period has been described as a "sensitive period," during which attachment is facilitated by the parents' opportunity to see, touch, hold, and care for their baby. What happens when the mother is unable to be with her baby, because of infection, for example, or because she is too ill to care for him? Does this missed opportunity affect her initial attach-ment to her baby? Does it affect her long-term relationship?

Mercer[14] describes a mother with idiopathic thrombocytopenic purpura who went into shock a few hours after delivery and subsequently underwent surgery for a retroperitoneal hematoma. Postoperatively she spent 4 days in an intensive care unit and was then transferred to a surgical unit. During this time she had no contact with her baby. Mercer's conversations with the mother indicate the mother's focus of attention on her own physical problems.

Rubin[20] has noted that even well mothers have a need for normal body function before they begin to "mother." This behavior on the part of the mother, while appropriate to the circumstances, is a barrier to mothering.

An additional barrier is the physical separation of mother from baby. Rules should be bent whenever possible to minimize the time of physical separation. In the interim, pictures of the baby that the mother can keep with her and

661

frequent discussions with the mother that emphasize her baby's individuality can help to facilitate her attachment.

Our records should indicate her progress toward attachment. When does she refer to the baby by his sex, calling the infant "him," for example, rather than "the baby"? When does she call him by name? Is she concerned about infant care in a specific way for her baby? When she has no opportunity to "mother," i.e., to feed and hold and dress the baby, these questions may not arise.

Mercer[14] reports on a follow-up visit to the mother described above when her baby was 9 months old. Even then, she never referred to her son by name. She talked much about herself but had to be questioned about her son. Although generalizations cannot be drawn from a single incident, the experience of even one family indicates the need for nurses to be aware of the potential implications of postpartum complications.

PHYSIOLOGIC COMPLICATIONS DURING THE PUERPERIUM

Postpartum Hemorrhage

Normal blood loss following separation and expulsion of the placenta is 200 to 400 ml. Postpartum bleeding of more than 500 ml. is considered excessive and is defined as *postpartum hemorrhage*. When the bleeding occurs within the first 24 hours following delivery, it is considered *early* or *immediate* postpartum hemorrhage. *Late* or *delayed* postpartum hemorrhage occurs from 24 hours to 3 weeks following delivery.

Although the potential for postpartum hemorrhage exists in all women, mothers who are anemic prior to labor or who have prolonged labor, fluid loss and dehydration during labor, pre-

eclampsia or eclampsia, or traumatic labor are especially at risk.

The principal causes of postpartum hemorrhage and the specific interventions are summarized in Table 21–1.

Whatever the cause, certain principles of care are important.

1. Hemorrhage is always frightening to the mother and whoever is with her. For emotional as well as physiologic reasons, she should not be left alone.

2. Massage the fundus, as described in Chapter 13.

3. Notify the physician.

4. Blood and fluids are given to replace lost volume and to maintain urinary output.

5. Monitor vital signs (including central venous pressure, if possible) and urinary output.

6. In severe hemorrhage, compression of the aorta just above the bifurcation between one's fist (or heel of the hand) and the vertebrae may slow bleeding. Because of the diastasis of the rectus abdominis muscle, this is easily achieved in the postpartum mother.

Puerperal Infection

Puerperal infection is a term that encompasses all bacteria-caused infections of the reproductive organs during labor or the puerperium. Synonyms include *puerperal sepsis, puerperal fever,* and *childbed fever*.

Prior to the twentieth century, puerperal sepsis was the major cause of maternal death. Many of our current practices that are now being questioned—the rigid separation of mothers and babies from other family members, for example—developed in the attempt to control puerperal sepsis.

Historical Perspective. Allegemeines Krankenhaus in Vienna was the largest maternity hospital in the late

Table 21–1   POSTPARTUM HEMORRHAGE

Type	Cause	Intervention
EARLY	Vaginal laceration Cervical laceration Tears of vaginal varicose veins	Direct suture of laceration Packing of vagina
	Uterine atony	Massage of fundus Oxytocic drugs Packing uterus (if above inadequate) Hysterectomy (if above inadequate)
	Retained placenta	Removal Curettage
	Placenta accreta (placenta firmly adherent to myometrium) Placenta increta (placental tissues infiltrate myometrium)	Hysterectomy
	Laceration or rupture of uterus	Hysterectomy (Chapter 14)
	Inversion of uterus	Manual replacement and oxytocic drugs Laparotomy to reposition uterus (if above inadequate) Prophylactic antibiotics
	Coagulation defects	Treatment of cause Heparin Fibrinogen (see Fibrinogenopenia, Chapter 10)
LATE	Retained placenta	Curettage
	Subinvolution of the uterus	Depends on cause (see text) Curettage Antibiotic drugs Oxytocic drugs
	Endometritis	Penicillin therapy Curettage (if no response to above)

eighteenth and early nineteenth centuries. In 1840 the maternity service was divided. In one section, instruction was given to and care was given by medical students; in the other, midwives were taught and they gave the care. Although the medical students used cadavers in their studies, the midwives only used mannequins. By 1846, four times as many women on the wards where mothers were delivered by medical staff were dying as on the wards where midwives cared for mothers. The maternal mortality for the medical students' ward was 9.9 per 100 mothers, although 2 and 3 decades earlier the maternal mortality rate for the entire hospital had been only 1.3 per 100 mothers.

In 1846, Ignaz Philipp Semmelweis

became assistant director of the medical students' clinic and began to search for the cause of the high rates of maternal mortality. He found that (1) infections were far more common in women with labors lasting more than twenty-four hours and (2) sepsis was rare in women who delivered at home.

While Semmelweis pondered the possible significance of these facts, a friend cut his finger during an autopsy and subsequently died after a course of illness very similar to puerperal sepsis. Semmelweis was then able to recognize infection carried from the dissecting rooms to the mothers as the source of puerperal sepsis.

In 1847 Semmelweis asked medical students to scrub their hands with chloride of lime before they examined women who were pregnant. By 1848 the maternal mortality rate (which had risen to 11.4 per cent in 1846) was 1.27 per cent, lower even than that of the midwives (1.33 per cent in 1848). Nevertheless, Semmelweis and his ideas were ridiculed by most of his colleagues, and Semmelweis became embittered and mentally ill before his death in 1865.

A generation later, in 1879, Pasteur demonstrated the relationship between bacteria (the existence of which was unknown until 1863) and puerperal sepsis.

Meanwhile in the United States in 1843 Oliver Wendell Holmes was also suggesting that physicians might be a causative factor in puerperal fever, an idea no more welcome to the American medical community than that of Semmelweis to his European colleagues. Holmes, however, became the Dean of the Harvard Medical School and in a publication in 1855 titled *Puerperal Fever as a Private Pestilence* was able to win his point. Maternal mortality improved significantly, but the isolation of mother and baby from the contaminated outside world (including fathers) also became an increasingly frequent practice.

Etiology. The anatomic and physiologic changes of pregnancy and of delivery leave the reproductive tract of the woman recently delivered particularly susceptible to infection. In addition, certain women are at increased risk, including:

1. Women with untreated local infections during pregnancy.

2. Women with prolonged labor (more than 24 hours) or difficult labor and/or delivery.

3. Women with anemia.

4. Women in whom lacerations of the reproductive tract occur.

5. Women who require uterine exploration following delivery (for example, exploration for a retained placenta).

Infection may develop from organisms already present in the reproductive tract (endogenous or autoinfection) or, more commonly, from organisms introduced from other individuals or the environment (Table 21-2).

Infections are also classified by site. Common sites include the vulva *(vulvitis)*, the vagina *(vaginitis)*, the endometrium *(endometritis)*, connective tissue in the pelvis *(pelvic cellulitis)*, and the pelvic cavity *(peritonitis)*. Local infections may lead to septicemia, bacterial invasion of the bloodstream, and thrombophlebitis (inflammation of the veins of the pelvis and legs).

Common causative organisms include streptococci (particularly beta hemolytic streptococci), *Escherichia coli,* staphylococci (particularly *S. aureus* and *S. albus*), and bacteroides.

Symptoms. A temperature of 100.4°F. (38°C.) after the first 24 hours following delivery that remains elevated for more than 24 hours strongly

Table 21-2   GENERAL CLASSIFICATION OF PUERPERAL INFECTIONS

Type	Source	Predisposing Factors	Comments
Endogenous infection	Bacteria in the genital tract	Excess bruising of tissue due to prolonged labor	Usually mild; rarely fatal
	Septicemia	Traumatic delivery	
	Sepsis in adjacent organ	Instruments used in labor or in delivery	
		Retained placenta, membranes, or clots of blood	
		Exhaustion superimposed on trauma	
		Hemorrhage superimposed on trauma	
		Severe anemia	
		Malnutrition	
Exogenous infection	Organisms from nurses, physicians, and other caretakers	Same as for endogenous infection	Most common type of infection
	Environment		
	Marital partner (gonorrhea and syphilis)		
	Patient's hands		

suggests the possibility of puerperal sepsis. Other signs, more specific to the varying types of sepsis, are summarized in Table 21-3.

Treatment: General Principles. The treatment of puerperal sepsis is similar to that of all infections. Antibiotics, specific to the causative organism once the results of cultures are known, have made a remarkable difference in treatment.

Nursing measures remain important, nevertheless. A high fluid intake is encouraged, usually from 3000 to 4000 ml. per day. If the mother is unable to take adequate fluids orally, parenteral fluids are given.

Rest is a major component of care. A semi-Fowler's position may be recommended to promote the flow of lochia; keeping the mother comfortable in this position is part of the nursing challenge.

Keeping the uterine muscle contracted, by fundal massage and administration of oxytocics, will slow the spread of bacteria through the walls of the uterus and aid in the expulsion of clots or membranes that facilitate infection.

Ideally the nurse who cares for mothers with an infection should not care for other mothers. This is not practical in every setting. Scrupulous handwashing along with other isolation precautions can protect other mothers, however.

The policies of most hospitals will not allow mothers with sepsis to hold and care for their babies. Many of the organisms that cause infection in the mother, the beta hemolytic streptococci, for example, are highly dangerous for newborns (Chapter 18) and can be a cause of death. It becomes our respon-

Table 21-3 PUERPERAL SEPSIS IN VARIOUS SITES

Infection	Cause	Symptoms	Treatment
Vulvitis; vaginitis	Trauma Infection during labor	Inability to urinate Local pain from swelling	Removal of sutures to effect drainage Sitz baths Perineal heat lamp Antibiotics
Endometritis		Slight chills Temperature above 100.4°F. (38°C.) Rapid pulse Uterus relaxed and tender Foul-smelling or profuse lochia Malaise Vomiting and diarrhea (as infection progresses)	Appropriate antibiotics for organism involved
Pelvic cellulitis	Lacerations of the cervix, lower uterine segment, or vagina	Tender unilateral swelling of cervix that spreads laterally Temperature above 100.4°F. (38°C.) for more than 24 hours; may be several degrees higher	Bed rest Antibiotics Maintain hydration Blood transfusion if hemoglobin level drops

sibility to talk with the mother about her baby and in as many ways as possible to facilitate bonding during the time mother and baby must be separated (above).

Table 21–3 summarizes specifics of treatment.

Breast Complications

Breast complications occur on a continuum. The least serious complications are the most frequent; the most serious are relatively rare. Moreover, proper attention to the less serious consequences will often prevent more serious problems.

Potential breast complications are sore nipples (Chapter 20), cracked or bleeding nipples, engorgement (Chapter 20), a clogged milk duct, mastitis, and breast abscess.

A part of the nursing care plan for mothers who are breast-feeding is teaching them to recognize early signs of these complications so that they can be promptly treated, and less severe complications will not become more severe.

Clogged Milk Duct. When one section of the breast is tender, with a small sometimes reddened area, it is possible that the milk duct in that area has become clogged. Untreated, a clogged milk duct may become infected.

The principle of treatment of a clogged duct is keeping the breast as nearly empty as possible and the milk

Table 21–3 PUERPERAL SEPSIS IN VARIOUS SITES *(Continued)*

Infection	Cause	Symptoms	Treatment
Pelvic peritonitis	Spread of infection from genital organs	Acute local pain Temperature above 100.4°F. (38°C.) for more than 24 hours Rapid pulse Frequent vomiting Abdominal distention (usually subsequent to above symptoms) Rapid and tender abdomen during acute attack	Same as for cellulitis
Thrombophlebitis	Thrombi at placental site become infected; inflammation spreads to deep pelvic veins and may extend to femoral veins	Usually do not occur until approximately 1 week after delivery Tenderness and warmth of leg Vein feels hardened Edema, beginning in foot and moving toward thigh Chills Temperature elevation	Bed rest Elevation of leg Heat to leg (leg is never massaged; embolus may result) Antibiotics Anticoagulants (heparin) Maintain hydration
Septicemia	Septic invasion of the bloodstream	Acute onset during first 3 postpartum days Rapid pulse in absence of blood loss High temperature Scant or absent lochia in overwhelming septicemia	Antibiotics Fluids Bed rest

flowing. The baby is nursed frequently (every 2 to 3 hours) and always on the affected side first, so that that breast will be more completely emptied. After each feeding, any milk remaining in the affected breast is expressed by hand. The mother should make sure that her bra is not too binding or too tight in any area, since this may place pressure on a part of the duct system. She can also be sure that any dried secretions covering the nipple are rinsed away (they may need prior soaking to loosen them) so that the milk flows freely.

Mastitis. There are several potential routes by which a mother may develop mastitis. If her baby has become colonized with staphylococci in a hospital nursery, he may transmit the organism to her breasts. The mother's own hands or the hands of hospital personnel may introduce the organism. If nipples are cracked or fissured, if breast tissue is bruised, or if a duct is clogged, the potential for infection is higher. Therefore early recognition of these predisposing factors is important.

SYMPTOMS. Initial symptoms of mastitis may be one or more of the following: headache, an elevated temperature with or without chilling, malaise, aching and other "flu-like" symptoms, and a rapid pulse rate. The breast may be engorged, reddened, very hard and hot to the touch, and tender and/or painful.

TREATMENT. The treatment of mastitis includes rest for the mother local heat to the affected breast, and keeping the breast as empty as possible. Specific suggestions to the mother include the following:

1. Rest in bed as much as possible; a prone (face down) position is preferable.

2. Apply warm, lightweight, wet compresses to the affected breast. Clean washcloths are fine. Cover the compresses with Saran Wrap to hold the moisture. Change every 2 hours.

3. Nurse your baby frequently; every 2 to 3 hours. Nurse on the affected side first to empty that breast more completely. (At one time the mother with mastitis was told to discontinue nursing or to discard the milk from the affected breast. This is no longer believed to be necessary, in that the causative organism is probably already in the baby's nose and mouth. Nor will the antibiotics that may be prescribed for the mother harm the baby.)

4. A firm bra will support the mother's breasts and make her more comfortable.

5. One aspirin-phenacetin-caffeine (A.P.C.) tablet may be taken prior to nursing.

If the mother has a fever, penicillin may be prescribed (penicillin G, 250,000 units, every 4 hours is a usual recommendation).

Early treatment usually resolves mastitis in a short period, often in 2 to 3 days, and the mother is able to continue breast-feeding as long as she desires. In the rare instance when a mother has repeated mastitis, we must help her examine handwashing practices, her methods of laundry, and so on.

Breast Abscess. A breast abscess is a localized complication of a more generalized infection (mastitis), in which pus accumulates in a local area. The treatment for an abscess is an antibiotic and may also include surgical incision and drainage of the abscess.

When an abscess occurs, the mother should discontinue nursing on the affected side, but she should express milk by hand from that breast and discard it until the abscess heals. Meanwhile, she can continue to nurse on the unaffected breast.

Subinvolution

Subinvolution is the term that describes the failure of the uterus to return to postnatal size and consistency within the usual period of time. Two common reasons are retention of placental fragments or fragments of the fetal membranes or infection of the endometrium (endometritis).

In checking the height of the fundus each day and the color and amount of the lochia, the nurse may suspect subinvolution. The fundus will be higher than expected and the lochia more profuse and red.

The treatment will depend upon the cause; it may include curettage to remove retained fragments, antibiotics for infection, and an oxytocic preparation to stimulate contraction of the uterine muscle.

Complications of the Urinary Tract

The effect of labor and delivery on the bladder was described in Chapter 19. When measures are not taken to assure adequate voiding, *cystitis,*, due to residual urine and/or bladder trauma, may result. The mother may complain of frequent, painful voiding or of suprapubic or perineal pain. She may recognize the fact that she has not emptied her bladder completely. Frequently she has a slight temperature elevation (100° to 101°F. or 37.8° to 38.3°C.). Urine examination reveals bacteria, pus, and, frequently, red blood cells.

Upper urinary tract infection (e.g., pyelitis, pyelonephritis) is suspected when there is flank tenderness (i.e., tenderness in the area of one or both kidneys). Other symptoms include frequency of urination, an elevated temperature that may be accompanied by chills, and nausea and vomiting. As in any infection, malaise may be present. Bacteria and pus are found in the urine.

Treatment of both lower and upper urinary tract infections includes specific antibiotic therapy, 3000 to 4000 ml. of fluid per day, and emptying of the bladder. The mother usually remains in bed.

EMOTIONAL COMPLICATIONS DURING THE PUERPERIUM

Just as physiologic problems during the puerperium can interfere with family integration, maternal emotional problems can restrict mothering and affect every member of the family.

Considerable ambiguity clouds discussion of emotional complications during the puerperium. There is often no clear distinction made between disorders precipitated by childbirth and disorders occurring in the postpartum period but not critically related to childbirth. Some postpartum reactions may begin during pregnancy; others after delivery.

Some reactions appear to be caused by immediate difficulties of motherhood; others seem to be based on deepseated conflicts concerning femininity, motherhood, or sexual and reproductive roles. Nevertheless, there seem to be basic areas of agreement that can be helpful both in clinical nursing practice and in developing nursing research.

Like all emotional illness, emotional complications of the puerperium can be divided into psychoses and neuroses. Psychotic illness is far less frequent, estimated to occur in 1 or 2 women per 1000 deliveries. Neurotic illness, chiefly depression, is estimated to occur in 1 to 3 of every 100 postpartum women, or approximately 10 times more frequently. In addition, less marked symptoms occur in a larger number of women; some estimate this incidence to be as high as one out of four women in the postpartum year. (Estimates vary considerably, depending upon the definition of illness.)

Postpartum Neuroses

Neurosis is the term often used to describe all mental illness of a nonpsychotic nature. Neuroses, which restrict the individual's functioning and disturb her well-being, include anxiety states, phobias, obsessions, hypochondriasis, and depression. In the postpartum period, depression has repeatedly been found to be the most common neurosis.

Postpartum neuroses cannot be viewed as a specific entity, but rather as part of the health-illness continuum. At one end of the continuum are mothers who exhibit symptoms of postpartum blues (Chapter 19), which are considered a part of normal emotional lability in the first days following pregnancy. At the opposite end of the continuum are women with symptoms sufficiently severe to require hospitalization or intensive treatment. This group represents from 1 to 3 per cent of women who have delivered.

Between these two extremes are a large number of women who exhibit some symptoms, such as despondency, tearfulness, feelings of inadequacy or inability to cope, hypochondria, irritability, undue fatigue, decrease in appetite, difficulties in sleeping, decreased libido, and fears for the baby's health.

Since these symptoms are very general and since many of them may, and usually do, occur at one time or other in most new mothers, the recognition of illness is obviously more a matter of degree. For example, all mothers have periods of fatigue (lack of sleep is a frequent hazard of new parents), but chronic fatigue that is unrelieved by rest may indicate illness. There are days when each new mother may feel inadequate to cope—days when the baby seems to cry incessantly, for example—but the mother who has a constant feeling of inadequacy needs professional counseling.

Characteristics of Mothers Who Develop Postpartum Neuroses. Is it possible to predict which mothers will have postpartum neuroses and thereby to give them special attention and perhaps even to prevent their symptoms or alleviate their severity? In a very specific sense the answer is no, although certain factors in common do appear in the research literature.

In both prospective and retrospective studies,[16, 17] a past history of neurosis was found to be the single most important factor in predicting neurotic reactions during or after pregnancy.

Bardon[2] found unconscious conflicts about assuming the roles and responsibilities of mothering to be the most frequent and most important stress factor. He suggests that real or fantasized difficulties between a child and her parents—an unhappy relationship or unmet dependency needs, for example—are transferred to her own child. As the child of the mother becomes the mother of the child, she sees herself in her child and her mother in herself. Kaij and Nilsson[13] suggest that women with poor or unsatisfactory relations with their mothers during infancy and adolescence; women insufficiently informed about sexual matters, especially menarche; and women with early sexual experience and more than one sexual partner are more likely to have a negative attitude toward pregnancy and to develop postpartum neurosis.

Tod, in a prospective study of 700 consecutive pregnancies, found 20 mothers (2.9 per cent) with postpartum depression (1958 to 1963).[24] He described all of them as having "inadequate personalities" (introverted and with symptoms of neuroses). Other characteristics included: abnormal psychiatric history: 55 per cent; abnormal marital history: 55 per cent; abnormal obstetric history: 60 per cent; anemia: 40 per cent; previous medical problems: 20 per cent; and previous stillbirth or baby with a congenital defect: 25 per cent. Tod found that neither social class nor age was significant.

The presence or absence of "postpartum blues" does not appear to be indicative of future emotional problems. Behavior during the brief period of hospitalization that may indicate abnormality includes a lack of interest in the child (failure to name him or call him by name, disinterest in feeding and holding him, and so on) and a marked concern about the problems to be faced by the mother when she returns home.

Barglow and associates[3] found that

25 percent of women with postpartum mental illness had a recurrence in a subsequent pregnancy.

Contributing Factors. In addition to factors within the mother's personality, other variables have been suggested as possible contributors to postpartum neuroses.

Hormonal factors, particularly the postnatal fall in progesterone, have been postulated as contributing to neurosis.

Tod has questioned the role of folic acid as a causative factor. From 1958 to 1963, he found an incidence of depression of 2.9 per cent in 700 women.[74] In a retrospective study of 700 women who delivered between 1965 and 1970, only 0.9 per cent of the second group were depressed. He suggests that the fall may be related to the routine administration of folic acid during pregnancy during the second time span. Folic acid has been shown to be related to mental disturbance in some other conditions, including tropical sprue, pernicious anemia, and postgastrectomy anemia.[22, 23]

Cone found the incidence of depression to be lower in mothers who delivered at home than in mothers who delivered in hospital.[7] Her study, done in Cardiff, Wales, where home deliveries are common, may reflect differences in mothers who choose home versus mothers who choose hospital (mothers were matched for parity and mode of delivery) or may suggest factors in the hospital environment, an idea worth exploring further.

Other areas that have been investigated, with no conclusive findings, include age, social status, parity, and specific genetic factors.

Symptoms. The most common symptoms of postpartum neuroses are summarized in Table 21–4.

Treatment. The treatment will vary with the specific diagnosis. Antidepressive drugs, psychotherapy, and allowing the mother to express her distress and incompletely acknowledged hostilities are major principles of treatment.

Bardon[2] suggests that when hospital admission is necessary, admitting both mother and infant will enable them to have good experiences together, rather than confirming the mother's existing doubts and feelings of inadequacy.

Untreated, symptoms may persist for a year or more, with potentially devastating consequences for the entire family.

Postpartum Psychoses

As noted above, psychoses are far less common than neuroses, but the impact of a psychotic mother on her family can be monumental.

Symptoms of puerperal psychosis include mixed or rapidly changing affects; a clouding of consciousness; hypochondriacal delusions; hallucinations; erroneous beliefs that the child is dead, malformed, or severely ill; and general anxiety.

The duration of illness may range from a few days to a year to a chronic state lasting many years. Kaij and Nilsson[13] report about 20 per cent of the women recovering within 1 month; 40 per cent having a course of illness lasting 6 months or longer, and 15 per cent becoming chronically ill. When the illness is chronic, there is some question as to whether it is a true postpartum psychosis or a pre-existing condition that becomes more evident when the mother is faced with new responsibilities.

Although for many women the postpartum psychosis represents a single, discrete event, as many as 30 per

Table 21–4   COMMON SYMPTOMS OF POSTPARTUM NEUROSES

Symptom	Characteristics	Comments
Depression	Varies from mild and transitory to deep and long-lasting	Most common symptom Prenatal depression lasting several months may recur postpartum
Neurasthenia	Extreme fatigue Sleeplessness Emotional lability Irritability	May last from several months to a year May be incapacitating
Anxiety	Pronounced Mother may feel abandoned by short absences of husband	May become chronic if not appropriately cared for at early stage
Phobias	Fear of infanticide Fear of insanity	Often a single episode; except in schizophrenia (a psychosis), the risk of infanticide is not present
Sexual difficulties	Decreased libido Incapacity for orgasm	More pronounced than during pregnancy
Psychosomatic complaints	Frequent and varied complaints of physical symptoms	Distinguish carefully from physical symptoms

cent may have further psychotic episodes. The ratio of risk of a subsequent postpartum psychosis occurring has been estimated to be as high as 1:7, although some researchers suggest only a slightly increased risk.

Treatment is directed toward the specific psychotic symptoms.

FOURTH TRIMESTER CARE

Two generations ago, when mothers remained in the hospital from 10 days to 3 weeks, assessment of potential complications was not difficult. Today, however, with mothers returning home from 1 to 3 days after delivery, the opportunity for close assessment no longer exists. We have already noted that many mothers leave the health care system when they are discharged. Few will fail to seek medical attention for a dramatic symptom, such as a marked hemorrhage or a high fever. But without follow-up, many women particularly those without a private physician, may not seek care for less obvious problems, either physical or emotional.

One of the immediate challenges to our system of nursing care is a *systematic* way to provide care during the "fourth trimester." Donaldson[8] describes a follow-up program at Hoag Memorial Hospital-Presbyterian in California that includes:

1. Initial telephone contact with families after they return home.

2. Assessment of needs.

3. Reinforcement of teaching.

4. Repeated calls, home visits, and referral to other agencies when necessary.

5. Communication with appropriate staff and agencies.

Mothers know, and are reminded during the telephone calls, that they may call the maternity unit at any time, 24 hours a day.

In many communities in England, home visits by community health nurses are frequent for several weeks after delivery for all patients.

Nurses everywhere need to evaluate the fourth trimester care in their communities to better meet the needs of childbearing families.

REFERENCES

1. Assali, N., and Brinkman, C. (eds.): *Pathophysiology of Gestation.* Vol. 1, Maternal Disorders. New York, Academic Press, 1972.

2. Bardon, D.: Puerperal Depression. *In* Morris, N. (ed.): *Psychosomatic Medicine in Obstetrics and Gynecology.* Basel, S. Karger, 1972.

3. Barglow, P., Wilson, J., and Shipman, W.: The Nature of Post Partum Mental Illness. *In* Morris, N. (ed.): *Psychosomatic Medicine in Obstetrics and Gynecology.* Basel, S. Karger, 1972.

4. Barnard, M.: Supportive Nursing Care for the Mother and Newborn Who are Separated from Each Other. *MCN, 1*(2):107, 1976.

5. Brown, W.: A Prospective Study of Post Partum Psychiatric Disorders *In* Morris, N. (ed.): *Psychosomatic Medicine in Obstetrics and Gynecology.* Basel, S. Karger, 1972.

6. Charles, D., and Klein, T.: Postpartum Infection. *In* Charles, D., and Finland, M. (eds.): *Obstetric and Perinatal Infections.* Philadelphia, Lea & Febiger, 1973.

7. Cone, B.: Puerperal Depression. *In* Morris, N. (ed.): *Psychosomatic Medicine in Obstetrics and Gynecology.* Basel, S. Karger, 1972.

8. Donaldson, W.: Fourth Trimester Follow-up. *American Journal of Nursing, 77*:1176, 1977.

9. Eiger, M., and Olds, S.: *The Complete Book of Breastfeeding.* New York, Bantam Books, 1972.

10. Grossman, E.: Helping Mothers to Nurse Their Babies. *GP, 31*(4):78, 1965.

11. Holmes, O. W.: Contagiousness of Puerperal Fever. *New England Quarterly Journal of Medicine and Surgery, 1*:503, 1842–1843.

12. Holmes, O. W.: *Puerperal Fever as a Private Pestilence.* Boston, Ticknor and Fields, 1855.

13. Kaij, L., and Nilsson, A.: Emotional and Psychotic Illness Following Childbirth. *In* Howells, J. (ed.): *Modern Perspectives in Psycho-Obstetrics.* New York, Brunner/Mazel, 1972.

14. Mercer, R.: Postpartum: Illness and Acquaintance-Attachment Process. *American Journal of Nursing, 77*:1174, 1977.

15. Newton, M., and Newton, N.: The Normal Course and Management of Lactation. *Child and Family, 9*(2):102, 1970.

16. Nilsson, A.: Para-natal Emotional Adjustment. *Acta Psychiatrica Scandinavica,* Suppl.:220, 1970.

17. Nilsson, A., Kaij, L., and Jacobson, L.: Postpartum Mental Disorder in an Unselected Sample. The Importance of Unplanned Pregnancy. *Journal of Psychosomatic Research, 10*:341, 1967.

18. Pitt, B.: Psychiatric Illness Following Childbirth. *Hospital Medicine 2*:815, 1968.

19. Pitt, B.: Neurotic (or Atypical) Depression Following Childbirth. *In* Morris, N. (ed.): *Psychosomatic Medicine in Obstetrics and Gynaecology.* Basel, S. Karger, 1972.

20. Rubin, R.: Puerperal Change. *Nursing Outlook, 9*:753, 1961.

21. Schwarz, R.: *Handbook of Obstetric Emergencies.* Flushing, N.Y., Medical Examination Publishing Co., 1973.

22. Smith, A.: Megaloblastic Madness. *British Medical Journal, 2*:1840, 1960.

23. Strachan, R., and Henderson, J.: Psychiatric Syndromes Due to Avitaminosis B_{12} with Normal Blood and Marrow. *Quarterly Journal of Medicine, 34*:303, 1965.

24. Tod, E.: Puerperal Depression. *In* Morris, N. (ed.): *Psychosomatic Medicine in Obstetrics and Gynecology.* Basel, S. Karger, 1972.

25. The Womanly Art of Breastfeeding. Franklin Park, Ill., La Leche League, 1963.

Chapter 22

THE FAMILY OF THE HIGH RISK NEWBORN

Becoming parents under even the most ideal of circumstances involves major changes in lifestyle. Consider, then, what monumental changes a couple or a single mother must face when the birth, or the baby, differs from normal. Perhaps he is born before term and must be in an intensive care nursery. There may be an obvious birth defect, such as a cleft lip or a meningocele. Or a condition with long-term implications, such as Down's syndrome, may be suspected.

Nurses can help parents begin to cope with their feelings and make plans for their baby who is ill or who has a problem that will exist for many years. Before they can do this, nurses must:

1. Recognize their own feelings about infants who are ill.

2. Cope with their own feelings.

3. Recognize characteristic behavior in parents of babies who are ill.

4. Be aware of the kinds of nursing intervention that may be helpful to parents.

A second problem of families with high risk babies is the separation caused by the care these infants receive, often in a medical center many miles from home. This separation can inter-

fere markedly with the bonding and attachment process described in Chapter 20. Thus another aspect of nursing care is assessing the attachment behavior in parents of high risk newborns and facilitating that attachment.

It is with these topics that this chapter is concerned.

RECOGNIZING OUR FEELINGS ABOUT ILL BABIES

Consider this situation: You are working in the nursery when a baby, newly delivered, arrives. His father will be coming to the nursery shortly to see his first-born son. Normally this is a joyful occasion; you get a great deal of satisfaction from "showing" babies to their parents for the first time. But in the middle of this baby's back is a large meningocele. How do you feel about showing this baby to his father? Threatened? Anxious? Helpless? Sad? Would you like to position the baby so that the father will not see the defect? Are you angry about being placed in the position of having to show the baby?

None of these feelings is unusual. They are shared not only by student

674

nurses but by many other members of the health team. To recognize that we sometimes feel this way is the beginning of developing an ability to cope with the reality of a high risk baby and his parents.

The Sources of Our Feelings

Our own experiences, both professional and personal, influence the way in which we will view the problems of a particular baby and his family. For example, if we have seen very good results in the repair of cleft lips in babies, we find we can talk quite comfortably with parents, giving this realistic assurance. Moreover, and perhaps even more important, we can handle the baby easily and affectionately. Parents are quick to perceive our reactions to their baby; our positive feelings toward them and their baby will help them to react in a positive way as well.

Nurses and other health team members may also have negative feelings toward babies who are critically ill or handicapped. One student nurse, for example, whose brother had been brain damaged at the time of birth and eventually placed in an institution, found it particularly difficult to care for babies and families who appeared to have similar problems.

Just as parents detect positive attitudes, they may even more quickly perceive negative feelings toward themselves and their baby. How do we hold their baby? Do we hide him in the corner of the nursery? Do we avoid spending time with the mother and father? Because of their own feelings of guilt and anger and disappointment (see below), they are usually supersensitive to any indication that we reject their baby. Even a chance remark overheard in a corridor may be taken as evidence of our rejection.

Learning to explore and deal with our feelings about sick or handicapped babies can be painful. Nurses sometimes choose maternity and newborn nursing as an area of practice because they feel it involves happy people—joyful parents and healthy babies—in contrast to many other areas of health care. But because joy is the expectation, coping with sadness is even more difficult than it might be under different circumstances. To be an effective nurse for pregnant families, we must have the resources to help parents cope with unexpected grief as well as with happier moments.

Somewhat different kinds of feelings may surface in the nursery concerning decisions about how much treatment is given to a particular baby. We may feel angry about the aggressive treatment given to one infant who we feel has little chance of survival ("Why don't they let him die in peace?"). On the other hand we may feel just as hostile about failure to treat a baby who we believe would have a good chance of surviving. Part of the frustration for nurses comes from the feeling that we have no choice in the decisions that are made; we need to recognize this. Part of the *result* of that frustration may involve subtle (and usually unconscious) manipulation of parents to one's point of view. Needless to say, this is very destructive behavior. Parents of newborns who are ill have to cope with multiple problems and feelings; our care must be supportive.

What can be done to help staff (nurses, physicians, and other professional and nonprofessional workers) deal with these kinds of feelings? Frequent opportunities for all nursery staff to meet together in multidisciplinary conferences seem to be the most helpful approach. The opportunity for each person to share his or her ideas can tremendously enhance care. Such sessions are of little value, of course, if they are authoritarian or defensive.

Not every hospital has reached the point of being comfortable with interdisciplinary conferences. Although this is the ideal, and a goal toward which every institution should be working, nursing conferences oriented toward discussion of feelings and frustrations can also be very helpful.

In looking at our feelings about babies who are sick or malformed, we also need to be aware of the ways in which we cope with those feelings. For many nurses, detachment is a frequent means of coping. We are not going to allow our emotions to get involved with that baby and his family. We tend to call all babies "he" regardless of sex, or else refer to the infant as "it." This is very distressing to parents who will frequently have to correct us in the course of conversation.* We wonder if this is just habit or if this is a way of keeping our distance—of not seeing the baby as a particular person whose loss might hurt us, but merely as a baby. Once we recognize the baby as a boy or girl and call the baby by name we are "hooked," and then must grieve, not only should the baby die, but also to a degree when we, who have cared for him during the first days and become "attached," must give him up to the parents.

INITIAL COMMUNICATION WITH PARENTS

The moment at which parents are first told that their infant is dead or critically ill or has a birth defect is a very difficult one for parents, nurses, physicians, and other health team members. The situation raises a number of questions. Who should tell the parents? Who should be told—the father first, the mother, both parents together? What if the father is not available? How should the parents be told? What should they be told? These questions have concerned us for many years, but changes in other aspects of maternity care have caused us to think again about the way we answer them.

Several decades ago, when many mothers were asleep at the time their infants were delivered and for some time afterward, and when fathers were kept in distant waiting rooms, "telling" was often postponed. Today, in a growing number of hospitals, the mother is watching the delivery with her husband beside her. Such postponement is not possible under these circumstances. Occasionally, a father may be asked to leave the delivery room when a complication is suspected. We have to consider whether such a practice offers psychologic protection to the delivery room personnel rather than to the father. If there is a serious problem to be faced, it would seem that the support the mother and father would offer to one another would be of real value. There are probably individual exceptions to this concept, but they should be exceptions and not the rule.

A second traditional practice that is fortunately on the decline (but hardly eradicated) is explaining the baby's condition to the father or some other member of the family but withholding part or all of the truth from the mother. The assumption here is that the father is better able to cope with reality and to make decisions than the mother who has recently delivered. Aside from the fact that this assumption is, at best, questionable and that it places a tremendous burden on a new father, the delay not only doesn't fool the mother but adds to her anxiety. Her energy is

---

*The supreme importance of the baby's sex is underscored by the virtually universal first question asked at birth—"Is it a boy or a girl?"

drained in wondering what is wrong, why she hasn't seen her baby, why the nurses and perhaps her husband are avoiding her, and why no one answers her questions. Moreover, if we are less than honest with either parent in the hours after a problem is first recognized, they may easily doubt what we tell them later, wondering if we are still "putting them off."

What is initially said to parents will depend, of course, on the baby's condition. In every instance it is important to be honest. However, even when the baby is quite ill, honesty can often be combined with a note of optimism, such as "many babies as sick as your baby do get well." Some optimism is helpful in encouraging parents to develop an attachment to their baby (see below).

At this time parents need some idea of the tests and procedures that may be carried out; we must get their written permission for those procedures. Talking with both parents together, as soon as the baby's problem is recognized, is nearly always the most helpful course. In this way, the same information is given to both parents. The physician or midwife who delivered the baby should be present; he or she may be the only member of the team who has known the parents, and is known to them, prior to delivery. A nurse who will be caring for the mother in the first days following delivery should also be present, not only for support, but so that she, also, will know what the parents have been told. Nursing notes should include the basic information given to the family, so that everyone who subsequently cares for this family will be better able to support them.

After the parents have been told about their baby's condition, we need to be available to them. We can stay nearby, perhaps hold the mother's hand if it seems to be the right thing to do

(particularly if the father is not there). Most of us feel at a loss for words, but words are not really necessary. "Hit and run," in which the parents are "hit" with distressing information about their baby and then we "run" away, leaving them to deal with what has been told them in solitude should be unthinkable.

The initial shock of their baby's condition will block out much that is told parents at this time. Some written information about the nursery in which their baby will receive care should be given to them; they will turn to it in the hours and days that follow, and it will help to remind them of what we have said in these first minutes. An example of one such information sheet, explaining perinatal care at the North Carolina Baptist Hospital, Winston-Salem, North Carolina, follows:

At North Carolina Baptist Hospital a perinatal team of obstetricians, pediatricians, nurses, respiratory therapists and social workers cares for mothers and infants who require constant, comprehensive medical and nursing attention.

At the request of their physicians, mothers may be admitted for several days or weeks before delivery for specialized care, or babies may be admitted to the Intensive Care Nursery following delivery.

THE INTENSIVE CARE NURSERY

Staffed by our specially trained team, the Intensive Care Nursery contains equipment specifically designed to assure tiny babies of receiving the most advanced medical and nursing care. Only with this team can your baby receive the around the clock intensive care that he/she needs. Different members of this team will be talking with you about your baby at different times.

VISITING

Parents are encouraged to visit their baby in the Intensive Care Nursery as soon as possible and as often as they wish. At times, however, you may be asked to wait because of events occurring in the unit, even though these events do not directly concern your baby.

On your first visit one of the nurses will show you how to wash your hands thoroughly with a special soap, in order to protect your baby from infection. You should do this each time you come into the nursery.

At first your baby may be in an isolette or another kind of specially warmed bed. You will be able to touch him and hold his hand. As your baby's condition improves, you will be able to hold him and to feed him. In order to further protect your baby from infection, we will ask you to wear a gown when you do this. If you wish to breast feed your baby, please talk with us about this. Many times this is possible.

You will see a great deal of equipment in the nursery, which may seem frightening. We will try to explain each piece to you. Some of this equipment tells us how your baby is doing (for example, how fast his heart is beating). Other equipment is used to help your baby (to help him breathe more easily, for example).

We understand your concern about your baby. We want you to be fully informed about his condition, and about the care he is receiving. Please ask whatever questions you have; parents' questions are always important to us.

Because of distance many parents are unable to visit as often as they wish. You are welcome to keep in touch with us by telephone. Our telephone number is (919) 727-4784 or 727-4785.

A SPECIAL NOTE

If you have a cold, a sore throat, a fever, or an open skin sore, you should not come into the nursery. Tiny babies catch infections very easily. We will be happy to talk with you on the telephone until you are well again.

Most important, this early time of communication should give parents the feeling that we are concerned about them and about their baby and that we will be available to answer their questions or just to listen whenever they wish us to do so. We want them to know we will be honest and open in trying to answer their questions.

If the baby is to be transferred to another hospital (e.g., from a community hospital to a medical center with an intensive care nursery), the reasons should be explained to the parents in a way they can understand. Parents should *see and touch* their baby before the transfer. This is particularly true of the mother who, because of her own hospitalization, may not be able to see her baby for several days—critically important days in terms of maternal attachment.

If the baby is to remain in the same hospital, the parents should have early and frequent opportunities to visit him in the nursery. Helping the parents to cope during these visits is discussed later in this chapter.

This initial period of communication is not a time to discuss every complication that may occur. For example, the preterm baby may develop hyperbilirubinemia in 2 to 3 days, but this can be dealt with later. To bring out too much initially will raise a barrier to attachment.

PARENTS' REACTIONS TO THEIR HIGH RISK BABY

Although every parent will have individual emotions when a child is born who in some way appears less than perfect to them, there are patterns of reactions that seem to appear. These emotions, which are the emotions of the grief process associated with death and dying, occur even when the defect is one that to us may appear relatively minor and repairable (a cleft lip, for example), as well as when the problem is major, life-threatening, or terminal. The grief process is not only common; it seems essential that the parents grieve for the lost baby of their imagination before they can accept their baby as he really is.

Mrs. Andrews' third child was a full-term healthy newborn with a unilateral cleft lip that extended into the naris. The first night after the baby was born, Mrs. Andrews cried frequently and was obviously very sad. However, on subsequent days she learned to feed him and seemed very comfortable with him, cuddling him and talking to him. She wanted her 19 year old daughter to see the baby prior to the lip repair, which was done when the baby was 5 days old, so that her daughter too would accept him as he was.

Her behavior on the morning of surgery, when she came to the nursery early to hold him before he went to the operating room, indicated to us that she had formed a strong bond with her son, even prior to a successful surgical repair. She told us, "At first all I could do was cry, but now he seems no different from my other children."

Shock and disbelief are usual first reactions—"Why me?"—"Why us?" they ask. Denial is one way of coping with the shock. "I don't believe it . . . I can't believe it . . . I won't believe it." Sometimes denial leads to behavior by parents that nurses view as very inappropriate. Their baby is critically ill, yet they seem unconcerned; they may even be laughing. Only gradually does the full impact of their baby's problem become real for them.

A second group of feelings, normal to this situation, are those of *shame, embarrassment, loss of self-esteem,* and *feelings of personal inadequacy.* "What caused this?" they ask, which may often be translated, "What is wrong with us that we couldn't have a normal child?"

A seemingly routine request may thus bring a sharp response. As noted in Chapter 2, it is customary to karyotype the chromosomes of both the mother and father of a baby suspected of having Down's syndrome in order to determine the type of chromosomal problem and assess the risk of recurrence. When this was explained to one father, he angrily answered, "There's never been anything like that on my side of the family."

His wife was not present when he made the statement. Had she been, he might not have said what he did, but he most certainly would have thought it. We need to be ready to accept such feelings and to let parents know that other parents also feel this way under similar circumstances.

Guilt about the origin of an anomaly or prematurity is another frequent response to abnormality. Is it something we did? Our long-standing beliefs about sin and punishment, a part of our heritage for many centuries, leave the nagging fear that this is a punishment for some deed, or for some thought. Perhaps the pregnancy was originally undesired—many are, even when the baby is later accepted. Maybe an abortion was contemplated, or even attempted; the feeling of guilt here can be almost overwhelming. Guilt feelings, unresolved, may lead to depression.

Parents are *anxious* for many reasons. What will become of this child? How will we care for him—physically, emotionally, financially? Can we love him as we love our other children? Will this child hurt our other children? A particularly important question is—will future children run the risk of a similar defect?

Anger, also common, is probably the hardest of all the grief-related emotions for us to deal with, because so often we, the nurses, are the target of that anger, and it seems so unjustified. We wonder, what did *we* do to deserve this? It isn't *our* fault that the baby is ill or malformed. Of course it isn't. But anger is a part of the grief process. If we can accept this idea, the anger, even when directed at us, should not really upset us.

Why are parents angry? They are angry that this happened to them. Even though they know it is irrational, they are often angry at the baby. They may be angry at each other. And they feel guilty because they are angry. The anger will come out in many ways. The bath water is too hot, the bed is too hard, or the food is terrible.

Family Disruption

Since we know that the birth of a normal, healthy infant brings changes to a family's style of life, it is reasonable to expect that the birth of a high risk baby will be even more disruptive. In addition, the strong individual emotions that accompany a high risk birth—anger, guilt, and the like—may further cause family disruption.

The Shutt family, both mother and father, traveled over 100 miles every day from the time of the baby's birth until his death 7 months later, to visit their infant son in the hospital. During all this time, a 7 year old daughter was at home with her grandmother.

If the baby is obviously sick at the time of birth or during the first days afterward, family problems may appear early. When the disorder is not diagnosed until later, disruption may be evident from the time of diagnosis.

A first example is of a family that had apparently been well adjusted prior to the diagnosis of cystic fibrosis in their baby, who was 9 months old. The same types of behavior, however, may be evident in families of children with neonatal problems.

Quarrels between parents concerning interpersonal psychosexual behavior and genetic prognosis had ensued almost immediately thereafter. Both parents had turned to their own parents to air their grievances.[17]

Tips also noted that the three older children had been informed by classmates of the complex family situation. The behavior and social and academic standing of the children had deteriorated as a consequence.[17]

A second example describes a family with two unaffected children and a third and fourth child with congenital spastic paraplegia of genetic origin.

Immediately after receiving the adverse and distasteful genetic prognosis, the parents had become concerned about their interpersonal relationships. Nocturnal arguments had ensued and the mother had developed severe dyspareunia. She had become overly concerned with the management of the affected children and had neglected the older children who developed behavioral disturbances and began failing in school. The father, previously dominant, had withdrawn and assumed a passive role in the family circle . . .

During the consultation, the parents refused to communicate with one another, but both were excessively free in the discussion of family problems with all team members. As the family history was discussed, both parents overtly degraded the other's family. Each parent also strongly suspected the other of extramarital affairs.[17]

In both instances counseling enabled the parents to identify their concerns, to talk about them more realistically, and ultimately to resolve them.

Acceptance is the final step in the grief process. We need to realize that it will be many months, even a year or more, before that acceptance comes. Nurses who care for the infant and his family at the time of birth do not often see parents at this point. We must not expect acceptance in the 3 to 5 day period that mothers remain on the obstetric unit, or even in the weeks that the baby is in the nursery.

There are, however, clues, even in the first days, that may indicate eventual outcome. Caplan's research, summarized in Table 22–1, suggests several.[2]

Our Role in Helping Parents Cope

Although nurses, physicians, and social workers, as well as other family members, may feel inadequate to help the grieving parents of a high risk baby

Table 22–1 SOME PARENTAL RESPONSES TO PRETERM BIRTHS*

Responses Suggesting Healthy Outcome	Responses Suggesting Unhealthy Outcome
Parents obtain as much information as possible about the infant's condition—ask frequent questions, request specific information	Parents do not seek information about the baby
Parents aware of negative feelings and able to express them and accept help from family and friends	Parents deny negative feelings; unable to accept help from family and friends
Parents appropriately anxious about infant's condition	Parents deny infant's life in jeopardy; converse about less threatening subjects

*After Caplan: *Psychiatry,* 23:365, 1960.

there are specific ways in which we can help them work through the grief process to arrive at the kind of healthy acceptance that is essential for their own well-being, as well as that of their baby. Several have already been discussed in the preceding pages.

Showing Acceptance. The importance of our own attitude toward the baby has already been mentioned. The baby, despite any defect that he may have, should not be hidden in a corner of the nursery. The baby can be talked to, and about, as a baby. The parents should be encouraged to name the infant, and his name should then be placed on his bed, so that we can refer to him by name.

Explaining Equipment. How did you feel when you walked into the intensive care nursery for the first time? If you were in a medical center, with monitors, respirators, alarms, intravenous lines, and the like, you may have thought, "I could never work in a place like this." If nurses who are familiar with hospitals feel this way (and many registered nurses do), consider how parents must feel in an intensive care nursery for the first time, with *their* baby as a patient.

How can we help them cope with such an overwhelming experience?

Even before they enter the doors for the first time, we can describe what they will see—the reason for each piece of equipment, about the way it is helping their baby—and also tell them something about the way their baby will look. Then we can accompany them to their baby's bed, again explaining everything carefully, for much of what we have previously said will not be comprehended. Continuing explanations are necessary.

Continuing Communication. Parents need to feel welcome each time they telephone or come to the nursery. Increasingly, parents are allowed to visit intensive care nurseries as frequently and as long as they desire (as we become more knowledgeable about the importance of attachment in infant care), although they may be asked to leave briefly during certain procedures involving their own or other babies.

Many questions about their baby and his care will be asked more than once; answers may not have been understood or may have been forgotten in the stress surrounding the family. These questions should be answered with patience and care each time.

Good communication among nurses, physicians, and other workers in the nursery is also essential to good communication with parents. Nothing can be more confusing or distressing to parents than to hear different stories from different people. Major information communicated to parents should be documented and easily accessible to everyone caring for the baby. A check sheet can be one aid in this area, as well as being a help in assessing attachment (below).

Equally as important as knowing what parents have been told is knowing what they understand about what they have heard. We need to listen for clues about their understanding or lack of it. For example, when the father of a baby with serious brain damage talks about his son as a future Little Leaguer, communication has certainly been ineffective for some reason. It may be that this father is not psychologically ready to accept what he has heard. Or we may have been unclear about what we said to him. An important question to ask about each family each day is "Where are they in their understanding of their baby's condition?"

In addition to picking up clues in conversation, we can ask them what they have been told. For example, if a mother says, "How much longer will my baby need to have that needle in his head (intravenous line)?" we might first ask her what information she has already been given. Many parents will ask a question of several nurses and physicians, just to see if they will get the same answer. It is a way of looking for assurance, but it can certainly be very hard on staff if our own communication is not good.

ATTACHMENT BETWEEN PARENTS AND THEIR HIGH RISK BABY

The steps by which parents form attachments to their healthy newborn babies were discussed in Chapter 20. Attachment is equally important for the parents of the high risk baby. Studies indicate that approximately one-third of all infants who are battered or "fail to thrive" in the absence of physiologic disease were either preterm babies or babies who were ill in the period following birth. The common denominator was separation from their parents during the early days when attachments are formed. Facilitating the attachment of high risk babies and their parents is obviously highly important.

Attachment is equally important if the baby is expected to die. Parents will grieve, regardless of whether or not they have formed an attachment. It is far healthier for them to grieve for a specific, tangible baby than for a vague entity they have never known. Normal grief can be resolved. Undefined grief may linger—as anger or sadness or in some other form—for a very long time.

It is not surprising that parents are reluctant to form attachments to their sick or malformed baby. Their problem is then compounded by the guilt they experience about not feeling love for their baby.

As with healthy term babies, attachment formation with high risk babies involves seeing, touching, and caretaking. Many parents who will eagerly caress a term baby may shrink from a preterm infant or a child with a defect. This is one more reason why we need to be with them the first times they visit, and we should always remain close by. We may have to encourage their touch. "Would you like to hold your baby's hand?" we can say. Sometimes if we hold his hand or stroke his head or leg while we are talking, we can encourage parents to be less fearful. Fathers often need a great deal of encouragement to handle tiny babies, although in some families the father may be less reluctant than the mother.

It is more difficult to involve parents in caretaking with a very sick baby than with the term baby. At first parents may not be able to feed their baby or bathe or diaper him, but we can assure them that their gentle stroking and talking to him play a real role in his care (Fig. 22–1). We can also use our ingenuity to involve the parents in as many ways as possible. For example, if the baby is to have a gavage feeding, we might insert the tube and be sure of its position; the mother might then pour the premeasured formula into the syringe. As the baby's condition improves, the parents can assume a more active role in his care.

The centralization of high risk newborns in medical centers, although obviously offering significant advantages from the standpoint of physiologic care, presents some real barriers to attachment. Parents may live 50 or 100 miles from the hospital in which their baby receives care; they may even live in a different state. Many times they lack transportation to travel back and forth except on weekends. Often there are other children at home who also need care. How do we foster attachment on a long distance basis? No one has final answers to this question, but attempts are being made to deal with the problem.

The telephone is an important means of communication for parents. It gives us a chance to tell them how much their baby has gained, how he is eating, and little personal bits of information such as, "He opened his eyes while I was bathing him," that not only mean a lot to most parents but contribute to their feelings of attachment. An ideal situation is a telephone number that can be called long distance at no charge to the family. Many parents cannot afford long distance calls each day; some have no access to telephones at all.

Letters and photos from the hospital can be helpful if the mother and

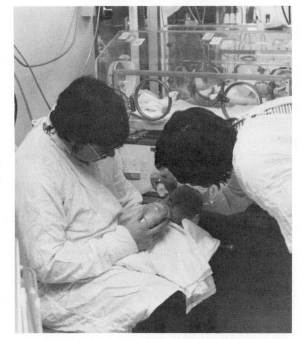

Figure 22–1 Even though Todd still requires some oxygen, his father can feed him while his mother holds the tubing carrying oxygen close to his face.

father are unable to come for several weeks at a time.

Contact through public health nurses in the parents' home area, if for some reason it is difficult to reach the parents themselves, is another avenue of communication. Certainly the public health nurse should be contacted before the baby is discharged so that she may come to know the family and be available to them for teaching and counsel.

The concept of "back-transfer," that is, sending the baby back to the hospital nearer to his home community for intermediate level care before discharge, is growing in popularity. Not only is the baby nearer his family, which facilitates their visiting and their learning to care for him, but local care is often less expensive.

The Assessment of Attachment

The criteria for assessing attachment in high risk families are very much like those for assessing attachment behavior in families with healthy newborns described in Chapter 20. It is normal, however, for attachment behavior to proceed more slowly. As we have already noted, the mother and father may touch the infant more slowly. Monitors and other equipment attached to the baby may make it difficult to caress his body. Moreover, the baby will not be able to respond to his parents in the way that a healthy baby does.

The frequency of parental visiting or calls may indicate something of the level of attachment. The previously mentioned check sheet gives one way of quickly ascertaining when parents have failed to have any contact with the baby or hospital for a period of several days. There may be other reasons than lack of interest in the baby, but these families need follow-up. Ideally, some-

one should call and say something such as, "We hadn't heard from you in several days; is there anything wrong that we can help you with?"

HELPING THE FAMILY COPE

As we have already noted, one of the most difficult aspects of the care of high risk infants is facing the reality that many of our patients will not recover. Duff and Campbell[6] suggest that two philosophies underlie the way in which we care for these babies and their families:

1. A "disease-oriented" philosophy which sees death only in a highly negative context of failure.

2. A "person-oriented" philosophy which recognizes that under some circumstances death is not only inevitable but is not necessarily the worst of fates.

The way in which we have traditionally treated the dying newborn and his family is not much different from the way in which the American culture in general, and the nursing and medical subcultures that preside over our dying have dealt with death at any age. With few exceptions (the baby with anencephaly or the baby of less than 25 weeks' gestation, for example), we make heroic efforts to save the baby. However, if we fail, we then feel we have done all we can and frequently withdraw from the baby and family, emotionally if not physically.

Some newborns die in spite of anything we can do. For others, life may be prolonged, but not necessarily saved, by a variety of means. The intensity and duration of care given to a particular baby must take into account not only medical factors but family feelings as well. We find great satisfaction working in a nursery in which the understanding and feelings of parents are discussed along with laboratory values and respiratory status on daily rounds.

Consider the difference that the feelings of parents made in the care of two infants who happened to be in the same intensive care nursery at the same time. Baby A was able to breathe only in 100 per cent oxygen; Baby B required a tracheostomy and continual ventilation. During week after week of intensive care, repeated attempts were made to help both babies become able to breathe normally in room air. Careful studies were undertaken to discover the underlying cause of each baby's problem. Both mothers and fathers visited every day; their attachment was evident. Baby A was entered in her church's "beautiful baby contest" via photographs. Baby B had his sister's picture taped to his isolette along with mobiles and music boxes.

Gradually, it became evident to the staff that neither baby was likely to ever breathe independently, and the information was shared with the parents. Over the next few days the parents of Baby A decided, along with staff, that their baby would receive no more oxygen. We could continue to feed her and care for her in every other way for as long as she was able to live. They continued to visit her each day and brought her 2 year old sister so that she, too, might see her. In a few days, Baby A died.

Baby B's parents continued to believe that he would recover until the time of his death. Because of their wishes, the baby was ventilated via a respirator throughout his life.

Different families deal with death in different ways; in these instances including the parents in the decision-making resulted in two different courses of action. What is helpful for one family may not be so for a second.

One aspect worth noting in the behavior of both of these families, and in the one below as well, is the involvement of siblings. Because small children are often jealous of a brother or sister, particularly one who separates them from their parents for the long periods of time that hospital visits require, they may wish that the baby dies, so that their parents will become available to them once again. Since for a small child wishing something to happen is hard to differentiate from causing it to happen, there may be a great deal of guilt when the baby does, in fact, die. Often parents, wrapped up in their own grief and their concern for the baby, need some help in realizing that their other children need support through this difficult period. A question such as, "What does your child (children) say about the baby?" will remind parents to be sensitive to their other sons and daughters.

Can we make the death of an infant, despite the inevitable sorrow, a positive experience for families? We submit the following as evidence that we can:

A premature infant was believed to have a hopeless prognosis. The parents and doctor, with the agreement of the medical and nursing staff, decided to stop all heroic measures. The parents informed their healthy 3 year old daughter that her brother probably could not live, and, on her request, she was brought to see the baby.

Later, after contemplating autopsy and plans for disposition of the baby's body (both discussed at their request), the parents were asked which they preferred—to leave; to be beside their baby's incubator; or to have the baby, with all his tubes and apparatus removed, brought to them in a private room. Immediately, they chose the last. In the company of the doctor, they held their infant for 55 minutes while he died. During this time, they wept, talked to their daughter about him, found humor in some incongruities, or were silent. The mother cradled the baby to her bosom most of the time, while the father stroked his wife and baby.

He told us that the scene of mother and dying child was one of sublime beauty despite its occurrence in the midst of tragedy. He later said he believed that the time interval spent in intimacy with their baby was about 2 hours, not 55 minutes. She told us, "We had to say hello to him before we could say goodbye."

They came to think of this experience as a fitting funeral from which they gained greater strength for living. They helped each other. They also helped their daughter over the ensuing weeks as she overcame her abnormal fears of dying and openly dealt with her guilt for feeling that her bad wishes had killed her brother.

REFERENCES

1. Benfield, D., Leib, S., and Reuter, J.: Grief Response of Parents after Referral of the Critically Ill Newborn to a Regional Center. *New England Journal of Medicine, 294*:975, 1976.
2. Caplan, G.: Patterns of Parental Response to the Crisis of Premature Birth. *Psychiatry, 23*:365, 1960.
3. Christensen, A.: Coping with the Crisis of a Premature Birth. *MCN, 2*(1):33, 1977.
4. Donnelly, E.: The Real of Her. *JOGN Nursing, 3*(3):48, 1974.
5. Dubois, D.: Indications of an Unhealthy Relationship between Parents and Premature Infant. *JOGN Nursing, 4*(3):21, 1975.
6. Duff, R., and Campbell, A.: On Deciding the Care of Severely Handicapped or Dying Persons: With Particular Reference to Infants. *Pediatrics, 57*:487, 1976.
7. Dunn, D., and Lewis, A.: Some Important Aspects of Neonatal Nursing Related to Pulmonary Disease and Family Involvement. *Pediatric Clinics of North America, 20*:481, 1973.
8. Goodman, M.: Two Mothers' Reactions to the Deaths of their Premature Infants. *JOGN Nursing, 4*(3):25, 1975.
9. Klaus, M., and Kennell, J.: *Maternal-Infant Bonding: the Impact of Early Separation or Loss on Family Development.* St.Louis, C. V. Mosby Co., 1976.
10. Johnson, S., and Grubbs, J.: The Premature Infant's Reflex Behaviors: Effect on the Maternal-Child Relationship. *JOGN Nursing, 4*(3):15, 1975.
11. Kallop, F.: Working with Parents Through a Devastating Experience. *JOGN Nursing, 2*(3):36, 1973.
12. Lynch, H., Krush, T., Krush, A., et al.: Psychodynamics of Early Hereditary Deaths. *American Journal of Diseases of Children, 108*:605, 1964.
13. MacKeith, R.: The Feelings and Behavior of Parents of Handicapped Children. *Developmental Medicine and Child Neurology, 15*:524, 1973.
14. Mercer, R.: Responses of Mothers to the Birth of an Infant with a Defect. *ANA Clinical Sessions, 1974.* New York, Appleton-Century-Crofts, 1975.
15. Millington, M., Gravez, J., and Coffee, M.: For High-Risk Infants and their Parents: Postnatal Discussion Groups and Well-Baby Clinics Operate in Storefront. *JOGN Nursing, 4*(1):42, 1975.
16. Penfold, K.: Supporting Mother Love. *American Journal of Nursing, 74*:464, 1974.
17. Tips, R., Smith, G., Lynch, H., et al.: The "Whole Family" Concept in Clinical Genetics. *American Journal of Diseases of Children, 107*:67, 1964.
18. Young, R.: Chronic Sorrow: Parents' Response to the Birth of a Child with a Defect. *MCN, 2*(1):38, 1977.

Chapter 23

ISSUES IN CONTEMPORARY CHILDBEARING

Because childbearing, along with childrearing, is essential to the ongoing of society, vital issues surround our practice in which we care for childbearing families. Many of these issues have been explored in this text. Some issues that produced major debates just a few years ago (for example, the presence of fathers in labor and delivery rooms) have been resolved for many families.

In an increasing number of hospitals, families are no longer separated from their infants, and even siblings may join their mother for a part of the day. In contrast to a decade ago, when most mothers were asleep under general anesthesia at the time their child was born, many parents today participate actively in birth.

We, as nurses, have played major roles in the changes in childbearing practices, by broadening our knowledge based on research from biologic and behavioral sciences and from our own nursing research. Thus we have become increasingly better prepared for the role.

Society, however, continues, and will always continue in a state of change. New issues arise as old issues are moved toward resolution. Several

issues that are particularly important today are discussed in this chapter.

THE PROBLEM OF MORTALITY

Infant Mortality

Infant mortality is considered an important index of a nation's health care. Thus it was disappointing to learn in the late 1950's and early 1960's that rates of infant mortality in the United States were higher than rates in many other nations.

Moreover in the decade between 1955 and 1965, infant mortality rates were decreasing more rapidly in many other nations than in the United States. Thus the United States ranked eighth among countries with the lowest infant mortality in 1955, eleventh in 1960, and sixteenth in 1965. In the following decade, 1965 to 1975, infant mortality rates in the United States began to drop more rapidly, although the 1975 rate of 16.1 deaths per 1000 live births was for the first time lower than that of Sweden and the Netherlands in *1960* (Tables 23–1 and 23–2).

When rates for white infants are

687

separated from rates for all others (Tables 23-3 and 23-4), the white infant mortality rate in the United States in 1975 (14.2 per 1000 live births) is still far higher than the rates in 1973 for six other nations (Table 23-1). The mortality rate for all infants other than white in 1975 (24.2) is higher than that of many nations in 1973 (Table 23-1).

Mortality rates vary widely from one part of the United States to another. In 1975 Hawaii had the lowest rate of infant mortality (12.9 per 1000 live births), while Mississippi was the state with the highest rate (22.3). The infant mortality in Washington, D. C. in 1975 was 29.0. Infant mortality is highest in the South (17.8 in 1975) and lowest in the West (14.1 in 1975) with rates for the north-central states (15.8 in 1975) being similar.

THE HEALTH CARE SYSTEM AND MORTALITY

Why should a wealthy nation, with access to all of the world's knowledge, have a rate of infant mortality greater than that of many other nations? Obviously there is no single answer.

One major factor in infant mortality is the number of babies born who weigh less than 2500 grams. Improved care for these babies after birth (as described in Chapter 18) is important in reducing mortality, but reducing the number of low birth weight babies delivered is also significant. Page and associates[19] suggest that if all of the existing knowledge of prenatal management were applied to all pregnancies and if all pregnant women were to cooperate fully, the frequency of infants weighing

Table 23-1   INFANT, NEONATAL, AND PERINATAL
MORTALITY IN SELECTED NATIONS*

Country	Year	Infant Mortality[1]	Neonatal Mortality[2]	Perinatal Mortality[3]
Sweden	1974	9.2	7.1	12.9
Finland	1973	10.0	–	–
Japan	1973	11.3	7.4	18.0
Denmark	1973	11.5	8.7	14.6
Netherlands	1973	11.5	8.5	16.4
Norway	1973	11.9	8.5	16.8
France	1973	15.5	–	–
New Zealand	1973	16.2	–	–
Australia	1973	16.5	11.8	22.4
England/Wales	1973	16.9	11.1	21.3
United States	1973	17.6	–	–
"	1974	16.7	–	–
"	1975	16.1	–	–
Scotland	1973	19.0	13.0	22.7
Northern Ireland	1973	21.0	15.0	25.9
Greece	1973	24.1	17.3	25.8
Poland	1973	26.1	16.4	21.3
USSR	1973	26.4	–	–

*Source: World Health Statistics Annual, 1973–1976. Geneva, World Health Organization, 1976.
[1]Infant mortality represents deaths per 1000 live births under 1 year of age.
[2]Neonatal mortality represents deaths per 1000 live births under 4 weeks of age.
[3]Perinatal mortality represents deaths per 1000 live births between 28 weeks' gestation (late fetal deaths) and the end of the first week of birth.

Table 23–2   INFANT MORTALITY RATES FOR SELECTED YEARS 1955–1973*†

Country	1955	1960	1965	1973
Sweden	17.4	16.6	13.3	9.2‡
Netherlands	20.1	16.4	14.4	11.5
Norway	21.3	20.0	16.4	11.9
Australia	22.0	21.5	18.5	16.5
New Zealand	24.5	22.6	19.5	16.2
United States	26.5	25.6	24.7	17.6

*Sources: *Statistical Yearbook, 1973.* New York, United Nations Publishing Service, 1974; *Vital Statistics of the United States, Vol. II Mortality.* Rockville, Md., National Center for Health Statistics, U.S. Dept of Health, Education and Welfare, 1972; *World Health Statistics Annual, 1973–1976.* Geneva, World Health Organization, 1976; Final Mortality Statistics Report: *Monthly Vital Statistics Report,* 24:11, Feb. 3, 1976, Rockville, Md., National Center for Health Statistics, U.S. Dept. of Health, Education and Welfare, 1976.
†Per 1000 live births.
‡1974 infant mortality rate.

less than 2500 grams at birth could be reduced by 25 per cent.

A number of studies support the relationship between inadequate prenatal care and an increased incidence of low birth weight babies.[13, 23] Thus it seems important to examine the way in which health care for childbearing families is delivered. In fact, the delivery of all health care is germane, because long-term malnutrition and other health problems can present barriers to successful childbearing even when prenatal care is excellent.

A general examination of the health care delivery systems of other nations or of our own nation is beyond the scope of this book. We propose here to examine some of the ways in which nurses, through the development or expansion of extended roles, are improving not only mortality rates for newborns but the quality of care for childbearing families.

One concept is particularly important as we consider the functions of nurses in expanded roles, i.e., that the financial status of the patient should not be the criterion for judging whether a woman is cared for primarily by a nurse in an expanded role (who is responsible to a physician for the *medical aspects* of patient care) or whether she is cared for primarily by the physician. The best way to utilize the time of health professionals in order to achieve

Table 23–3   INFANT MORTALITY IN THE UNITED STATES BY RACE, 1974–1975*†

	1974	1975	Per Cent Decrease
Total	16.7	16.1	3.6
White	14.8	14.2	4.1
All others	24.9	24.2	2.8

*Source: Final Mortality Statistics Report. *Monthly Vital Statistics Report,* 24:11, Feb. 3, 1976, Rockville, Md., National Center for Health Statistics, U.S. Dept. of Health, Education and Welfare, 1976.
†Per 1000 live births.

Table 23–4   NEONATAL AND INFANT MORTALITY IN THE UNITED STATES
BY RACE AND SEX, 1975*†

	Neonatal Mortality	Infant Mortality
All females	10.2	14.2
All males	12.9	17.9
White (male and female)	10.4	14.2
White males	11.7	15.9
White females	9.0	12.3
All others	16.8	24.2
All other males	18.2	26.2
All other females	15.3	22.2

*Source: Final Mortality Statistics Report. *Monthly Vital Statistics Report*, 24:11, Feb. 3, 1976, Rockville, Md., National Center for Health Statistics, U.S. Dept. of Health, Education and Welfare, 1976.
†Per 1000 live births.

quality care would be to provide nursing supervision of the patient with a basically normal course of pregnancy and to allow more intensive medical supervision of mothers considered high risk patients. Nurses have a great deal to offer high risk patients, as well as women with no complications, but women with a high risk pregnancy *also* need more intensive medical supervision. Because low income people often have more health problems, such a division of labor could result in increased nursing supervision of middle and upper class patients and increased physician care of patients with limited incomes.

The Certified Nurse-Midwife

Midwife is derived from the Middle English *mid-wif,* meaning "with woman." Even in the 1970's the word midwife brings to some persons an image of a toothless granny delivering a baby in a dark cabin. The certified nurse-midwife resembles that image about as closely as the present-day graduate of an American medical school resembles the barber-surgeon of the fourteenth century.

Nurse-midwives first practiced in the United States in 1925 in the Frontier Nursing Service (FNS), which was

organized in Kentucky by Mary Breckenridge, a nurse who continued as the active director of the FNS until her death in 1965. Because there was no school of midwifery in the United States, British nurse-midwives or American nurses educated in England or Scotland served as midwives in rural Kentucky.

When the Second World War began in Europe in 1939, this transatlantic exchange was no longer possible, and the Frontier Graduate School of Midwifery was started that year.

It was not, however, the first school for nurse-midwives in the United States. That distinction belongs to the Maternity Center Association in New York City, where the first program was established between 1931 and 1933.

A third school opened at Tuskegee Institute in Alabama in 1941, but because neither professionals nor the community was ready for the nurse-midwives, it closed in 1946. During those few years, however, fetal mortality in that area of Alabama dropped from 45.9 per 1000 live births to 14.0 per 1000 live births.

Catholic University was the first university to grant a degree in midwifery, and in 1955, the American College of Nurse-Midwives was founded.

In many areas of the world, care for pregnant mothers and infants who have no complications is conducted almost totally by nurse-midwives. Several of these countries, such as the Netherlands and Norway, have rates of infant mortality below the rates of the United States. Although there are other variables, it appears obvious that nurse-midwives can be a valuable part of the team caring for childbearing families.[14]

Studies in the United States have also proved the value of the nurse-midwife. Levy and his associates compared rates of prematurity and neonatal mortality and prenatal care in a rural California county before, during, and after a 3 year demonstration program in rural California. During the program, prenatal care increased and prematurity and neonatal mortality decreased. After the demonstration project ended, prenatal care decreased while prematurity rose from 6.6 to 9.8 per cent and neonatal mortality rose from 10.3 to 32.1 per 1000 live births. After searching for any other factors that may have influenced these changes, it was concluded that nurse-midwives were the major factor in change.

In Mississippi the infant death rate in 1965 was 41.5 per 1000 live births (compared with a national rate of 24.7), and maternal mortality was double the national rate. In less than 3 years (1968 to 1971) in one large county in Mississippi the Midwifery Program of the University of Mississippi Medical Center was able to reduce infant mortality to 21.3 per 1000 live births.[10]

Preparation of the Nurse-Midwife. There are two routes by which nurse-midwives are prepared. One type of program, which leads to certification as a nurse-midwife upon satisfactory completion of the course and a national certification examination, is open to any registered nurse; such a program lasts from 8 months to a year. Other programs, which lead to a master's degree, require the registered nurses who enter to have a bachelor of science degree; these programs last from 1 to 2 years.

A current list of programs is available from The American College of Nurse Midwives, 1000 Vermont Ave., N.W., Washington, D. C. 20005. The American College also publishes *Statements of Standards, Functions, and Qualifications for the Practice of Nurse Midwifery;* a journal, *Journal of Nurse Midwifery;* and other information about nurse-midwifery.

Curricula include both theory and practice in prenatal, intrapartum, and postpartal care and in family planning. A master's program may also include courses in statistics, research, group dynamics, teaching, administration, and curriculum development. Nurse-midwives prepared at the master's level may themselves become teachers of nurse-midwifery.

Practice of the Nurse-Midwife. A nurse-midwife is always responsible to a physician for her practice; she consults with him or her whenever necessary. Usually the nurse-midwife assumes responsibility for low risk maternity patients during the antepartal, intrapartal, postpartal, and often interpartal periods. She delivers the infant and evaluates him, as well as his mother, during their stay in the hospital. Teaching, counseling, and provision for family planning are a part of her care, as is the return postpartum examination.

Gatewood and Stewart[10] described the incorporation of two nurse-midwives into their private obstetric practice in rural Georgia. In the first year of team practice (two obstetricians and two nurse-midwives), the team delivered 436 women vaginally and 31 by cesarean section. Nurse-midwives delivered 61 per cent of the mothers who had vaginal deliveries, taught preparation-for-childbirth classes (previously unavailable in the community), alternated with the obstetricians for prenatal care, examined and taught postpartal patients, and provided family planning information.

The authors emphasize that every team member is involved in the care of each patient. Couples appear to respond enthusiastically to their team approach.

The Clinical Nurse-Specialist

The clinical nurse-specialist has a master's degree in nursing; if she cares for childbearing families, her master's degree will be in maternal and child health nursing. The role of the clinical specialist will vary from one practice setting to another, but she usually is involved in patient care, in staff development, and in research. The clinical specialist is likely to have a flexible schedule to meet the needs of patients and staff.

Some activities of the clinical specialist include:

1. Developing nursing care plans.
2. Developing and evaluating literature for patients.
3. Conducting nursing research.
4. Initiating or revising patient classes.
5. Evaluating patient teaching.
6. Implementing staff development in formal and informal ways.
7. Serving as a role model for patient care.
8. Acting as a change agent to improve care.

Nurse-Practitioner Programs and Roles

Several types of nurse-practitioner programs prepare registered nurses to function in expanded roles. These programs commonly involve several months of intensive training followed by a preceptorship, i.e., a specified period of practice under the direct supervision of a preceptor, who is usually a physician.

Other nurse-practitioner programs are part of advanced degree nursing programs.

The programs and roles described below are examples of some nurse-practitioner and nurse associate programs and of various roles related to childbearing. Specific programs may change, but we believe the concepts discussed here are a part of contemporary nursing.

States vary in mandating the laws that govern the practice of nurse-practitioners—whether they may write medical orders, for example.

The Maternal-Child Nurse-Practitioner. During pregnancy, a maternal-child nurse-practitioner functions in much the same way as the nurse-midwife, with the exception of delivering the infant. However, the maternal-child nurse-practitioner will continue to care for mother and child during the childbearing years (and care for the mother, should she again become pregnant). Thus a continuity of care is provided that is lacking not only for women and children in public clinics but for many patients in the private sector as well, who must seek an obstetrician or obstetric clinic for maternity care and a pediatrician or pediatric clinic for child care.

A pilot program for the preparation of maternal-child nurse-practitioners at the University of Colorado consists of 4 months of intensive preparation, including classroom and clinical teaching. Clinical experience in obstetrics and gynecology includes developing skills in pelvic examination, the fitting of diaphragms, the insertion of intrauterine devices, assessment of fetal growth, and the performance of Leopold's maneuvers. In pediatric clinical practice emphasis is on assessment by history and physical examination.

Graduates may work in a rural health clinic, a public health agency, an outpatient clinic, or a private obstetric-pediatric clinic. They may follow the mother from the clinic into the hospital, where they offer support and teaching and counseling during labor, delivery, and the immediate postpartum period, and then follow her again into the community setting.

An Obstetric-Gynecologic Nurse Associate Program. The obstetric-gynecologic nurse associate program at Rush-Presbyterian-St. Luke's Medical Center in Chicago is designed to prepare nurses to function in an expanded role in ambulatory settings, giving care to women in prepregnancy, pregnancy, and postpartum periods and giving gynecologic health maintenance care.

In a 24 week period, the curriculum includes clinical skills (e.g., pelvic and vaginal examinations); lectures (e.g., principles of intrapartum care); and discussions of referrals, techniques of counseling and guidance, and evaluation of social and family systems.

A Pediatric Nurse-Practitioner in a Hospital Setting. Most nurse-practitioner programs prepare nurses to function in ambulatory settings or in combinations of ambulatory and inhospital settings, as they follow their patients from one environment to another.

Schuman describes another role, that of the pediatric nurse-practitioner in a hospital setting, who has primary responsibility for physical examination and day-to-day follow-up of "well"infants and for communication with parents.[24] During her day the pediatric nurse-practitioner may:

1. Discuss the importance of follow-up visits with a postpartum mother.

2. Perform newborn physical examinations.

3. Encourage the mother with a preterm or sick baby to see and touch her baby and if the baby's condition permits, to hold and feed him.

4. Explain the reason for detention in the nursery for babies who will not be discharged with their mothers.

5. Serve as a liaison to other departments, such as the prenatal clinic or social services.

6. Teach parents and staff in formal and informal ways.

7. Write medical orders as determined by the nurse-practitioner and the chief of the department, commonly for laboratory work, X-rays, discharge, and so forth.

Childbirth Educator

The term childbirth educator is used by many people—nurses; other health professionals, such as physical therapists; and lay-persons—to describe themselves in a variety of roles that prepare parents for the experience of birth, and sometimes for parenting as well. Childbirth education has been described in Chapter 9.

For many nurses (nurses employed in prenatal clinics, for example) childbirth education is a part of regular practice.

Other nurses contract with couples to teach psychoprophylactic preparation or the Bradley method. These nurses may undertake specialized training leading to certification. For example, the American Society for Psychoprophylaxis in Obstetrics (ASPO) has a national teacher-training program and a national certification program. Candidates attend seminars, observe certified teachers, have a period of student teaching, prepare a bibliography and syllabus, and take a national examination. Postpartum reports written by mothers taught by the candidate (who must be an R.N. or a physical therapist) are also submitted as part of the accreditation process. The ASPO also conducts continuing education programs for members.

Standards for Nurses in Expanded Roles

With the exception of the certified nurse-midwife, for whom there are standards and a national examination for certification, there are no national standards for nurses practicing in an expanded role.* Nurses with similar titles and similar functions may have varying degrees of preparation and responsibility.

We believe that one of nursing's tasks in the coming decade will be to establish some standards for nurses in new roles. Such standards will not only serve the public interest but will enable nurses to evaluate programs before they commit time and money to enrollment.

Recognition of Excellence: Certification in Maternal-Child Nursing

When a nurse is graduated from an accredited school and passes a state board examination, she meets the criteria for entry into practice. Through her professional nursing experience and through continuing education, she will grow in expertise in the practice of nursing. How can that growth be recognized?

In 1975 the American Nurses Association, Division of Maternal and Child

---

*As noted above, the American Society for Psychoprophylaxis in Obstetrics has a certification process, but this practice varies somewhat from the usual understanding of an expanded role.

Health Nursing Practice (ANA/MCH) and the Nurses Association of the American College of Obstetricians and Gynecologists (NAACOG) Certification Corporation established a certification program in maternal-gynecological-neonatal nursing practice in order to formally recognize individual achievement and superior performance in nursing. A Joint Committee on Certification in Maternal-Gynecological-Neonatal Nursing was established to implement the program.

Registered nurses who immediately prior to the time of certification have at least two consecutive years of practice in the care of mothers and infants or of women with gynecologic problems are eligible to begin the certification process.

The Process of Certification. Each candidate first describes her education and clinical experience on the initial application, which begins the certification process.

There are two major components to the process. Each applicant must first take a two-part multiple choice examination. The first part of the examination covers a common core of knowledge, including psychosocial aspects of childbearing, parenting, growth and development, health maintenance, the health care delivery system, the nursing process, and patient assessment.

Each applicant then chooses one area in which to be tested in Part II. The areas include ambulatory women's health care, nursing care in labor and delivery, postpartal nursing care, or neonatal nursing care.

Those applicants who pass the examination then complete several documents: a description of their clinical setting and practice, a case study and two abstracts that demonstrate the nursing process, and the ANA-MCH Standards of Practice. Three references are also submitted.

The process of certification is in its infancy, and there will undoubtedly be changes as it evolves. It is one avenue for achieving, and receiving recognition for, excellent care of childbearing families.

THE HOME BIRTH MOVEMENT

A growing, although still very small, number of families in the United States are choosing to deliver their babies at home, rather than in hospitals. To a large extent nurses and physicians have felt very negative about the home birth movement. Nurses need to be aware of the:

1. Reasons families choose home birth.
2. Potential dangers weighed against the potential advantages.
3. Possibility of compromise.
4. Role of nursing in the home birth movement.

Why do Families Choose Home Birth?

Why do families choose a home birth (a birth that most professionals in the United States feel is potentially dangerous for mother and baby) over a hospital birth (a birth that the professionals believe is much safer)?

The parents who choose home birth are not uncaring, unconcerned mothers and fathers. Although for a minority home birth may be a part of a communal lifestyle (Chapter 4), many parents who opt for home birth are well educated and have given the issue serious consideration.

They see delivery of a baby, under most circumstances, as a natural part of family life. They object to the impersonal, often assembly line atmosphere of the hospital, and they object to the enforced separation from family and friends that often accompanies hos-

pitalization. Most couples who choose home birth recognize that there may be risks, but they believe that there are also risks in hospital births and that with adequate precautions the level of risk can be minimal.

The cost of hospital services has been an issue for some parents. As the cost of maternity care climbs to over $1000 in many sections of the country, some couples feel financially unable to afford hospital delivery. Conversely, home delivery may be more expensive for some patients because their hospitalization insurance will not cover the costs.

Professional Reaction

Some health professionals, including certain nurses, nurse-midwives, and physicians, have been supportive of the home birth movement. Some physicians will attend home births to intervene, should the need arise. The majority of the health care community, however, has reacted with disdain. Anger has been particularly directed toward the couple who initially rejects hospital services and then seeks those services when complications arise.

Dangers versus Advantages

The greatest concern of those who oppose home birth is the danger of unexpected complications, such as prolapse of the umbilical cord or maternal hemorrhage, complications that cannot be anticipated from prenatal assessment.

The risk of complications can be lowered by endeavoring to convince mothers with a potentially greater risk of complications that even if home birth is safe for some mothers, it is not advisable for them (see box) and that even for low risk mothers all risk cannot be eliminated.

SOME CONTRAINDICATIONS TO
HOME BIRTH

1. Maternal diabetes mellitus
2. Maternal heart disease
3. Maternal kidney disease
4. Any acute or chronic maternal health problem (e.g., anemia)
5. Rh incompatibility
6. Active herpes simplex virus
7. Symptoms of pre-eclampsia and/or eclampsia
8. Antepartum bleeding
9. Hydramnios
10. Maternal age less than 20 or greater than 35 years
11. Complication in previous pregnancy
12. Previous cesarean section

13. Small pelvis (cephalopelvic disproportion)
14. Abnormal presentation
15. History of large infants or increase in the size of subsequent infants
16. History of small for gestational age (SGA) babies
17. More than four previous deliveries
18. Inadequate nutrition
19. Lack of prenatal care
20. Lack of access to emergency care
21. Multiple pregnancy
22. Gestation of less than 36 weeks or greater than 42 weeks

A major argument against home birth has been that maternal and infant mortality in the United States has decreased as the number of hospital births has increased. As we compare mortality figures at the beginning of the twentieth century with corresponding figures today, this change is obvious. A number of contributing factors have changed as well. Both the general economic level of our population and the level of general education have risen. Antibiotics have been introduced. There is more awareness of nutrition, and diets are more varied. The birth rate has decreased. These factors have probably also contributed to improved outcomes.

Another comparison that is only partly relevant (because the different populations involved are not necessarily equivalent) is with certain European countries in which home birth remains popular but infant mortality is low, lower than in the United States. In the Netherlands, where infant mortality in 1973 was 11.5 per 1000 live births (compared with a rate of 17.6 in the United States) approximately 40 per cent of deliveries during that year were supervised by midwives at home.

The largest body of home birth data in the United States is that of the Frontier Nursing Service (FNS) in Kentucky. FNS nurse-midwives delivered approximately 10,000 babies in rural, predominantly substandard homes between 1925 and 1955; maternal mortality rates for white women were approximately 75 per cent lower than rates for white women in the remainder of the United States.

On the other hand, we are personally aware of infant mortality and morbidity in home birth that might have been prevented by hospital delivery.

Hospital deliveries may subject mothers and infants to a different kind of risk, iatrogenic risks from oxytocics, for example. The danger of hospital-type infection is a potential hazard. Infection may be a potential hazard in home delivery as well, if proper techniques are not observed. However, given the same technique, the home is a safer place from a bacteriologic standpoint because the mother is immune to organisms in her own home; hospital organisms, to which she may not be immune, are far more resistant.

Potential Advantages

A major advantage of home birth, frequently cited by consumers, is the opportunity to deliver their baby in a familiar and secure environment, surrounded by friends and family. There is no transfer from labor room to delivery table. The baby may be held and nursed at the mother's breast immediately after birth, an act not permitted in many hospitals although probably ideal in terms of attachment behavior (Fig. 23–1). The mother is not separated from her other children for a period of several days. Perhaps most significant, the mother and father take an active role in the delivery of their baby, rather than a passive "acted-upon" role.

At home the mother may be about her usual activities for a longer period of time, which often makes labor seem to be shorter. Moreover, in walking about and changing her position, uterine contractions may be more effective (as noted in Chapter 13) and less frequent. If she is less anxious because she is home, her relaxation will contribute to her comfort during labor.

The opportunity to choose a position for delivery is probably a physiologic as well as an emotional advantage. The traditional dorsal position with legs spread apart, although convenient for the obstetrician, is probably the worst of all possible positions for the mother. At home the mother may squat or sit or lie on one side.

Birth Attendants at Home Birth

Home birth may be attended by a physician, a certified nurse-midwife, a lay-midwife, or perhaps no attendant other than family and friends.

Physician. Although many physicians strongly oppose home births,

Figure 23–1 The baby may nurse prior to the delivery of the placenta to stimulate the release of oxytocin. (From Edwards, M.: *AJN*, 73:1332, 1973.)

others are positively supportive. There is an organization of physicians and families, the American College of Home Obstetrics, with an interest in making home birth a safe experience (address in appendix). The physician may not deliver the baby but is available in case of emergency.

Certified Nurse-Midwife. The preparation and role of the certified nurse-midwife has been described in this chapter. This nurse's role in home birth varies according to state law. Some certified nurse-midwives support home birth and deliver infants at home; others do not because of philosophy and/or law.

Lay-Midwife or Lay Birth Attendant. A lay-midwife is a lay-person who is essentially self-taught or taught by other lay-persons, although sympathetic physicians and nurse-midwives may also teach lay-midwives. Home delivery with a lay-midwife appears to be most common among families with alternate lifestyles (Chapter 4). In some states, a lay-midwife may become licensed. Lay-midwives conduct prenatal classes and examinations in some areas of the country.

Alternatives to Home Birth

Both advocates and adversaries of home birth may tend to view the controversy as an either/or situation. We suggest that both groups have an important message and that from their various perspectives we can plan for better health care.

Most of the desires of the home birth advocates could be met in hospitals or in special birth clinics. In this way much of the safety of the hospital can be combined with the emotional needs of the parents (below).

Back-up systems could be designed

that would afford greater safety to couples who still preferred home birth.

Homelike Delivery in a Medical Facility. A number of major medical centers (Booth Maternity Center in Philadelphia, Family Hospital in Milwaukee, New York Medical College-Flower and Fifth Avenue Hospitals, and Mount Zion Hospital in San Francisco are some examples) have developed facilities that combine the atmosphere of home with the safety of medical center care.

At the New Life Center, Family Hospital, Milwaukee, physical facilities include a carpeted early labor lounge for the mother and her family, which is furnished with books and magazines, games and a game table, and television and music facilities. There is a family snack lounge nearby and a waiting room for friends and family.

Perhaps even more important than comfortable physical facilities is the philosophy that allows the parents to make choices concerning their labor. For example, the New Life Center allows the mother (and father) to decide if she wishes to deliver in a traditional delivery room or in a private labor room, if she would like to give birth in a semi-sitting position, if she would like to hold or breast-feed her baby immediately after birth, and if she would like to tape record or photograph the birth, as well as many other aspects of her care. Mothers continue to have options during the postpartum period and after their return home.

At the Childbearing Center in New York City, birth occurs in a comfortable townhouse only minutes away from a medical center. Friends and family may be present; there is a kitchen for preparing food and a comfortable living room (Fig. 23–2). The mother labors and delivers in the same bed (Fig. 23–3) in a room not much different from a bedroom

Figure 23–2 The living-room of the Childbearing Center of the Maternity Center Association, where couples may spend the early hours of labor. (Courtesy of the Maternity Center Association, New York, N.Y.)

at home. Following birth she and her infant may return home after 12 hours if the pediatrician's examination finds the baby healthy. Nurses make two home visits following discharge.

Some hospitals have plans for early discharge, often within a few hours after birth, for low risk mothers and infants. Although the delivery itself is in the hospital, the time of separation from family, and of separation of mother and baby, is minimal.

Another type of approach is that of the "back-up squad." In Great Britain, when an emergency arises during delivery, a call from the home to the hospital brings two physicians, via ambulance, along with blood and equipment for transfusion and anesthetic equipment.[22]

Early Discharge and Perinatal Home Care. Hospital delivery followed by discharge as early as 12 hours postpartum is an alternative offered to some families at certain American and European hospitals. Yanover and colleagues[31] compared 44 families cared for under such a plan with 44 families receiving conventional care at the same hospital and found no significant difference in outcome.

The key elements of the plan described by Yanover included:

1. Collaborative perinatal care by

Figure 23–3 A cheerful, comfortable room for labor *and* delivery at the Childbearing Center of the Maternity Center Association. (Courtesy of the Maternity Center Association, New York, N.Y.)

the obstetrician, pediatrician, nurse-practitioner, and paramedical personnel.

2. Continuity of care throughout the prenatal, intrapartal, and postpartal phases.

3. Prenatal education, including special classes in preparation for early discharge.

4. Discharge as soon as mother and infant were assessed to be ready.

5. Daily home visits by the perinatal nurse-practitioner for 4 days to assess mother and baby. (After experience with a larger number of babies following the completion of the study, 3 days appeared to be an adequate period of time for daily home visits.)

Following delivery, mother and baby are closely observed during the first 6 hours. The mother and baby are then together for rooming-in. During the next 6 hours the mother is examined by the perinatal nurse-practitioner for problems related to postpartum hemorrhage, subinvolution of the uterus, abnormality at the episiotomy site, urination, breasts, phlebitis, and infection. The infant is also examined for jaundice, signs of infections, and any other deviation from normal. Appropriate specimens of blood are obtained from mother and baby.

Discharge prior to 24 hours is *not* allowed if:

1. The mother's membranes were ruptured for more than 24 hours.

2. Labor was less than 3 hours.

3. Maternal blood pressure exceeded 140/90 or, following delivery, was less than 90/60.

4. Maternal body temperature exceeded 38°C. (100.4°F.) during or following labor.

5. Vaginal bleeding was excessive.

6. The mother had any difficulty voiding or with ambulation.

7. The infant's birth weight was less than 2700 grams (6 pounds) or greater than 4050 grams (9 pounds).

8. The infant's gestational age was less than 38 weeks or greater than 42 weeks.

9. The infant's Apgar score was 7 or less at 1 minute.

10. The infant's vital signs fell within the following parameters: heart rate less than 110 or greater then 150 beats per minute, respiratory rate less than 30 or greater than 60 respirations per minute, temperature less than 36.1°C. or greater than 37.2°C. (97 to 98°F.).

11. The Coombs' test was positive.

12. The infant's hematocrit was less than 45 or greater than 65 per cent.

13. The infant had not voided.

14. The infant was not feeding well.

Nursing and the Home Birth Movement

What is nursing's role in the home birth movement? We can be aware of the desires of couples who find current hospital care unsatisfactory and recognize that in many respects it does indeed fail to meet needs. We can work to change the care that is given in hospitals, so that parents feel their needs can be met within the hospital setting. Even if we support the idea of home birth for some couples, it is important to improve hospital care because a number of women, for medical reasons described above, will never be able to be safely delivered at home. For women who do deliver at home, we can urge adequate back-up facilities.

And finally, research concerning mortality, morbidity, attachment, family dynamics, and other facets of home birth deserves our attention.

THE CRISIS OF A PROBLEM PREGNANCY

Any nurse who spends even a few weeks with potential mothers and fathers will come in contact with women and men to whom pregnancy, for any one of a number of reasons, presents a problem, either physical or emotional. By no means will all nurses formally become problem-pregnancy counselors. But all of us need to know enough about the process to talk with women and men in a way that is both informed and helpful and to make the best possible referrals.

Problem-pregnancy counseling is that which the phrase implies: counseling women (and their mates when it is at all possible) who have a pregnancy that either they, or sometimes we, see as a problem. Problem-pregnancy counseling is *not* abortion counseling, although abortion may be an alternative that is discussed. It is *not* a service only for, or even primarily for, the single woman. It may include genetic counseling or a referral for genetic counseling. At some point it will probably include discussion of responsible sexuality and contraceptive information.

Counselors may be nurses, physicians, family counselors, clergymen, or lay-persons with special training. In addition to a basic understanding of the counseling process, those who counsel women with troubled pregnancies must be fully aware of the resources that their own and other communities offer.

Ideally the initial counselor for a woman or couple with a troubled pregnancy should *not* be attached to an agency to which a patient might later be referred. For example, if the counselor works in an abortion clinic, no matter how objective he or she is in dealing with the alternatives open to the woman, the counselor's own position seems to suggest that he or she thinks highly of abortion as a solution. A counselor who works with an adoption agency, highly cognizant of the current shortage of adoptable babies, may unconsciously put this solution in a favorable light. Counselors working with some groups will not even suggest abortion as an alternative.

It is difficult for any of us to be totally objective, but the more successful we are in our attempt at objectivity, the better able we will be to help each woman. Counselors have no right to force their own wishes and views on women, or even to suggest them.

Mace describes the role of the problem-pregnancy counselor as accepting and supporting each woman as she struggles to reach the decision that is right for her.[15] If we can do this well, the crisis of a problem pregnancy can become, despite the misery, a chance for personal growth.

A particular pregnancy may be a problem for varied reasons:

1. The health of the mother may be threatened. Examples are the mother with serious heart pathology, diabetes that is poorly controlled, or major kidney disease. She may be mentally ill or feel that emotionally she cannot cope with the infant.

2. Previous children or one of the parents may have a major hereditary defect that makes the prospect of another child both emotionally and financially difficult. The family with one or more children with cystic fibrosis, for example, may be very threatened by another pregnancy.

3. A couple may feel that financially they just cannot care for another child, or even for a first child.

4. A couple may feel that they do not wish to add to the world's population. Many younger couples today (and some who are not so young) take the concept of zero population growth both seriously and personally.

5. The mother may be single and not wish to bear a child.

Options for the single woman with a problem pregnancy were discussed in Chapter 4. Genetic counseling was discussed in Chapter 2. Here we will explore the alternative of elective abortion.

ELECTIVE ABORTION

Of all the realities of maternity nursing, elective abortion may be the most difficult for many nurses. In certain hospitals a nurse may be asked to give life-saving care to a 27 week preterm infant on one day and assist in the abortion of a 24 week fetus on the next.

The issue of elective abortion is multifaceted. Nurses must deal with their own feelings about the ethical considerations involved and their proper professional response. Nurses must be aware of possible reactions of women to abortion, and they must understand the various procedures that result in the termination of pregnancy.

The Ethical Problem of Abortion

For most people, lay-persons as well as professionals who give health care, the issues surrounding abortion require careful thought. What are the major concerns? What are the arguments for and against abortion?

Opposition to Abortion

The Fetus as a Human Being. Most people who oppose abortion believe that a unique being with a life of its own exists from the moment of conception. They point out that the zygote has, encoded in its DNA, all the potential for full development as a person. There will never again be another being exactly like this being. Therefore, to destroy this life at any point is to kill a human being. It is suggested that allowing judgments about who should live and who should die in one area of life is no different from deciding who lives and dies under any circumstances (if abortion, why not infanticide, for example?).

Opponents argue that although the embryo has human potential, he is not yet a person.

The Rights of the Fetus. Closely related is the issue of the right of the fetus to live. If indeed the zygote-embryo-fetus is a human being, he then has basic rights, including the right to life.

Most opponents agree that the fetus does have rights, but these rights must be balanced against the rights of the mother and perhaps also of the father, other members of her family, and even the society as a whole.

Support for Abortion

Support for abortion is embodied in several arguments: population control, financial resources, the rights of women, and the hazards of illegal abortion are four reasons discussed frequently.

Population Control. The hazards of overpopulation were documented in Chapter 5. There are those who fear that without liberal, legal abortion, adequate population control will be impossible. Abortion is not advocated as the principal means of limiting population but as an adjunct to other methods.

Those who disagree suggest that there are better means of population control available.

Financial Resources. Some women choose abortion because they feel they cannot financially support the child. From the societal standpoint, the cost of abortion versus the cost of supporting a child whose family is unable to care for him financially is cited by some as a reason not only for abortion but for abortion supported by state and/or federal funding. It is argued that no state would be able to afford the cost of caring for those children who would result from pregnancies that are now aborted.

The same argument, opponents point out, could also be made for disposing of the elderly, the mentally retarded, and others in society who are supported by the society rather than contributing to the society.

Rights of Women. In recent years one of the most frequent arguments for abortion has been in terms of the right of a woman to control her own body. This freedom would include the right to decide whether she wishes to bear a child she has conceived.

Opponents argue that the zygote is not a part of her body but is a separate entity. Although the ovum was formerly part of her body, once it has been released by the ovary, it has its own independent life. They zygote is the equal contribution of man and woman. It has its own combination of genes, different from the combination of either the man or woman. On the other hand, it cannot grow without the protection and nourishment of the mother's body. (This may be possible some day but not currently.)

Hazards of Illegal Abortion. The argument here is not for abortion per se but for *legal* abortion. It is suggested that there have always been and will always be abortions, and in order to make them as safe for women as possible, they should be legal and available to all women.

Elective Abortion and Nursing Practice

Nurses, as well as all persons in the society, need to carefully consider the arguments for and against abortion. In an attempt to help nurses to practice within the framework of their own decisions, the Nurses Association of the American College of Obstetricians and Gynecologists (NAACOG) approved the following statement on abortion (and sterilization) on May 31, 1972. The statement attempts to protect both the right of the nurse to hold and practice her own ethical standards and the right of patients whose ethical decisions may differ from those of the nurse.

The Nurses Association of the American College of Obstetricians and Gynecologists recognizes that current knowledge of human behavior, population pressure and changes in medical technology challenge the position traditionally held regarding interruption of pregnancy.

We are aware of our nursing role in relation to operating with team members in meeting the health care needs of the woman seeking an abortion or sterilization. Genuine concern and compassion for this woman is strongly urged. However, there may be concern regarding nursing practice and participation in this particular area of health care. It is therefore our aim to recommend that an individual's rights must be maintained and safeguarded by written policies.

The Association recommends the following principles and guidelines:

1. Nurses have the responsibility to provide nursing care.

2. Nurses have the right to refuse to assist in the performance of abortions and/or sterilization procedures in keeping with their moral, ethical and/or religious beliefs, except in an emergency when a patient's life is clearly endangered, in which case the questioned moral issue should be disregarded. This refusal should not jeopardize the nurses' employment nor should they be subjected to harassment or embarrassment because of their refusal.

3. Nurses, in dealing with such patients, should not impose their views on the patients or personnel.

4. Nurses have the right to expect their employers to describe to them the hospital's policies and practices regarding abortions and sterilizations.

5. Nurses have the obligation to inform their employers of their attitudes and beliefs regarding abortions and sterilizations.

Just as patients need opportunities to express their feelings in a nonjudgmental milieu, so too must nurses and others who care for patients have an opportunity to share their feelings. The convictions of nurses who choose not to participate in abortions should be respected, not only for the sake of the nurse but for the sake of the patient. Hostile or disapproving attitudes have a way of surfacing in subtle ways—in failure to provide fresh water or to answer a call light, for example.

Counseling Prior to Abortion

Mace[15] suggests that prior to any abortion each woman should be counseled in such a way that she:

1. Understands the meaning of abortion and is sure that this is what *she* desires.

2. Is not coerced by others (boyfriend, husband, parents, friends, counselor).

3. Has considered her conscience and her values.

4. Has considered alternatives (adoption, for example).

5. Is knowledgeable about effective contraception.

The counseling process itself should give each woman an opportunity to tell her story in her own words and to express her feelings. Often she may not be in touch with her true feelings at first, but self-recognition is important before a decision is made. Options are then explored (Chapter 4). As a result each woman will be able, we hope, to take the responsibility for a decision that is in accord with her own values.

The Reactions of Women to Elective Abortion

Although it is conceivable that any individual woman may exhibit none of the feelings that observers have found common to women who have had abortions, nurses need to watch for signs of each of these, recognizing when their expression is within the range of normal and when additional counseling may be helpful.

Anger, guilt, fear, and sadness are emotions common to women both prior to and following induced abortion. Anger may be expressed at oneself ("I was dumb to let this [i.e., pregnancy] happen") or at the mate. If the mate is also the husband, the anger may influence many aspects of their relationship.

Some degree of guilt is not uncommon. The accompanying discomfort (there is always at least some discomfort that is somewhat equivalent to menstrual cramps) in the days that follow can reinforce feelings of guilt.

Fear may be related to fear of the procedure (see below), fear of pain, fear of after-effects, and/or fear that the fact of her abortion will become known.

Sadness is sometimes expressed in statements such as "I sometimes wonder what the baby might have been like."

On the more positive side, relief, gratitude that the abortion could be experienced with some degree of dignity, and new self-understanding are achieved by some women. Both positive and negative emotions often coexist in the same individual. How much some of these emotions, particularly the more negative ones, are due to the influence of a culture that for so many generations has considered not only abortion but sex outside of marriage (for females, at any rate) as sin is unclear at this point in history.

Nor is how long such feelings are likely to persist following abortion well documented. It can be a long time for some women. A counselor tells of a woman who considered an abortion nearly 20 years ago. She rejected the idea and bore, raised, and loved her son, now a young man. When the issue of abortion became widely discussed in her community recently, all of her old feelings came to the surface. She could no longer look at her son without feeling guilt for the abortion had had *only contemplated*. Although this mother's reaction and her guilt are probably extreme, her predicament does emphasize how much we have to learn about an issue that amounts to much more than a simple 5 minute procedure.

When a woman presents herself for the actual abortion procedure, she will have experienced, and may be continuing to feel, all of the emotions we have mentioned. Even the woman who feels very sure that this is the right thing for her to do may be anxious about the procedure itself. We can help this anxiety somewhat by a careful explanation of exactly what will happen in some detail. For example, if she is to have a saline instillation, she can be told that the solution used to prepare her abdomen will feel cold to her. One reason we as nurses need to be quite familiar with the procedures ourselves is so that we can prepare the patient for what to expect and answer her questions in an accurate and knowledgeable way.

Patients for induced abortion often have a very low tolerance for frustration. They have made their decision, and now they want the matter concluded as quickly as possible. Sometimes there must be a period of waiting, for the results of laboratory work, for example. The very least we can do in these instances is to acknowledge how difficult this must be for the woman. "I know how hard waiting must be for you;

it usually takes about 30 minutes for these reports to be ready," may be helpful.

Rules, too, may be particularly hard to accept at this time. Even though rules have been explained (such as the necessity for having nothing by mouth for the patient who is to have general anesthesia), they may need to be discussed a second and third time. Patients who are preoccupied and anxious do not learn readily; explanations are easily forgotten. For this reason, too, the period before the abortion procedure is not a good one for teaching about contraception or any other material we expect the patient to retain.

The degree of formality that is a part of the relationship between the nurse and the abortion patient (or any patient) will vary considerably. Adolescent patients usually welcome a very informal relationship in which they are called by their first name and "mothered" with warmth and acceptance. This kind of approach can be offensive to a mature professional woman. Acceptance and concern for her may be more readily appreciated when it is expressed in quiet competence.

Regardless of what we attempt, some patients who come for abortion will be hostile because of their own high level of anxiety. Being able to understand and accept these feelings is a part of their nursing care.

Physical Preparation for Abortion

Physical preparation for an induced abortion includes ascertaining the medical history and performing a number of laboratory tests and general and gynecologic examinations.

Medical history is one significant factor in deciding on the type of procedure most appropriate for an individual patient and also where it might best be performed. Induced abortion in an out-

patient clinic is not suitable for women with a number of conditions, including cardiac, pulmonary, hematologic, or metabolic disease. Physical conditions that should be noted in the medical history include anemia; sickle cell disease; liver, kidney, or heart disease; diabetes, and epilepsy. Any intrauterine surgery, including hysterotomy or cesarean section, should be recorded, as should allergies to medications. A respiratory tract infection will usually contraindicate the use of general anesthesia. On the other hand, general anesthesia may be advisable for very young or very anxious patients.

Obstetric history, including the date of the last menstrual period and previous pregnancies, is part of this record.

The time during which a nurse is recording the medical history gives her an opportunity to assess undue anxiety or ambivalence, which could indicate a need for more intensive counseling.

Laboratory work commonly includes a pregnancy test, urinalysis, complete blood count, serology, blood group and type, and sickle cell screening. When indicated, A RhoGAM crossmatch is done; the administration of immune globulin to Rh-negative women following induced abortion is just as significant in the prevention of hemolytic disease of the newborn as the administration following delivery (see Chapter 10).

Pap smears (and in some clinics gonococcal smears) are done at the time of the pelvic examination.

A thorough general and gynecologic examination, in most instances by a physician, completes the physical preparation.

Abortion Procedures

Aspiration. During the first 12 weeks following the last menstrual period vacuum aspiration (also termed suction curettage) is considered the safest method of terminating pregnancy.

Following a paracervical block or general inhalation anesthesia, the cervix is dilated. With the vacuum off, a vacurette is inserted into the dilated internal os; the vacuum is applied, and the tube is withdrawn gently. The uterine contents, trapped in a special container, are examined by the physician and may then be sent to a pathologist.

The patient may receive intravenous Pitocin during the procedure to reduce blood loss. Often she rests for a few minutes in the operating room before returning to the recovery suite.

Variations in the procedure may include:

1. Omitting dilatation very early in pregnancy when smaller bore evacuation tubes may be adequate.

2. Inserting a cylinder made from the stem of dry seaweed *(Laminaria digitata)* on the evening prior to the aspiration. The seaweed expands as it absorbs moisture and dilates the cervix. However, it may migrate in the cervix and become difficult to remove.

Abortion by aspiration is frequently done on an outpatient basis, with the woman remaining at the clinic for approximately 6 hours. This allows time for counseling and teaching, both before and after the procedure, as well as close observation of the woman.

After the twelfth week of pregnancy the technique of abortion becomes more complex.

Saline or Glucose Injection. When hypertonic saline or glucose is injected into the uterine cavity, severe damage results to both the placenta and fetus, and fetal death occurs. Hypertonic saline is used more often than glucose in this procedure because of the increased rate of infection associated with glucose. Hypertonic saline may not be given to the mother with heart disease.

Abortion by saline instillation is performed by:

1. Antiseptic skin preparation and draping.

2. Infiltration of the abdominal wall with a local anesthetic (such as 1 per cent lidocaine).

3. Insertion of a spinal needle into the intrauterine space through a site about midway between the umbilicus and the symphysis pubis, and the subsequent withdrawal of 200 cc. of amniotic fluid.

4. Instillation of 200 cc. of 20 per cent sodium chloride (or 50 per cent glucose). The sodium chloride may be injected manually or via drip infusion.

A major maternal danger of this procedure is the risk that the hypertonic sodium chloride will enter the woman's circulation, causing death from acute hypernatremia or causing neurologic or cardiopulmonary damage. The chances of this are felt by some to be less when a drip infusion is used. The infusion bottle can be lowered to check for a clear return flow, indicating that the needle is not in a blood vessel.

Complaints of headache or thirst by the patient also suggest direct intravenous injection; the infusion should be stopped immediately.

Menstrual Extraction. Menstrual extraction is the term used in a Supreme Court decision of January 1973 to describe a procedure in which a flexible polyethylene catheter, with two openings at its distal end, is inserted through the cervix into the uterus. Suction is applied, by syringe, or a hand or foot controlled pump, or electric vacuum apparatus, and the lining of the uterus that would normally be shed in menstruation is aspirated.

Although forerunners of this type of procedure, which is called by a number of names (menstrual regulation, menstrual aspiration, mini-abortion, menstrual induction, and several others) date back to 1927, it has become relatively common only in the 1970's.

By strict definition menstrual extraction is not abortion, in that it is most commonly performed in the fourth to sixth week following the last menstrual period, a time during which pregnancy tests are not reliable. It is a method of establishing nonpregnancy for the woman who *may* be pregnant and does not wish to be. Some studies indicate that as many as half of the women having a menstrual extraction were not pregnant and were, therefore, undergoing an unnecessary procedure. At least one physician has suggested that delaying menstrual extraction until from 6 to 8 weeks after the last menstrual period could eliminate these unneeded procedures.

Most reports indicate that the procedure itself has many advantages over other types of pregnancy termination. In the few studies that have been done, complications were far lower than with other types of first trimester abortions. It is an outpatient procedure that is brief and requires no general anesthesia. This contributes to a far lower cost to the patient. Menstrual extraction failed to terminate pregnancy in less than 2 per cent of patients.

It has been suggested that paramedical personnel (including nurses) could perform menstrual extraction after specialized training. Some women's groups have advocated the use of this technique by women in their own homes. No one is sure whether there might be a danger in repeated menstrual extractions in the same woman, although most agree that it should not be a substitute for contraception. Further research seems important before these issues can be resolved.

Prostaglandins. Prostaglandins are fatty acids of a number of varieties that occur in many human tissues. Human semen alone contains 13 varieties. In obstetrics prostaglandins are being used to induce both abortion and labor, although this use is still largely experimental. In 1974 the Food and Drug Administration approved one prostaglandin family product (Dinoprost, Prostin F-2 Alpha) for the termination of second trimester pregnancy.

Intravaginal or intrauterine (via injection into the amniotic sac) administration of prostaglandins can interrupt pregnancy as early as the first week after a missed menstrual period or at any time during the first 2 trimesters, although these substances currently appear most effective after the sixteenth week. Prostaglandins may also be given intravenously, but larger doses are required and the incidence of side effects is increased. Prostaglandins induce abortion by stimulating contractions of the uterine smooth muscle. In most instances, expulsion of the uterine contents occurs within 24 hours.

Because these substances stimulate the smooth muscle of the gastrointestinal tract as well as of the reproductive tract, nausea, vomiting, abdominal cramps, and diarrhea are the principal undesired reactions. Prochlorperazine (Compazine) may be given for nausea and meperidine (Demerol) for pain, but aspirin should not be used because it inhibits the body's synthesis of natural prostaglandins and thus prolongs abortion time. Special care in the use of prostaglandins is necessary for women who have asthma, epilepsy, hypertension, or glaucoma because of occasional side effects: bronchospasm, convulsions, and transient blood pressure elevation.

Some early researchers using prostaglandins hoped that they could play a major role in contraception in vaginal tampon form. They would be packaged along with a pregnancy testing kit. However, because they are not totally effective and because of the side effects, this has not yet become practical.

15-Methyl-E₂-Analog. A synthetic substance, 15-methyl-E$_2$-analog, which can be administered intramuscularly, has been found to equal the success rates and time required for intra-amniotic abortion. Intramuscular administration makes it more widely useful. A unique side effect of this preparation is the patient's feeling of being cold, accompanied by shivering, which may appear within 15 minutes after injection and may last as long as an hour. Since her temperature may also rise during that period, these symptoms may originate in the thermal regulation centers of the central nervous system.

Commercial Abortion Agencies

With the growth of legitimate abortion agencies it was probably inevitable that some commercial agencies would develop solely for profit. One example is the commercial referral agency. The agency may advertise on radio or television or in newspapers, particularly campus newspapers. The patient calls a designated phone number and is told, "Your abortion will cost $200; bring or mail $50 down-payment or deposit and we will arrange an appointment for you." After the patient has made this payment she is referred to a clinic, which may be a highly reputable clinic that knows nothing of the referral group and charges a customary fee of $150.

A second possibility is that the clinic itself is in collaboration with the referral agency and receives a "kickback" from the fee charged for the abortion.

Nurses can prevent such practices. Awareness of the fees normally charged by legitimate clinics and alertness to the possibility of such referral services are two ways of doing this. Referral through family planning clinics and other health agencies can be made available and then publicized. When patients come for abortion referral, we can be sure that they are treated in such a way that alternative referrals will not seem more desirable. For example, the college student who fears that her request for abortion through campus health facilities will be a difficult, uncomfortable procedure may seek an alternate route. Questionable referrals are most likely to continue when they fulfill a woman's need for sympathy and individualized concern.

SUMMARY

Issues, such as those described in this chapter, influence and impinge upon our nursing practice. Today's issues will be supplanted by new issues tomorrow. But nurses must always be actively involved in those arenas in which decisions are made if we are to give the best possible care to childbearing families.

POSTLOGUE

You have finished this text, and perhaps a course, but you have only started to learn about childbearing families. There has never been a day in our professional lives in which there was not an opportunity to learn—from a woman or a family, from a newborn or a preterm infant, from a colleague, from a student, from a friend, and from our personal experiences in childbearing.

Learning, sharing that learning, and using the information to continually improve the care of families fill nursing with an excitement and joy possible in few other professions.

REFERENCES

1. Bean,M.: The Nurse Midwife at Work. *American Journal of Nursing, 71*:949, 1971.
2. Bracken, M., Grossman, G., Hachamovitch, M., et al.: Abortion Counseling: An Experimental Study of Three Techniques. *American Journal of Obstetrics and Gynecology, 117*:10, 1973.
3. Brown, M., O'Meara, C., and Krowley, S.: The Maternal-Child Nurse Practitioner. *American Journal of Nursing, 75*:1298, 1975.
4. David, H.: Abortion in Psychological Perspective. *American Journal of Orthopsychiatry, 42*:61, 1972.
5. *Demographic Yearbook, 1975.* New York, United Nations, 1976.
6. Edwards, M.: Unattended Home Birth. *American Journal of Nursing, 73*:1332, 1973.
7. Final Mortality Statistics Report. *Monthly Vital Statistics Report, 24*:11, February 3, 1976. Rockville, Md., National Center for Health Statistics, U. S. Dept. of Health, Education and Welfare.
8. Fitzgerald, D., Herman, E., Ventre, F., et al.: *Home Oriented Maternity Experience.* Takoma Park, Md., H.O.M.E. Inc., 1976.
9. Fonseca, J.: Induced Abortion: Nursing Attitudes and Action. *American Journal of Nursing, 68*:1022, 1968.
10. Gatewood, T., and Stewart, R.: Obstetricians and Nurse Midwives: The Team Approach in Private Practice. *American Journal of Obstetrics and Gynecology, 123*:35, 1975.
11. Hogan, A.: A Tribute to the Pioneers. *Journal of Nurse-Midwifery,* Summer, 1975.
12. Keller, C., and Copeland, P.: Counseling the Abortion Patient is More than Talk. *American Journal of Nursing, 72*:102, 1972.
13. Kohl, S.: *Perinatal Mortality in New York City.* Cambridge, Harvard University Press, 1955.
14. Levy, B., Wilkinson, F., and Marine, W.: Reducing Neonatal Mortality Rate with

Nurse Midwives. *American Journal of Obstetrics and Gynecology, 109*:50, 1971.
15. Mace, D.: *Abortion: The Agonizing Decision.* Nashville, Abingdon Press, 1972.
16. NAACOG Statement on Abortions and Sterilizations. *JOGN Nursing, 1*(1):57, 1972.
17. Nunnally, D., and Bird, J.: The Clinical Specialist—Link between Theory and Practice. *JOGN Nursing, 4*(2):40, 1975.
18. Olrig, A.: A Nurse-Midwife in Practice. *American Journal of Nursing, 71*:953, 1971.
19. Page, E., Villee, C., and Villee, D.: *Human Reproduction: The Core Content of Obstetrics, Gynecology and Perinatal Medicine.* 2nd Edition. Philadelphia, W. B. Saunders Co., 1976.
20. Personal Experience at a Legal Abortion Center. *American Journal of Nursing, 72*:110, 1972.
21. *Population and Vital Statistics Report,* New York, The United Nations Statistical Office.
22. Ritchie, C., and Swanson, L.: Childbirth Outside the Hospital—The Resurgence of Home and Clinic Deliveries. *MCN 1*(6):372, 1976.
23. Schwartz, S., and Vineyard, J.: Prenatal Care and Prematurity. *Public Health, 80*:237, 1965.
24. Schuman, H.: A Pediatric Nurse Practitioner in the Neonatal Unit. *JOGN Nursing, 2*(6):42, 1973.
25. *Statistical Yearbook, 1973,* New York, United Nations Publishing Service, 1974.
26. *Vital Statistics of the United States, Volume II Mortality.* Rockville, Md., National Center for Health Statistics, U. S. Dept. of Health, Education and Welfare, 1972.
27. *What is a Nurse-Midwife?* Washington, D.C., American College of Nurse-Midwives.
28. Whitley, N.: Second Trimester Abortion: A Program of Teaching and Counseling. *JOGN Nursing, 2*(5):15, 1973.
29. Wilson, R.: *Problem Pregnancy and Abortion Counseling.* Saluda, N. C., Family Life Publications, 1973.
30. *World Health Statistics Annual, 1973–1976.* Geneva, World Health Organization, 1976.
31. Yanover, M., Jones D., and Miller, M.: Perinatal Care of Low Risk Mothers and Infants. *New England Journal of Medicine, 294*:702, 1976.

APPENDIX A

HEMOGLOBIN, HEMATOCRIT, AND LEUKOCYTE VALUES DURING THE FIRST
6 WEEKS OF POSTPARTUM LIFE (TERM INFANT)*

Age	Hemoglobin† (Grams %)	Hematocrit† (%)	Leukocytes‡
BIRTH			
Mean	19.0	61	18,000
Range	16.8–21.2	53.6–68.4	9,000–30,000
7 DAYS			
Mean	17.9	56	12,000
Range	15.4–20.4	46.6–65.4	5,000–21,000
14 DAYS			
Mean	17.3	54	12,000
Range	15.0–19.6	45.7–62.3	5,000–21,000
6 WEEKS			
Mean	11.9	36	—
Range	10.4–13.4	31.2–40.8	—
3 MONTHS			
Mean	11.3	33	12,000
Range	10.4–12.2	29.7–36.3	6,000–18,000

*Standards will vary slightly from one laboratory to another.
†Range represents 1 standard deviation in study by Matoth: *Acta Paediatrica Scand., 60*:317, 1971.
‡After Oski and Naiman: *Hematologic Problems in the Newborn.* 2nd Edition. Philadelphia, W. B. Saunders Co., 1972.

APPENDIX B

ENGLISH–METRIC CONVERSION: POUNDS AND OUNCES TO GRAMS

POUNDS	\ OUNCES 0	1	2	3	4	5	6	7	8	9	10	11	12	13	14	15
0	—	28	57	85	113	142	170	198	227	255	283	312	340	369	397	425
1	454	482	510	539	567	595	624	652	680	709	737	765	794	822	850	879
2	907	936	964	992	1021	1049	1077	1106	1134	1162	1191	1219	1247	1276	1304	1332
3	1361	1389	1417	1446	1474	1503	1531	1559	1588	1616	1644	1673	1701	1729	1758	1786
4	1814	1843	1871	1899	1928	1956	1984	2013	2041	2070	2098	2126	2155	2183	2211	2240
5	2268	2296	2325	2353	2381	2410	2438	2466	2495	2523	2551	2580	2608	2637	2665	2693
6	2722	2750	2778	2807	2835	2863	2892	2920	2948	2977	3005	3033	3062	3090	3118	3147
7	3175	3203	3232	3260	3289	3317	3345	3374	3402	3430	3459	3487	3515	3544	3572	3600
8	3629	3657	3685	3714	3742	3770	3799	3827	3856	3884	3912	3941	3969	3997	4026	4054
9	4082	4111	4139	4167	4196	4224	4252	4281	4309	4337	4366	4394	4423	4451	4479	4508
10	4536	4564	4593	4621	4649	4678	4706	4734	4763	4791	4819	4848	4876	4904	4933	4961
11	4990	5018	5046	5075	5103	5131	5160	5188	5216	5245	5273	5301	5330	5358	5386	5415
12	5443	5471	5500	5528	5557	5585	5613	5642	5670	5698	5727	5755	5783	5812	5840	5868
13	5897	5925	5953	5982	6010	6038	6067	6095	6123	6152	6180	6209	6237	6265	6294	6322
14	6350	6379	6407	6435	6464	6492	6520	6549	6577	6605	6634	6662	6690	6719	6747	6776
15	6804	6832	6860	6889	6917	6945	6973	7002	7030	7059	7087	7115	7144	7172	7201	7228
16	7257	7286	7313	7342	7371	7399	7427	7456	7484	7512	7541	7569	7597	7626	7654	7682
17	7711	7739	7768	7796	7824	7853	7881	7909	7938	7966	7994	8023	8051	8079	8108	8136
18	8165	8192	8221	8249	8278	8306	8335	8363	8391	8420	8448	8476	8504	8533	8561	8590
19	8618	8646	8675	8703	8731	8760	8788	8816	8845	8873	8902	8930	8958	8987	9015	9043
20	9072	9100	9128	9157	9185	9213	9242	9270	9298	9327	9355	9383	9412	9440	9469	9497
21	9525	9554	9582	9610	9639	9667	9695	9724	9752	9780	9809	9837	9865	9894	9922	9950
22	9979	10007	10036	10064	10092	10120	10149	10177	10206	10234	10262	10291	10319	10347	10376	10404

APPENDIX C

TABLE OF FAHRENHEIT AND CELSIUS (CENTIGRADE) TEMPERATURE
EQUIVALENTS*

94.0–34.4	97.0–36.1	100.0–37.8
94.2–34.6	97.2–36.2	100.2–37.9
94.4–34.7	97.4–36.3	100.4–38.0
94.6–34.8	97.6–36.4	100.6–38.1
94.8–34.9	97.8–36.5	100.8–38.2
95.0–35.0	98.0–36.6	101.0–38.3
95.2–35.1	98.2–36.8	101.2–38.4
95.4–35.2	98.4–36.9	101.4–38.5
95.6–35.3	98.6–37.0	101.6–38.6
95.8–35.4	98.8–37.1	101.8–38.7
96.0–35.5	99.0–37.2	102.0–38.8
96.2–35.6	99.2–37.3	102.2–39.0
96.4–35.7	99.4–37.4	102.4–39.1
96.6–35.8	99.6–37.5	102.6–39.2
96.8–36.0	99.8–37.6	102.8–39.3

*To convert Fahrenheit to Celsius (Centigrade), subtract 32 from the Fahrenheit reading and multiply by $5/9$.

APPENDIX D

American Nurses' Association—Standards of Maternal-Child Health Nursing Practice*

The development of standards of practice is important in every profession. The following *Standards of Maternal-Child Health Nursing Practice* was developed by the Executive Committee and the Standards Committee of the Division on Maternal-Child Health Nursing Practice of the American Nurses' Association in 1973. These standards are process standards.

A booklet discussing maternal-child health standards in more detail is available from the American Nurses' Association, 2420 Pershing Road, Kansas City, Missouri, 64108, for $1.00.

Maternal and Child Health Nursing Practice is based on the following premises:
1. Survival and the level of health of a society is inextricably bound to Maternal and Child Health Nursing Practice.
2. Maternal and Child Health Nursing Practice respects the human dignity and rights of individuals.
3. Maternal and Child Health Nursing Practice is family-centered.
4. Maternal and Child Health Nursing Practice focuses on the childbearing, child-rearing phases of the life cycle which include the development of sexuality, family planning, interconceptual care and child health from conception through adolescence.
5. Maternal and Child Health Nursing makes a significant difference to society in achieving its health goals.
6. Man is a total human being. His psychosocial and biophysical self are interrelated.
7. Human behavior shapes and is shaped by environmental forces and as such sets into motion a multitude of reciprocal responses.

---

*Reprinted by permission of the American Nurses' Association, Inc., 2420 Pershing Road, Kansas City, Missouri 64108.

8. Through his own process of self-regulation the human being attempts to maintain equilibrium amidst constant change.
9. All behavior has meaning and is influenced by past experiences, the individual's perception of those experiences, and forces impinging upon the present.
10. Growth and development is ordered and evolves in sequential stages.
11. Substantive knowledge of the principles of human growth and development, including normative data, is essential to effective Maternal and Child Health Nursing Practice.
12. Periods of developmental and traumatic crises during the life cycle pose internal and external stresses and have a positive or negative effect.
13. Maternal and Child Health Nursing Practice provides for continuity of care and is not bound by artificial barriers and exclusive categories which tend to restrict and delimit practice.
14. *All* people have a right to receive the benefit of optimal health services.

Maternal and Child Health Nursing Practice is aimed at:
1. Promoting and maintaining optimal health of each individual and the family unit.
2. Improving and/or supporting family solidarity.
3. Early identification and treatment of vulnerable families.
4. Preventing environmental conditions which block attainment of optimal health.
5. Prevention and early detection of deviations from health.
6. Reducing stresses which interfere with optimal functioning.
7. Assisting the family to understand and/or cope with the developmental and traumatic situations which occur during childbearing and childrearing.
8. Facilitating survival, recovery and growth when the individual is ill or needs health care.
9. Reducing reproductive wastage occurring at any point on the continuum.
10. Continuously improving the quality of care in Maternal and Child Health Nursing Practice.
11. Reducing inequalities in the delivery of health care services.

STANDARD I

Maternal and child health nursing practice is characterized by the continual questioning of the assumptions upon which practice is based, retaining those which are valid and searching for and using new knowledge.

Rationale: Since knowledge is not static, all assumptions are subject to change. Assumptions are derived from knowledge of findings of research which are subject to additional testing and revision. They are carefully selected and tested and reflect utilization of present and new knowledge. Effective utilization of these knowledges stimulates more astute observations and provides new insights into the effects of nursing upon the individual and family. To question assumptions implies that nursing practice is not based on stereotyped or ritualistic procedures or methods of intervention; rather, practice exemplifies an objective, systematic and logical investigation of a phenomenon or problem.

STANDARD II

Maternal and child health nursing practice is based upon knowledge of the bio-physical and psychosocial development of individuals from conception through the childrearing phase of development and upon knowledge of the basic needs for optimum development.

Rationale: A knowledge and understanding of the principles and normal ranges in human growth, development and behavior are essential to Maternal and Child Health Nursing Practice. Concomitant with this knowledge is the recognition and consideration of the psychosocial, environmental, nutritional, spiritual and cognitive factors that enhance or deter the biophysical and psychological maturation of the individual and his family.

STANDARD III

The collection of data about the health status of the client/patient is systematic and continuous. The data are accessible, communicated and recorded.

Rationale: Comprehensive care requires complete and ongoing collection of data about the client/patient to determine the nursing care needs and other health care needs of the client/patient. All health status data about the client/patient must be available for all members of the health care team.

STANDARD IV

Nursing diagnoses are derived from data about the health status of the client/patient.

Rationale: The health status of the client/patient is the basis for determining the nursing care needs. The data are analyzed and compared to norms.

STANDARD V

Maternal and child health nursing practice recognizes deviations from expected patterns of physiologic activity and anatomic and psychosocial development.

Rationale: Early detection of deviations and therapeutic intervention are essential to the prevention of illness, to facilitating growth and developmental potential, and to the promotion of optimal health for the individual and the family.

STANDARD VI

The plan of nursing care includes goals derived from the nursing diagnoses.

Rationale: The determination of the desired results from nursing actions is an essential part of planning care.

STANDARD VII

The plan of nursing care includes priorities and the prescribed nursing approaches or measures to achieve the goals derived from the nursing diagnoses.
Rationale: Nursing actions are planned to promote, maintain and restore the client/patient's well-being.

STANDARD VIII

Nursing actions provide for client/patient participation in health promotion, maintenance and restoration.
Rationale: The client/patient and family are provided the opportunity to participate in the nursing care. Such provision is made based upon theoretical and experiential evidence that participation of client/patient and family may foster growth.

STANDARD IX

Maternal and child health nursing practice provides for the use and coordination of all services that assist individuals to prepare for responsible sexual roles.
Rationale: People are prepared for sexual roles through a process of socialization that takes place from birth to adulthood. This process of socialization, to a large extent, is carried out within the family structure. Social control over child care increases in importance as humans become increasingly dependent on the culture rather than upon the family unit. The culture of any society is maintained by the transmission of its specific values, attitudes and behaviors from generation to generation. Attitudes and values concerning male and female roles develop as part of the socialization process. Attitudes toward self, the opposite sex and parents will influence the roles each individual assumes in adulthood and the responsibilities accepted.

STANDARD X

Nursing actions assist the client/patient to maximize his health capabilities.
Rationale: Nursing actions are designed to promote, maintain and restore health. A knowledge and understanding of the principles and normal ranges in human growth, development and behavior are essential to Maternal and Child Health Nursing Practice.

STANDARD XI

The client's/patient's progress or lack of progress toward goal achievement is determined by the client/patient and the nurse.
Rationale: The quality of nursing care depends upon comprehensive and intelligent determination of the impact of nursing upon the health status of the client/patient. The client/patient is an essential part of this determination.

STANDARD XII

The client's/patient's progress or lack of progress toward goal achievement directs reassessment, reordering of priorities, new goal setting and revision of the plan of nursing care.
Rationale: The nursing process remains the same, but the input of new information may dictate new or revised approaches.

STANDARD XIII

Maternal and child health nursing practice evidences active participation with others in evaluating the availability, accessibility and acceptability of services for parents and children and cooperating and/or taking leadership in extending and developing needed services in the community.
Rationale: Knowledge of services presently offered parents and children is the first step in determining the effectiveness of health care to all in the community. When it is recognized that needed services are not available, accessible or acceptable, the nurse takes leadership in working with consumers, other health disciplines, the community and governmental agencies in extending and/or developing these services. Services must be continually evaluated, expanded and changed if they are to improve the health and well-being of all parents and children within our society.

APPENDIX E

The Nurses Association of the American College of Obstetricians and Gynecologists—Obstetrics, Gynecologic and Neonatal Nursing Functions and Standards*

The Nurses Association of the American College of Obstetricians and Gynecologists (NAACOG) has developed a guide to nursing functions in obstetric and gynecologic nursing, along with standards and procedures by which they are performed which are intended to serve as guides for the improvement of patient care. These standards are structure standards. The following statements are taken from these standards. The complete document is available from NAACOG, One East Wacker Drive, Suite 2700, Chicago, Illinois, 60601.

ADVANCEMENT OF THE SPECIALTY

The obstetric-gynecologic neonatal health care system is experiencing an increased demand for quality and quantity of health care. To meet this demand and to function as a more effective member of the health care team, the nurse has had to expand her role.

New categories of nursing personnel are being developed, but specific national standards for the preparation and responsibilities of these new categories of nurses have not yet been established. No matter what national standards may be developed, administrative, medical, and nursing staffs in each health care institution should collaborate in developing their own application of standards for the OGN nurse.

As the knowledge and technology for better health increase rapidly, it is imperative that the OGN nurse take every opportunity to increase her professional knowledge and skills. Such continuing education may be in the form of broadened clinical experience, seminars or other hospital organized programs, reading journals and

*Reprinted by permission of the Nurses Association of the American College of Obstetricians and Gynecologists, One East Wacker Drive, Chicago, Illinois, 60601.

books, participation in nursing organizations, or enrolling in formal university level courses. It is essential that all members of the health care team be aware of this rapid increase in technical knowledge and the changing interrelationships it has encouraged among professionals involved in the delivery of health care. The expanded role of the nurse is a developing concept and all health care professionals must be prepared to alter their traditional views of the practicing OGN nurse.

GENERAL STANDARDS

PERSONNEL

The department of nursing must determine an appropriate ratio of staff to patients to cover requirements of patient care. All health care team members should participate in an organized orientation and in-service program related to the OGN specialty. Nursing administrators will take an active role in this phase of staff development and in the assignment of health care personnel.

Job descriptions should be written for all personnel and should include educational requirements, anticipated responsibilities and duties.

POLICIES AND PROCEDURES

Departmental policies and procedures should be established by representatives from the administrative, medical and nursing staffs and reviewed annually.

Nursing policies, procedures and protocols should be evaluated on a regular basis and revised as needed.

There should be cooperation and communication between medical and nursing staffs and other related services through patient care committees.

NURSING CARE PLAN AND EVALUATION

It is incumbent upon all members of the health care team to provide a safe, comfortable and therapeutic environment which will meet the physical, psychologic and spiritual needs of the patient.

Individual plans for patient care should be based upon an assessment of the patient's total needs. Provision must be made to evaluate nursing care rendered.

PROFESSIONAL RESPONSIBILITY

The professional nurse must assume the responsibility of maintaining competence in her practice. She is accountable for the implementation and direction of nursing care rendered. It is her responsibility to continue her education to keep abreast of the most modern and current trends in health care.

PATIENT EDUCATION

Patient education is an important function of the OGN nurse and it must be an integral part of all nursing activities. The OGN nurse should be specifically prepared for her role as a teacher and as one skilled in interpersonal relations. She should have educational as well as other resources available for her patients. For effective patient education, collaboration among all members of the OGN health team is essential and must conform to the information the patient is getting from her physician.

FACILITIES AND EQUIPMENT

It should be the responsibility of the personnel on the unit to identify and set standards for care of the facilities and equipment and to make referrals to the appropriate departments, such as Anesthesia, Pharmacy, Housekeeping, Maintenance, etc., for implementation.

For provision of quality health care, nursing personnel must play an active role in planning for the facility, in the selection and evaluation of equipment and supplies and in the evaluation and the coordination of maintenance needs.

APPENDIX F

Arizona Nurses' Association—Perinatal Nursing Standards*

The following standards were developed by the Committee for Preparation of Standards of Perinatal Nursing Practice, Arizona Nurses Association, in 1977. The objective of these Perinatal Nursing Standards is to give structure, direction, and a more formal recognition to the maternal-fetal and neonatal nursing practice, education, and evaluation. Perinatal nursing integrates the interdependent normal and high risk segments of maternal-fetal and neonatal health care and includes the care of all pregnant women and neonates and their families.

A complete copy of these standards, including assessment factors, is available from the Arizona Nurses Association, 4525 North 12th Street, Phoenix, Arizona, 85014, for $1.50.

STANDARD I

Perinatal nursing practice is characterized by the continual questioning of the assumptions upon which practice is based, retaining those which are valid and searching for and using new knowledge.

STANDARD II

Perinatal nursing practice is based upon knowledge of the normal and abnormal biophysical and psychosocial development of the pregnant woman, her fetus/ newborn and her family.

STANDARD III

Nursing diagnoses are based upon the collection of data about the health status of the mother/fetus/newborn.

---

*Reprinted by permission of the Arizona Nurses' Association, 4525 North 12th Street, Phoenix, Arizona 85014.

STANDARD IV

The plan of nursing care includes priorities and the prescribed nursing approaches or measures to achieve the goals derived from the nursing diagnosis.

STANDARD V

The plan of nursing care contains a nursing history. The care plan expresses assessment of the patient/family, defines health care goals and nursing actions. This process is recorded, communicated and accessible.

STANDARD VI

Perinatal nursing practice provides for the use and coordination of all perinatal health care services within the region.

APPENDIX G

Journals Useful to Nurses Who Care for Childbearing Families

American Journal of Diseases of Children, American Medical Association, 535 North Dearborn Street, Chicago, Illinois, 60610.

American Journal of Nursing, American Journal of Nursing Company, 10 Columbus Circle, New York, New York, 10019.

American Journal of Obstetrics and Gynecology, C. V. Mosby Company, 11830 Westline Industrial Drive, St. Louis, Missouri, 63141.

American Journal of Orthopsychiatry, 49 Sheridan Avenue, Albany, New York, 12210.

American Journal of Public Health, 1015 Eighteenth Street, N.W., Washington, D.C., 20036.

Archives of Disease in Childhood, British Medical Association, Tavislock Square, London, England.

*Birth and Family Journal, 110 El Camino Real, Berkeley, California, 94705.

*Briefs, Maternity Center Association, Publication Office, 6900 Grove Road, Thorofare, New Jersey, 08086.

The Canadian Nurse, 50 The Driveway, Ottawa, Ontario, Canada.

Child and Family, P. O. Box 508, Oak Park, Illinois, 60303.

Children Today, Superintendent of Documents, U.S. Government Printing Office, Washington, D.C., 20402.

*ICEA News, International Childbirth Education Association, P. O. Box 20852, Milwaukee, Wisconsin, 53220.

International Journal of Nursing Studies, Headington Hill Hall, Oxford, OX3 OBU England.

*JOGN, Journal of Obstetric, Gynecologic and Neonatal Nursing, Nurses Association of the American College of Obstetricians and Gynecologists, Harper and Row, Publishers, 2350 Virginia Avenue, Hagerstown, Maryland, 21740.

Journal of the American Dietetic Association, 430 North Michigan Avenue, Chicago, Illinois, 60611.

---

*These journals are primarily devoted to childbearing topics.

Journal of Nurse Midwifery, 1000 Vermont Avenue, N.W., Washington, D.C., 20005.

Journal of Pediatrics, C. V. Mosby Company, 11830 Westline Industrial Drive, St. Louis, Missouri, 63141.

Keeping Abreast Journal, Box 6459, Cherry Creek Station, Denver, Colorado, 80206.

Maternal-Child Nursing Journal, 3505 Fifth Avenue, Pittsburgh, Pennsylvania, 15213.

MCN: The American Journal of Maternal Child Nursing, American Journal of Nursing Company, 10 Columbus Circle, New York, New York, 10019.

Nursing, (77) (78), etc., Intermed Communications, 132 Welsh Road, Horsham, Pennsylvania, 19044.

Nursing Clinics of North America, W. B. Saunders Company, West Washington Square, Philadelphia, Pennsylvania, 19105.

Nursing Digest, 12 Lakeside Park, 607 North Avenue, Wakefield, Massachusetts, 01880.

Nursing Mirror, Surrey House, 1 Throwley Way, Sutton, Surrey, SM1 400, England.

Nursing Outlook, American Journal of Nursing Company, 10 Columbus Circle, New York, New York, 10019.

Nursing Research, American Journal of Nursing Company, 10 Columbus Circle, New York, New York, 10019.

Nursing Times, Little Essex Street, London, WC 2R 3LF, England.

Nutrition Reviews, 665 Huntington Avenue, Boston, Massachusetts, 02115.

Obstetrics and Gynecology, Journal of the American College of Obstetrics and Gynecology, 2350 Virginia Avenue, Hagerstown, Maryland, 21740.

Pediatrics, American Academy of Pediatrics, Evanston, Illinois, 60204.

APPENDIX H

Audiovisual Resources Related to Childbearing

Unless otherwise indicated, resource is a 16 mm. film. Asterisk* indicates appropri ate for parents and/or other lay-groups as well as for professional nurses. The addres ses of companies supplying these audiovisual resources follow this listing.

Abortion: A Rational Approach, Audio Visual Narrative Arts, Inc. Two filmstrips with audiocassette tapes or 33⅓ RPM records discussing abortion and the Supreme Cour decision of 1973.
About Conception and Contraception, Canadian Film Institute. Describes reproduc tive physiology, sexual intercourse, conception, and contraception.
Adapting to Parenthood, 1975, Polymorph Films. New parents discuss their initia adjustments.
The Amazing Newborn, Ross Laboratories.
Anemia in the First Week of Life, 1973, National Medical Audiovisual Center. Slides audiocassette, and guide.
Are You Ready for the Postpartum Experience? 1975, Parenting Pictures. Include discussion of husband-wife relationships, sleep deprivation, breast- and bottle feeding, depression, and satisfaction.
Birth Atlas Slide Series, Maternity Center Association. A series of 22 slides, adapte from the *Birth Atlas,* and guide.
Breast Feeding: Prenatal and Postpartum Preparation, Health Sciences Communicatio Center, Case Western Reserve University.
The Beat of a Different Drummer, 1976, Nurse Midwife Program, College of Nursing Medical University of South Carolina. Black adolescents share their feelings abou marriage, abortion, birth control, and the experience of labor and delivery.
The Biological Aspects of Sexuality, Harper and Row. 35 mm. slides and audiotap cassette.
Birth without Violence, 1976, New Yorker Films. The Leboyer method of infar delivery.
Blueprint for Life, Milner-Fenwick, Inc. Describes chromosomes, meiosis, mitosis fertilization, and genetic counseling.

726

*The Bonding Birth Experience, 1977, Parenting Pictures. Includes coping techniques during labor, fetal monitoring, the father's role, bonding, family adjustment, and breast-feeding.

Bottle Babies, International Film Center. Discusses the implications of the use of commercial baby food in underdeveloped nations.

Brazelton Neonatal Behavioral Assessment Scale, Educational Development Center, Inc. A series of three films that describe the assessment of neonatal behavior; the third film is a self-scoring examination.

*The Case against Rubella, National Foundation—March of Dimes. Describes the effects of maternal rubella infection during pregnancy and the development of rubella vaccine.

*The Cesarean Birth Experience, 1977, Parenting Pictures. Experiences of cesarean delivery.

Changing Concepts: The Nursing Care of the Newborn, Health Media Corporation. A series of slides, audiocassette tapes, and guides: (1) Introduction of Newborn Nursing, (2) The First 12 Hours of Life, (3) Fetal Circulation, (4) Transitional Circulation, (5) Assessing Cardiac Status, (6) Forces of Labor, (7) Fetal Heart Rate Monitoring, and (8) Forces of Labor and Fetal Heart Rate Monitoring.

Contraception: A Matter of Choice, Audio Visual Narrative Arts, Inc. Two filmstrips with audiocassette tapes or 33^{1}/$_{3}$ RPM records discussing the history of fertility control, state laws, and medically-accepted means of contraception.

The Crisis of Loss, The American Journal of Nursing Company. Filmstrip with audiotape cassette or 33^{1}/$_{3}$ RPM record. Examines loss and mourning within the framework of crisis theory. Not specifically concerned with infant death but concepts applicable.

Death of a Newborn, Ross Laboratories. Parents and physician discuss feelings 2 months after the death of their child.

*Diagnosis Before Birth, National Foundation—March of Dimes. Discusses the prenatal and postnatal diagnosis of birth defects and genetic counseling.

The Distressed Newborn, Network for Continuing Medical Education. Videotape.

Early Complications of Pregnancy, Medcom Press. Slides, audiocassette, and guide.

Facilitating Self-Disclosure, The American Journal of Nursing Company. Filmstrip with audiocassette tape or 33^{1}/$_{3}$ RPM record. Examines skills that facilitate a patient's or parent's expression of feelings in both psychiatric and nonpsychiatric clinical settings.

*Family Planning, Trainex Corporation: 35 mm. filmstrip with audiotape cassette or 33^{1}/$_{3}$ RPM record in English or Spanish for patient teaching; discusses six methods of contraception and problems when contraception is not used.

Fetal Growth and Development, Mead Johnson Laboratories. 16 mm. film or videotape with study guide.

First Breath, Childbirth Education Films, Inc. For health professionals; describes the benefits of prepared childbirth through interviews with psychiatrists, pediatricians, and obstetricians.

*From Generation to Generation: Genetic Counseling, National Foundation—March of Dimes. Filmstrip or slides with audiocassette or record discussing genetics in easily understood terms.

Hospital Maternity Care: Family Centered, The American Journal of Nursing Company. Describes family-centered care for childbearing families.

*How Babies Begin, The American Journal of Nursing Company. Filmstrip describing reproduction and contraception in simple terms; for use in patient teaching.

*How Many Children Do You Want? The American Journal of Nursing Company. A series of three filmstrips with audiotape cassettes or 33¹/₃ RPM record for patient teaching: (1) How Babies Begin, (2) Drugstore Methods and Least Effective Methods of Birth Control, and (3) Doctor Methods of Birth Control.

Human Embryology, W. B. Saunders. Slides of illustrations from the book Human Embryology by Keith L. Moore, published by W. B. Saunders Company.

*Hunger in America, Parts I and II, CBS Reports Program, Carousel Films. Emphasizes the effects of malnutrition and starvation on mothers, babies, and children in varied areas of the United States.

Hydatidiform Mole, Oxford Tape-Slide Series. Slides, audiocassette, and guide.

Hypoglycemia, National Foundation–March of Dimes. Slides, audiocassette tape, and guide.

I'm Seventeen, Pregnant and Don't Know What To Do, Children's Home Society of California. Filmstrip.

*Inside My Mom, National Foundation–Supply Division. Filmstrip or slide set with audiocassette or record describing nutrition as basic to life in cartoon style.

Introduction to Congenital Heart Disease, National Medical Audiovisual Center. Series of slides, audiocassette tapes, and guides: (1) Perinatal Circulation, (2) General Background, (3) Common Acyanotic Lesions, (4) Common Cyanotic Lesions, and (5) The Large USD in Infancy.

Jaundice in the Newborn, 1973, National Medical Audiovisual Center. Slides, audiocassette, and guide.

Maternity Nursing, The American Journal of Nursing Company. A series of 15 classes, 44 minutes each, available as 16 mm. film, videotape, or audiotape cassettes.

*More Than Love, National Foundation–March of Dimes. Filmstrip, record, and guide discussing prenatal care and birth defects.

Neonatal Infections: Diagnosis and Prevention, Mead Johnson Laboratories. 16 mm. film or videotape with study guide.

Neurological Evaluation, Health Sciences Communication Center, Case Western Reserve University. Describes and demonstrates neurological examination of the newborn.

The Neurologically Suspect Infant, 1973, National Medical Audiovisual Center. Slides, audiocassette, and guide.

*Newborn, 1972, West Glen Films. Focuses on the experience of a mother and father and their first child.

Normal Puerperium, Oxford Tape Slide Series. Slides, audiocassette, and guide.

Nutrition in Pregnancy, Jay Hathaway Productions, Inc.

Nutritional Support of the Premature, Mead Johnson Laboratories. 16 mm. film or videotape with study guide.

*The Only Kid on the Block, National Foundation–March of Dimes. Describes the impact of a serious birth defect on a boy, his family, and neighbors.

The Perinatal Assessment of Maturation, 1973, National Medical Audiovisual Center. Slides, audiocassette, and guide.

Physical Examination of the Newborn, Medcom Press. Slides, audiocassette, and guide.

Postpartum Haemorrhage, 1976, Parts I and II, Oxford Tape-Slide Series in Obstetrics and Gynecology. Slides, audiocassette, and guide.

Poverty in Rural America, United States Department of Agriculture. A graphic presentation of lifestyles in mountain hollows and along dirt roads.

Purposes of Family Planning, Canadian Film Institute. Describes the positive purposes of family planning for consumers of all ages and income levels.

Respiratory Distress Syndrome, 1973, National Medical Audiovisual Center. Slides, audiocassette, and guide.

Respiratory Distress Syndrome, Mead Johnson Laboratories. 16 mm. film or videotape with study guide.

Resuscitation of the Newborn, Mead Johnson Laboratories. 16 mm. film or videotape with study guide.

Resuscitation of the Newborn, 1977, ACOG Film and Video Service. Discusses resuscitation from the perspectives of prenatal assessment, intrapartum monitoring, and recognition and care of the depressed baby.

Thermal Regulation of the Neonate, Mead Johnson Laboratories. 16 mm. film or videotape with study guide.

The Story of Eric, Centre Films, Inc. Describes preparation for labor and labor and delivery using the Lamaze method.

Tomorrow Happens Today, National Foundation–March of Dimes. Filmstrip with record or cassette and guide discussing prenatal care and protection of the unborn child.

The Use of Nasal CPAP, 1976, Health Sciences Communication Center, Case Western Reserve University. Principles of CPAP, techniques of administration, characteristics of the infant with RDS, and related therapies are included.

Wednesday's Child, Human Betterment League, N.C., Inc. Describes biologic, emotional and social aspects of genetic disease and genetic counseling.

ADDRESSES FOR FILMS

ACOG Film and Video Service, P. O. Box 299, Wheaton, Illinois, 60187.

The American Journal of Nursing Company, Educational Services Division, 10 Columbus Circle, New York, New York, 10019.

Audio Visual Narrative Arts, Inc., P. O. Box 398, Pleasantville, New York, 10570.

Canadian Film Institute, 303 Richmond Road, Ottawa, Ontario, Canada.

Carousel Films, 1501 Broadway, Suite 1503, New York, New York, 10036.

Centre Films, Inc., 1103 North El Centro Ave., Hollywood, California, 90038.

Childbirth Education Films, Inc., 648 Riverside Road, North Palm Beach, Florida, 33408.

Children's Home Society of California, 3100 West Adams Boulevard, Los Angeles, California 90018.

Educational Development Center, Inc., Distribution Center, 39 Chapel Street, Newton, Massachusetts, 02160.

Harper and Row, Media Department, 10 East 53rd Street, New York, New York, 10022.

Health Media Corporation, P. O. Box 167, Tulsa, Oklahoma, 74101.

Health Sciences Communication Center, Case Western Reserve, University Circle, Cleveland, Ohio, 44106.

Human Betterment League of North Carolina, Inc., P. O. Box 3036, Winston-Salem, North Carolina, 27102.

International Film Center, 33 Sixth Ave., New York, New York, 10014.

Jay Hathaway Productions, Inc., 4349 Tujunga Avenue, North Hollywood, California, 91604.

Maternity Center Association, 48 East 92nd Street, New York, New York, 10028.

Mead Johnson Laboratories, Evansville, Indiana, 47721.

Medcom Press, 2 Hammarskjold Plaza, New York, New York, 10017.

Milner-Fenwick, Inc., 3800 Liberty Heights Avenue, Baltimore, Maryland, 21215.

National Foundation–March of Dimes, Supply Division, Box 2000, White Plains, New York, 10602.

National Medical Audiovisual Center, Washington, D.C., 20409.

Network for Continuing Medical Education, 15 Columbus Circle, New York, New York, 10023.

New Yorker Films, 43 West 61st Street, New York, New York, 10023.

Oxford Tape-Slide Series in Obstetrics and Gynecology, Pretest Service, Inc., 71 South Turnpike, Wallingford, Connecticut, 06492.

Parenting Pictures, R. D. 1, Box 355B, Columbia, New Jersey, 07832.

Polymorph Films, 331 Newbury Street, Boston, Massachusetts, 02115.

Ross Laboratories, 585 Cleveland Avenue, Columbus, Ohio, 43216.

Trainex Corporation, Subsidiary Medcom, Inc., P. O. Box 116, Garden Grove, California, 92642.

United States Department of Agriculture, Washington, D.C., 20250.

W. B. Saunders Company, West Washington Square, Philadelphia, Pennsylvania, 19105.

West Glen Films, West Glen Communications, Inc., 565 Fifth Avenue, New York, New York, 10017.

APPENDIX I

Organizations Concerned with Childbearing

American Academy of Husband-Coached Childbirth, P. O. Box 5224, Sherman Oaks, California, 91413.
American Academy of Pediatrics, P. O. Box 1034, Evanston, Illinois, 60204.
American College of Home Obstetrics, c/o Gregory White, M.D., 2821 Rose Street, Franklin Park, Illinois, 60131.
American College of Nurse Midwifery, 330 West 58th Street, New York, New York, 10019.
American Diabetes Association, Inc., 1 West 48th Street, New York, New York, 10020.
American National Red Cross, 17 and D Street, N.W., Washington, D.C., 20006.
The American Nurses' Association, 2420 Pershing Road, Kansas City, Missouri, 64108.
American Society for Psychoprophylaxis in Obstetrics, 1523 L St., N.W., Washington, D.C., 20005.
Child Study Association of America, 9 East 89th Street, New York, New York, 10028.
The Couple to Couple League, P.O. Box 11084, Cincinnati, Ohio, 42511 (natural family planning).
International Childbirth Education Association, P. O. Box 5852, Milwaukee, Wisconsin, 53220.
La Leche League International, Inc., 9616 Minneapolis Avenue, Franklin Park, Illinois, 60131.
Maternity Center Association, 48 East 92nd Street, New York, New York, 10028.
National Family Planning Federation of America, Inc., 1221 Massachusetts Avenue, N.W., Washington, D.C., 20005.
The National Foundation—March of Dimes, 1707 H Street, N.W., Washington, D.C., 20006.
National League for Nursing, 10 Columbus Circle, New York, New York, 10019.
Nurses Association, American College of Obstetrics and Gynecology, One East Wacker Drive, Chicago, Illinois, 60601.
Parents Without Partners, 80 Fifth Avenue, New York, New York, 10011.
Planned Parenthood Federation of America, Inc., 810 Seventh Avenue, New York, New York, 10019.

APPENDIX J

The Pregnant Patient's Bill of Rights*

The American Hospital Association has developed a Patient's Bill of Rights that is increasingly recognized as a standard of care.

Because the woman who is pregnant represents two patients, herself and her fetus, she should be recognized as having additional rights. The following Pregnant Patient's Bill of Rights has been suggested by Doris Haire and was published in the *Journal of Nurse Midwifery*, 20:29, 1975.

1. *The Pregnant Patient has the right*, prior to the administration of any drug or procedure, to be informed by the health professional caring for her of any potential direct or indirect effects, risks or hazards to herself or newborn infant which may result from the use of a drug or procedure prescribed for or administered to her during pregnancy, labor, birth or lactation.

2. *The Pregnant Patient has the right*, prior to the proposed therapy, to be informed, not only of the benefits, risks and hazards of the proposed therapy but also of known alternative therapy, such as available childbirth education classes which could help to prepare the Pregnant Patient physically and mentally to cope with the discomfort or stress of pregnancy and the experience of childbirth, thereby reducing or eliminating her need for drugs and obstetric intervention. She should be offered such information early in her pregnancy in order that she may make a reasoned decision.

3. *The Pregnant Patient has the right*, prior to the administration of any drug, to be informed by the health professional who is prescribing or administering the drug to her that any drug which she receives during pregnancy, labor and birth, no matter how or when the drug is taken or administered, may adversely affect her unborn baby, directly or indirectly, and that there is no drug or chemical which has been proven safe for the unborn child.

4. *The Pregnant Patient has the right*, if cesarean section is anticipated, to be informed prior to the administration of any drug, and preferably prior to her hospitalization, that minimizing her and, in turn, her baby's intake of nonessential preoperative medicine, will benefit her baby.

---

*Reprinted by permission of the *Journal of Nurse-Midwifery*.

732

5. *The Pregnant Patient has the right*, prior to the administration of a drug or procedure, to be informed if there is *no* properly controlled follow-up research which has established the safety of the drug or procedure with regard to its direct and/or indirect effects on the physiological, mental and neurological development of the child exposed, via the mother, to the drug or procedure during pregnancy, labor, birth or lactation—(this would apply to virtually all drugs and the vast majority of obstetric procedures).

6. *The Pregnant Patient has the right*, prior to the administration of any drug, to be informed of the brand name and generic name of the drug in order that she may advise the health professional of any past adverse reaction to the drug.

7. *The Pregnant Patient has the right* to determine for herself, without pressure from her attendant, whether she will accept the risks inherent in the proposed therapy or refuse a drug or procedure.

8. *The Pregnant Patient has the right* to know the name and qualifications of the individual administering a medication or procedure to her during labor or birth.

9. *The Pregnant Patient has the right* to be informed, prior to the administration of any procedure, whether that procedure is being administered to her for her or her baby's benefit (medically indicated) or as an elective procedure (for convenience or teaching purposes).

10. *The Pregnant Patient has the right* to be accompanied during the stress of labor and birth by someone she cares for, and to whom she looks for emotional comfort and encouragement.

11. *The Pregnant Patient has the right* after appropriate medical consultation to choose a position for labor and for birth which is least stressful to her baby and to herself.

12. *The Obstetric Patient has the right* to have her baby cared for at her bedside if her baby is normal, and to feed her baby according to her baby's needs rather than according to the hospital regimen.

13. *The Obstetric Patient has the right* to be informed in writing of the name of the person who actually delivered her baby and the professional qualifications of that person. This information should also be on the birth certificate.

14. *The Obstetric Patient has the right* to be informed if there is any known or indicated aspect of her or her baby's care or condition which may cause her or her baby later difficulty or problems.

15. *The Obstetric Patient has the right* to have her and her baby's hospital medical records complete, accurate and legible and to have their records, including Nurses' Notes, retained by the hospital until the child reaches at least the age of majority, or, alternatively, to have the records offered to her before they are destroyed.

16. *The Obstetric Patient*, both during and after her hospital stay, has the right to have access to her complete hospital records, including Nurses' Notes, and to receive a copy upon payment of a reasonable fee and without incurring the expense of retaining an attorney.

It is the obstetric patient and her baby, not the health professional, who must sustain any trauma or injury resulting from the use of a drug or obstetric procedure. The observation of the rights listed above will not only permit the obstetric patient to participate in the decisions involving her and her baby's health care, but will help to protect the health professional and the hospital against litigation arising from resentment or misunderstanding on the part of the mother.

GLOSSARY

abortion, elective: interruption of pregnancy at the choice of the woman for reasons other than her own physical safety.

abortion, habitual: three or more consecutive spontaneous abortions.

abortion, incomplete: spontaneous abortion in which only part of the products of conception are expelled.

abortion, induced: deliberate interruption of pregnancy.

abortion, inevitable: spontaneous abortion with bleeding, uterine contractions, and progressive cervical dilatation.

abortion, missed: abortion in which the fetus dies but is retained in the uterus for 8 weeks or longer following death.

abortion, septic: abortion in which infection occurs in the endometrium and the products of conception.

abortion, spontaneous: the process by which a nonviable fetus is expelled from the uterus.

abortion, threatened: transcervical bleeding in a gravida when the fetus is less than 20 weeks' gestational age.

abortus: fetus of less than 20 weeks' gestation or 500 grams.

abruptio placentae: premature separation of a normally implanted placenta; may be complete or partial.

acini cells: milk-producing cells of the alveoli in the breast.

acme: highest point (as in the acme of a contraction).

acrocyanosis: peripheral cyanosis of the hands and feet, common in newborns.

afterbirth: term used by laymen to describe placenta and membranes expelled following delivery.

AGA: appropriate for gestational age; babies with birth weights between the tenth and ninetieth percentiles.

agalactia: failure of the secretion of milk.

agenesis: failure of an organ to develop; e.g., renal agenesis—failure of the kidneys to develop.

alae nasi: the nostrils.

albuminuria: detectable amounts of albumin present in the urine.

alleles: contrasting forms or states of a gene.

alpha-fetoprotein (AFP): the major circulating protein of the early human fetus; highly elevated levels of AFP in amniotic fluid are associated with neural tube defects (e.g., spina bifida, hydrocephalus).

amenorrhea: the absence of menstruation.

amniocentesis: process by which amniotic fluid is withdrawn from the amniotic sac through a needle inserted through the abdominal and uterine walls.

amnion: inner of two fetal membranes forming the amniotic sac.

amnionitis: infected amniotic fluid.

amniotic fluid: fluid surrounding the fetus within the amniotic sac.

amniotomy: the artificial rupture of the membranes.

anaerobic metabolism: metabolism occurring in the absence of oxygen; utilizes body compounds to produce energy.

analgesia: a substance that relieves pain.

android pelvis: narrow "male-type" of pelvis.

anencephalus: absence of the cranial vault, due to a failure of the anterior end of the neural tube to close.

anesthetic: a substance that causes loss of sensation, with or without the loss of consciousness.

anomaly: malformation.

anoxia: absence of oxygen.

antenatal: before birth.

antepartal: before labor.

anthropoid pelvis: pelvis in which the anteroposterior diameter equals or is greater than the transverse diameter.

antibody: a substance produced by the body that is antagonistic to a specific antigen.

antigen: any substance capable of causing the production of an antibody; may be an invading organism, a foreign protein, and so forth.

Apgar scoring: a method of rapid assessment of the newborn in the delivery room, originally suggested by Virginia Apgar, M.D.

apnea: temporary absence of respiration.

Apt test: differentiates maternal blood from fetal blood.

areola: pigmented area surrounding the nipple.

artificial insemination: instrumental injection of semen into the vagina for the purpose of fertilization.

Aschheim-Zondek test: a pregnancy test involving the injection of urine from a woman into a mouse. After 5 days the mouse is sacrificed; if the mouse's ovaries are enlarged, the test is positive. Used less frequently today than in past decades.

asphyxia: a condition of an organism in which oxygen is decreased or carbon dioxide is increased.

atelectasis: a condition of the lungs in which many of the alveoli are collapsed.

atresia: absence of a passage normally present in the body; e.g., esophageal atresia.

auscultation: assessment by listening to sounds within the body.

autosomes: all of the chromosomes except the sex chromosomes.

axis: a real or imaginary line that runs through the center of a body; e.g., pelvic axis.

bag of waters: amniotic sac (lay term).

ballottement: a sign elicited by the examiner when two fingers are placed in the vagina; the fetus is felt to "bounce."

Bandl's ring: thickened muscle tissue between the upper and lower segments of the uterus.

Barr body: a chromatin mass derived from one of the X chromosomes. The number of Barr bodies is one less than the number of X chromosomes.

Bartholin's glands: two small glands near the vaginal orifice with ducts opening between the edge of the hymen and the labia minora.

bicornuate uterus: an anomaly of the uterus.

bilirubin: a product formed by the breakdown of red blood cells.

biopsy: removal of a small segment of tissue for examination.

- - - blast: a suffix designating a developing cell; e.g., neuroblast, a developing nerve cell.

blastocyst: an early stage of embryologic development.

Braxton Hicks contractions: intermittent uterine contractions occurring during pregnancy.

Brazelton assessment: a set of criteria assessing the interactional behavior of a newborn.

breech presentation: buttocks or feet as presenting part. Complete breech: buttocks and feet present. Footling breech: one or both feet present. Frank breech: buttocks present; hips flexed.

bregma: the area of the anterior fontanel.

brown fat: source of energy for heat production in newborns.

bruit, uterine: the sound of the passage of blood through the uterine blood vessels; sometimes mistaken for fetal heart rate.

Candida vaginitis: a vaginal infection accompanied by intense burning and itching.

caput: occiput of the fetal head presenting at the vaginal opening prior to birth.

caput succedaneum: edema of the superficial tissues that overlie the bone of the part of the head presenting first at delivery.

caul: fetal membranes covering the head during delivery.

centromere: the point at which the strands of a chromosome are joined.

cephalhematoma: collection of blood between a cranial bone and the overlying periosteum.

cephalic presentation: when the head is the presenting part.

cephalopelvic disproportion (CPD): when the size or shape of the fetal head is too large to pass through the maternal pelvis.

cervix: the segment of the uterus between the corpus and the external os.

cesarean section: an operative procedure by which an infant is delivered through an incision in the abdominal and uterine walls.

Chadwick's sign: a bluish-violet color of the vagina during pregnancy due to increased vascularity.

chloasma: pigmentation of the face during pregnancy; "the mask of pregnancy."

choanal atresia: a congenital defect in which there is a bony or membranous obstruction of the posterior nares.

chorioamnionitis: infection in the amniotic membranes.

chorion: the outer layer of fetal membranes.

chorion frondosum: becomes the fetal component of the placenta.

chromosomes: rod-shaped bodies within a cell, on which genes are located (visible under the microscope).

circumcision: surgical excision of the foreskin (prepuce) of the penis.

cleft lip: congenital fissure of lip, called hare-lip by laymen.

cleft palate: failure of the palate to fuse during embryonic life; may involve hard and/or soft palate.

climacteric: a period of time, usually several years, during which ovarian function becomes less and less responsive to the stimulation of the gonadotropic hormones.

clitoris: erectile tissue at the anterior end of the vulva; homologous to the male penis.

coccyx: last four bones of the spinal column.

coitus: sexual intercourse.

colostrum: yellowish fluid secreted from the breasts prior to the secretion of milk.

complement: a natural property of blood that is a factor in the destruction of bacteria.

conceptus: the embryo or fetus, the fetal membranes, the amniotic fluid, and the fetal portion of the placenta.

confinement: the period of birth and the early puerperium.

congenital: occurring during intrauterine life.

conjugate, diagonal: distance from the sacral promontory to the point at which the lower margin of the symphysis pubis rests on finger inserted in the vagina.

conjugate, true: anteroposterior diameter of the pelvic inlet; cannot be measured directly but is derived by subtracting 1.5 to 2.0 cm. from the diagonal conjugate.

conjunctiva: mucous membrane lining the eyelid, which is reflected onto the eyeball.

conjunctivitis: inflammation of the conjunctiva.

contraception: prevention of conception.

copulation: sexual intercourse.

corona radiata: follicular cells bordering the ovum.

corpora cavernosa: (1) two cylinders of spongy tissue within the penis, (2) tissue within the clitoris.

corpus albicans: the term for the corpus luteum during the final portion of the regressive phase.

corpus luteum: the follicle after the ovum has been extruded; so called because the follicle is filled with a yellow material.

corpus spongiosum: a cylinder of spongy tissue within the penis.

cotyledon: one lobule of the placenta.

Couvelaire uterus: "boardlike" uterus due to hemorrhage within the myometrium following abruptio placentae.

CPAP: continuous positive airway pressure; one method of treating respiratory distress syndrome.

craniotabes: softening of localized areas in the cranial bones.

creatinine: a body chemical found particularly in blood and muscle; measurements of creatinine in mother's urine correlate with the amount of fetal muscle mass and thus with fetal size.

Credé prophylaxis: instillation of silver nitrate ophthalmic solution in the newborn infant's eyes to prevent ophthalmia neonatorum.

crowning: the appearance of the presenting part at the entrance of the vagina.

cul-de-sac of Douglas: peritoneal pouch between the anterior wall of the rectum and the posterior wall of the uterus.

curettage: scraping of the uterine endometrium with a curette.

cyesis: pregnancy.

cystocele: herniation of the bladder into the vagina.

decidua: the endometrium during pregnancy.

decidua basalis: maternal side of the placenta.

decidua capsularis: the decidua surrounding the chorionic sac.

decidua vera: the decidua other than that of the placenta.

decrement: decline or decrease, as in a contraction.

deletion: a piece of one chromosome that breaks off and is lost.

ΔOD_{450} (read delta OD_{450}): a measurement of the optical density of amniotic fluid in the evaluation of Rh_D sensitized mothers.

dextrocardia: having the heart on the right side of the body.

DHEA (dehydroepiandrosterone): an estrogen precursor; significant in the measurement of estrogens as a test of fetal well-being.

diaphoresis: profuse perspiration.

diaphragmatic hernia: congenital anomaly in which the diaphragm does not form completely, allowing abdominal organs to be displaced into the thoracic cavity.

diastasis rectus: condition in which the abdominal rectus muscles separate at the midline.

dilatation: the process by which the cervix dilates to 10 cm. in diameter.

dizygotic: from two zygotes, as dizygotic twins.

DNA (deoxyribonucleic acid): protein that contains genetic information.

dominant inheritance: inheritance requiring a gene from one parent only.

Down's syndrome: a condition in which there are three number 21 chromosomes (trisomy 21).

Dubowitz assessment: set of criteria used in the assessment of gestational age of the newborn infant.

Duncan's mechanism: delivery of the placenta with the maternal surface outermost.

ductus arteriosus: an anatomic connection between the pulmonary artery and the aorta, normally patent during fetal life but closing shortly after birth.

ductus venosus: an anatomic connection between the umbilical vein and the inferior vena cava, allowing most blood to bypass the liver during fetal life but closing shortly after birth.

dura (dura mater): the outer covering of the brain and spinal cord.

dysmenorrhea: difficult menstruation.

dyspareunia: difficult or painful intercourse.

dystocia: difficult labor.

ecchymosis: bruising.

eclampsia: occurrence of one or more convulsions, not attributable to other cerebral conditions, in a woman with pre-eclampsia.

ectoderm: outer layer of embryo from which skin, hair, nails, and so forth develop.

ectopic: in an abnormal position.

ectopic pregnancy: implantation of the fertilized ovum outside of the uterine cavity.

EDC: estimated date of confinement; the date the baby is expected to be born.

effacement: the process by which the cervical canal becomes shorter and thinner.

effleurage: light massage with the fingertips.

ejaculation: expulsion of semen from the urethra.

embryo: the developing conceptus from 2 to 8 weeks following fertilization.

embryologic age: the age of the embryo-fetus dated from the time of conception.

endometriosis: condition occurring when patches of endometrium are found outside the uterus.

endometrium: mucous membrane lining the inner surface of the uterus.

engagement: the status of the fetus when the largest part of the presenting part has passed the pelvic inlet and entered the true pelvis.

engorgement: vascular congestion, resulting in distention, as in breast engorgement.

entoderm: inner layer of the embryo from which internal organs develop.

epicanthus: fold of skin extending from the nose to the median aspect of the eye, covering the inner canthus; characteristic of Oriental persons; may occur in persons with Down's syndrome.

episiotomy: an incision made in the perineum, using blunt scissors.

epispadias: opening of the urethra on the dorsal aspect of the penis.

epithelial pearls (Epstein's pearls; Bohn's nodules):   raised white areas of epithelial cells on the hard palate or gums.

Erb-Duchenne paralysis: paralysis of the upper arm resulting from injury to the fifth and sixth cervical nerves during delivery.

erythema toxicum: a rash of unknown etiology occurring in the newborn; resolves spontaneously.

erythroblastosis fetalis: hemolytic disease of the newborn due to incompatibility between the blood group of the mother and the blood group of the fetus.

estradiol: an estrogen.

estriol: the oxidized end product of estradiol and estrone; formed in the liver.

estrogens: hormones secreted by the cells of the ovarian follicle, the corpus luteum, and, during pregnancy, by the placenta.

estrone: an estrogen.

estrus: period of sexual activity in mammals other than primates.

exchange transfusion: replacement of 75 to 80 per cent of recipient's blood with donor blood by withdrawing and replacing small amounts at a time.

extension: the stretching-out of a limb or part; the opposite of flexion.

fallopian tubes (uterine tubes):   tubes extending laterally from each side of the uterus to the area of the ovary.

ferning: the branching pattern that cervical mucus exhibits just prior to ovulation when it is allowed to dry on a glass slide.

fertilization: penetration of the ovum by a sperm.

fetal death: death of a fetus weighing 500 grams or less or of 20 weeks' gestation or less.

fetal heart rate, baseline fetal heart rate: the rate between contractions. Baseline fetal heart rate variability: fluctuations normally present in baseline fetal heart rate.

fetal mortality rate: number of fetal deaths per 1000 births.

fetus: the term given to the conceptus from 8 weeks after fertilization until birth.

fibrin: an elastic substance, deposited in fine threads, that causes the blood to clot.

fibrinogen: a protein that is changed to fibrin during the process of clot formation by the action of thrombin.

fibrinogenopenia: a deficiency of fibrin and fibrinogen.

fibroid: a tumor consisting of fibrous and muscular tissue.

fimbria: any fringelike structure; e.g., the fringelike extension at the distal end of the fallopian tube.

FiO₂ (fraction of inspired oxygen):   the amount of oxygen an individual is receiving.

fissure: a groove.

fistula: an abnormal tubelike passage; e.g., tracheoesophageal fistula, an abnormal passage between the trachea and esophagus.

flexion: bending or being bent; the opposite of extension.

follicle: a small excretory duct or tubular gland (see also graafian follicle).

follicle-stimulating hormone (FSH): hormone that stimulates the maturation of the graafian follicle; produced by the anterior pituitary gland during the first half of the ovarian cycle.

fontanel: space at the intersection of the sutures on the fetal head.

fontanel, anterior (bregma): diamond-shaped space at the junction of the frontal, sagittal, and coronal sutures.

fontanel, posterior: triangular space at the junction of the sagittal and lambdoid sutures.

foramen ovale: opening in the septa between the atria of the heart during fetal life; normally closes shortly after birth.

foreskin (prepuce): fold of skin covering the glans penis.

fornices of the vagina: anterior and posterior spaces formed by the protrusion of the cervix into the vagina.

fornix: an arched structure (plural, fornices).

fossa: a shallow depression.

fourchette: a band or fold of mucous membrane connecting the posterior ends of the labia minora.

fraternal twins (dizygotic twins): twins that result when two ova are fertilized.

frenulum: a membranous fold connecting parts or restricting their separation.

frenulum clitoridis: frenulum joining the inner labia minora on the undersurface of the clitoris.

frenulum linguae: frenulum from the lower gum to the root of the tongue.

frontum: forehead.

fundus: upper portion of the uterus between the point of attachment of the uterine tubes.

galactorrhea: excessive secretion or flow of milk.

galactosemia: a condition in which the infant cannot metabolize lactose and galactose due to lack of a specific enzyme; inherited as an autosomal recessive trait.

gametes: sex cells.

gastroschisis: a defect in the abdominal wall at the base of the umbilical stalk.

gavage: feeding through a tube passed into the stomach.

genes: determiners of hereditary traits.

genotype: genetic composition of an individual; e.g., possessing a gene for cystic fibrosis.

gestation: pregnancy, the period of pregnancy.

gestational age: the age of the embryo-fetus dated from the time of the last menstrual period.

gestational diabetes: diabetes that occurs only during the period of pregnancy.

glabella: smooth area above the nose between the eyebrows.

glans penis: smooth, round head of the penis.

glycosuria: presence of glucose in the urine.

gonad: sex gland; the ovary or testis.

Goodell's sign: softening of the cervix in the second month of gestation.

graafian follicle (vesicular follicle): mature ovarian cyst containing the fully developed ovum that will be released at ovulation.

gravid: pregnant.

gravida: a pregnant woman.

grunt: sound made by the closing of the glottis to prolong expiration and thus keep the alveoli from collapsing.

gynecoid pelvis: the typical female pelvis in which the inlet is round.

gynecology: the study of the diseases of the female reproductive tract and associated structures.

harlequin sign: momentary variance in color between right and left sides of body; of no pathologic significance.

Hegar's sign: softening of the lower uterine segment during the second and third months of pregnancy.

hematocrit: the volume of red blood cells per unit of circulating blood.

hematoma: a collection of blood in tissue.

hemoglobin: a component of blood consisting of globin, a protein, and hematin, an organic compound of iron.

hemorrhagic disease of the newborn: bleeding disorder in the first days of life related to a deficiency of vitamin K.

hermaphrodite: possessing genital and sexual characteristics of both sexes.

heterozygous: having different alleles for a trait on each gene of a pair; e.g., a genotype Dd.

histogenesis: the process by which tissues differentiate.

homoiotherm: an animal that can maintain its internal temperature at a specific level regardless of the environmental temperature.

homozygous: having the same alleles for a trait on each gene of a pair; e.g., a genotype DD.

human chorionic gonadotropin: a hormone produced by the trophoblast; the basis of testing for pregnancy.

human chorionic somatomammotropin (HCS): a hormone produced by the placenta; basis of one test of fetal well-being. Also called human placental lactogen (HPL).

human placental lactogen (HPL): human chorionic somatomammotropin.

hyaline membrane disease (HMD): a disease primarily of preterm newborns, characterized by a lack of surfactant in the alveoli of the lungs; also termed respiratory distress syndrome (RDS).

hydatidiform mole: a developmental anomaly of the placenta in which some or all of the chorionic villi degenerate into transparent vesicles.

hydramnios: amniotic fluid in excess of 2000 ml.

hydrocele: serous fluid in a saclike cavity, such as the cavity that surrounds the testicle.

hydrocephalus: a condition in which excessive cerebrospinal fluid leads to rapid head growth.

hydrops fetalis: describes the fetus of a sensitized Rh_d (negative) mother with intrauterine anemia and congestive heart failure.

hymen: a pinkish membrane of elastic and collagenous tissue at the entrance of the vagina. An *imperforate hymen* has no opening.

hymenal tag: hymenal tissue protruding from the floor of the vagina.

hymenotomy: surgical incision of the hymen.

hyperbilirubinemia: excess of unconjugated bilirubin in the blood.

hypercapnia: excessive carbon dioxide in arterial blood.

hyperemesis gravidarum: prolonged, severe nausea during pregnancy.

hypermagnesemia: excessive serum magnesium; may occur following the administration of magnesium sulfate.

hyperplasia: increase in the number of cells.

hypertensive states of pregnancy: hypertensive disease occurring during pregnancy, including pre-eclampsia and eclampsia.

hypertrophy: increase in the size of cells.

hypofibrinogenemia: deficiency of fibrinogen; may occur following a missed abortion or abruptio placentae.

hypogalactia: insufficient milk secretion.

hypogastric plexus: a large plexus of motor fibers formed above the promontory of the sacrum near the bifurcation of the aorta.

hypoglycemia: in the newborn, blood glucose level below 40 mg. per 100 ml. after 72 hours; blood glucose level below 30 mg. per 100 ml. prior to 72 hours.

hypomagnesemia: low serum magnesium; may occur following blood transfusion.

hypoplasia: the underdevelopment of an organ.

hypospadias: a condition in which the urethra opens on the ventral surface of the penis.

hypoxemia: inadequate level of oxygen in the blood.

hypoxia: inadequate level of oxygen in the body.

hysterectomy: surgical removal of the uterus.

hysterectomy, abdominal: removal of the uterus through an abdominal incision.

hysterectomy, pan- - -:   removal of the entire uterus, the ovaries, and the tubes.
hysterectomy, subtotal: surgical removal of the fundus and body of the uterus, but not the cervix.
hysterectomy, total: removal of the entire uterus, but not the ovaries and tubes.
hysterectomy, vaginal: removal of the uterus through the vagina.
hysterotomy: surgical incision into the uterus.

iatrogenic: medically caused; e.g., an iatrogenic condition would be caused by the treatment, such as blindness in a preterm infant due to high levels of arterial oxygen concentration.
icterus: jaundice.
idiopathic: of unknown cause.
idiopathic respiratory distress syndrome: see respiratory distress syndrome or hyaline membrane disease.
IDM: infant of a diabetic mother.
IgA: primary immunoglobulin of colostrum.
IgG: immunoglobulin that crosses the placenta and confers passive immunity to those infections to which the mother is immune (e.g., diphtheria, measles, and so forth).
IgM: first immunoglobulin made by infant after birth (or before birth if there is intrauterine infection).
impetigo contagiosa: a contagious staphylococcal infection of the skin.
implantation: attachment of the fertilized ovum, normally occurring in the uterine mucosa.
impotence: inability to participate in sexual intercourse; term usually refers to male partner.
inborn error of metabolism: hereditary deficiency of a specific enzyme resulting in a problem in metabolism; e.g., galactosemia, phenylketonuria.
incompetent cervix: inability of cervix to remain closed throughout pregnancy, resulting in spontaneous abortion or preterm delivery.
increment: increase, as in the increment of a contraction until the acme is reached.
induction: (1) intervention to cause labor to begin, (2) in embryology, the process by which one tissue transmits a stimulus that leads to the development of neighboring tissues.
inertia: inactivity; e.g., the absence of uterine contractions during labor.
infant mortality rate: number of deaths in the first year of life per 1000 live births.
innominate bone: hip bone.
interstitial cell-stimulating hormone (ICSH):   stimulates the production of testosterone by the interstitial cells of Leydig in the testes; corresponds to luteinizing hormone (LH) in the female.
intertuberous diameter: distance between ischial tuberosities; measures the plane of the pelvic outlet.
intervillous space: areas filled with maternal blood in the maternal portion of the placenta, where maternal-fetal exchange takes place.
intrathecal: within the subarachnoid space.
introitus: entrance; e.g., of the vagina.
intromission: insertion of one object into another; e.g., insertion of the penis into the vagina.
inversion of the uterus: when the uterus is turned inside out; may be caused by pulling on the umbilical cord before the placenta has detached.
inverted nipple: a condition in which the nipple does not protrude from the breast.
involution: the process by which the reproductive organs return to their normal size and function.
ischium: posterior and inferior part of the lower portion of the innominate bone.
IUD (intrauterine device):   devices placed within the uterus as a means of contraception.
IUGR (intrauterine growth retardation):   failure of the fetus to grow properly, because of intrauterine infection, placental pathologic processes, and so forth.

jaundice (icterus): yellow discoloration of tissues due to the deposition of unconjugated bilirubin.
jaundice, breast milk: jaundice that occurs when pregnanediol in mother's milk inhibits the conjugation of bilirubin by interfering with the enzyme glucuronyl transferase.
jaundice, pathologic: any jaundice that is not physiologic.
jaundice, physiologic: jaundice occurring in an otherwise healthy newborn more than 24 to 36 hours of age.

karyotype: systematic arrangement of photographed chromosomes in order to demonstrate structure and number.
Kegel exercise: exercise for the muscles surrounding the vagina.
kernicterus: brain damage due to the deposit of unconjugated bilirubin in brain cells.
ketosis: the accumulation of ketone bodies (e.g., acetone) in the body as a result of incomplete metabolism of fatty acids.

labia: lips or liplike.
labia majora: the large, outer lips of the vulva.
labia minora: the thin, pink, hairless inner lips of the vulva.
laceration: a cut or tear.
lactase: the enzyme necessary for lactose digestion.
lactation: refers to (1) the secretion of milk or (2) the period during which milk is secreted.
lactiferous ducts: ducts through which milk travels from the lactiferous sinus to the nipple.
lactiferous sinus: located beneath the edge of the areola of the breast, the sinus holds milk and must be compressed by the baby's lips to send milk through the lactiferous duct to the nipple opening.
lactogenic hormone: hormone produced by the anterior pituitary; stimulates the growth of breast tissue and the process of lactation (also called prolactin, luteotropin).
lactose: the sugar in human milk.
lambdoidal suture: the suture between the occipital and parietal bones.
laminaria tent: a cone of *Laminaria* (dried seaweed), which swells when it becomes moist; may be used to dilate the cervix in an induced abortion.
lanugo: fine, downy hair covering the fetus from 20 weeks until birth.
laparotomy: abdominal incision.
let-down reflex: response to oxytocin that allows milk in the alveoli of the breast to flow into the milk ducts.
leukorrhea: white or yellow-white mucus discharged from the cervix or vagina; may be physiologic or pathologic.
levator ani: a broad muscle helping to form the floor of the pelvis.
LGA: large for gestational age; babies with birth weights greater than the ninetieth percentile.
libido: sexual drive.
lie: the relationship between the long axis of the fetus and the long axis of the mother.
lightening: the descent of the uterus when the baby's presenting part becomes fixed in the pelvis.
linea nigra: pigmented line seen from the umbilicus to the pubes in some women during pregnancy.
linea terminalis: divides the upper or false pelvis from the lower or true pelvis.
lithotomy position: lying on one's back with thighs flexed upon the abdomen and lower legs flexed upon the thighs.
lochia: vaginal discharge during the puerperium.
lochia alba: yellowish or whitish lochia after the second postpartum week.
lochia rubra: dark red vaginal discharge during the first 3 to 4 days following delivery.

lochia serosa: pink or serous brown-red lochia, usually occurring from 4 to 10 days following delivery.

low forceps delivery (outlet forceps): forceps are applied after the fetal head is crowning.

L/S ratio (lecithin/sphingomyelin ratio): a test to assess lung maturity in the fetus by measuring the phospholipids in amniotic fluid; a ratio of 2.0 or better usually indicates mature lungs.

luteinizing hormone (LH): hormone that stimulates ovulation and the development of the corpus luteum; produced by the anterior pituitary gland.

luteotropic hormone (LTH): hormone believed responsible for the maturation of the corpus luteum; produced by the anterior pituitary gland (see also lactogenic hormone).

macerated: softened by steeping in fluid; e.g., a macerated fetus.

macroglossia: enlarged tongue.

macrophages: monocytes in tissues and human milk; important in resistance to infection.

macrosomic: of large body size, as in some infants of diabetic mothers.

malpresentation: abnormal fetal presentation.

mastectomy: surgical removal of part or all of a breast.

mastitis: infection of breast tissue.

meconium: odorless, viscid first stools after birth; from dark green to black in color.

meconium ileus: paralysis of the lower gastrointestinal tract due to thick, putty-like meconium; a neonatal sign of cystic fibrosis.

meconium staining: condition of a newborn with hypoxia in utero.

mediastinum: the folds of the pleura and intervening space between the right and left lung.

meiosis: the process by which ova and sperm divide.

- - -melia: refers to a limb; e.g., phocomelia, absence of part of a limb.

menarche: first menstruation.

meningocele: congenital malformation of the spine in which the meninges protrude through a defect in the vertebrae.

menopause: the cessation of menstruation.

menorrhagia: profuse or excessive menstrual flow.

menses (menstruation): periodic vaginal discharge.

mentum: chin.

mesoderm: middle layer of embryo from which muscle, bone, and connective tissue develop.

metritis: inflammation of the uterus.

metrorrhagia: bleeding between menstrual periods.

microcephalus: a small head resulting from failure of the skull and brain to grow.

micrognathia: abnormally small jaw.

midforceps delivery: forceps are applied when the head is engaged but has not yet reached the perineal floor.

midwife: a person who delivers infants.

midwife, certified nurse (CNM): a registered nurse who has graduated from a nurse-midwifery program and passed a national certification examination.

midwife, "granny": a woman with no formal training who delivers infants, usually in a rural area.

midwife, lay: a person, usually a woman, who delivers infants but is not a nurse-midwife or a physician.

milia: tiny white papules seen on the face of newborns that disappear spontaneously.

miscarriage: lay term for spontaneous abortion.

mitosis: the process by which all cells divide, except the sex cells, after the stage of the primary oocyte and primary spermatocyte.

molding: the process by which the shape of the fetal head changes to fit the pelvis during labor.

Mongolian spot: pigmentation in the area of the lower back and buttocks, usually seen in nonwhite infants, which fades as the child grows older.

moniliasis: fungal infection of skin or mucous membrane.

monocytes: white blood cells important in resistance to infection.

monozygotic: originating from a single fertilized ovum; e.g., monozygotic twins.

mons pubis (mons veneris): fatty tissue covering the bony pubic symphysis.

monstrosity: major congenital abnormality (derived from the Latin *monstrare* [to show] because of the ancient belief that the birth of deformed infants was a sign from the gods).

montrice: an individual trained in psychoprophylactic methods who supports women during labor.

morbidity: disease or abnormal condition.

Moro reflex: reflex normally present in term newborn involving extension and then embracing movements of arms and flexion of knees and thighs.

morphogenesis: the process by which organs of the body and the body itself take shape.

mortality: death.

mortality, fetal: death of a fetus weighing 500 grams or more or of 20 weeks' gestation or more.

mortality, infant: death in the first year of life.

mortality, maternal: death of a woman during pregnancy and for a varying period following delivery.

mortality, neonatal: death of a newborn who has shown any sign of life within 28 days following birth.

mortality, perinatal: fetal mortality plus neonatal mortality; i.e., death from 20 weeks' gestation (or 500 grams weight) until 28 days after birth.

mortality rate: number of deaths per a specific population; e.g., deaths per 1000 births.

mortality rate, fetal: number of fetal deaths per 1000 births (or live births).

mortality rate, infant: number of deaths in the first year of life per 1000 births.

mortality rate, maternal: the number of maternal deaths per 100,000 births.

mortality rate, neonatal: number of neonatal deaths per 1000 births (or live births).

mortality rate, perinatal: the sum of the fetal mortality rate plus the neonatal mortality rate.

morula: a ball of cells in the very early development of the embryo.

mosaicism: condition in which there are different chromosomal patterns within the cells of a single organism.

mucous membrane: specialized mucus-secreting tissue lining many body structures.

mucus: fluid secreted by mucous membranes.

multigravida: a woman pregnant for the second or subsequent time.

multipara: a woman who has delivered two or more viable infants.

multiple pregnancy: pregnancy involving more than one fetus; e.g., twin pregnancy.

mutation: change in a gene.

myelomeningocele: congenital malformation of the spine in which the meninges and spinal cord protrude through a defect in the vertebrae.

myoepithelial cells: contractile cells surrounding the alveoli in the breast, which contract and express milk from the alveoli into the mammary ducts.

Nägele's rule: method of estimating the expected date of confinement (EDC). Count back 3 months from the first day of the last menstrual period and add 7 days.

navel: umbilicus.

necrotizing enterocolitis: a condition believed to result from lack of oxygenation to the bowel and infection, resulting in necrosis of the bowel wall.

neonate: an infant from birth to 28 days of age.

neonatal death: see mortality, neonatal.

neonatal death rate: see mortality rate, neonatal.

neonatologist: a physician with special training in the care of the newborn.

neonatology: the study of the neonate.

nevus: a congenital area of pigmentation in the skin (mole).

nevus flammeus: port wine stain; an area of discoloration of the face and neck.

nevus vasculosus (strawberry hemangioma): elevated area consisting of immature capillaries and endothelial cells; slowly regresses over a period of several years.

nidation: implantation of the fertilized ovum in the endometrium.

nonshivering thermogenesis: the process by which newborns produce heat by increasing their metabolic rate.

nucleotide: single segment of the helical strand of DNA.

nulligravida: a woman who has never been pregnant.

nullipara: a woman who has never delivered a viable infant (20 weeks' gestation or more).

nurse-practitioner: a registered nurse with additional education who practices in an expanded role.

occiput: back part of the head.

oligohydramnios: abnormally small amount of amniotic fluid; may indicate a defect of the fetal urinary tract.

oliguria: diminished secretion of urine.

omphalitis: infection of the umbilical stump.

omphalocele: congenital defect in which the abdominal wall fails to close and the abdominal contents herniate through the navel.

oogenesis: the process by which oogonia develop into mature ova.

oogonia: the forerunners of the mature ova.

oophorectomy: surgical removal of an ovary.

ophthalmia neonatorum: gonococcal infection of the newborn's eyes.

opisthotonos: an arched, hyperextended position of the body.

orgasmic platform: the congested walls of the lower vagina during intercourse.

orifice: opening, as in vaginal orifice.

os: mouth, as in uterine os.

ovary: gland that contains ova (in many stages of development) and that also produces estrogen and progesterone.

ovulation: discharge of the ovum from the ovary.

ovulation method of family planning: a method based on observation of changes in cervical mucus and abstinence during the days surrounding ovulation.

ovum: egg; female germ cell.

oxytocic: a pharmacologic agent that stimulates uterine contractions.

oxytocin: hormone from the posterior pituitary gland; stimulates uterine contractions and the let-down reflex during breast-feeding.

oxytocin challenge test: a test of fetal well-being in which the mother is given a small dose of oxytocin to stimulate contractions, and the fetal heart rate is monitored.

PaCO_2: the partial pressure of carbon dioxide in arterial blood.

palpation: physical examination using the fingers or palms.

PaO_2: amount of oxygen that has diffused through the alveoli into the arterial blood.

Papanicolaou test: a test for cervical cancer that involves "scraping" the ectocervix, the endocervix, and the vaginal pool.

para: a term describing the number of pregnancies in which an infant of more than 20 weeks' gestation was delivered (whether alive or dead).

paracervical nerve block: administration of a local anesthetic into the pelvic plexus.

parametritis: inflammation of the parametrium.

parametrium: smooth muscle, fatty tissue, and connective tissue extending laterally from the uterus between the layers of the broad ligaments.

parenteral: any route other than oral through which medications or nutrients are administered.

parity: number of live or stillborn infants of more than 20 weeks' gestation that a woman has delivered.

parturient: woman in labor.

parturition: process of giving birth.

patent: open.

pathogen: a substance or organism capable of producing disease.

pathogenic: productive of disease.

pathognomonic: characteristic symptom of a disease that helps to differentiate that disease from others.

pedigree: a diagram of the genetic history of a particular trait.

PEEP: positive end expiratory pressure; a modality used in conjunction with a ventilator in the treatment of respiratory distress.

pelvic inlet: upper margin of the pelvic cavity.

pelvic outlet: inferior margin of the pelvic cavity.

pelvimeter: instrument used in measuring pelvic diameters.

pelvimetry: process of measuring pelvic diameters to assess capacity for vaginal delivery.

pelvis, false: that portion of the pelvis above the linea terminalis and the symphysis pubis.

pelvis, true: that portion of the pelvis below the linea terminalis.

peridural anesthesia: the injection of an anesthetic into the extradural space; anesthetic does not penetrate the dura or the spinal cord.

perinatal mortality: see mortality, perinatal.

perinatal mortality rate: see mortality rate, perinatal.

perinatologist: an obstetrician with special interest in the perinatal period, with particular interest in high risk mothers and infants.

perineum: area between the vulva and the anus, made up of skin, muscle, and fascia.

periodic breathing: brief periods of apnea without cyanosis common in the respiration of preterm infants.

pessary: supportive device placed inside the uterus.

petechiae: minute hemorrhages.

pH: the chemical symbol for hydrogen ion concentration; the greater the number of hydrogen ions, the more acidic the solution and the lower the pH.

phagocyte: a white blood cell that destroys micro-organisms.

phagocytosis: ingestion and digestion of bacteria and particles by phagocytes.

phenotype: genetically expressed characteristics of an individual; e.g., hair color, presence of hemophilia.

phenylketonuria (PKU): an inborn error in metabolism; the infant cannot metabolize phenylalanine, an essential amino acid.

phimosis: tightness of the foreskin of the penis, so that the foreskin cannot be pushed back over the glans penis.

phlebitis: inflammation of a vein.

phlegmasia alba dolens: "milk leg"; thrombophlebitis resulting in blanching, swelling, and pain in the thigh and leg.

phototherapy: the use of light as a treatment for hyperbilirubinemia.

pica: nonfood substances that are eaten.

pinna: cartilage of the ear.

placenta: organ through which fetal-maternal exchange of gases (oxygen and carbon dioxide), nutrients, and wastes occurs.

placenta accreta: invasion of the uterine muscle by the placenta; separation of the placenta thus becomes impossible in most situations.

placenta, battledore: insertion of the umbilical cord into the margin of the placenta.

placenta circumvallata: a raised white ring at the edge of the placenta.

placenta previa: abnormal implantation of the placenta in the lower uterine segment.

placenta, retained: condition in which part or all of the placenta remains in the uterus following delivery.

placenta succenturiata: an accessory placenta.

placentae, abruptio: see abruptio placentae.

placental infarct: hard, whitish area on the fetal or maternal side of the placenta.

platypelloid pelvis: oval pelvis with a shortened anteroposterior diameter.

plethoric: of a deep, beefy red color.

pneumomediastinum: accumulation of air in the mediastinum.

pneumopericardium: air in the pericardial sac.

pneumothorax: air in the thoracic cavity.

podalic version: shifting the position of the fetus to bring the feet to the pelvic outlet.

polycythemia: increased erythrocytes.

polydactyly: an extra finger or toe.

polygenic inheritance: traits controlled by more than one gene.

polyhydramnios: see hydramnios.

polymorphonuclear leukocytes (polys): white blood cells important in the resistance to infection.

polyuria: excessive secretion of urine.

position: relationship between the presenting part and the mother's pelvis.

post-term infant: an infant with a gestational age of more than 42 weeks; also termed postmature.

precipitate delivery: rapid labor and delivery.

pre-eclampsia: hypertension with proteinuria, edema, or both, occurring after the twentieth week of pregnancy.

prepuce (foreskin): fold of skin covering the glans penis.

presenting part: the part of the fetus that first enters the vagina.

preterm infant: an infant with a gestational age of less than 38 weeks; also termed premature.

primigravida: a woman during her first pregnancy.

primipara: a woman who has delivered one viable infant.

prodromal: early symptoms of a disease.

progesterone: hormone secreted by the corpus luteum and, during pregnancy, by the placenta.

projectile vomiting: expulsive vomiting.

prolactin: see lactogenic hormone.

prolapse of the umbilical cord: condition in which the umbilical cord is at or below the level of the presenting part.

proliferative phase of the menstrual cycle: precedes ovulation.

prophylaxis: prevention.

prospective study: a study of events that are expected to occur after the study is initiated.

prostaglandin: a biologic substance present within the body that plays a role in many body processes, including contraction of the uterus.

proteinuria: protein in the urine; one symptom of pre-eclampsia.

pruritus: itching.

pseudocyesis: a condition in which a woman believes she is pregnant but is not (false pregnancy).

psychoprophylaxis: a method of preparation for labor.

ptyalism: excessive salivation.

puberty: the period of life during which the reproductive organs mature.

pudendal nerve block: administration of a local anesthetic into the pudendal nerves on the right and left of the perineum.

puerperal sepsis: infection of the pelvic organs during the puerperium.

puerperium: the period of time from the completion of the third stage of labor until the complete involution of the uterus, usually occurring 6 weeks later.

pulmonary oxygen toxicity (POT): a condition that occurs in some infants who have received too much oxygen at too much pressure for too long a period of time; also termed bronchopulmonary dysplasia, chronic lung disease.

pulse pressure: the difference between systolic and diastolic blood pressure.

pyelonephritis: inflammation of the kidney and its pelvis.

quickening: fetal movement perceived by the mother.

radioimmunoassay: a test for pregnancy that measures an antigen-antibody reaction by a radioisotope technique.

rales: sounds heard as air passes through fluid in the bronchi and alveoli; classified as dry or moist.

recessive inheritance: inheritance requiring genes from both parents.

rectocele: herniation of the rectum into the vagina.

rectovaginal fistula: an opening between the rectum and vagina.

residual urine: urine remaining in the bladder after voiding.

respiratory distress syndrome (RDS): a disease primarily of preterm newborns, characterized by a lack of surfactant in the alveoli of the lungs; also termed hyaline membrane disease (HMD).

restitution: at delivery, the rotation of the presenting part of the fetus after it emerges from the vagina.

retroflexion of the uterus: condition in which the body of the uterus is tipped posteriorly but the position of the cervix remains unchanged.

retrolental fibroplasia: a condition caused by oxygen given in too high concentration to the immature infant, resulting in blindness.

retrospective study: a study of events that occurred before the study was initiated.

retroversion of the uterus: condition in which the body of the uterus is tipped posteriorly with the cervix pointing anteriorly; uterine displacement.

Rh$_D$ factor: a factor in blood that is a possible antigen when the mother lacks the factor (Rh$_D$ negative) but the fetus has the factor (Rh$_D$ positive).

rhythm method: a method of contraception in which the couple abstains from intercourse on days prior to and following ovulation.

Ritgen maneuver: method of controlling the delivery of the fetal head.

RNA: ribonucleic acid; a protein within each cell.

Rubin test: a test for patency of the uterine tubes by the insufflation of carbon dioxide.

rugae: folds or creases (e.g., rugae of the vagina).

sacrum: bone comprised of five fused vertebrae located between the fifth lumbar vertebra and the coccyx.

saddle block: injection of medication into the conus of the dural sac; anesthetizes the area that would come in contact with a saddle while riding a horse.

sagittal suture: membranous space between the parietal bones from the anterior fontanel to the posterior fontanel.

scaphoid abdomen: "sunken" abdomen; e.g., the abdomen of a newborn infant with diaphragmatic hernia.

scapula: shoulder blade.

Schultze's mechanism: delivery of the placenta with the fetal surface outermost.

sclerema: hardening of the skin and subcutaneous tissue.

secretory phase of the menstrual cycle: follows ovulation.

semen: secretion from the male urethra in which sperm are transported.

SGA: small for gestational age; babies with birth weights below the tenth percentile.

Shake test: a test to assess lung maturity in the fetus by measuring the phospholipids in amniotic fluid; more rapid and less complex than the L/S ratio.

significant other(s): individual(s) who have a close, meaningful relationship with a particular person.

simian crease: a single abnormal transverse crease in the palm of the hand.

Skene's ducts: paraurethral ducts, found on each side of the urethral meatus.

smegma: cheeselike secretion around the labia minora.

souffle: soft blowing sound heard on auscultation.

souffle, funic: sound produced by fetal blood rushing through the umbilical vessels; synchronous with fetal heart rate.

souffle, placental: sound produced by blood flow in placenta; synchronous with maternal pulse rate.

souffle, uterine: sound produced by blood in the arteries of pregnant uterus; synchronous with maternal pulse rate.

spermatic cord: cord from which the testis is suspended; contains blood vessels, nerves, muscle fibers, and the vas deferens.

spermatogenesis: the process by which spermatogonia develop into sperm.

spermatogonia: forerunner of mature sperm.

spina bifida occulta: congenital malformation of the spine in which the posterior portions of the vertebrae fail to close.

spinnbarkeit: a property of cervical mucus that enables it to make a thread when placed between two glass slides.

station: the level of the presenting part in relation to the pelvis.

station zero: when the presenting part is at the level of the ischial spines (engaged).

strabismus: crossed eyes.

striae gravidarum: red, slightly depressed streak marks on the abdomen, and occasionally on the breasts, during pregnancy; "stretch marks."

stridor: harsh, high-pitched respiratory sound.

subinvolution: failure of the uterus to return to normal size and state following pregnancy.

subluxation: incomplete dislocation; e.g., congenital subluxation of the hip.

supernumerary nipples: excessive number of nipples, usually located along an embryologic nipple-line.

supine hypotensive syndrome: hypotension caused by the interference with the flow of blood returning to the heart via the inferior vena cava; due to the weight of the uterus on the inferior vena cava when the mother is supine.

suppuration: formation of pus.

surfactant: a substance formed by Type II cells in the alveoli of the lungs that reduces surface tension and prevents the alveoli from collapsing.

sutures: membranous spaces between the bones of the cranium in a fetus or newborn infant.

symphysis pubis: area where pubic bones join at the midline.

syndactyly: webbing of the fingers or toes.

tachypnea: rapid respiration (in newborn, a respiratory rate greater than 60 per minute).

talipes calcaneovalgus: a congenital condition in which the foot is flexed and deviates laterally.

talipes equinovarus: a congenital condition in which the foot is extended and deviates medially.

teratogen: any environmental factor, chemical or physical, that affects the embryo-fetus adversely.

term infant: an infant with a gestational age from 38 weeks to 42 weeks.

testicle: a gland in the male scrotum that produces sperm and the hormone testosterone.

testosterone: hormone secreted by the interstitial cells of the testes.

tetanic contraction: a contraction that exceeds 90 seconds in duration.

tetany: a state of excessive muscle tone.

thermoneutral environment: environment that allows a baby to maintain a body temperature of 36.5°C. (97.7°F.) with a minimum use of energy.

thromboembolus: obstruction of a blood vessel by a clot that has migrated from the site of formation.

thrombophlebitis: inflammation of a vein with subsequent formation of a clot.

thrombus: blood clot obstructing a blood vessel.

thrush: an infection caused by the fungus *Candida albicans*.

tine test: screening test for tubercular infection.

tonic: prolonged muscular contraction.

TORCH organisms: refers to toxoplasmosis, other (syphilis), rubella, cytomegalovirus, and herpes simplex, organisms that may injure the embryo-fetus in utero.

toxemia: term previously used to describe hypertensive states of pregnancy, including pre-eclampsia and eclampsia.

tracheoesophageal fistula: congenital anomaly in which there is a connection between the trachea and esophagus.

traditional societies: societies in which cultural change occurs slowly, so that there is minimal change from one generation to the next.

transient tachypnea of the newborn: rapid respiratory rate for several days following birth due to fluid in lungs that clears spontaneously as fluid is absorbed.

transition: the last phase of the first stage of labor, from the time the cervix is approximately 8 cm. dilated until complete dilatation.

translocation: refers to a piece of one chromosome that breaks off and subsequently attaches itself to another.

trauma: physical or psychologic injury.

Trichomonas vaginalis: a protozoan causing a vaginal infection, Trichomonas vaginitis.

trimester: three month period.

trisomy: the presence of three chromosomes rather than the usual two. Example: trisomy 21 (i.e., three of the number 21 chromosome) results in Down's syndrome.

trophoblast: outer layer of cells of the developing blastocyst.

tubercles of Montgomery: small papillae that appear on the surface of the nipples and the areolae; secrete a lipoid substance that lubricates the nipples.

tunica albuginea: tight fibrous sheath enclosing each testis.

ultrasonography: a technique by which high frequency sound waves are beamed into the body.

umbilical cord: the structure linking fetus and placenta, normally containing two umbilical arteries and one umbilical vein.

umbilical hernia: protrusion of the bowel at the umbilicus through a defect in the abdominal wall.

umbilicus: navel.

urinary frequency: a frequent need to void.

uterine tubes (fallopian tubes): tubes extending laterally from each side of the uterus to the area of the ovary.

vagina: tube between the uterus and the vaginal orifice.

vaginismus: intense spasm of the muscles surrounding the vagina.

varices: varicose veins; distended veins.

vas deferens: tubelike structures through which spermatozoa leave the testes.

vasectomy: a surgical procedure in which the vas deferens is severed and tied, blocking the passage of sperm.

vernix caseosa: a fatty secretion of fetal sebaceous glands and dead epidermal cells that covers fetal skin during the second half of pregnancy.

version: an attempt to "turn" the baby in a transverse "lie" to a longitudinal "lie." Version may be *external* or *internal podalic.*

vertex: top of head.

vertex presentation: presentation in which the head, either flexed or neither flexed nor extended, is the presenting part.

viable: capable of living, as a viable fetus, a fetus of 28 weeks' gestation or more.

villi: small vascular protrusions on a membranous surface; e.g., chorionic villi.

vulva: the collective term for the external female genitalia.

vulvectomy: surgical removal of the external female genitalia.

Wharton's jelly: a jelly-like substance surrounding the umbilical arteries and vein within the umbilical cord.

womb: uterus.

X-linked inheritance: inheritance through genes located on the X chromosome.

zona pellucida: the covering of the discharged ovum.

zygote: fertilized ovum.

INDEX

Note: Page numbers in *italics* refer to illustrations.
Page numbers followed by the letter *t* refer to tables.